The Queer
Encyclopedia
of Film & Television

Also edited by Claude J. Summers:

The Queer Encyclopedia of Music, Dance & Musical Theater

The Queer Encyclopedia of the Visual Arts

The Queer Encyclopedia of Film & Television

Claude J. Summers

Editor

CLEIS
PRESS

Published in the United States by Cleis Press Inc.,
P.O. Box 14697, San Francisco, California 94114.

Printed in the United States.
Cover design: Scott Idleman
Cover photograph: Photograph of Marlene Dietrich my John Kobal Foundation/Hulton Archives and used with kind permission of Peter Riva. Photograph of Paul Lynde used with kind permission of Michael Airington. Photograph of Ellen DeGeneres used with permission of WireImage.
Book design: Karen Quigg
Cleis Press logo art: Juana Alicia
First Edition.
10 9 8 7 6 5 4 3 2 1

Archives, libraries, service bureaus, and individuals have been indispensable in providing access to the images that illustrate *The Queer Encyclopedia of Film & Television*. These organizations and individuals deserve particular thanks. Archiv für Sexualwissenschaft for granting access to the still from *Anders als die Andern* on page 125. Algonquin Books for providing the image of Tab Hunter on page 177. Barbarahammerfilms.com for providing the image of Barbara Hammer on page 169. Beach Front Bookings for providing the image of Kate Clinton on page 181. Robert Benevides for providing the image of Raymond Burr on page 57. Clipart.com for providing the image of Jean Cocteau on page 75, the image of Marlene Dietrich on page 92, and the image of Errol Flynn on page 152 (Copyright © 2003-2005, Clipart.com). The office of Bill Condon for providing the image of him on page 77. Department 56 for providing the image of Sandra Bernhard on page 47. Arthur Dong for providing the image of himself and Robert Shepard on page 98 and the image of himself on page 100. Lynne Fernie for providing the animation still from *Apples and Oranges* on page 121. Bruce LaBruce for providing image of himself on page 194. Library of Congress Prints and Photographs Division for providing the image of Dorothy Arzner and Marion Morgan on page 33, the image of Montgomery Clift on page 73, the image of Greta Garbo on page 158, the image of Rock Hudson on page 176, the image of Charles Laughton on page 197, the image of Jean Marais on page 208, the image of Agnes Moorehead on page 214, the image of Mauritz Stiller on page 265, and the image of Andy Warhol and Tennessee Williams on page 286. The office of Richard Hatch for providing the image of him on page 14. Jack Nichols for providing the image of himself, Frank Kameny, and George Weinberg on page 11. François Orenn for providing the image of Jean-Daniel Cadinot on page 62. Special thanks to Stathis Orphanos for providing the image of Clive Barker on page 45, the image of James Broughton on page 55, the image of Mart Crowley on page 81, the image of George Cukor on page 83, the image of James Bridges and Jack Larson on page 140, the image of John Schlesinger on page 250, and the image of Gavin Lambert on page 252. Panacea Entertainment for providing the image of Richard Chamberlain on page 67. Ken Phillips Publicity Group for providing the image of Margaret Cho on page 72. Patricia Rozema for providing the image of herself on page 245. RuCo, Inc. for providing the image of RuPaul on page 248. TLA Releasing for providing the promotional poster art for *Bulgarian Lovers* on page 180. Ulrike Ottinger Filmproduktion for providing the image of Ulrike Ottinger on page 227. The office of Christine Vachon for providing the image of her on page 278. The office of John Waters for providing the image of him on page 289. Andrea Weiss for providing the image of herself on page 293. William Morris Agency for providing the image of Craig Lucas on page 202.

LIBRARY OF CONGRESS CATALOGING-IN-PUBLICATION DATA

The queer encyclopedia of film and television / Claude J. Summers, Editor.
   p. cm.
   Includes bibliographical references and index.
   ISBN 1-57344-209-7 (pbk. : alk. paper)
  1. Gays in the performing arts—Biography—Dictionaries. 2. Gays—Biography—Dictionaries.
  I. Summers, Claude J.
     PN1590.G39Q44 2005
     790.2'086'64—dc22
            2005015928

For Ted, again;

and for Wik, the "onlie begetter,"

and for Robert Herndon and Linda Rapp

ACKNOWLEDGMENTS

A collaborative project of the scope of *The Queer Encyclopedia of Film & Television* necessarily depends on the kindness and cooperation of numerous individuals, including especially the authors of the articles.

I owe most to Andrew "Wik" Wikholm, President of glbtq, Inc., whose vision and commitment and enthusiasm have made this book possible. Ted-Larry Pebworth has been a supportive partner and collaborator in many ways beyond the indexing and copyediting skills that he has deployed in this project. Linda Rapp, friend and assistant, has generously contributed her time, energy, and expertise.

I am grateful to all those who offered advice and made suggestions, especially as to topics and contributors. Gary Morris, Patricia Juliana Smith, and Mark McLelland have been especially helpful as members of the www.glbtq.com advisory board. Michael Tanimura, production manager at glbtq, discovered a number of inconsistencies and errors and knew how to correct them. Betsy Greco, glbtq project administrator, has been unfailingly efficient and cheerful. The sharp-eyed and informed staff at Cleis Press has been a joy to work with. I am especially grateful to Mark Rhynsburger.

Work on this project has been sustained by the interest and support of numerous friends, including Roberts Batson, Albert Carey, Barry Cazaubon, Neil Flax, Robert Herndon, George Koschel, and Robert McCabe. I am also grateful to my friends John Edward and Willene Hardy and Gary and Mary Ann Stringer, who provided shelter from Hurricane Katrina and facilitated the final preparations of this book.

CONTENTS

Introduction

*T*HE *QUEER ENCYCLOPEDIA OF FILM & TELEVISION* introduces a remarkably rich and varied cultural achievement. It surveys the contributions of gay, lesbian, bisexual, transgender, and queer people to film and television and also their representation in and sometimes vexed relationship to these media. That is, this work is interested in glbtq individuals not only as actors, directors, screenwriters, television performers, and producers, but also as subjects, objects, and consumers of the popular arts. There are articles on Film Spectatorship as well as on Film Sissies, on Stereotypes as well as on American Television Situation Comedies.

As Mark Finch writes in the overview of Film included in this volume, "It is a part of popular cultural mythology that homosexuals are meant to be obsessed with Hollywood—all those queens crying for Judy, dykes swooning for Garbo. What is much less remarked upon is precisely the reverse: Hollywood's obsession with homosexuality." Among other topics, this book is interested in popular culture's varied and evolving constructions of homosexuality.

The history of the representation of sexual minorities by film and television and other popular entertainments is a fascinating subject. Such a history not only reveals the majority's complex, ambiguous, and shifting attitudes toward sex and sexual minorities, but it also witnesses to the myriad ways in which gay men and lesbians alternately absorbed, resisted, challenged, and modified the prejudices of the dominant society, while also utilizing popular culture as a means of queer engagement, finding in it opportunities for identity building and subcultural exchange.

Presenting more than 160 articles, ranging from broad surveys of film and television genres to succinct accounts of topics and individuals, *The Queer Encyclopedia of Film & Television* offers a revisionist history of these arts by seeing them through a queer lens. It places the achievements of gay, lesbian, bisexual, transgender, and queer actors, directors, screenwriters, and set and costume designers in historical contexts and privileges the representation of subjects that have traditionally been censored or marginalized.

Celebrating the richness and variety of queer contributions to the popular arts, this book presents that achievement as an invaluable cultural legacy to be celebrated and treasured.

Gay, lesbian, and bisexual actors and actresses have been among the elite members of the theatrical and film community, which has generally welcomed the sexually unorthodox, yet only recently have many enjoyed the luxury of openness, and their achievements been seen in light of their sexuality. Some hid behind "lavender marriages" or fake biographies in order to "pass" as heterosexual, while others lived under threat of exposure and consequent loss of livelihood. Indeed, most of the actors whom we recognize as gay or lesbian were outed posthumously or, as in the case of many, including Sir John Gielgud and Rock Hudson, by scandal and illness, or came out only after their careers had faded, like Tab Hunter and Richard Chamberlain.

Notwithstanding some notable exceptions such as Ellen DeGeneres, Lily Tomlin, Rupert Everett, Nathan Lane, and Sir Ian McKellen, even today gay and lesbian film and television actors tend to remain closeted because they believe that coming out would limit the kinds of roles they are offered. Today, the question of an actor's homosexuality tends to center on whether the public will accept an openly gay actor in a heterosexual role, especially as a romantic lead. The question, of course, is less whether a gay or lesbian actor can play such roles convincingly (obviously they can, as examples from Valentino to Chamberlain richly attest) than whether knowledge of their sexuality would inhibit audience identification.

There is real value in isolating queer contributions to popular culture in order to see them in their own terms as expressions of a multifaceted queer artistic impulse and as documentations of the variety and diversity of queer experience. Indeed, not to do so perpetuates stereotypes and contributes to a distorted image of homosexuals by ignoring or denying the achievements of a beleaguered minority.

Queer art and achievement have so often been denigrated, suppressed, or robbed of their specificity and roots in efforts to render them "universal" that they have very infrequently been seen whole and in the contexts that gave them life. The aim of *The Queer Encyclopedia of Film & Television* is to help remedy the effects of an old but still active, homophobic project of exclusion and denial, by in fact presenting queer art and accomplishment whole and in the multiple contexts that helped shape them. Doing so yields new insight into the creative impulse and increases our understanding of a wide range of achievements.

Recovering and Reclaiming Our Heritage

Recovering our cultural heritage is a crucially important endeavor for everyone, but it is especially significant for gay men, lesbians, and others who have grown up in families and societies in which their sexual identities or gender expressions have been ignored, concealed, or condemned. They often come to a realization of their difference with little or no understanding of alternative sexualities beyond the negative stereotypes that pervade contemporary society, and they usually feel isolated and frightened at the very time they most need reassurance and encouragement.

Not surprisingly, a staple of the gay and lesbian coming-out story is the trip to the local library, where the young homosexual, desperate for the most basic information, is usually utterly confused or bitterly disappointed by what he or she discovers, for even now our society does not make it easy for young people to find accurate information about alternative sexualities. Only later is the radical loneliness of young people who have accepted their sexual identity assuaged by the discovery of a large and varied cultural heritage, one that speaks directly to the experience of contemporary men and women in the West but that also reflects other forms of same-sex love and desire in different times and places.

This volume is at once a documentation and reclamation of that cultural legacy and also a contribution to it. It participates in a long endeavor by queer men and women to recover a social and cultural history that has frequently been deliberately distorted and censored.

For centuries, educated and literate homosexuals living in eras that condemned homosexuality have looked to other ages and other societies in order to find cultural permission for homosexual behavior, to experience some relief from the incessant attacks on their self-esteem, and to penetrate the barriers of censorship that precluded open discussion of the love that dared not speak its name. Such attempts range from the ubiquitous lists of famous homosexuals in history to more elaborate and sophisticated historical research, such as that of Jeremy Bentham in the eighteenth century and of Edward Carpenter and John Addington Symonds at the end of the nineteenth century, as well as the recurrent attempts by gay and lesbian artists and writers to discover traditions and languages through which to express themselves.

Too often, however, attempts to document the gay and lesbian cultural legacy paid little attention to historical differences and tended to make few distinctions between different kinds of homosexualities, equating the emergent homosexual of the nineteenth century with the ancient Greek pederast, the medieval sodomite, and the Native North American *berdache*, for example, as though all four phenomena were merely minor variations on the same pattern.

The Queer Encyclopedia of Film & Television is motivated by the same impulse to understand the past and to recover the (often suppressed or disguised) artistic expressions of same-sex love that propelled earlier projects. But as the beneficiary of a more open climate and a recent explosion of knowledge about homosexuality in history, it is in a far better position to discover a usable past. The new understanding of sexuality in history and culture that emerged in the 1980s and 1990s has in fact enabled this particular enterprise. Without the gay, lesbian, and queer studies movement, this and the other volumes in this series would not have been possible.

Gay, Lesbian, Queer Studies Movement

In entering the academic mainstream, gay, lesbian, and queer studies have enlarged our understanding of the meaning of sexual identities, both in our own culture and in other times and places. They have challenged naive, uninformed, and prejudiced views, and, perhaps most important, have discovered and recovered significant artifacts and neglected artists and other individuals of note.

Queer studies in film, theater, and the performing arts have also reclaimed established and celebrated creators and performers, revealing the pertinence and centrality of (frequently disguised or previously misinterpreted) same-sex relationships and queer experience to understanding canonical works. They have viewed celebrated achievements through a queer lens, in the process discovering aspects of the world's artistic heritage that either had not been noticed or had been suppressed.

But though gay, lesbian, and queer studies have enriched the academic study of history and culture, they still tend to be ghettoized in elite universities, often in women's studies programs that are themselves frequently isolated. Meanwhile, standard cultural histories continue all too often to omit or discount gay and lesbian representations, fail to supply relevant biographical information about gay, lesbian, bisexual, and transgender artists, and foster the grievously mistaken impression that the world's artistic traditions are almost exclusively heterosexual.

The Queer Encyclopedia of Film & Television aims to redress these deficiencies. It seeks to place portrayals of same-sex desire in historical context, to provide accurate biographical information about performers and filmmakers who have contributed to queer culture, and to explore important questions about the presence of homoeroticism in popular culture.

How does the homosexuality of an artist affect his or her work even when that work has nothing specifically to do with homosexuality? How does one decipher the "coding" of works in which the homosexual import is disguised? Is there such a thing as a gay sensibility? Are some film genres more amenable to homoeroticism than others? What is the enduring appeal of film sissies? Why is Judy Garland such an icon of gay men of a certain age? Why is transvestism generally treated only as the stuff of comedy in mainstream movies? How do the distinct cultures and sexual traditions of Asia color the queer representations of Asian film? What is the New Queer Cinema? These are some of the questions asked and variously answered in this book.

Relationship to Previous Volumes

The Queer Encyclopedia of Film & Television is the fourth of four volumes, edited by Claude J. Summers, mining the resources of www.glbtq.com, the online encyclopedia of gay, lesbian, bisexual, and transgender culture. The first volume, published before www.glbtq.com was launched in 2003, is *The Gay and Lesbian Literary Heritage* (New York: Henry Holt, 1995; revised edition, New York: Routledge, 2002); the second volume is *The Queer Encyclopedia of the Visual Arts* (San Francisco: Cleis Press, 2004); the third, *The Queer Encyclopedia of Music, Dance & Musical Theater* (San Francisco: Cleis Press, 2004). There is some overlap between the concerns of this volume and these previous ones.

Entries on dramatic literature and on playwrights may be found in *The Gay and Lesbian Literary Heritage*. While there are entries in the present volume on writers such as Mart Crowley, Ivor Novello, Craig Lucas, and Paul Rudnick, they are included by virtue of their subjects' contributions in the area of performance and screenwriting rather than as playwrights *per se*.

There is, however, some duplication of entries that were included in *The Queer Encyclopedia of Music, Dance & Musical Theater* and in *The Queer Encyclopedia of the Visual Arts*.

For example, while Michael Bennett and Tommy Tune are not included in this volume since they are known almost exclusively for their contributions to musical theater, figures such as Marlene Dietrich, Judy Garland, Nathan Lane, Vincente Minnelli, and Arthur Laurents, who have contributed to film and theater more generally as well as to musical theater, are included in both volumes. In addition, some overviews that were included in *The Queer Encyclopedia of Music, Dance & Musical*

Theater, such as the entry Set and Costume Design, are included in the present volume as well.

Some entries that might have been appropriate for this volume, but that are included in one of the previous volumes, are omitted here for reasons of space. For examples, Sir Cecil Beaton, who was a set and costume designer as well as a photographer, is included in *The Queer Encyclopedia of the Visual Arts;* Sir Noël Coward, who occasionally acted in films and who wrote some screenplays, is included in both *The Gay and Lesbian Literary Heritage,* where he is considered primarily as a playwright, and *The Queer Encyclopedia of Music, Dance & Musical Theater,* where he is discussed primarily as a composer and nightclub entertainer; and David Geffen, who is a film producer, is included in *The Queer Encyclopedia of Music, Dance & Musical Theater* by virtue of his greater fame as a music industry executive.

Finally, there are some entries in this volume that consider individuals who are also profiled in previous volumes, but from different perspectives. For example, the entries on Jean Cocteau and Harvey Fierstein in *The Gay and Lesbian Literary Heritage* and the entry on Andy Warhol in *The Queer Encyclopedia of the Visual Arts* are quite different from the entries on those subjects in this volume. Whereas in the previous volumes Cocteau and Fierstein were considered as writers and Warhol as a visual artist, in this volume Cocteau and Warhol are evaluated as filmmakers and Fierstein primarily as an actor.

Theoretical Issues

The study of the representation of alternative sexualities in culture must inevitably confront a variety of vexed issues, including basic conceptual questions of definition and identity. Who, exactly, is a homosexual? What constitutes sexual identity? To what extent is sexuality the product of broadly defined social forces? To what degree do sexual object-choices manifest a biological or psychological essence within the desiring individual? These questions are not only problematic for the historical study of homosexuality and of queer art, but also reflect current controversies about contemporary and historical sexual roles and categories, and they resist glib answers.

Although contemporary North Americans and Western Europeans typically think in terms of a dichotomy between homosexuality and heterosexuality, and between the homosexual and the heterosexual, with vague compartments for bisexuality and bisexuals, such a conception is a historically contingent cultural construct, more revealing of our own age's sexual ideology than of actual erotic practices even today. The range of human sexual response is considerably less restricted than these artificial classifications suggest, and different ages and cultures have interpreted (and regulated) sexual behavior differently.

Because human sexual behavior and emotions are fluid and various rather than static or exclusive, the sexologist Alfred Kinsey and others have argued that the terms *homosexual* and *heterosexual* should more properly be used as adjectives rather than nouns, referring to acts and emotions but not to people. Moreover, the conception of homosexuality and heterosexuality as essential and exclusive categories has historically operated as a form of social control, defining the person who responds erotically to individuals of his or her own sex as the "Other," or, more particularly, as *queer* or *unnatural*.

But though it may be tempting to conclude that there are no such entities as homosexuals or heterosexuals or bisexuals, this view, which so attractively stresses the commonality of human beings and minimizes the significance of sexual object-choices, poses its own dangers. Human sexuality is simply not as plastic as some theorists assert, and to deny the existence of homosexuals, bisexuals, and heterosexuals—or the pertinence of such categories—is to deny the genuineness of the personal identities and forms of erotic life that exist today. It is, indeed, to engage in a process of denial and erasure, rendering invisible a group that has had to struggle for recognition and visibility.

For most people, sexual orientation is not merely a matter of choice or preference but a classification that reflects a deep-seated internal, as well as social, reality. However arbitrary, subjective, inexact, and culture-bound the labels may be, they are impossible to escape and they affect individuals—especially those in the minority categories—in profound and manifold ways.

The most painful and destructive injustice visited upon people of alternative sexuality has been their separation from the normal and the natural, their stigmatization as *queer*. Yet the internalization of this stigma has also been their greatest strength and, indeed, the core of their identity in societies that regularly assign individuals to ostensibly exclusive categories of sexual desire. The consciousness of difference both spurred and made possible the recent creation of a homosexual minority—a gay and lesbian community—in the Western democracies, a process that involved transforming the conception of homosexuality from a "social problem" and personal failing to an individual and collective identity.

Quite apart from the fact that it facilitates identity politics, however, an acceptance of otherness, whether defined as lesbian, gay, bisexual, transgender, or the umbrella term *queer*, is also often personally empowering. Fostering qualities of introspection and encouraging social analysis, it enables people who feel excluded from some of the core assumptions and rituals of their society to evaluate themselves and their society from an ambiguous and often revealing perspective.

Homoerotic desire and behavior have been documented in every conceivable kind of society. What varies are the meanings that they are accorded from era to era and place to place. In some societies, homosexuality is tolerated and even institutionalized, whereas in others it is vilified and persecuted. In every society, there are undoubtedly individuals who are predominantly attracted to members of their own sex or who do not conform easily to gender expectations, but the extent to which that sexual attraction or gender nonconformity functions as a defining characteristic of these individuals' personal and social identities varies considerably from culture to culture.

Thus, any transhistorical and transcultural exploration of the queer artistic heritage must guard against the risk of anachronism, of inappropriately imposing contemporary culture-bound conceptions of homosexuality on earlier ages and different societies. Sexual categories are always historically and culturally specific rather than universal and invariant.

On the other hand, however, the recognition of cultural specificity in regard to sexual attitudes need not estrange the past or obscure connections and continuities between historical periods and between sexual ideologies. For instance, modern North American and Western European male homosexuality, which is predominantly androphilic (that is, between adult men), egalitarian, and socially disdained, is in many crucial respects quite different from ancient Greek male homosexuality, which was predominantly—though by no means exclusively—pederastic, asymmetrical in power, and socially valorized; but awareness of those differences does not obviate the similarities that link the two distinct historical constructs.

Neither does the acknowledgment of the distinctions between ancient Greek homosexuality and modern homosexuality entail the dismissal of the enormous influence that classical Greek attitudes toward same-sex love exerted on the formation of modern Western attitudes toward homosexuality. For many individuals in the early modern and modern eras, ancient Greek literature, philosophy, and art helped counter the negative attitudes toward same-sex eroticism fostered by Christian culture. Ancient Greek literature and art have provided readers, writers, and artists of subsequent centuries a pantheon of heroes, a catalogue of images, and a set of references by which same-sex desire could be encoded into their own representations and through which they could interpret their own experiences.

Nor should our sensitivity to the cultural specificity of sexual attitudes cause us to rob individual artists of individual perspectives or to condescend toward the past. All artists exist in relation to their time and must necessarily create from within their world views, or, as philosopher Michel Foucault would say, the *epistemes* of their ages. But the fact that artists are embedded in their cultures does not mean that they lack agency and individuality.

Artists tend to be more independent than their contemporaries, not less; and though they may express the tendencies and suppositions of their societies, they also frequently challenge them, even if those challenges are themselves facilitated and contained by societal beliefs. Hence, it is a mistake to assume that artists of earlier ages, before the general emergence of a modern homosexual identity, could not share important aspects of that consciousness, including a subjective awareness of difference and a sense of alienation from society. One of the rewards of studying the queer cultural heritage is, in fact, the discovery of a queer subjectivity in the past and of the affinities as well as differences between earlier and later homosexualities.

A Beginning, Not an End

For all its considerable heft, *The Queer Encyclopedia of Film & Television* has no pretensions to comprehensiveness.

There are some notable omissions of topics and artists, due variously to lack of space, an absence of available information and research, a difficulty in finding qualified contributors, and a continuing fearfulness on the part of many performers and creators to acknowledge their sexuality, even in fields that would seem to be queer friendly. Moreover, *The Queer Encyclopedia of Film & Television* is undoubtedly biased in favor of American popular culture, even as it also provides a great deal of information about other traditions and cultures.

The point that needs emphasis, however, is that as the first comprehensive work of its kind, this encyclopedia is an important beginning, not an end. It introduces readers to a wealth of achievement in the areas of film, television, and performance, making accessible the fruits of the intense study that has recently been focused on queer culture.

How to Use *The Queer Encyclopedia* *of Film & Television*

SIR FRANCIS BACON DIVIDED BOOKS INTO THREE TYPES. "Some books are to be tasted, others to be swallowed, and some few to be chewed and digested: that is, some books are to be read only in parts; others to be read, but cursorily; and some few to be read wholly and with diligence and attention." This book aspires to all three categories.

We certainly believe that *The Queer Encyclopedia of Film & Television* is inviting and rewarding enough to entice readers into diligent and attentive study. At the same time, however, we hope that the book will also invite browsers, who will dip into it repeatedly over time for pleasure and enlightenment. In addition, we hope that it will also serve as a valuable reference tool for readers who need to find particular information quickly.

The essays in the *Encyclopedia* are presented alphabetically, an arrangement that should encourage browsing. They are generally of three types: overviews of broad areas such as Australian Film or British Television; essays on genres, topics, or movements of particular significance for queer film and television; and entries on individuals who have contributed to queer film and television. The A-to-Z List of Entries provides a convenient, alphabetical guide to the entries.

The entries on individuals are diverse, varying from succinct accounts to in-depth critical analyses of major figures. The most important criterion in determining whether an individual was assigned an entry is his or her contribution to the queer cultural tradition.

Another criterion had to do with departmental considerations and copyright restrictions: For example, many of the entries for playwrights and screenwriters, such as Tennessee Williams and Tony Kushner, are included in the literature department of www.glbtq.com and were not available for publication in this volume. They may be accessed online at www.glbtq.com or found in *The Gay & Lesbian Literary Heritage,* ed. Claude J. Summers (New York: Routledge, 2002). Topics particularly related to musical theater and film and individuals such as Tommy Tune and Michael Bennett whose primary contributions to the queer theatrical tradition are in the area of musical theater are included in *The Queer Encyclopedia of Music, Dance & Musical Theater*, ed. Claude J. Summers (San Francisco: Cleis, 2004) and may be found there or online at www.glbtq.com.

In any case, the lack of an individual entry for a director, writer, producer, or performer does not mean that the individual is not significant to the glbtq heritage or is not discussed in the volume. For example, there are no entries for screenwriters Gavin Lambert and Ron Nyswaner, but both are nevertheless discussed in the volume. Even playwrights like Williams and Kushner, whose full-scale entries are in *The Gay & Lesbian Literary Heritage,* are featured in the volume. Discussions of artists who are not accorded individual author entries can most conveniently be found via the Index of Names.

The frequent cross-references should be helpful for readers interested in related topics or in finding further discussions of particular authors. At the end of nearly all the articles, readers are urged to "see also" other entries.

Each article is followed by a brief bibliography. With some exceptions, the bibliographies emphasize secondary rather than primary material, pointing the reader to other studies of the topic or individual.

Finally, the volume's two indexes should be of help in maneuvering through this large collection. The Topical Index conveniently groups entries that are related to each other in various ways, such as sharing the same profession or participating in the same medium. One can tell at a glance, for example, what actors, screenwriters, or directors are included or which entries discuss bisexuality or transgender issues.

The Index of Names should be especially valuable in enabling readers to discover discussions of individuals, some of whom are discussed in several entries in addition to—or in lieu of—their own entries.

A-to-Z List of Entries

Topical Index

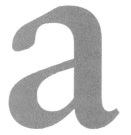

Akerman, Chantal   (b. 1950)

BELGIAN FILMMAKER CHANTAL AKERMAN MADE HER first film, *Saute ma ville* (1968), a short, Chaplinesque tragicomedy, at the age of eighteen. Since that time, she has created numerous films that address various themes, but are most frequently centered on women, often lesbians. Akerman's films explore women at work and at home, women's relationships with men, women, and children, as well as such perennial topics as food, love, sex, romance, art, and storytelling.

Chantal Akerman was born to Polish Holocaust survivors in Brussels in 1950. At the age of fifteen, she decided to make films after watching Jean-Luc Godard's landmark film *Pierrot le fou* (1965). In 1967, she enrolled in the Belgian film school INSAS, after which she attended the Université Internationale du Théâtre in Paris. She soon left school because she was more interested in making films than sitting in a classroom.

She saved money from clerical and waitressing jobs to make her first film. *Saute ma ville,* though it was seen primarily at film festivals, brought her to the attention of critics who admired its innovativeness.

Akerman moved to New York in 1972 to further her filmmaking career. She returned to Europe in 1973, but her first stay in New York was crucial to her development as a filmmaker. Since that time, she has lived in New York, Brussels, and Paris, where she currently resides.

During her teenage years, Akerman decided to make films that would present scenes and characters to the viewer in a personal and immediate way. Viewers of Akerman's films gain intimate knowledge of the people and places that she presents. Ironically, however, the characters rarely speak. In Akerman's films the space created by silence is more important than dialogue in the revelation of personality.

Akerman's first feature film, *Je, tu, il, elle* (1974), is paradigmatic of her work. It can be interpreted as a study of the shifting boundaries of identity and sexuality. Based on a story Akerman wrote in Paris in 1968, the film is divided into three sections: "Time of Subjectivity," "Time of the Other," and "Time of Relationship."

In "Time of Subjectivity," the main character Julie, played by Akerman, is presented in solitude in a bleak, stripped-down room. Julie performs a series of repetitive activities—such as moving a bed around the room—that are completely without context. Julie, therefore, lacks any type of social placement. This creates discomfort for her, and she externalizes her emotions by removing all objects from the room and taking off her clothes.

"Time of the Other" shows Julie hitchhiking. When a trucker gives her a ride, she is intensely curious about him. She listens carefully to the story he tells about the changes he has experienced in his sexual desire for his wife and daughter. When he requests that Julie bring him to orgasm with her hand, she complies. When Julie masturbates herself, the trucker acknowledges the complexity of Julie/Akerman's identity. While Julie is outside the frame, the trucker looks directly at the camera, briefly confirming Akerman's double role as character and director.

During "Time of Relationship," Julie arrives at the apartment of a young woman. Although the woman at first refuses Julie's sexual advances, the woman feeds her and then makes love with her. During the lengthy love-making scene, both women are naked and presented frontally to the camera. Afterward, Julie exits the frame and is heard singing in the shower.

The lesbian sex scene at the end of *Je, tu, il, elle*, filmed in an uncomfortably direct yet distanced manner, investigates issues related to voyeurism, exhibitionism, and the female image on screen. Ostensibly erotic and potentially voyeuristic, the scene is flattened out and drained of any pornographic interest by the detachment of the medium-long shot and by framing that crops the sexually active areas of the actors' bodies. Since the camera never moves, all elements in the scene, from the bedsheets to the women's breasts, are presented as equal.

Je, tu, il, elle successfully undermines the concept of fixed identity. In the "Time of Relationship" section, Akerman addresses the complexity of her dual role as director and character; the distanced shots during the lovemaking scene situate Akerman both in front of and behind the camera. Finally, the film's title (in English: I, you, he, she) points to the shifting nature of personal and sexual identity.

Akerman's extensive filmography includes *Les Rendez-Vous d'Anna* (1978), which documents the journey of a female filmmaker through Western Europe, and *Window Shopping* (1985), a wacky musical that takes place in a Parisian shopping mall. *Jeanne Dielman, 23 Quai du Commerce, 1080 Bruxelles* (1975), her most famous film, is an exhaustively detailed study of a Belgian widow who commits murder when a man disrupts her regimented life. Each of Akerman's films presents a different world to the viewer, one that deserves to be fully explored and carefully analyzed.

One of the most innovative filmmakers of her generation, Akerman is intent not so much on telling traditional stories as on using a particular cinematic language and style to explore people and places.

—*Joyce M. Youmans*

BIBLIOGRAPHY

Benkov, Edith J. "Chantal Akerman." *Gay & Lesbian Biography*. Michael J. Tyrkus, ed. Detroit: St. James Press, 1997. 10–11.

Bergstrom, Janet. "Keeping a Distance." *Sight and Sound* 9.11 (November 1999): 26–28.

Indiana, Gary. "Getting Ready for the Golden Eighties: A Conversation with Chantal Akerman." *Artforum* 21.10 (Summer 1983): 55–61.

Margulies, Ivone. *Nothing Happens: Chantal Akerman's Hyperrealist Everyday*. Durham, N.C.: Duke University Press, 1996.

Peranson, Mark. "The Many Faces of Chantal Akerman." *Varsity Review* (March 5, 1998): www.varsity.utoronto.ca/archives/118/mar05/review/many.html

SEE ALSO

European Film; Film; Film Directors

Almendros, Néstor   (*1930–1992*)

ACADEMY AWARD–WINNING CINEMATOGRAPHER NÉSTOR Almendros achieved his greatest renown working with such directors as Eric Rohmer and François Truffaut, but he also directed several films himself, including the blistering indictment of the persecution of homosexuals in Castro's Cuba, *Improper Conduct* (*Mauvaise conduite*, 1984).

Almendros was born and grew up in Barcelona. Always an avid moviegoer, he joined a film society in 1946. The films that he saw there made him realize that movies could be an art form, not merely a source of entertainment. He later recalled his experience at the film society as his "entry into the world of cinema, my first moment of awareness."

In 1948, he left Spain for Cuba, where his father had been living since going into exile after the Fascist victory in the Spanish Civil War in 1939. The young Almendros was delighted to discover the wide variety of international films shown in Cuba but disappointed by the absence of film societies and scholarly criticism. He therefore started the country's first film society. Among the other founding members were Guillermo Cabrera Infante, who went on to a career as a writer, and Tomás Gutiérrez Alea, who became a filmmaker.

Almendros and several other members of the society aspired to a career in cinema but found the closed nature of the local media unions to be an obstacle. In any event, they hoped to make more serious films than the musicals and melodramas being produced in Cuba. In 1949, Almendros and Gutiérrez Alea made their first attempt at independent filmmaking with *Una confusión cotidiana* (*A Daily Confusion*), based on a story by Kafka.

Almendros soon realized that he would need more training to succeed at his chosen profession. He enrolled in the Institute of Film Techniques at City College of New York. He was frustrated by the school's lack of resources, however, and in 1956 decided to pursue his studies at the Centro Sperimentale in Italy, but there he was disappointed by the quality of the instructors and their conservative views on cinematographic technique.

Unwilling to return to the repressive political climate of either Batista's Cuba or Franco's Spain, Almendros went back to New York, where he got a job as a Spanish instructor at Vassar College. With the savings from his modest salary he bought a 16mm camera and began experimenting with the use and effect of light.

Working in Castro's Cuba

In 1959, Almendros returned to Cuba after the success of Castro's revolution. Although he eventually became bitterly disillusioned with Castro's policies, he initially embraced the hope that the new regime would bring positive changes.

Almendros found a job with ICAIC, the Cuban government's department of cinematographic productions. He worked as a cameraman and as a director on propagandistic films with political or educational themes.

Not satisfied with the nature of his official work, Almendros undertook an independent documentary project entitled *Gente en la playa* (*People at the Beach*). He experimented with the use of light, from the brilliant illumination of the sun at the beach to the relatively obscure interior of a crowded bus.

Almendros was not reticent in expressing his ideas about film technique, which led to clashes with those in power at ICAIC. As a result, the materials for *Gente en la playa* were seized to prevent him from completing it. Eventually he was able to retrieve them, finish the editing, and sneak the film past the bureaucrats by retitling it *Playa del pueblo* (*The Beach of the People*). The film was later banned because it had been made without official sanctions.

As a result of Castro's embrace of Communism, the films being shown in Cuba came almost exclusively from the Soviet bloc. Moreover, Cuban film criticism was based on politics, rather than artistic merit. Almendros found this atmosphere stifling, and he again became an exile.

Career in Cinematography

Almendros went to France, where he showed a smuggled copy of *Gente en la playa* at various film festivals. It was well received but did not lead to any offers of work. In 1964, Almendros was about to give up his dream of a career in cinema when he had a lucky break. He happened to be present when the director of photography on Eric Rohmer's *Paris vu par...(Paris Seen By...)* quit. Almendros volunteered for the job. The producer, Barbet Schroeder, offered him a one-day trial, and then, pleased with his results, retained him.

At that time, Rohmer was working for French educational television. Knowing that Almendros needed work, he got him a job making educational documentaries. Between 1965 and 1967 Almendros made some two dozen such films.

In 1966, Rohmer gave Almendros his first opportunity to be the director of photography on a feature film. *La collectionneuse*, which won a Silver Bear award at the Berlin Film Festival, brought Almendros to the attention of critics. He would go on to work on over fifty more films. Rohmer was the director of seven of these, including *Ma nuit chez Maud* (*My Night at Maud's*, 1969), *Le genou de Claire* (*Claire's Knee*, 1970), and *Die Marquise von O.* (*The Marquise of O.*, 1975), which won the jury prize at the Cannes film festival in 1977.

Almendros also had the opportunity to work on nine films with François Truffaut, whom he had long admired. Their first collaboration was on *Domicile conjugal* (*Bed and Board*, 1970). In the years to come, they would work together on such films as *Histoire d'Adèle H.* (*The Story of Adèle H.*, 1975), *L'homme qui aimait les femmes* (*The Man Who Loved Women*, 1977), and *Le dernier métro* (*The Last Métro*, 1980), which was awarded the César prize for photography by the French Academy of Film Arts and Techniques.

Almendros's work as a director of photography took him to Hollywood as well, where he was employed on a wide variety of projects, including Terence Malick's *Days of Heaven* (1976), which won him an Academy Award for best photography, Robert Benton's *Kramer vs. Kramer* (1978), Randall Kleiser's *The Blue Lagoon* (1979), Alan J. Pakula's *Sophie's Choice* (1982), and Robert Benton's *Places in the Heart* (1984).

In his work as a cinematographer, Almendros was concerned above all with the question of light. Even in his earliest amateur filmmaking days, he studied and experimented with the use of natural available light. Critics have described him as painterly in his attention to light, color, and composition. This painterliness, combined with his willingness to take risks and attempt solutions to difficult lighting problems, made his work particularly attractive to *nouvelle vague* directors such as Rohmer and Truffaut, who sought verisimilitude rather than artificial effects in the appearance of their films.

Rohmer praised Almendros for his precision and meticulousness, characteristics that are reflected in Almendros's discussion of his cinematographic work in his autobiography, *A Man with a Camera* (1984). With an artist's awareness, he explains what went into creating the ambience needed for various scenes in his movies, always in the context of the director's vision of the story to be told. At the same time, he shows considerable technical expertise and ingenuity in meeting the challenges put to him.

Documentaries on Repression in Cuba

In 1984, Almendros realized a project that combined several of his roots in filmmaking—directing, documentaries, and Cuba. *Improper Conduct* (*Mauvaise conduite*) uses filmed interviews with twenty-eight Cuban exiles who had been interned in UMAP (Military Units to Aid Production) concentration camps. The former prisoners had been jailed for what the Castro regime considered dissidence, running afoul of the institutionalized homophobia of Cuban law. Almendros used this film as a vehicle to expose the persecution of gays, but he expressed the hope that viewers would understand that "this is only an aspect, perhaps the most absurd, of a greater repression."

Critical reaction to the film was extremely positive. *Improper Conduct* was hailed as a powerful and important political documentary. It won several awards, including the Human Rights Grand Prix in Strasbourg. As an exposure of the Castro regime's brutal treatment of its homosexual citizens, *Improper Conduct* anticipates such works as writer Reinaldo Arenas's powerful account of his own persecution and imprisonment in Cuba, *Before Night Falls* (1993).

In 1988 Almendros codirected another documentary about repression in Cuba, *Nobody Listened* (*Nadie escuchaba*). Once again, the film drew its power from its directness—real people telling their horrifying stories in their own words. To Almendros, the words themselves and the expressive faces of the people uttering them were the most important elements of the film. He deliberately eschewed "arty lighting effects" and background music.

An intensely private man, Almendros conducted his emotional and sexual life with great discretion. In his autobiography, he does not even mention his homosexuality.

Almendros died at the age of sixty-one of AIDS-related lymphoma. He will be remembered as a master of using light to bring realism to films and using films to bring harsh reality to light.

—*Linda Rapp*

BIBLIOGRAPHY

Almendros, Néstor. *A Man with a Camera.* Rachel Phillips Belash, trans. New York: Farrar, Straus and Giroux, 1984.

———. "Nobody Listened—Story of Cuban Repression." *American Cinematographer* 69.5 (May 1988): 44–48.

———, and Orlando Jiménez-Leal. "Improper Conduct." *American Film* 9 (September 1984): 18, 70–71.

Bailey, John. "Memories of Almendros." *American Cinematographer* 80.8 (August 1999): 120–122.

Greenbaum, Richard. "Improper Conduct." *Films in Review* 35 (November 1984): 528–529.

Honan, William H. "Nestor Almendros, Cinematographer, Dies at 61." *New York Times*, March 5, 1992.

Mira, Alberto. "Almendros, Néstor." *Who's Who in Contemporary Gay and Lesbian History.* Robert Aldrich and Garry Wotherspoon, eds. London: Routledge, 2001. 12.

Revault d'Allonnes, Fabrice. "L'art moderne de la lumière." *Cahiers du cinéma* 454 (April 1992): 74.

Rohmer, Eric. "Nestor Almendros, naturellement." *Cahiers du cinéma* 454 (April 1992): 72–73.

Smith, Paul Julian. *Vision Machines: Cinema, Literature, and Sexuality in Spain and Cuba, 1983–1993.* London: Verso, 1996.

Strick, Philip. "Nestor Almendros." *Sight & Sound* 3.2 (February 1993): 29–30.

Truffaut, Laura. "Renaissance Exile." *Film Comment* 30.1 (January 1994): 15–17.

SEE ALSO

Documentary Film; Film Directors

Almodóvar, Pedro   (b. 1949)

PEDRO ALMODÓVAR IS THE MOST SUCCESSFUL FILM director to have emerged from post-Franco Spain. In works that always bear his distinct cinematic and narrative style, Almodóvar presents absurd situations tightly framed by the trappings of everyday life.

An average-looking nun who methodically seduces "lost women" (*Dark Habits*, 1983), a modest housewife who discusses her sadomasochistic desires during sewing class (*Pepi, Luci, Bom and the Other Girls from the Heap,* 1980), and a priest who is slightly disturbed by the return of his altar boy lover as a voluptuous transsexual (*The Law of Desire*, 1987): These are the forms of queerness that Almodóvar presents as just plain ordinary.

The brilliance of the director's cinematic style, however, lies not merely in the amusing creativity of these situations, but also in the yawning gap between their queerness and their everyday context. In fact, Almodóvar's success resides in his ability to stretch the divergence of this queerness and its normalizing context to an extreme without compromising the believability of either. Although he denies that this strategy has anything to do with his being gay or with gay cinema in general, with it he manages to achieve a radical queering of vision.

Much of Almodóvar's success has come through a conscious adjustment and marketing of his own image. Therefore, the line between fact and fiction has often blurred in his frequent autobiographical reflections.

What seems clear is that the director was born in Calzada de Calatrava, a small village in Castilla La Mancha, where his father worked as a mule-driver. Almodóvar claims that poverty forced his miraculous self-education in writing and cinema; in fact, however, he was educated at a prestigious Salesian seminary located in the city of Cáceres. Upon completing his college degree in 1967, Almodóvar moved to Madrid, where he worked at the state telephone company by day and in a rock band by night.

At this time, he began writing screenplays and novels, all of which reflected the increasingly punk style of his music. With the death of Spain's repressive dictator

Francisco Franco in 1975, Almodóvar found the freedom to produce one of his feature-length screenplays as *Pepi, Luci, Bom*, which was finally released in 1980. Although this film clearly reflects the punk or *Movida* movement of which Almodóvar was a significant part, its plot focuses on the places where this subculture and the general culture meet.

The merging of the subculture and the general culture is defined most specifically in the relationship of Luci, a fortysomething housewife, and Bom, a sadistic female punk musician for whom Luci leaves her policeman husband. That Luci ultimately returns to her far more sadistic husband suggests the normality of her lesbian relationship as opposed to her "perverse" marriage. Almodóvar renders this reversal particularly comic by making Luci and her marriage initially seem so ordinary as compared to Bom's transgressive world of punk.

Similar reversals of extreme normality and transgression appear in *Dark Habits*, where a convent populated by lesbian and heroin-addicted nuns takes in a "lost" stripper, and *The Law of Desire*, where a gay film director and his transsexual sibling form a family that is quite normal when compared to the mad world around them.

Although Almodóvar's later films, including *Tie Me Up, Tie Me Down* (1989), perform these reversals of transgression and "normality" less smoothly, they nonetheless ground themselves in the queer ways of seeing pursued by early American gay films, such as Kenneth Anger's *Scorpio Rising* (1963) or James Bidgood's *Pink Narcissus* (1971).

Indeed, it is precisely the amusing way that Almodóvar makes queerness so central and inviting that renders his films so much more broadly appealing than their American precedents.

The broad appeal of Almodóvar's films was underlined when *All About My Mother* (1999) won an Academy Award as Best Foreign Film and the Spanish Oscar equivalent, the Goya, for Best Spanish Film. The director's latest works, *Talk to Her* (2002), perhaps his most complex narrative, and *Bad Education* (2004), have solidified his reputation as a significant filmmaker, while revealing new warmth and emotion.

—*Andres Mario Zervigon*

BIBLIOGRAPHY

García de Léon, María Antonia, and Teresa Maldonado. *Pedro Almodóvar, la otra españa cañí (sociologia y crítica cinematográficas)*. Cuidad Real: Diputacion de Ciudad Real-Area de Cultura, 1989.

Smith, Julian. *Desire Unlimited: The Cinema of Pedro Almodóvar*. London: Verso, 1994.

———. *Laws of Desire: Questions of Homosexuality in Spanish Writing and Film, 1960–1990*. Oxford: Clarendon Press, 1992.

Vernon, Kathleen, and Barbara Morris, eds. *Post-Franco, Postmodern: The Films of Pedro Almodóvar*. Westport, Conn.: Greenwood Press, 1995.

SEE ALSO

Film; Film Directors; Transvestism in Film; Anger, Kenneth

American Television: Drama

DESPITE A STEADY INCREASE IN THE NUMBER OF "big-screen" queer characters and queerly themed movies, by comparison the overt presence of gay men and lesbians on the American small screen has been, and continues to be, far more limited. Recently, however, television dramatic series such as NBC's *ER* and subscriber network Showtime's *Queer As Folk* have seen a noticeable rise in prominent and recurring queer characters.

Compared to the cable networks, the "big three" broadcast television networks (ABC, CBS, and NBC) have been timid in tackling homosexuality in its multifarious forms. However, long before the advent of cable, broadcast networks were tentatively exploring homosexuality.

Early Representations

The early explorations of homosexuality were accomplished largely by inserting into dramatic television series stereotypically gay characters. As Edward Alwood has explained, from 1968 to 1974 homosexuals on television were recognizable in programs such as *Kojak*, *M*A*S*H*, *Police Woman*, and *Hawaii Five-O* because of their routine representation as limp-wristed, effeminate drag queens who walked with a swish and talked in a high-pitched voice.

Further, as Kylo-Patrick R. Hart has noted, a 1973 episode of ABC's prime-time series *Marcus Welby, M.D.* portrayed homosexuality as a serious illness that subjects gay men to unfulfilling lives, even though this view was strongly challenged the same year by the American Psychiatric Association.

In the face of these stereotyped representations, however, the 1970s also saw the rise of TV movies or MOWs (the broadcast industry slang for "movie of the week") that portrayed homosexuals in a more positive light. These made-for-television movies, promoted as special "events," were specifically themed to address controversial subject matters that otherwise would not be seen in regular programming.

The first TV movie to deal with gay subject matter was ABC's 1972 drama *That Certain Summer*, which explored a teenage boy's reaction to finding out that his father is gay. *That Certain Summer* starred Hal Holbrook as the father and Martin Sheen as his lover, and it garnered much critical acclaim, including a Best Supporting Actor Emmy Award for Scott Jacoby, who played the teenage son.

In 1978, lesbian love was the subject of NBC's *A Question of Love*. Gena Rowlands and Jane Alexander starred in the poignant story of a lesbian mother and her lover, whose "dirty secret" is discovered by Rowlands's ex-husband. He initiates legal proceedings against the pair, and an ugly custody battle ensues.

Another type of battle ensued in ABC's 1985 drama *Consenting Adult*, starring Marlo Thomas and Martin Sheen. Thomas and Sheen portrayed parents trying desperately and, in Sheen's case, unsuccessfully, to deal with their son Jeff's (Barry Tubb) nascent homosexuality.

The Age of AIDS

With the emergence of AIDS on the national scene, the television landscape altered significantly.

NBC broadcast the landmark 1985 TV movie *An Early Frost*, featuring Aidan Quinn as Michael Pierson, an aspiring lawyer and closeted gay man who, unknown to his family, lives with his lover, Peter (D. W. Moffett). Michael not only discovers that Peter has been unfaithful to him, but also, because of this infidelity, that Michael has been infected with the AIDS virus. This discovery threatens to tear apart his relationships with Peter and with his family as well. As Rodney Buxton has explained, the fragile veneer of the Pierson family's stability bursts apart when Michael learns that he has AIDS, exposing all the resentments that various family members had repressed.

Paradoxically, *An Early Frost*, in spite of drawing respectable audience ratings, was a victim of its own success, at least to the extent that it opened the door for new portrayals of homosexuality and AIDS. Many advertisers believed the subject matter was either too controversial or too depressing. Further AIDS-related TV movie projects were also shelved because of the perception that *An Early Frost* had effectively addressed the issue for television audiences.

In 1986, however, Showtime premiered its adaptation of William M. Hoffman's highly regarded Broadway play *As Is*. As Hart has observed, *As Is* is structurally less complex than *An Early Frost*. Nevertheless, its graphically honest depictions of AIDS served a profound educational purpose. Not only did *As Is* dispel several popular misconceptions about the disease, such as methods of contraction through casual contact or by air; it also drew attention to the diversity of AIDS sufferers.

Despite advertiser resistance to the disease as an inherently depressing subject, by 1987 AIDS had begun surfacing in the plots of several prime-time television shows—though, as Emile Netzhammer and Scott Shamp have pointed out, the fact that regular characters must be around for next week's episode usually prevents central characters from becoming infected with a disease that will probably kill them. In order to circumvent this quandary, network executives featured AIDS on individual episodes of shows, including *21 Jump Street, The Equalizer,* and *Midnight Caller,* but in doing so created a causal link between AIDS and gay men.

For example, the 1988 episode of *21 Jump Street* entitled "A Big Disease with a Little Name" shows Officer Tom Hanson (Johnny Depp) assigned to guard from peer harassment an AIDS-stricken hemophiliac male teenager. This Ryan White–type AIDS-scare scenario alters when Hanson discovers that the teen is not hemophiliac. Instead, the teen reveals to Hanson that he is gay and refers obliquely to the "real reason" he has AIDS: unsafe sex.

Although TV movies such as PBS's *Andre's Mother* (1990), HBO's *And the Band Played On* (1990), and ABC's *Our Sons* (1991) attempted to cast AIDS sufferers as noble victims, the connection between gay men and their sexual practices nevertheless remained firmly in place.

Andre's Mother, the Emmy Award–winning adaptation of gay playwright Terrence McNally's drama, aired in 1990 as part of the *American Playhouse* series. The show's conflict revolved around the refusal of the eponymous Andre's mother (Sada Thompson) to accept her late son's sexual identity, even as Andre's lover, Cal (Richard Thomas), battles continually for this acceptance.

Andre's Mother is particularly important because it shifted the "AIDS outsider" dynamic away from the deceased Andre, who is reverently remembered by friends and Cal alike. Instead, Andre's mother becomes the outsider, shut out by both her son's gayness and his disease, before reluctantly moving toward acceptance as the movie ends.

It remains unclear how much these televised depictions of AIDS resulted in an increase in AIDS awareness and in greater compassion and understanding for those most affected by the epidemic. However, as a result of increased AIDS awareness and a shift in AIDS demographics away from gay men, television portrayals of homosexuals began to break new representational ground.

Gays Enter the Television Mainstream

But even before the specter of AIDS rose in media prominence, another landmark event occurred on a prime-time series. In 1981, television audiences for the wildly popular ABC show *Dynasty* were introduced to Steven Carrington (Al Corley from 1981 to 1982 and again in 1991, and Jack Coleman from 1982 to 1989), the first openly bisexual, and later gay, recurring character in a dramatic television series.

Steven weathered traumas typical of a nighttime soap opera: bisexual liaisons resulting in an out-of-wedlock pregnancy, widely circulated rumors about his homosexuality, and gay lovers murdered by his outraged father, oil baron Blake Carrington. Although deeply conflicted at the outset, Blake finally recognized and supported Steven. In 1991's *Dynasty Reunion*, the father embraced Steven and his partner, telling his son that "I am so glad to see that you have someone who loves you as much as I do."

Steven Carrington notwithstanding, *Dynasty* long maintained a marked queer appeal. The show effortlessly combined the trappings of glamorous opulence with scheming, backstabbing characters who exuded an appealing amorality.

Dynasty episodes were further highlighted with moments of gloriously high camp, particularly in the memorable catfights between the two leading ladies, Krystle (Linda Evans), Blake's present wife, and Alexis (Joan Collins), Blake's former wife. Both straight and queer TV audiences quickly came to expect, if not demand, a weekly hair-pulling, furniture-throwing, name-calling, dress-shredding showdown between the two otherwise impeccably dressed and well-mannered (if not always well-behaved) society scions.

Following the demise of *Dynasty*, producer Aaron Spelling (who had created and produced *Dynasty*) debuted *Melrose Place* in 1992. *Melrose Place* began as a spin-off from another popular Spelling production, *Beverly Hills 90210*, a teen-oriented show that featured many different, though incidental, gay characters during its ten-year network run (1990–2000).

Departing from its teen cousin, *Melrose Place* focused on the lives of a group of young professionals who all shared the same Los Angeles apartment complex. The series also featured a recurring gay male character, Matt Fielding (Doug Savant), who was alternately praised as a revolutionary step forward for gay men on television or reviled as a representational nobody.

Much of the criticism surrounding Matt's character resulted from the deliberate downplaying of his homosexuality. Hart has commented that, particularly in the show's first two seasons, so much of Matt's social life took place off camera that the series failed to explore very effectively the realities associated with gay male life. Matt was tapped, instead, to provide emotional support to his fellow apartment denizens.

By the third season, however, the show's writers and producers began exploring Matt's gay life on a regular basis, though these explorations were couched in the same soap opera–style melodrama seen in *Dynasty*. Matt found himself involved in a variety of dysfunctional relationships, ranging from one with a closeted naval officer who later discloses that he is HIV-positive to another with a gay policeman turned obsessed stalker and, finally, one with a physically abusive therapist.

Matt was also fired from his job on two separate occasions because of his sexual orientation and developed an uncontrollable drug habit before moving to San Francisco in the show's sixth season, thus effectively ending his tenure on *Melrose Place*.

The Rise of Prime-Time Lesbianism

At about the same time that Matt's role on *Melrose Place* was waning, a new star and a new show was finding adherents. In September 1995, *Xena: Warrior Princess* debuted on the USA cable network. Fashioned after mythical Amazon warriors, Xena (Lucy Lawless) and her cohort Gabrielle (Renee O'Connor) were an immediate hit with both straight and queer audiences who wanted something different from the usual prime-time network offerings.

Clad in leather and chain mail, sporting an almost fearless insouciance, Xena exuded difference, and became a model for strong women who would not be cowed by (usually male) opponents. Even though Xena was not a lesbian, *per se*, her ambiguous relationship with the softer, more feminine Gabrielle certainly hinted at a barely sublimated lesbianism that the show's writers played up at every opportunity.

Indeed, the sympathetic lesbianism seen in *Xena: Warrior Princess* illustrates the sharp contrast in portrayals of lesbians and gay men that has existed, and continues to persist, in television drama. *Dynasty*'s Steven Carrington and *Melrose Place*'s Matt Fielding exhibited the stereotypical promiscuity and dysfunctionality of gay male relationships, while the bond between Xena and Gabrielle was marked by loyalty, devotion, and commitment.

These traits, in fact, have media antecedents stretching back to 1989, with the pathbreaking feminist medical drama, ABC's *Heartbeat*. This show, which lasted for only one season, featured Gail Strickland as nurse-practitioner Marilyn McGrath, the first recurring openly lesbian character in prime time. Speaking to *People* magazine interviewer Susan Toepfer, *Heartbeat* writer Sara Davidson has remarked that audiences should see McGrath as a terrific person first, then find out that she had a private life that, at its core, was no different from anyone else's.

Heartbeat introduced a relationship plot for McGrath's character almost immediately, a romantic interest played by Gina Hecht, but the series' short-lived network run effectively ended the recurring lesbian presence on a prime-time dramatic show until the advent of *Xena*. However, corresponding with the rise of *Xena* came the 1995 NBC TV movie *Serving in Silence: The Margarethe Cammermeyer Story*, which directly addressed the U.S. military's "Don't Ask, Don't Tell" policy regarding open declarations of homosexuality.

Serving in Silence told the story of Colonel Margarethe Cammermeyer (Glenn Close), a twenty-eight-year Army veteran who, after applying to the Army War College, "admitted" in response to a direct question posed by an investigating officer that she was a lesbian. Because of this declaration, the Army began proceedings leading to her immediate discharge, and Cammermeyer instituted legal proceedings in response. The movie, which was produced by Barbra Streisand, garnered respectable audience ratings but drew fire on the eve of its premiere because of a discreet kiss between Close and her onscreen lover, Judy Davis.

Kissing to Be Clever

The furor over the discreet kiss shared by Close and Davis was hardly unexpected, given the backlash from previous televised expressions of homosexual affection. In February 1991, two female attorneys on the NBC series *L.A. Law*, C. J. Lamb (Amanda Donohoe) and Abby Perkins (Michele Greene), engaged in what has become famous as the first lesbian kiss on network television.

Larry Gross has observed that in the last few episodes of the 1991 season, the recipient of the famous kiss, Abby Perkins, seemed eager to push things even further, only to have the bisexual C. J. hold back and declare that Abby was not really ready. Thus viewers would have to wait until the next season to find out if network television was ready to permit two women to express sexual desire for each other. But the answer never came. Michele Greene left the show over the summer and C. J., after being given a one-episode lesbian lover, soon embarked on an affair with a straight man.

Although the kiss between Abby and C. J. was actually just a quick peck on the lips viewed from behind one of the women, it was enough to reignite the furious debate over depictions of same-sex desire on television that began in 1989. On November 7, 1989, ABC aired the "Strangers" episode of the yuppie series *thirtysomething*, in which the series' two main gay characters, Peter (Peter Frechette) and Russell (David Marshall Grant), are introduced and, in due course, fall into bed together.

Joe Wlodarz has noted that the most sensational and controversial aspect of the episode is the physical enactment of the men's desire for each other (both insinuated and visually confirmed) as they share a postcoital moment in bed and talk about their experience of losing friends to AIDS.

However, according to Richard Kramer's script, the bedroom scene was to be preceded by a seduction scene in which Russell kisses Peter and to be concluded with an affectionate embrace in bed. The viewing audience never witnessed these two moments, prompting gay author Armistead Maupin to observe that the gay kiss—and particularly the gay male kiss—can only be imagined to be "repulsive to most viewers because they have been systematically denied sight of it."

A similar censoring befell a proposed kiss for *Melrose Place*'s hapless Matt Fielding during the 1994 season finale. In the final episode, the visiting best friend of main character Billy Campbell (Andrew Shue) falls for Matt, and a scene was shot in which the two characters kiss before they retire to separate beds. However, as Larry Gross notes, conservative critics chimed in with protests and threats of boycotts. In response, the network altered the scene. Instead of kissing, the men shook hands, exchanged a meaningful glance and moved toward each other, before the camera cut away to Billy looking through the blinds of his apartment with a shocked expression on his face.

However, while gay male expressions of sexual desire remained firmly in the closet, lesbian kisses appeared more frequently and with less fanfare. On January 11, 1997, an episode of the ABC series *Relativity* showed a close-up, ten-second kiss between Rhonda Roth (Lisa Edelstein) and her girlfriend Suzanne (Kristin Dattilo). Surprisingly, no network affiliates pulled the episode from their schedule, even though ABC heavily marketed the show's content.

Speaking with *Advocate* columnist Robert Pela, GLAAD (Gay and Lesbian Alliance Against Defamation) spokesperson Alan Klein noted that the lack of negative response to the show was clearly a sign that times and perceptions are changing.

Changing Perceptions and Breakthrough Representations

Despite changing social and media perceptions, however, there is still a lingering reticence on the part of broadcast network executives to televise overt displays of homosexual affection and desire. It is unlikely that broadcast networks will ever reach the levels of queer representational acceptance that cable and subscriber networks have shown recently, but there have nevertheless been changes even on broadcast networks, such as the coming-out in 2000 of Dr. Kerry Weaver (Laura Innes) on NBC's *ER* and Willow's (Alyson Hannigan) getting a girlfriend on the WB's *Buffy the Vampire Slayer* in the 2000–2001 season.

Nonetheless, cable and subscriber networks have in recent years been far more pathbreaking in their depictions of homosexual content. For instance, the broadcast networks would not have dared attempt what subscriber network Showtime executed in 2000 with the debut of *Queer As Folk*. Billed in 1999 as the first all-gay soap opera, *Queer As Folk* exploded on Britain's Channel 4 before being transplanted, for U.S. viewers, to Pittsburgh.

Produced by life partners Ron Cowen and Daniel Lipman (who also created the series *Sisters* and 1985's television movie *An Early Frost*), *Queer As Folk* offers an unflinching, no-holds-barred slice of queer life, including foam parties, nipple piercing, and recreational drug use. There is also no shortage of erotically charged same-sex lovemaking scenes, usually between amoral lothario Brian Kinney (Gale Harold) and his much younger boyfriend, Justin Taylor (Randy Harrison).

Yet, despite the rampant hedonism, the show also provides a balance of sympathetic characters who search for and achieve meaningful—if tenuously held—relationships. In the show's first season, Michael Novotny (Hal Sparks), whose best friend is Brian, becomes intimately involved with a chiropractor, Dr. Dave Cameron (Chris Potter); and though this relationship ends at the conclusion of season one, Michael soon finds a longer-term partner in HIV-positive literature professor Ben Bruckner (Robert Gant). Best friends Emmett Honeycutt (Peter Paige) and Ted Schmidt (Scott Lowell) also do a turn as lovers in season three.

Living among Queer As Folk's predominantly gay male cadre is a lesbian couple, Lindsay Peterson (Thea Gill) and Melanie Marcus (Michelle Clunie), who serve as dual mothers to Gus, the infant offspring of Lindsay and Brian. The two women have the show's longest-running relationship.

Lindsay and Mel helped pave the way for another Showtime series, the steamy lesbian hit The L Word, which premiered in January 2004. Although The L Word has been widely praised, it has also drawn criticism similar to that received by Queer As Folk. Constance Reeder, columnist for the lesbian publication off our backs, has complained that The L Word is not groundbreaking TV, but is, instead, "Queer As Folk with breasts."

However, queer theorist Eve Kosofsky Sedgwick has noted that, while the show is certainly not "edgy" in its "relation to reality or political process," it is nevertheless "absurdly luxurious" in its exploration of the "portrayal of generational dynamics in this group of women, even if only between thirtysomethings and twentysomethings."

Like its predecessor Queer As Folk, The L Word has thrived on controversy. While Queer As Folk will end its run in 2006, The L Word was renewed for a second season only two weeks after its debut. The eagerly anticipated season two began airing in February 2005.

Another cable dramatic series that features queer characters is HBO's Six Feet Under, which debuted to critical acclaim in 2001. Developed, written, and frequently directed by Alan Ball, who won a 1999 Academy Award for his screenplay for the film American Beauty, the show focuses on a family who own and operate a funeral home in Los Angeles.

Younger son David Fisher (Michael C. Hall) came out to his family in an early episode, and the show frequently follows his attempts to find a replacement for his former lover Keith Charles (Matthew St. Patrick), an L.A. police officer who broke up with David because he was not honest about his homosexuality. In casting the gay son as the "stable" member of the dysfunctional family and in treating the interracial relationship between David and Keith sympathetically and matter-of-factly, Six Feet Under normalizes homosexuality.

In May 2004, producers of another HBO television drama, The Sopranos, announced that Joseph Gannascoli, who plays Vito Spatafore on the hit show, would come out as a gay mobster. Gannascoli explained that he relished the chance to play a gay character, and said that he wanted to be "effeminate but knockaround."

But perhaps the most significant achievement in glbtq representation in American television drama came in December 2003, when HBO premiered a six-hour, $60 million presentation of Tony Kushner's pathbreaking AIDS epic Angels in America, directed by Mike Nichols. Angels, which featured an all-star cast including Meryl Streep, Emma Thompson, and Al Pacino, received rave reviews and garnered an astonishing eleven Emmy Awards.

Emma Thompson, in an Advocate interview about her response to the play, remarked "I opened the play, read the first couple of pages, rang Mike [Nichols], and said 'I'll do it.' The writing has that effect on you. It's so remarkable."

Television portrayals of homosexuals have made significant strides since the homophobic images seen in the late 1960s and early 1970s. In time, perhaps, there will be an all-queer series appearing on a broadcast network, so stay tuned.

—*Nathan G. Tipton*

BIBLIOGRAPHY

Alwood, Edward. *Straight News: Gays, Lesbians, and the News Media.* New York: Columbia University Press, 1996.

Berlant, Lauren. "Sex in Public." *Critical Inquiry* 24.2 (1998): 547–567.

Buxton, Rodney. "An Early Frost." *The Museum of Broadcast Communications* website. www.museum.tv

Doty, Alexander. *Making Things Perfectly Queer: Interpreting Mass Culture.* Minneapolis: University of Minnesota Press, 1993.

————, and Corey K. Creekmur, eds. *Out in Culture: Gay, Lesbian, and Queer Essays on Popular Culture.* Durham, N.C.: Duke University Press, 1995.

Dyer, Richard. *The Matter of Images.* New York: Routledge, 1993.

"Gannascoli Plays 1st Gay 'Sopranos' Capo." *UPI News Track,* May 3, 2004.

Giltz, Michael. "Faces of Angels." *Advocate,* December 9, 2003, 38.

Gross, Larry. "Don't Ask, Don't Tell: Lesbian and Gay People and the Media." *Images that Matter: Pictorial Stereotypes in the Media.* Paul Martin Lester, ed. Westport, Conn.: Praeger, 1995. 149–159.

Hart, Kylo-Patrick R. "Representing Gay Men on American Television." *Journal of Men's Studies* 9.1 (2000): 59–79.

Hensley, Dennis. "Inside Queer As Folk." *Advocate,* November 21, 2000, 47.

Joyrich, Lynne. "Epistemology of the Console." *Critical Inquiry* 27 (Spring 2001): 439–467.

Kaye, Lori. "Where Are the Funny Girls?" *Advocate*, January 16, 2001, 85.

Maupin, Armistead. "A Line That Commercial TV Won't Cross." *New York Times*, January 9, 1994.

Netzhammer, Emile C., and Scott A. Shamp. "Guilt By Association: Homosexuality and AIDS on Prime-Time Television." *Queer Words, Queer Images: Communication and the Construction of Homosexuality*. R. J. Ringer, ed. New York: New York University Press, 1994. 91–106.

Pela, Robert L. "Rating TV Ratings." *Advocate*, February 18, 1997, 33.

Pilipp, Frank, and Charles Shull. "TV Movies of the First Decade of AIDS." *Journal of Popular Film & Television* 21.1 (1993): 19–26.

Reeder, Constance. "The Skinny on The L Word." *off our backs* 34.1–2 (2004): 51-52.

Sedgwick, Eve Kosofsky. "'The L Word': Novelty in Normalcy." *Chronicle of Higher Education*, January 16, 2004, B10.

Signorile, Michelangelo. *Queer in America: Sex, the Media, and the Closets of Power*. New York: Random House, 1993.

Skeggs, Beverly, Leslie Moran, Paul Tyrer, and Jon Binnie. "Queer As Folk: Producing the Real of Urban Space." *Urban Studies* 41.9 (2004): 1839–56.

Toepfer, Susan. "Is Prime Time Ready For Its First Lesbian? Gail Strickland Hopes So—and She's About to Find Out." *People*, April 25, 1988, 95.

Wlodarz, Joe. "Smokin' Tokens: thirtysomething and TV's Queer Dilemma." *Camera Obscura: Feminism, Culture, and Media Studies* 33–34 (1995): 193–211.

See also

American Television: News; American Television: Reality Shows; American Television: Situation Comedies; American Television: Soap Operas; American Television: Talk Shows

American Television: News

A S IN THE MAINSTREAM PRINT MEDIA, GAY PEOPLE AND issues pertaining to them have been inadequately covered by American television news. Some of the reasons for this underreporting have to do with the nature of television news in general. The medium favors highly dramatic, visually exciting content (fires, tornadoes, car chases, and so on) over substantive reportage and reasoned analysis. Television's inherent conservatism can also be blamed. After all, the medium's primary function is not to inform, or even entertain, viewers, but to deliver an audience to advertising sponsors.

Apart from those occasions when prominent women such as Ellen DeGeneres, k.d. lang, and Rosie O'Donnell have publicly acknowledged their homosexuality, lesbians have been even less visible in television news reports than their gay male counterparts. Unfortunately, this, too, is unsurprising, given America's patriarchal culture, in which women are all too often not paid serious consideration.

For most of television's history, news coverage of gay people and relevant issues, if it existed at all, was usually negative. Frequently, gay achievement was ignored; it was not unusual, for example, for television news reports of the 1973 election of Elaine Noble to the Massachusetts state legislature to fail to identify her as an openly lesbian politician. Even major news stories such as the outbreak of the AIDS epidemic were downplayed. By the beginning of 1983, the three major networks combined had dedicated a total of only thirteen minutes to this escalating international health crisis.

Important First Steps

In the 1960s and 1970s, the bulk of the attention accorded to gay people in television news reports was in sensational documentary specials. Few openly gay individuals appeared on camera, and when they did, it was customary for their faces to be obscured. In a 1966 Florida television news program aired on Miami's WJTV, Richard Inman purported to represent the gay viewpoint, but said he had given up homosexuality four years earlier and giggled when asked if he thought gay couples could live happily together over a long term.

A special episode of *CBS Reports*, aired on March 7, 1967, almost certainly exposed the largest television audience up to that time to the existence of openly gay people. Hosted by Mike Wallace, "The Homosexuals" was the product of two years' work and debate by members of the CBS news staff. The first version of the documentary was extensively revised for fear that it could be construed as an endorsement of homosexuality.

In the end, the CBS report mainly represented the traditional view of homosexuality as an illness, and emphasized the outsider status of gay people. However, it at least suggested that other viewpoints were possible. Still, nervous advertising sponsors would not touch it; the commercial breaks were filled by public service announcements.

"The Homosexuals" showed footage of Washington activists Frank Kameny, Jack Nichols, Lilli Vincenz, and others picketing in front of the White House and at other strategically chosen locations. In an interview segment, Nichols appeared under an alias ("Warren Adkins") to spare his father embarrassment.

"Adkins" was one of a few positive gay role models who appeared in the documentary to declare their satisfaction with their own homosexuality. Unconsciously anticipating later arguments by gay activists that homosexuality is not a choice, "Adkins" said he couldn't conceive of renouncing his homosexuality and compared it to the color of his hair or skin.

The day after "The Homosexuals" aired on CBS, Nichols was fired from his job in a Washington hotel.

Most viewers agreed with psychiatrist Charles Socarides, who opined for the camera that homosexuality precluded the possibility of living a happy, productive life. (Years later, Socarides's own son, Richard, would become an openly gay staff member in the Clinton White House.)

"The Homosexuals" remains a landmark of American television news because of its articulation, however minimal, of dissenting views. James Braxton Craven, a federal district court judge from North Carolina, appeared on the program to question the legal sanctions against those who engaged in consenting homosexual acts. "The Homosexuals" also addressed gay influence in the arts.

Noted author and political commentator Gore Vidal defended gay playwright Edward Albee's 1962 classic, *Who's Afraid of Virginia Woolf?* Along with his fellow dramatists Tennessee Williams and William Inge, Albee had been criticized in the *New York Times* and elsewhere for writing women characters who were supposedly gay men in drag. Vidal countered this nonsense by emphasizing the popularity of Albee's play. "Obviously it's popular because what he has to say about married couples speaks to everybody," Vidal told Mike Wallace.

An (Unwitting?) Agent of Backlash

As gay people began to demand their rights, television news often became an agent of backlash. Gay protesters were frequently defined, often unintentionally, as troublemakers or—at best—as embattled parties to ludicrous "debate." Television news clips showed Anita Bryant denouncing homosexuals as unfit for the company of children. (It has frequently been observed that no other minority group is ever subjected to such defamatory characterizations on television news programs.)

Among activists, there was an increasing dissatisfaction with the inadequate representation of gay people on television news. Mark Segal, a young gay man from Philadelphia, staged several high-profile protests of shows such as *Today* and news figures such as Walter Cronkite, typically chaining himself to a desk or a camera. At his 1974 trial for trespassing, Segal seemed to make some headway with Cronkite; and coverage of gay news by CBS, Cronkite's employer, increased in the following year.

Subsequent news documentaries on the subject of homosexuality, however, were even more problematic.

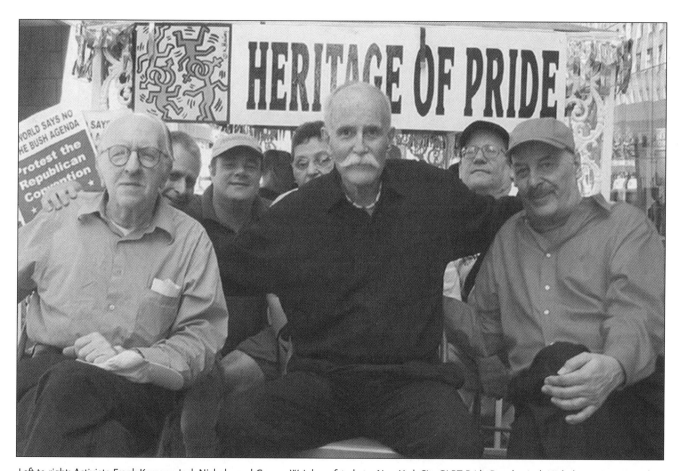

Left to right: Activists Frank Kameny, Jack Nichols, and George Weinberg feted at a New York City GLBT Pride Parade. Jack Nichols was interviewed on the news program *CBS Reports* in 1967. The program also showed footage of Washington activists including Frank Kameny. George Weinberg coined the term *homophobia*. Photograph by Craig Houser.

In 1979, ABC News *Close-Up* presented an hour-long documentary (again, with no sponsors) emphasizing gay promiscuity and suicide. In April 1980, *CBS Reports* took a step backward from "The Homosexuals" when it aired "Gay Power, Gay Politics." An ostensible look at the influence of the gay voting bloc in San Francisco, the program emphasized sadomasochism (using footage shot at a heterosexual club) within the gay community.

Dianne Feinstein, then mayor of San Francisco, told the CBS news crew to leave her office after she was asked, "How does it feel to be mayor of Sodom and Gomorrah?" Less than six months after "Gay Power, Gay Politics" aired, the National News Council cited CBS for dubious news practices such as stereotyping and false implications in connection with the program. This, of course, was less widely reported.

Winds of Change

In 1978, PBS offered an unprecedented look at the breadth and diversity of the gay community when it aired the documentary *Word Is Out: Stories of Some of Our Lives*. Peter Adair and the Mariposa Film Group spent five years making this sensitive work, which explored gay history and options for the present.

There were other occasions for hope, including several episodes of Phil Donahue's talk show, on which openly gay guests were invited to speak out on issues and entertain questions from viewers. (In October, 1982, noted activist Larry Kramer was one of Donahue's guests.) At their best, Donahue's shows took on the seriousness and importance, if not the nominal mantle, of television news, giving viewers access to information that remained unavailable elsewhere.

As they had done many times before, frustrated gay people took matters into their own hands and, in 1992, created *In the Life*. Although it began as a variety entertainment show, *In the Life* soon became more news-oriented, offering informed reports on protest marches, the ongoing AIDS epidemic, and other issues. Produced by a not-for-profit agency, the series was offered free of charge to all public television stations.

When it began airing in 1992, *In the Life* was broadcast on six stations. In the early years of the new millennium, it was airing on 120 stations. However, many stations still refuse to carry it despite the fact that its production values rival the best of television news anywhere.

At the time of this writing, public television continues to surpass the networks in the quality of its depiction of gay people and their concerns. Although it may not command an audience as large as the networks—each episode of *In the Life*, for example, is seen by an estimated million viewers, as compared with the multiple millions who tune in to the commercial networks—PBS is more than equal to network television in importance.

For example, an extraordinary documentary by openly gay filmmaker Arthur Dong, titled *Licensed to Kill*, aired on public television in 1998. In this hard-hitting work, Dong traveled to various prisons to interview inmates who had been convicted of murdering gay men. By asking a varied group of killers why they targeted homosexual men, Dong highlighted the pernicious influence of religious and political figures who have used their prominent positions as bully pulpits from which to denounce homosexuality.

All too often, such "leaders" have been allowed to make their damaging statements in forums provided by television news programs. Media watchdog groups such as GLAAD (the Gay and Lesbian Alliance Against Defamation), however, have been increasingly effective in educating news organizations about issues involving the gay community.

One sign of the winds of change may be discerned in the episode of ABC's *Primetime Thursday* that aired on March 14, 2002, featuring Rosie O'Donnell and the issue of gay adoption. While the show included the obligatory antigay spokesperson, this time a Florida state representative who opposes gay adoption, the host, Diane Sawyer, subjected him to a withering cross-examination.

Moreover, the show exposed the dubious credentials of such "experts" on the issue as antigay activist Paul Cameron, the author of discredited studies that purport to demonstrate the unfitness of gays and lesbians as parents; and countered those studies with more respectable sociological research. Most importantly, it not only offered a forum for O'Donnell, but it also portrayed positively the loving household of gay parents Steven Lofton and Roger Croteau, who—because of Florida's ban on gay adoption—may have a ten-year-old boy taken from them despite their having raised him from infancy.

Perhaps the most important harbinger of change is the growth of niche broadcasting, especially the development of television that caters particularly to glbtq audiences. For example, Q Television Network, which launched in 2005, offers original programming that includes queer perspectives on news and culture. LOGO, a channel of MTV that is scheduled to launch in 2005, promises to offer a range of original series, documentaries, and specials, and to team up with CBS News to cover glbtq news stories in a "professional and authentic voice."

One of the pioneers in producing news shows aimed at glbtq audiences is *QTV Newsmagazine*, which debuted in 1995 as a local San Francisco public access offering. *QTV Newsmagazine* now airs on Comcast cable channels and is also available via the Internet. Hosted by Executive Producer Rahn Fudge, the newsmagazine offers programs that originate both in San Francisco and in Key West, Florida.   —*Greg Varner*

BIBLIOGRAPHY

Alwood, Edward. *Straight News*. New York: Columbia University Press, 1996.

Downie, Leonard, and Robert G. Kaiser. *The News About the News: American Journalism in Peril*. New York: Knopf, 2002.

Kaiser, Charles. *The Gay Metropolis*. Boston: Houghton Mifflin, 1997.

Loughery, John. *The Other Side of Silence: Men's Lives and Gay Identities*. New York: Henry Holt, 1998.

Varner, Greg. "A Look at the Dark Side: Documentarian Arthur Dong Asks Killers of Gay Men Why They Did It." *Washington Blade*, June 12, 1998.

www.inthelifetv.org

SEE ALSO

American Television: Talk Shows; Documentary Film; DeGeneres, Ellen; Dong, Arthur; *In the Life*; O'Donnell, Rosie

American Television: Reality Shows

IN 2000, WHEN SELF-DESCRIBED "FAT NAKED FAG" Richard Hatch emerged as the first-season winning contestant on the phenomenally popular network reality television show *Survivor*, he credited his survival success in large part to his homosexuality. According to Hatch, growing up gay, being part of a minority community—and thus subject to scrutiny by others—inspired him to be both introspective and egocentric. These dual poles of introspection and egocentrism are, in fact, key elements in understanding the important roles gay men and lesbians play within the confines of reality television shows, even as they present interpretive quandaries for hetero- and homosexual viewers alike.

In a typical reality television show, particularly one with game-show trappings such as CBS's *Survivor* and *Big Brother*, or ABC's *The Mole*, cast members as well as viewers regard introspection as suspicious behavior. Surely, the viewers surmise, something is being hatched under that quiet facade, and usually this supposition is proved correct. For these shows' gay and lesbian participants, however, the conflation of introspection with cunning and plotting too easily becomes connected to the unfortunate stereotype that gay men and lesbians are inherently crafty, conniving, and untrustworthy.

Even in ostensibly less competitive shows such as Bravo's *Boy Meets Boy*, Fox's *Playing It Straight*, and even MTV's "docusoap"—Sam Brenton and Reuben Cohen's neologism for a television show that seamlessly combines elements of documentary realism with soap opera-style plotting—*The Real World*, introspection is often seen as a negative attribute, indicating moodiness, insecurity, or simmering hostility.

At the opposite end of the emotional spectrum, egocentrism in gay and lesbian cast members or competitors is almost universally viewed in stereotypical terms. Egocentrism rehearses the well-worn cliché that gay men and lesbians are self-absorbed, narcissistic, and desperate to be on display. However, a more recent trend in reality television, "makeover" or "make-better" shows such as NBC/Bravo's *Queer Eye for the Straight Guy* and the Style Network's *The Brini Maxwell Show*, have effectively countered this stereotype.

Reality television continues to evolve, as do its gay and lesbian participants, who bring to these shows a powerful set of societal presuppositions. While too often the shows play directly into stereotyped expectations, gay men and lesbians have demonstrated repeatedly that these preconceptions can be overcome. In fact, reality television viewers have come increasingly to expect the appearance of gay men and lesbians in these shows because their presence helps further underscore the "reality" in reality TV.

Early Incarnations: Docudramas

The term *reality TV* properly entered the lexicon in the early 1990s with the rise of such gritty police and rescue programs as *Cops* and *Rescue 911*. However, the documentaryesque format of these shows, with their cinema verité, almost intrusive "slice of life" approach to observing, cataloging, and broadcasting human interactions, actually originated in the 1970s with the groundbreaking PBS series *An American Family*.

The series, broadcast initially in 1973 and rebroadcast in 1991, documented the real-life dysfunctional doings of the Loud family of Santa Barbara, California. In addition to showcasing bitter family arguments and revealing salacious family secrets such as a philandering husband and a crumbling marriage, *An American Family* was also groundbreaking in no small part because of eldest son Lance's onscreen coming out.

David Horowitz notes that, with his blue lipstick, dyed rooster-red hair, red eye shadow, and wildly exaggerated swish, Lance Loud (1952–2002) shocked television viewers of the 1970s by publicly proclaiming his homosexuality. Loud, who went on to become a regular columnist for *The Advocate* before succumbing to AIDS at age fifty, explained that while he thought the open declaration of his homosexuality would mark him as "incredibly unique," he realized quickly that he would forever be remembered only as "a famous fag."

In spite of their prominently displayed dysfunctionality and unraveling family dynamic, *An American Family* ensured the Louds a lasting place in the pop-culture vocabulary and an important part in the history of homosexuals on television. In 2002, PBS eulogized Lance Loud in the retrospective documentary *Lance Loud! A Death in an American Family,* and filmmakers Susan and Alan Raymond remarked that the broadcast history of onscreen gay men and lesbians can be traced directly back to Loud, noting that before *An American Family* there was not an accessible gay character on American television. Yet despite the fertile groundwork laid by Lance Loud and his American family, almost twenty years would elapse before gay men and lesbians would reappear in real-life situations played out on the small screen.

"This Is the True Story...": MTV's Real Cool World

When viewers tuned in to MTV in 1992, they were introduced to seven strangers chosen to share a house together for three months, who had their lives taped nonstop, with the end result of their communal experience broadcast to a nationwide audience in a series of thirteen episodes. This was the premise of MTV's runaway hit show and soon-to-be cultural icon *The Real World.*

The show's cast of seven strangers was diverse; it comprised three women and four men, two African Americans and five Caucasians, six heterosexuals and one homosexual, Norman Korpi. Korpi's presence in MTV's SoHo loft was not, however, greeted with the shock that Americans felt in response to Lance Loud's overt homosexuality. Instead, Korpi presented himself as a gay role model: politically active, intellectually astute, and perhaps most important, in the words of fellow cast member Julie, just everyday people.

MTV's decision to cast Korpi in the premiere season of *The Real World* set a precedent that MTV would adhere to closely, the conscious inclusion of gay men and lesbians in the "seven strangers" formula. Almost invariably the gay or lesbian cast members come across as the most "normal" of the seven cast mates, and very often they are the most involved in political causes.

In the New York season, for instance, Korpi cajoled other cast members into joining him at the March for Reproductive Rights in Washington, D.C. In 1993, Los Angeles *Real World*er Beth Anthony campaigned for gay marriage; and, shortly after taping ended for the season, she married her girlfriend, Becky. *Real World* New Orleans (2000) featured Danny Roberts, who, by announcing that his lover was in the military, brought to MTV viewers the debate over the military's "Don't Ask, Don't Tell" policy, dramatizing in richly human terms the cost such a policy exacts of those who are directly affected by it.

But the *Real World* cast member who left perhaps the most lasting, politically charged, and poignant impression on MTV audiences was Pedro Zamora (1972–1994), a resident in the 1994 San Francisco season. Zamora, an AIDS activist, was HIV-positive during the show's taping, and he used his appearance on the show to educate MTV viewers and the public at large about both the dangers of HIV/AIDS and the rights and dignity of people living with AIDS. Zamora died from AIDS complications on November 11, 1994, and was eulogized by President Bill Clinton.

MTV's *The Real World* continues to lure viewers into the lives of seven randomly chosen strangers each year, and every new season brings with it the promise of a new gay or lesbian character whom viewers will come to know, and with whom many can readily identify. Yet the formulaic elements of *The Real World* have been eclipsed by the recent ascension of more competitive, money-driven reality game shows such as *Survivor* and *The Amazing Race,* even as the gay and lesbian presence on these shows remains constant.

Game-Show Reality: Outwit, Outlast, Out There!

When Richard Hatch walked away with the $1 million prize for being the last Survivor standing, American television viewers sat up and took notice. Here was a hirsute, paunchy gay man seen by millions of Americans winning a test of raw physicality and brilliant cunning and being handsomely rewarded by a jury of his reality game-show peers.

Hatch was, of course, no one's idea of a gay role model, much less a network superstar, but according to

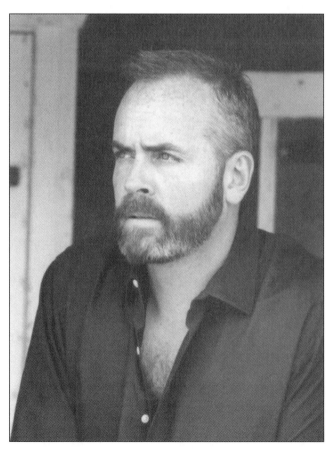

Richard Hatch, winner of the *Survivor* reality show in 2000.

Advocate columnist Erik Meers, his soap-operatic con-nivings were the best thing for CBS's ratings since 1980's prime-time soap-opera *Dallas* cliffhanger "Who Shot J. R. Ewing?" In fact, Hatch's popularity owed far more to his scheming than to his being openly gay, a fact that as the show progressed became incidental.

Like his reality show predecessors on MTV, Hatch's position in *Survivor* was simply a part of the reality TV formula, and increasingly gay men and lesbians began appearing regularly on the rapidly proliferating reality game shows. *Survivor: Africa* (2001) featured flamboy-ant competitor Brandon Quinton; *Survivor: Marquesas* (2002) offered castaway John Carroll; and ABC's show *The Mole* showcased two gay cast members, Jim Morrison and Jennifer Biondi, in its 2001 premiere season.

But perhaps the biggest boost for visibly gay and les-bian persons on television was the triumph by Reichen Lehmkuhl and Chip Arndt in CBS's *The Amazing Race* (2003). Like Richard Hatch, Lehmkuhl and Arndt gar-nered a $1 million prize for besting their competitors, and they did so while insisting that CBS caption them as "married" for the duration of the show.

Advocate writer Jon Barrett notes wryly that in a summer saturated with queer eyes and boys meeting boys, this "married" couple stole the show, won more than a few hearts, and took home the million-dollar prize. And they did it all the while looking so hot that even the straight guys on the show were flirting with them. Although Lehmkuhl and Arndt dissolved their relationship soon after the show ended, they remain close and still consider themselves a "team."

Love and Marriage

In 2002, Bravo took advantage of the controversy over same-sex marriage by producing an original reality miniseries entitled *Gay Weddings*. Exploring the trials and tribulations faced by four diverse gay couples as they plan and put together their dream weddings, *Gay Weddings* showcased four very different couples over five months as they coped with their own anxieties and hopes and contended with the attitudes and (sometimes surprising) reactions of others.

Featuring four disparate settings—a private backyard wedding in the high desert, a tropical beach party in Puerto Vallarta, an elegant Deco restaurant affair, and a Hollywood extravaganza—*Gay Weddings* chronicled the roller-coaster ride that is wedding planning from a decidedly nontraditional point of view. In the process, it underlined both the distinct concerns of gay and lesbian couples and their common aspirations for acceptance and recognition.

While Lehmkuhl and Arndt competed under the "married" banner on *The Amazing Race,* another muta-tion of the reality game shows featured gay men either

vying for each other's attentions or, ironically, trying to outsmart a woman into thinking they were straight. *Entertainment Weekly* columnist Mandi Bierly has termed this subgenre of reality television "Guess the Gay" games, and these shows feature gay men interspersed with straight male ringers competing for the affections of, alternatively, a woman (*Playing It Straight)* or another man (*Boy Meets Boy).*

Not surprisingly, these guessing-game competitions have attracted fierce criticism from the glbtq community, especially the shows' premise that gay men have distinc-tive physical features and/or mannerisms that mark them as homosexual. (In fact, however, the difficulty in distinguishing the gay and straight men on these shows effectively undercuts the offensive premise. If anything, the shows indicate how easy it is for gay men to pass as straight and for straight men to pass as gay.)

Since the dynamic of a gay man pretending to be straight in order to seduce a woman evokes painful memories of real-life experience for many gay men and straight women, *Playing It Straight* was especially sav-aged. These shows, while mildly entertaining, did not receive the high viewer interest of shows like *Survivor.* Fox, faced with criticism and low ratings, abruptly can-celed *Playing It Straight* halfway through its run.

Boy Meets Boy, which pioneered in showing gay courting rituals, was criticized by its own star, James Getzlaff. On learning that some of the show's contes-tants were actually straight, Getzlaff complained bitterly that the show had the very real potential of turning into a practical joke. He also worried that the show played on homophobic stereotypes by reinforcing the idea that gay men secretly like straight men, but have to hide it.

Still, *Boy Meets Boy* offered gay viewers an opportu-nity to test their "gaydar" while observing a bevy of handsome men competing for the affections of another handsome man, still a rarity on television.

All Things Just Keep Getting Better: Queer Eyes and Gay Guys

As reality television entered fully into the new millen-nium, the format of these shows changed once again, and yet another subgenre was spawned: the "makeover" or "make-better" show. The viewing public, seemingly growing tired of variations on the competitive elimina-tion reality game shows, turned increasingly to shows that provided an entertaining and learning experience. Thus was ushered in the era of the Queer Eye.

The legend started innocently enough. According to television producer David Collins, as quoted in the *Advocate,* a Boston woman was berating her husband for his slovenly appearance. Pointing at four smartly dressed, well groomed, and nicely mannered gay men, she complained that her husband did not look like them. As Collins notes wryly, "What she needed was a queer eye for her straight guy." Collins then related this story to his straight producing partner, David Metzler, and the two began the creation of an unscripted lifestyle-makeover show. Thus was born *Queer Eye for the Straight Guy*.

Queer Eye debuted on the Bravo network in the summer of 2003 and featured "The Fab Five," a team of gay experts who perform emergency transformations on hapless straight men who, somewhat surprisingly, eagerly submit themselves for an appearance on the show. Armed with rubber gloves, natural fabrics, pre-shave oils, and witty remarks, the Fab Five, now consisting of Kyan Douglas (hair and grooming), Thom Filicia (interior design), Jai Rodriguez (culture), Ted Allen (food and wine), and Carson Kressley (fashion), sweep down on a chosen straight man's dwelling and, in the space of a 60-minute episode, enact a total (mind, body, and soul) transformation of said straight man.

Quite often the transformations are so successful that the straight participants do not want the Fab Five to leave. David Collins observes that during the show the straight man bonds with the Fab Five, and this bonding generates a broader awareness of who gay men are and what it means to be straight and cool with themselves.

The Fab Five's expert knowledge, along with their broadly suggestive humor, makes the gap between straight and gay bridgeable; and, according to Kylo-Patrick R. Hart, the humorous exchanges make it clear to the straight subjects, as well to straight viewers at home, that gay men do not really pose threats to their sexuality or well-being. This is an important point and one that *Queer Eye for the Straight Guy* exploits at every turn: Gay men can help straight men lead better lives. David Collins summarizes the show's premise by explaining that *Queer Eye for the Straight Guy* is ultimately you, only better.

The Future of GLBTQ Reality Television

Even though *Queer Eye* has been in existence only for a short while, it has already generated immense and overwhelmingly favorable publicity. It has also provided the genesis for another queer "make-better" show, Style Network's *The Brini Maxwell Show*. Robert Philpot describes the show as Martha Stewart filtered through 1950s icon Donna Reed, but Brini Maxwell supplies an interesting twist within the confines of her retro-kitsch home-entertaining and decorating ideas. Brini Maxwell is actually Ben Sander, a glam transvestite who, as Lynette Rice relates, spent five years dispensing helpful hints on New York City's public access television before moving to the more upscale digs of the Style Network.

Reality television shows have already demonstrated the marketability and popularity of gay and lesbian participants, and as reality television expands its boundaries

even farther, encompassing a wider array of queer personalities, television viewers will increasingly and invariably get the message that queers are simply another variation on the people who might move in next door.

—*Nathan G. Tipton*

BIBLIOGRAPHY

Andreoli, Rick. "Party of Five." *Advocate*, July 22, 2003, 62.

Armstrong, Jennifer, Mandi Bierly, and Alynda Wheat. "If We Ran Reality TV: Paris, You're In. Trista, You're Out." *Entertainment Weekly*, May 21, 2004, 24.

Barrett, Jon. "Reichen and Chip: Reality Sets In." *Advocate*, October 28, 2003, 32.

Brenton, Sam, and Reuben Cohen. *Shooting People: Adventures in Reality TV*. London: Verso: 2003.

Hart, Kylo-Patrick R. "We're Here, We're Queer—and We're Better Than You: The Representational Superiority of Gay Men to Heterosexuals on 'Queer Eye for the Straight Guy.'" *Journal of Men's Studies* 12.3 (Spring 2004): 241–253.

Hatch, Rich. *101 Survival Secrets: How to Make $1,000,000, Lose 100 Pounds, and Just Plain Live Happy*. New York: Lyons Press, 2000.

Horowitz, Craig. "Reality Check." *People*, March 22, 1993, 61.

Johnson, Hillary, and Nancy Rommelmann. *MTV's The Real Real World*. New York: MTV Books, 1995.

Jones, Wenzel. "Lance Loud." *Advocate*, November 12, 2002, 60.

Meers, Erik. "Keeping It Real." *Advocate*, April 30, 2002, 38.

Philpot, Robert. "Underground TV: The Beauty of 'The Beast.'" *Knight Ridder/Tribune News Service*, July 10, 2004.

Pollet, Alison. *MTV's The Real World New Orleans Unmasked*. New York: MTV Books, 2000.

Rice, Lynette. "Alterna-TV." *Entertainment Weekly*, February 13, 2004, 65.

Sigesmund, B. J. "Boys R Us: Dating Games." *Newsweek*, July 21, 2003, 52.

SEE ALSO

American Television: Drama; American Television: News; American Television: Situation Comedies; American Television: Soap Operas; American Television: Talk Shows

American Television: Situation Comedies

EVEN THOUGH GAY AND LESBIAN CHARACTERS IN dramatic television shows have been sporadic, American situation comedies (known more popularly as sitcoms) have consistently featured a wide array of queer characters both in guest appearances and as recurring ensemble members.

Queer portrayals have been staples of hit television series ranging from the late-1970s soap opera spoof *Soap* to the mid-1990s lesbian phenomenon *Ellen*, and from the queerly inflected NBC sitcom *Frasier* to NBC's openly gay hit *Will and Grace*.

While television sitcoms have shared with their dramatic television counterparts a reliance on stock stereotypical characterizations of queers as, alternatively, wispy and effeminate or gossipy and ruthlessly backstabbing men or flannel-shirt-wearing, humorless women, these representations are by no means uniform. There has, in fact, been a positive shift in the depiction of gay men and lesbians in television sitcoms, concurrent with both a change in social attitudes and a rise in openly queer television comedy writers and sitcom stars.

Hiding in Plain Sight: The 1960s

Although most television sitcoms in the 1960s revolved around the well-established nuclear family motif, a discernible gay sensibility began making its presence known, however subtly, on the small screen. At a time when depictions of openly gay characters on television were unheard of, many identifiably queer characters nevertheless did appear in varying guises. These characters included oddball uncles, wicked mothers-in-law, or fey neighbors whose visits to the otherwise normative home usually caused no small amount of uproar. One show notable for its queerly inflected cast was the magically successful sitcom *Bewitched*, which debuted on ABC in 1964.

While the show itself was based on the antic interaction between Samantha (Elizabeth Montgomery), a witch who doubled as a suburban Connecticut housewife, and her mortal husband, Darrin Stephens (Dick York from 1964 to 1966 and Dick Sargent from 1966 to 1972), many of its recurring supporting characters had definite queer overtones.

Agnes Moorehead, widely rumored to be a lesbian, portrayed Samantha's worldly, witty, and bitchy mother, Endora, while "confirmed bachelor" Paul Lynde played Samantha's affected, practical-joking Uncle Arthur. In 1994, the series' leads reunited when Elizabeth Montgomery stood beside the second Darrin, Dick Sargent, as he announced that he was gay. The same year, the pair also served as Grand Marshals for the Los Angeles Gay Pride Parade.

Another queer presence surfaced on television the year after the debut of *Bewitched*. In 1965, the variety program *The Steve Lawrence Show* featured, as part of its ensemble, the comic talents of Charles Nelson Reilly. Reilly's extensive career, which began in the early 1960s, featured Broadway appearances in such shows as *Bye Bye Birdie* (in which he was understudy to Paul Lynde) and a Tony Award–winning turn in *How to Succeed in Business Without Really Trying* in 1961 as the nasty "corporate nephew" Bud Frump.

After similar award-winning success in the 1964 hit musical *Hello, Dolly!* Reilly nosed his way into televi-

sion on Lawrence's short-lived show. He quickly followed his success by securing a part in the memorably offbeat 1969 children's show *H. R. Pufnstuf* and its spinoff, the 1971 series *Lidsville*, before becoming a celebrity panelist on the long-running game show *The Match Game*, which first appeared in 1973. Much of *The Match Game*'s popularity derived from Reilly's outrageously sissified persona and his snappy put-downs of the other panelists.

In many ways, Paul Lynde's career trajectory and biting, sarcastic wit mirrored that of Reilly's. While he achieved recognition for his role on *Bewitched,* Lynde—like Reilly—garnered a fan following through his recurring appearances on a game show. From 1968 to 1979 and again from 1980 to 1981, Lynde occupied the center square on the long-running TV celebrity quiz show *Hollywood Squares*, and his wisecracking, quick-witted answers to host Peter Marshall's questions became a trademark of the show.

The center square became notorious because, after Lynde's tenure, subsequent guests occupying the center square followed Lynde's example and tended to be extravagantly flamboyant, if not openly gay. One of the celebrities occupying the center square was Wayland Flowers and his drag-queenesque puppet Madame, and Charles Nelson Reilly made frequent guest appearances. When *Squares* was revived as *The New Hollywood Squares* from 1986 to 1989, comedian Jim Jay Bullock took the center square and acted as the show's subhost. The show returned again in 1998 under its original name, and this time openly gay Hollywood columnist Bruce Vilanch ruled the square, thus leading many critics to dub the spot "the gay square."

Lynde's television appearances were not, however, limited to *Hollywood Squares*. After stints on *The Phyllis Diller Show* (1967), *The Jonathan Winters Show* (1967), *Dean Martin Presents the Golddiggers* (1968–1969), and two *Gidget* TV movies (1969 and 1972), Lynde starred in his own sitcom, *The Paul Lynde Show*. The show debuted on ABC in 1972 and featured Lynde as Paul Simms, a respectable attorney who lives a quiet life with his wife and two daughters. However, when Howie, the new husband of Simms's eldest daughter, takes up residence in the Simms household, Paul is driven to distraction.

Unfortunately *The Paul Lynde Show* had little chance to succeed. It was scheduled against formidable competition from NBC's police drama *Adam-12* and Carol Burnett's comedy-variety show on CBS. Moreover, viewers were uncomfortable with Lynde's over-the-top, outrageous onscreen behavior and wholly unbelievable portrayal of a "family man." The show lasted one season before being canceled.

While these queer stars did not play openly gay characters, nevertheless their presence in notable sitcoms and variety shows lent to television a palpable queer sensibility that audiences could see and tacitly accept, if not completely understand. This "covert openness" would, indeed, ultimately lead to more open portrayals of queer sitcom characters in subsequent decades.

First Sightings: The 1970s

In 1970, one year after the Stonewall riots in New York City, which heralded the advent of the gay liberation movement, the NBC comedy show *Rowan and Martin's Laugh-In* first acknowledged the subject of gay men and their lifestyle openly. As Kylo-Patrick R. Hart has pointed out, *Laugh-In* created the stereotypically effeminate character named Bruce, who was subjected to long strings of antigay jokes about gay men and gay liberation. The distinctly unfunny Bruce remained a part of the show's repertoire until *Laugh-In*'s demise in 1973.

In 1979, *Laugh-In* was revived and the show's writers replaced the outdated Bruce character with the campy comic duo of gay ventriloquist Wayland Flowers and his Phyllis Diller/Tallulah Bankheadesque puppet Madame, who dressed like a drag queen. By providing salacious show-business gossip and hilarious sexual double entendres to *Laugh-In*'s viewers, Madame was an instant hit and went on to host her own show, *Madame's Place*, in 1982. However, despite Flowers's self-evident (if backgrounded) homosexuality, much of Madame's routines typically relied on bitchy gay repartee and thus, for viewers, her humor implicitly reinforced stereotypical representations of queers, even as it also often satirized heterosexual duplicity and hypocrisy.

But even while queers were being played primarily for laughs, several sitcoms were quietly striving to move beyond stereotyped representations of homosexuals. In 1971, during its first season, *All in the Family* featured the bigoted Archie Bunker (Carroll O'Connor) learning that one of his best drinking buddies (and a retired professional athlete) was a happily well-adjusted gay man.

In 1973, *The Mary Tyler Moore Show* episode "My Brother's Keeper" revealed that the brother of Mary's longtime friend Phyllis Lindstrom (Cloris Leachman) was gay.

In the 1975 episode "Archie the Hero," *All in the Family* again featured a gay character, female impersonator Beverly LaSalle (Lori Shannon), whose life Archie saves before realizing that "classy dame" Beverly is really a male. Shannon twice reprised his/her role, first in the 1976 episode "Beverly Rides Again" and then in the memorable two-part 1977 episode "Edith's Crisis of Faith."

"Edith's Crisis of Faith" was both daring and disturbing because of its handling of homophobia and violence against gays. In the episode's first part, Beverly drops in to visit the Bunkers and invite them to her revue at Madison Square Garden. Archie is, predictably, uncomfortable attending a show featuring Beverly's "kind of people," but following some good-natured cajoling from Edith (Jean Stapleton) and Beverly, he grudgingly agrees to go. Flush with triumph, Beverly rushes out to get some celebratory champagne, but on the way to the liquor store she is attacked and killed by muggers.

Beverly's sudden, shocking death triggers Edith's crisis of faith, and the segment ends as Edith angrily asks God how He could allow a sweet and gentle soul like Beverly to die so needlessly and violently. Edith's obvious affection for and unblinking acceptance of Beverly give this episode special poignancy; it was nominated for an Emmy Award for Outstanding Writing in 1977.

For better or worse, 1977 was a watershed year for queer or queer-appearing sitcom characters. *Three's Company*, a comedy series about a man who pretended to be gay so he could share an apartment with two women, premiered on ABC. Some of the show's humor stemmed from banter between Jack Tripper (John Ritter) and landlord Stanley Roper (Norman Fell) that relied on stereotypical gay attributes and included lascivious, leering stares and epithets such as "Tinkerbell."

The underlying homophobia of *Three's Company* was only slightly counterbalanced by the rise of bisexual Jodie Dallas (Billy Crystal) on another ABC show, the absurdist soap-opera spoof *Soap*.

Jodie began his run on *Soap* by dating professional football player Dennis Phillips (Bob Seagren)—before discovering that Dennis is also dating women for image purposes. Distressed by this news, Jodie decides to have a sex change, but he is dissuaded by seductive nurse Nancy Darwin (Udana Power), who becomes the impetus of Jodie's first foray into heterosexuality.

Jodie's apparent conversion from gay man to transgendered person and then to straight man elicited considerable controversy from queer television viewers, forcing the show's producers to respond that Jodie did not convert to heterosexuality but was, instead, merely going through a very tumultuous time.

Although Jodie does not follow through with his gender reassignment, the "Once a Friend" episode of the popular *All in the Family* spinoff *The Jeffersons* during the same year showed George Jefferson (Sherman Hemsley) reuniting with Eddie Stokes (Veronica Redd), an old Navy buddy who had become Edie, a female. While this episode contained a great deal of stereotyping, it was among the first sensitive portrayals of a transgendered person on network television.

Another sitcom that routinely offered queer portrayals that rose above stereotypes was ABC's wry police comedy *Barney Miller*, which ran from 1975 to 1982. The show involved the day-to-day interactions between the detectives of New York City's 12th Precinct. The precinct was based in Greenwich Village, and through this location passed an unending array of colorful characters, among them two gay men, Marty (Jack DeLeon) and Daryl Driscoll (Ray Stewart), who made semiregular appearances on the show.

Barney Miller was also one of the first sitcoms to feature an onscreen coming-out. The "Inquisition" episode (air date September 13, 1979) featured the 12th Precinct receiving an anonymous letter that threatens to expose the homosexuality of one of its officers. The letter attracts attention at Headquarters, and the by-the-book Lieutenant Scanlon arrives at the 12th and begins a witch hunt to uncover the gay officer. In the midst of Scanlon's investigation, Officer Zitelli (Dino Natali) confides to Miller that he is gay, but Barney does not reveal this information to Scanlon. The show subsequently received critical praise for the respectful and discreet way in which Zitelli's declaration was handled.

As the 1970s drew to a close, broadly defined queer characters became more and more visible on the small screen. With this increased frequency came a discernible increase in audience acceptance. In fact, viewers began tuning in not merely to see gay stereotypes but to watch for the alternative forms of comedy that queer characters provided on various sitcoms. Indeed, armed with this sense of acceptance, many sitcom writers began fortifying queer roles by incorporating into these characters a marked awareness of current social issues. With the alarming rise of AIDS in the mid-1980s, this social awareness would become an integral part of many queer sitcom characters.

The Politics of Comedy: The 1980s

With the appearance of two transvestites on ABC's quirky 1980 sitcom *Bosom Buddies*, the 1980s began on an auspicious note. *Bosom Buddies* featured two friends, Kip (Tom Hanks) and Henry (Peter Scolari) who, after moving to New York, secure a great and cheap apartment that also happens to be in a hotel for women. In order to keep the apartment, Kip and Henry make a "slight adjustment": They dress in drag and take on female personas, Buffy and Hildegarde.

Although a few critics derided the show's flimsy premise, the chemistry, camaraderie, and comic timing shared between Hanks and Scolari surprised and delighted viewers, who gave the show high Nielsen ratings. After a few weeks, however, ABC inexplicably took the show off the air for a network hiatus, and when the show returned, the viewers did not. *Bosom Buddies* was renewed for a second season, but even in the face of over 35,000 letters of protest ABC canceled the show in 1982.

While the queerness of *Bosom Buddies* derived from its explorations of men in drag, in 1981 NBC presented a made-for-television movie revolving around the life of an openly gay man. *Sidney Shorr: A Girl's Best Friend*

was a seriocomic feature starring Tony Randall as an openly gay man who befriends a troubled single mother and her young daughter. NBC quickly adapted the movie into the sitcom series *Love, Sidney* but, because of pressure from conservative religious groups, just as quickly downplayed Sidney's homosexuality.

Larry Gross has noted that, as a result of this backpedaling, Sidney's sexuality tended to be so subtly coded that innocent viewers could readily misunderstand it. In fact, according to Gross, the only clues to Sidney's homosexuality were his crying at old Greta Garbo movies and having a photo of his dead lover, Martin, on the mantelpiece. Despite the network's attempts to conceal Sidney's sexual orientation, however, the show's writers continued to allude to it coyly in almost every episode. Precisely because of the show's clever writing, *Love, Sidney* became a favorite of television critics, though it failed to garner sizable audience ratings and was canceled in 1983.

Somewhat surprisingly, *Sidney*'s demise ushered in a new openness for queer sitcom characters. In 1984, subscriber network Showtime debuted *Brothers*, a comedy about three brothers, one of whom, Cliff Waters (Paul Regina), was unapologetically gay. *Brothers*, which ran for eight seasons, was the first weekly series on either cable or network television to showcase an openly gay recurring character portrayed sympathetically and nonstereotypically. The show was among the first to deal honestly with queer issues such as social prejudice, coming out, and self-acceptance. *Brothers* also addressed AIDS in the early years of the epidemic, and its sensitive handling of the disease in a comedic setting became a touchstone for later cable and network shows.

In television comedy as a whole, AIDS had a resoundingly profound effect. However, more often than not sitcoms encouraged the perception that gays were to blame for AIDS. Moreover, they frequently suggested that by spreading AIDS gay men were ruining the lives of everyone else.

In 1987, as part of its second season, CBS's Southern, woman-centered sitcom *Designing Women* explicitly drew the connection between heterosexual problem and homosexual culpability. The episode entitled "Killing All the Right People" had, as part of its dual storyline, twenty-four-year-old Kendall Dobbs (Tony Goldwyn) dying of AIDS and asking the women to plan his funeral. Kendall's disease ties in neatly with the second plot, in which series regular Mary Jo Shively (Annie Potts) has to defend condom distribution to the PTA of a local school.

However, Mary Jo argues for condoms only as a means of protecting children, not as a way to stop the spread of AIDS, which the episode tacitly connects with promiscuous homosexual behavior. Thus, as Emile Netzhammer and Scott Shamp observe, even though

Kendall is portrayed as sweet, well adjusted, and sympathetic, the episode subtly blames his homosexuality for his fatal condition.

Queer characters were not always brought on expressly to incorporate social awareness into a comedic setting. NBC's *The Golden Girls*, another woman-centered sitcom, included an episode dealing with lesbianism. The 1986 episode "Isn't It Romantic" featured Jean (Lois Nettleton), a gay college friend of Dorothy's (Bea Arthur) who drops in for a visit and subsequently falls in love with dimwitted series regular Rose (Betty White). Rose, who has no idea that Jean is a lesbian, is flattered when Jean reveals the nature of her affection. After some discussion, however, the two women decide that their friendship is sufficient.

A similar brush with lesbianism also took place on *Designing Women* in the 1990 episode "Suzanne Goes Looking for a Friend." The episode centers on ditsy Suzanne Sugarbaker (Delta Burke), who, with no one to accompany her to a charity benefit, digs through old beauty-pageant memorabilia in search of her "best girlfriend," Eugenia Weeks (Karen Kopins). After reuniting with Suzanne, Eugenia tells her about coming out, which Suzanne misinterprets as a debutante presentation to society. Only after a fun evening with Eugenia at the charity benefit does Suzanne discover that her coming-out was from the closet rather than into high society.

Even though these episodes contained substantial amounts of broad humor and were generally well-meaning and sympathetic in their portrayals of gay men and lesbians, they tended to become formulaic, as they spawned many variations well into the 1990s. A typical episode featured a heterosexual recurring character having trouble accepting a person who had just come out. Inevitably, by the end of the show, the straight character would do something magnanimous and, in so doing, overcome his or her homophobia.

Before long, audiences grew tired of these essentially monolithic portrayals of gay/straight interactions, and television writers began to explore new approaches to queer television representations.

Expressions of Openness: The Early 1990s

As Hart has noted, in the 1990s glbtq people achieved wider recognition and greater levels of social tolerance than in the past, and the major network prime-time shows began increasingly to represent diverse and inclusive characters who reflected the wide range of roles that queers occupy in American society.

In 1990, for example, CBS debuted the quirky dramatic comedy *Northern Exposure*, a show that followed the lives and loves of Cicely, Alaska's, eccentric residents. While most of the relationships on *Northern Exposure* were heterosexual, the show was notable for its "just folks" portrayal of queer characters. The 1992 episode "Cicely" explained that the town was named after one of the lesbian founders who, along with her lover Roslyn, transformed the backwater mud hole into what they termed the "Paris of the West."

In 1994, the episode "I Feel the Earth Move" presented television's first-ever gay wedding; characteristically, most of Cicely's residents found nothing unusual about the nuptials.

Although there was a slight controversy surrounding *Northern Exposure*'s gay wedding, in late 1995 another gay wedding on the popular ABC sitcom *Roseanne* was the center of a firestorm of protest. Queer viewers objected not to the episode, but to the network's decision to delay the episode's airing from prime time to a later, "adult" time period.

Leon (Martin Mull) and Scott's (Fred Willard) gay wedding on *Roseanne* was followed almost immediately by a lesbian wedding on the hit show *Friends*. In January 1996, the episode "The One with the Lesbian Wedding" showcased the marriage of Ross's ex-wife Carol (Jane Sibbett) and her partner Susan (Jessica Hecht). Candace Gingrich, the lesbian half-sister of conservative former Speaker of the United States House of Representatives Newt Gingrich, played the minister who presided over the ceremony. Unlike *Roseanne*'s gay wedding, however, the *Friends* episode generated little controversy. This was due in large part to the absence of any same-sex kisses.

You May Now (Not) Kiss the Bride

Although in the 1990s queer characters and queer situations in television comedies began to be more accepted by mainstream viewers, same-sex affection was rare and kissing was practically nonexistent. ABC executives refused to allow *Roseanne*'s gay couple, Leon and his lover Scott, to kiss because of boycott threats. This came as no surprise to the show's creator, Roseanne Barr, who had weathered similar protests over a same-sex kiss with Mariel Hemingway in the 1994 episode "Don't Ask, Don't Tell."

As a publicly funded entity, PBS found itself vulnerable to conservative criticism and pressure when, also in 1994, it aired the hugely popular miniseries *Tales of the City*. Based on gay author Armistead Maupin's fictional accounts of freewheeling 1970s San Francisco, *Tales* featured a fair amount of adult language, nudity, and sexual situations, both heterosexual and homosexual. The series' ratings soared predictably but, as Rodney Buxton has remarked, *Tales of the City* generated enough controversy that conservative forces were able to pressure CPB (the Corporation for Public Broadcasting) to withdraw funding for the sequel, *More Tales of the City*, which finally aired in 2001 on Showtime.

In the wake of the conservative backlash, Maupin commented in a *New York Times* article that letting the series' characters show affection was important. He had come to resent profoundly the way that the universal symbol of love, the kiss, had been reserved exclusively for heterosexuals on the television screen. Indeed, it would be six more years before viewers would witness, on the February 22, 2000, episode of NBC's *Will and Grace*, two gay male characters kissing in prime time.

However, as website columnist Alan Foster has noted, even though a same-sex male kiss occurred between Will (Eric McCormack) and Jack (Sean P. Hayes), the world hardly noticed, because NBC failed to give advance media notice for this gay milestone.

Although network television executives shied away from depicting overt expressions of queer affection, television viewers were nevertheless treated to an ever increasing array of same-sex embraces, including numerous male–male kisses. Because they mostly occurred within the boundaries of farce or satire, however, these displays of affection were explained away as "joke kisses." Still, it was impossible to ignore the increasingly affectionate nature of queerly inflected, if problematic, characters in both sitcoms and sketch comedy shows.

All the World's a Stage

In terms of queer portrayals in television comedy, sketch comedy shows such as NBC's long-running *Saturday Night Live* and Fox's urban showcase *In Living Color* have aired numerous depictions of hilariously bizarre queer characters (though too often the point seemed to be that being queer was itself hilariously bizarre).

Since its debut in 1975, *Saturday Night Live* has provided such recurring sketches as the cartoon superhero send-up "The Ambiguously Gay Duo," the weightlifting pair Hans and Franz (Dana Carvey and Kevin Nealon), who promised to "pump you up," and the sexuality-challenged, genderless creature Pat (Julia Sweeney). Sweeney's sketch "It's Pat!" ran from 1990 to 1994, and much of its humor derived from speculation about Pat's gender and sexuality. By tacitly extolling the acceptance of androgyny, the sketch's theme jingle added further fuel to speculation over Pat's gender identity.

Many cast members also appeared regularly in drag for such popular sketches as the organized religion spoof "The Church Lady" (Dana Carvey) and the Jewish chat show segment "Coffee Talk" (Mike Myers).

During the 1986–1987 season, *Saturday Night Live* boasted as part of its complement comic Terry Sweeney, who, by virtue of his recurring role on the show, became the first openly gay regular performer on network television.

Sweeney's stint, however, was short-lived. Speaking to *Advocate* columnist Mike Goodridge, Sweeney's partner and former *SNL* writer Lanier Laney remarked that the show had a very straight, homophobic atmosphere, and it was quickly apparent that, even though Terry was one of the most popular performers of the 1986 season, he was not going to last long.

A homophobic atmosphere can also be discerned in the troublesome broad sketch humor of Fox network's *In Living Color*. Flamboyant black queens Blaine Edwards (Damon Wayans) and Antoine Marywether (David Alan Grier) appeared in a recurring series of sketches titled simply "Men On…" and discussed topics ranging from film to art to vacation to football. Although the sketches were often very funny, the stereotyped depiction of two gay men as bitchy, mincing, and effeminate struck many viewers as offensive.

Still, *In Living Color* was one of the first television shows that featured openly gay black men and, paradoxically, paved the way for the appearance of "normal queer" Carter Heywood (Michael Boatman) on ABC's sitcom *Spin City*.

In contrast to the problematic queer portrayals seen on *Saturday Night Live* and *In Living Color*, the Canadian sketch show *Kids in the Hall* was filled with a positive mixture of broad satire and thoughtful, if subversive, humor. Formed in 1985 in Toronto, the *Kids* troupe consisted of five Canadian improvisational comics (Dave Foley, Bruce McCulloch, Kevin McDonald, Mark McKinney, and openly gay Scott Thompson) whose humor, according to *MacLean's* columnist Diane Turbide, routinely targeted middle-class suburban blandness, shark-like businessmen, and homophobia.

After four years playing comedy clubs in Toronto, the Kids moved to television with their eponymous weekly half-hour sketch series. From 1989 to 1994, *Kids in the Hall* aired simultaneously on the CBC (Canadian Broadcasting Channel) and subscriber network HBO, and it was later picked up by CBS and cable network Comedy Central.

Although the show was acclaimed for its irreverent humor, its notable trademark was the characters' use of drag. The joke, though, never came from them being in drag but, rather, from the situations in which they placed their characters. The Kids, in fact, made a conscious effort to be accurate and convincing in their portrayals of women, relying on the sketch's overall humor and their appearances *as females* rather than using drag as parody.

The cast members also routinely portrayed a variety of characters with differing sexual orientations, and although the characterizations were sometimes offensive, the troupe's verbal delivery, body language, and sheer comic momentum made up for occasional lapses into bad taste. Indeed, with an emphasis on more "normal" comic portrayals, *Kids in the Hall* signaled a new approach to queer comedy that would become commonplace by the late 1990s.

We're Here, We're Queer, We're Just Like You!

As the 1990s drew to a close, appearances by queer sitcom characters became more frequent and, gradually, more normalized. Rather than relying on stereotypes, television comedies began to portray queers more positively and more complexly.

In 1997, Michael Boatman's portrayal of openly gay mayoral aide Carter Heywood won particular praise from GLAAD, the Gay and Lesbian Alliance Against Defamation, which recognized Boatman's conscious efforts at steering Carter's character away from one-dimensionality and stereotype. But Boatman's achievement in 1997 was overshadowed by one of the single most defining moments in television history.

On April 30, 1997, millions of viewers tuned in to the ABC sitcom *Ellen* to witness the first "real-life," television coming-out—that of comedian Ellen DeGeneres. In a star-studded episode that combined elements of comedy and reality TV, the eponymous Ellen acknowledged that she was a lesbian. Culminating months of media speculation sparked by DeGeneres's teasing on- and offscreen innuendoes about her sexuality, her coming-out was predictably greeted with a mixture of harsh criticism from conservative groups and warm praise from the gay and lesbian community.

As Lynn Joyrich has noted, because of the self-conscious referentiality of the prolonged coming-out, queer-themed inside jokes were available to all viewers even before the character actually came out. However, after The Episode aired, *Ellen*'s humor was seemingly replaced by an increasing amount of political commentary, leading many viewers to seek out other comedic venues.

In an interview with *Mediaweek* columnist Alan James Frutkin, television producer Jeffrey Richman stated that once Ellen embraced the subject of homosexuality, the show seemed to hammer home the issue constantly, and all the stories became about the character of Ellen Morgan and her evident, identifiable gayness. Thus, while Ellen's coming out was a milestone for queers on television, it simply did not make for good television comedy. *Ellen*'s open expression of homosexuality, however, paved the way for NBC's *Will and Grace*.

Speaking to *Advocate* interviewer Lori Kaye, *Friends* cocreator David Crane noted that *Ellen* not only opened the closet door for *Will and Grace* but also helped identify the formula that has fueled its success. *Will and Grace*'s formula for success was to go slow and come out of the gate funny rather than emotional. By combining clever—if uneven—writing and a genuinely likable cast, the formula seems to have worked.

Cocreated and cowritten by openly gay writer Max Mutchnick and David Kohan, *Will and Grace* debuted in 1998 and showcased the innocuously codependent relationship between gay lawyer Will Truman (Eric McCormack) and straight interior designer Grace Adler (Debra Messing).

Much of the show's real humor, however, came from its supporting cast: shallow, self-centered queen Jack McFarland (Sean P. Hayes) and ultrabitch Karen Walker (Megan Mullally), whose biting banter often threatened to overshadow the show's main characters. *Will and Grace* also deployed many time-honored comedic methods such as slapstick and screwball comedy, leading gay author Andrew Holleran to complain that the show was in danger of becoming a bad episode of *I Love Lucy*.

However uneven and silly the show sometimes gets, it deserves credit for not shying away from topical issues. For example, in the episode "Girls, Interrupted" (air date May 2, 2000), Jack joins a gay-to-straight conversion group in order to meet the group leader, Bill (Neil Patrick Harris). After Bill gives Jack a sharply earnest speech chastising Jack's brazen attempts at seduction, he acquiesces to Jack's suggestion of a shower rendezvous, thus hilariously exposing the hypocrisy and absurdity of "conversion therapy."

The homophobic Christian organization Focus on the Family objected to this episode, stating that it made a mockery of the struggles of "ex-gay" men and women. Their protest gives credence to Andrew Holleran's declaration that *Will and Grace* is more than just a sitcom; it is *our* gay sitcom, fearless and tacky and lewd.

The success of *Will and Grace* has thus far spawned three more queer sitcoms, though none has captured the loyalty of glbtq viewers.

Fox's *Normal, Ohio* appeared in 2000 and starred John Goodman as William "Butch" Gamble. Goodman tossed aside the popular "body beautiful" gay television stereotype by appearing as a burly, beer-drinking, football-watching, almost stereotypically heterosexual man who just happened to be gay. Unfortunately, the show's writing depended too much on characters ridiculing Goodman's antics and dancing around complicated issues such as coming out and homophobia rather than confronting them directly. *Normal, Ohio* disappeared from television screens after its initial thirteen-episode run.

The second progeny of *Will and Grace* was the CBS sitcom *Some of My Best Friends*, which premiered in February, 2001, and starred Jason Bateman as Warren Fairbanks, a gay writer who needs someone to share his Greenwich Village apartment after his boyfriend moves out. The show was based on Tony Vitale's 1997 movie *Kiss Me, Guido*, and follows the movie's plot fairly closely. Warren places an advertisement in the local paper for a GWM (gay white male) roommate, and Bronx Italian hunk Frankie (Danny Nucci) responds— only he thinks that GWM stands for "guy with money."

Jason Bateman described the show as a contemporary *Odd Couple*, and though the show featured no shortage of stereotypes (the flamboyant Vern, played by Alec Mapa, and the dimwitted macho Italian Pino, played by Michael DeLuise), the lead actors consciously attempted to give their characters a sense of normalcy. After a midseason start, however, *Some of My Best Friends* was given a summer hiatus and never returned.

In fall 2003, amid the clamor of political pundits debating the pros and cons of same-sex marriage, ABC, the former home of TV's pathbreaking *Ellen*, launched *It's All Relative*, the network's version of *Will and Grace*, with a twist.

It's All Relative centered on a long-term committed gay couple whose highly intelligent, Harvard-educated daughter is determined to marry her working-class bartender boyfriend. Her boyfriend's father does not take kindly to gays, but for the sake of the kids, the future in-laws must figure out a way to get along. Craig Zadan, one of the show's coexecutive producers, noted that the show's humor came from the conflict between blue-collar and snooty people, rather than from the conflict between gays and straights.

According to the show's cocreator and cowriter Chuck Ranberg, *It's All Relative* traded on some degree of stereotyping for both gay and straight parents, but, as Zadan noted in an *Advocate* interview, the goal of *It's All Relative* was to use stereotypes and break them down, all the while making sure that these stereotypes were blended with corresponding amounts of humanity. In fact, one of the show's revolutionary qualities stemmed directly from breaking a powerful television stereotype by presenting a committed gay relationship normally and matter-of-factly, as an average, middle-class couple who cook, work, and pay the bills.

The show was also revolutionary for its casting of two openly gay actors, Christopher Sieber and John Benjamin Hickey, in the roles of the gay couple. Hickey remarked to the *Advocate* that the fact both men are gay really added to the on-set chemistry. Unfortunately, and despite its promise, *It's All Relative* suffered from low ratings and was not renewed for a second season.

Conclusion

Throughout their history, television sitcoms have held a mirror up to society, and in that mirror they have reflected the presence of gay, lesbian, bisexual, and transgendered people, often in distorted and unflattering ways, but occasionally in ways that acknowledge our humanity and complexity. Although sitcoms have long relied on problematic stereotypes for their humor, as the decades have progressed television viewers in general and queer viewers in particular have demanded a more varied palette of characters. By watching "classic TV" reruns alongside current television offerings, viewers can easily perceive crucial shifts in the representation of

homosexuality and homosexuals. In the future, increasingly funny and honest queer portrayals in television sitcoms are likely.

—*Nathan G. Tipton*

BIBLIOGRAPHY

Buxton, Rodney. "Sexual Orientation and Television." The Museum of Broadcast Communications website. www.museum.tv

Frutkin, Alan James. "Will Power." *Mediaweek,* September 11, 2000, 38.

Goodridge, Mike. "Believe the Hype." *Advocate,* October 24, 2000, 89.

_____. "Relatively Revolutionary: A Sitcom Featuring a Gay Couple with a Daughter—Shocking, or Just Good Business Sense? Both, Say Producers." *Advocate,* October 14, 2003, 52.

Gross, Larry. "What Is Wrong with This Picture? Lesbian Women and Gay Men on Television." *Queer Words, Queer Images: Communication and the Construction of Homosexuality.* R. J. Ringer, ed. New York: New York University Press, 1994. 143–156.

Hart, Kylo-Patrick R. "Representing Gay Men on American Television." *Journal of Men's Studies* 9.1 (2000): 59–79.

Holleran, Andrew. "The Alpha Queen." *Gay and Lesbian Review* 7.3 (2000): 65–66.

Joyrich, Lynne. "Epistemology of the Console." *Critical Inquiry* 27 (2001): 439–467.

Kaye, Lori. "Where Are the Funny Girls?" *Advocate,* November 21, 2000, 85.

McCormick, Patrick. "Out of the Closet and into Your Living Room." *U.S. Catholic* 63.4 (1998): 45–49.

Maupin, Armistead. "A Line That Commercial TV Won't Cross." *New York Times,* January 9, 1994.

Millman, Joyce. "Joyce Millman On Television: Queertoons." *Salon Online Magazine,* August 3, 1998. www.salon.com

Netzhammer, Emile C., and Scott A. Shamp. "Guilt By Association: Homosexuality and AIDS on Prime-Time Television." *Queer Words, Queer Images: Communication and the Construction of Homosexuality.* R. J. Ringer, ed. New York: New York University Press, 1994. 91–106.

Turbide, Diane. "TV Highs and Lows: New Canadian Series Soar and Stumble." *Maclean's,* October 30, 1989, 107.

SEE ALSO

American Television: Drama; Canadian Television; DeGeneres, Ellen; Flowers, Wayland; Lynde, Paul; Moorehead, Agnes; Sargent, Dick; Vilanch, Bruce

American Television: Soap Operas

TREATMENTS OF GAY RELATIONSHIPS ON NETWORK soap operas have always been limited; recently, however, gays and lesbians have created their own soap operas to tell the convoluted stories of lesbian and gay entanglements.

Serial dramas have been a part of American popular culture since the early days of radio, when they were labeled "soap operas" because their sponsors advertised detergent and other household products to the housewives who tuned in. Even then, the audience was more diverse than was widely admitted, and today those addicted to a daily dose of their "soaps" include college football players and retired businessmen as well as the stereotypical housewife.

In fact, although many still ridicule the melodrama of soaps and mock those who watch them, much of network programming has taken on a serial format, from the Fox network's *Buffy the Vampire Slayer* to NBC's *ER* to HBO's *The Sopranos*. In 2001, MTV introduced its own take on the soap opera with *Spyder Games*. The reason behind this evolution is simple: Cheap to produce and liberally saturated with commercials, soap operas are the most profitable of all network programming.

Early Programming

Although they usually have largely white casts and politically and socially conservative viewpoints, soap operas have traditionally enticed viewers with racy potboiler story lines featuring love triangles, scheming villains, and convoluted plots. However, more than any other television genre, soaps have also traditionally been written and produced by women and have revolved around the family and emotional issues that are of interest to women.

In 1968, ABC introduced a new kind of soap opera, which, while containing plenty of old-fashioned soap action, added a focus on relevant social issues of the day and a few recurring characters of color. The show was *One Life to Live,* and its success over the next decades encouraged other soap operas to tackle more serious issues. Along with such issues as abortion, homelessness, and domestic violence, soaps began to deal with homosexuality.

However, soap operas have remained largely white, and their treatment of serious issues has been marked by a certain shallowness. Accordingly, treatment of gay relationships on soaps has always been limited.

Although soaps began to feature the occasional gay character, these characters were always set within a finite story line and they disappeared after the conclusion of that story line. AIDS story lines became popular in the 1980s, but they almost invariably featured white women who did not contract the disease through gay sex.

More Recent Programming

Stories with a liberal point of view on the subject of homophobia appeared in the mid-to-late 1990s on *One Life to Live, General Hospital*, and *All My Children*—all involving good gay teachers falsely accused of bad things.

All My Children not only introduced the first lesbian character (played by Donna Pescow) in 1983, but is also the first soap where a member of a major cast family has come out as gay. Bianca Montgomery (played by Eden Riegel), sixteen-year-old daughter of longtime soap diva Erica Kane (Susan Lucci), came out as a lesbian in December 2000.

Although bringing ultra–femme fatale Erica's daughter out as a lesbian while still a teenager is a courageous act of soap-opera plotting, giving Bianca romantic happiness has been more problematic. Her coming-out relationship took place offscreen, and ended unhappily, and her next involvement was a hopeless crush on a straight woman. While these are not unrealistic stories in the life of a teenage lesbian, they do not paint a picture of a fulfilled life for lesbians on the soaps. In a medium where steamy sex scenes are the norm, gay characters are rarely allowed even to touch.

Camp Soaps

Camp has always been an arena where gay characters are allowed to thrive. The 1977 satire *Soap* included one of the most beloved gay characters ever to appear on television. Billy Crystal's Jodie brought a sweet humor and ironic dignity to his role as a gay man in a burlesque of soap operas that was both campy and sharp.

The late 1990s saw the introduction of science fiction/fantasy soaps (*Xena, Warrior Princess* and *Dark Angel*, for example) that combined lesbianism, martial arts, and high camp. Many lesbians follow these soaps cultishly, creating websites and attending gatherings of fans.

Gay Soaps

There are many who claim that gay life is like a soap opera. Tight communities that are always at least partly secretive may naturally inculcate complex webs of relationship that rival anything on network television. It is then, perhaps, no surprise that gay men and lesbians have created their own soap operas to tell the convoluted stories of lesbian and gay entanglements.

In 1988, Boston filmmakers Laura Chiten, Cheryl Qamar, and Rachael McCoullum made several episodes of *Two in Twenty (Because One in Ten Sounds Lonely)*, a soap about lesbian housemates and their friends interspersed with satirical commercial interruptions.

In the late 1990s, writer Russell Davies created the sexually graphic gay soap *Queer As Folk* for British television's Channel 4. The Showtime cable network remade it in 2000 for American television, where it has received mixed reviews from gays and straights alike. The success of *Queer As Folk* spawned a lesbian soap, *The L Word*, which premiered in 2004. Other soaps, with titles like *Pink Soap* and *Gay Daze* can be found on the Internet, where fans can participate interactively, voting for their preferred plot twists.

—*Tina Gianoulis*

BIBLIOGRAPHY

Anger, Dorothy. *Other Worlds: Society Seen Through Soap Opera.* Peterborough, Ont.: Broadview Press, 1999.

Behrens, Web. "You Better Sit Down, Erica." *Advocate,* December 19, 2000, 60.

Bell, Katherine. "Russell Davies: The PlanetOut Interview." www.planetout.com/pno/entertainment/interviews/2000/09/davies.html

Brunsdon, Charlotte. *The Feminist, the Housewife & the Soap Opera.* New York: Oxford University Press, 2000.

La Guardia, Robert. *From Ma Perkins to Mary Hartman: The Illustrated History of Soap Operas.* New York: Ballantine Publishing Group, 1977.

Logan, Michael. "Pine Valley Enters the Gay '90s." *TV Guide,* October 28, 1995, 42.

Miller, Karen K. "Search for TV's Tomorrow...Race, Gender, and Sexuality in Soapland." *Sojourner: The Women's Forum* 24.4 (December 1999): 12.

SEE ALSO

American Television: Drama; American Television: Situation Comedies; British Television

American Television: Talk Shows

TELEVISION TALK SHOWS ARE FOR MANY AMERICANS an embarrassingly guilty pleasure, especially since the genre has become a principal purveyor of trash television. These shows frequently feature guests whose shocking revelations of infidelity, promiscuity, kinkiness, and bad behavior of all sorts are abetted by shouted encouragements (or disparagements) from raucous audience members. The result is that they succeed in shaming all parties involved. Nevertheless, they undeniably possess a certain prurient appeal for many viewers.

For glbtq people, however, talk shows are both promising and problematic. Historically, they have been important in bringing glbtq people and issues to public awareness, though these shows have also exploited glbtq people, given voice to anti-gay sentiments, and presented glbtq people as stereotypes and freaks.

Joshua Gamson has noted that talk shows provide to sex and gender nonconformists both visibility and voice, but in a space that is distorted yet real, hollow yet gratifying. Perhaps most significant, talk shows help redraw the lines between the so-called normal and the abnormal.

Early Incarnations

Participatory talk shows have been in existence since the 1930s and 1940s, with radio shows such as *Truth or Consequences,* a radio staple from 1950 to 1958, featuring audience members answering questions mailed in by listeners. The show also provided an added bonus that, if the audience member answered the question incorrectly, a gratuitous public humiliation of some sort would ensue.

Television realized quickly the potential of this format and provided shows such as the campy audience-participation tearjerker *Queen For a Day* (1956–1964), which provided women a chance to compete for merchandise prizes by telling emotionally wrenching stories of need, the winner determined by audience response via an applause meter.

Although in the 1950s and 1960s a number of variety talk shows also appeared, these shows were premised on a devotion to light and casual conversation reflecting normative societal values. Hosted by figures as diverse as Gypsy Rose Lee, Dinah Shore, Virginia Graham, Dick Cavett, Mike Douglas, and Merv Griffin, these shows usually featured celebrity guests and were essentially daytime versions of *The Tonight Show.* Not only did they maintain a definite sense of formality and decorum, but little attention was paid to contentious issues of any kind and nonnormative presences were not permitted.

The one national talk show host of the period who frequently featured gay men and lesbians was David Susskind, whose show was broadcast by PBS. While Susskind's show was a precursor of every format from Jerry Springer to Charlie Rose, his exposure was limited by virtue of its placement on PBS, whose local affiliates frequently scheduled it late at night. Susskind's homosexual guests were often shot in shadow, sometimes wore masks, were frequently apologetic, and were often subjected to queries that now seem absurd and offensive.

Often, the experiences of gay men and lesbians were countered by "experts," though sometimes the reverse was true as well, as when, in a groundbreaking 1967 episode, Susskind featured antigay psychiatrist Lawrence Hatterer facing off with Dick Leitsch, president of New York City's chapter of the Mattachine Society. For all the indignities visited upon his glbtq guests, Susskind deserves credit for giving gay men and lesbians a voice. Susskind seemed to showcase gays so frequently that a contemporary cartoon parodied him by drawing a homosexual interviewing a group of David Susskinds.

The real breakthrough in the late 1960s was pioneered by a local television personality in Dayton, Ohio, named Phil Donahue. He began actively engaging and encouraging audience questions and participation; and in so doing he created a new talk format that proved amazingly popular. His local show soon went national and spawned a number of imitators and competitors.

Talking Back

While early Phil Donahue shows were concerned primarily with women's issues, he was not afraid to court controversy. Donahue soon began inviting such nonmainstream figures as atheists, feminists, Nazis, and homosexuals to join him in very vocal forums. Donahue pushed the envelope of what was then considered acceptable conversation on television by discussing such taboo topics as condoms, penis size, masturbation, gender reassignment surgery, and, of course, homosexuality.

Donahue's project of making visible ideas and subjects that had been previously invisible on television neatly coincided with the burgeoning, late-1960s gay rights movement. His show served as an invaluable format for public education about the different varieties of queer presence. His show helped "normalize" gay men and lesbians in the minds of millions of middle-class housewives, who were his primary audience.

A late-1970s *Donahue* episode, for example, featured sex researchers William Masters and Virginia Johnson, who talked with Phil and his audience about their book *Homosexuality in Perspective*. This show in particular provided scientific refutation of several myths about homosexuality, and asserted many similarities between heterosexuals and homosexuals.

Later *Donahue* shows would stress the need for tolerance, understanding, acceptance, and a respect for individuality, values that Donahue himself seemed to embrace. His show came to be viewed as a safe space for discussing homosexual issues such as coming out and homophobia. His show featured a gay wedding and discussed whether homosexuality might be transmitted genetically. His was also the first daytime show to focus attention on the mysterious disease that would later be known as AIDS.

This is not to say, however, that *Donahue* shows were always queer friendly. Sometimes Donahue would resort to sensationalism in order to provoke controversy. An episode about cross-dressing in which Donahue appeared in a pink and black skirt unleashed a torrent of criticism, both from conservatives who charged that he was glorifying transvestism and from queers who accused Donahue of sensationalizing and demeaning cross-dressers.

For the most part, however, Donahue demonstrated a genuine commitment to destroying stereotypes. Even though his show courted controversy, it never degenerated into the "freak shows" that would become the mainstay of talk shows in the 1980s and 1990s. According to Gamson, the show's producers sought guests from stigmatized groups who would present as normal and well-adjusted a face as possible.

Until the mid-1980s, Phil Donahue was the sole practitioner of audience-centered, issues-oriented talk on television. With the debuts of *Sally Jessy Raphaël* in 1985 and *The Oprah Winfrey Show* in 1986, television talk turned away from issues and focused more on titillation and personality. The approach of these shows leaned more toward public talk as personal confession and

therapy, and the emphasis turned from contentious debate to rancorous, hostile confrontation. This format became increasingly popular well into the 1990s, and led to the creation of what many television viewers considered trash TV.

Talking Trash

While Donahue's audience was, as he frequently declared, atypically liberal, the studio participants for shows like *Sally Jessy*, *Oprah Winfrey*, and the 1987 series *Geraldo*, hosted by former *20/20* reporter Geraldo Rivera, were often quite hostile and much less tolerant than the shows' hosts.

The guest format, however, initially remained unchanged, as gay and lesbian guests continued to be recruited through mainstream organizations. As the audiences became increasingly hostile and vocal, however, the shows' guests also became more outspoken and more outrageous.

In 1987, former radio talk show host Morton Downey Jr.'s combative program entered the airwaves. Downey, a right-wing conservative, had little time or patience for liberals of any stripe, routinely dismissing them as "scumbuckets" or "pablum pukers."

Angela Gardner, a spokesperson for the cross-dressing group Renaissance Education Association, appeared on the show in 1989 and described the experience as akin to "a root canal without an anesthetic." She noted that Downey craved controversy, openly turned his audience against the guests, and often threw guests off the set.

Although Downey's television show lasted only two years, he deserves the dubious credit of being considered the father of trash talk. His loud, raucous format dealt a fatal blow to informative talk shows such as *Donahue*. In Downey's wake, many of the previously low-key shows such as *Sally Jessy Raphaël* and *Geraldo* abruptly changed their approach and, in so doing, turned up the volume of their talk.

An early 1990s episode of *Sally Jessy Raphaël*, for instance, showcased a panel on the topic "My husband left me because he's gay." The wronged party in this show, the wife, described to a sympathetic audience how she became physically ill when she saw her husband with another man. She described her ex-husband's lover as "a flaming faggot" and accused her husband of being "a faggot and a liar." When the ex-husband tried to defend himself, both the studio audience and the host vilified him—explicitly for his deceit and implicitly for his sexuality.

According to Gamson, however, the ex-husband's lies were partly scripted by the show itself. While the cameras were rolling, guests were told to tell the truth, while off camera guests and audiences alike were encouraged to perform narrow and sometimes flat-out dishonest versions of themselves in order to fit the show's script.

Oprah Winfrey, whose show featured a scenario similar to that of *Sally Jessy Raphaël*, grew increasingly tired of talk show sensationalism and, in 1995, reverted to a format more in line with *Donahue*'s more decorous discussions. Oprah's ratings dropped in response to this format change.

By the mid-1990s, viewers had become accustomed to guests and audiences making lurid spectacles of themselves. Many shows depended on conflict as a major key to attracting viewing audiences, and, as Meredith Berkman has observed, much of this conflict was endorsed and indeed encouraged by the shows' corporate executives. These conflicts would typically occur in response to surprise revelations, and would usually degenerate into fistfights and profanity-laced verbal exchanges. But another type of conflict, the unexpected ambush, was to have deadly consequences.

On March 9, 1995, three days after appearing on an episode of *The Jenny Jones Show* that was ostensibly about secret admirers but was actually entitled "Secret Same-Sex Crushes," Jonathan Schmitz, a 24-year-old heterosexual, arrived at the mobile home of 32-year-old homosexual Scott Amedure. Within a matter of minutes, Schmitz shot Amedure twice at close range and killed him. Schmitz contended that the show had lied to him about the sex of his secret admirer, and his humiliation was so great when it was publicly revealed that Amedure was the admirer that Schmitz was driven to kill him.

Representing Schmitz in the wrongful death suit brought by Amedure's family, attorney Geoffrey Fieger argued that the motive for Amedure's murder was a case of homosexual panic and alleged that *The Jenny Jones Show* was at least partially responsible for the killing.

Although there was no scientific basis for this disturbing argument, psychologist Robert Cabaj has stated that many people find it understandable that a man would kill another man who professes a sexual attraction to him. Indeed, as Gamson has noted, what upset the public was not Amedure's death but, rather, his homosexuality.

Talking Backlash

In the wake of Amedure's murder and the subsequent $25 million award against *The Jenny Jones Show*, other purveyors of trash television have severely curtailed the appearances of glbtq people on their daytime talk shows.

The wildly popular *Jerry Springer Show* currently traffics almost exclusively in heterosexual relationships gone horribly awry. When Springer first appeared in 1991, however, his guest rosters routinely featured drag queens, drag kings, gay teenagers, transsexual lesbians, and club kids (young queers who frequent dance clubs and dress outrageously both in and out of the clubs).

Although Springer shares with his talk-show kin a semblance of tolerance toward sexual nonconformists, he has frequently wondered aloud why queers so often seem to flaunt their sexuality, almost to the point of exaggeration.

This sentiment is an accurate insight into the thinking of what Springer terms polite society. Indeed, talk shows are significant because they at once make sexual and gender nonconformity public and visible while providing venues for the societal anxieties and hostilities that sexual and gender nonconformists evoke.

As gay men and lesbians have increasingly been accepted as part of mainstream society, however, the need for talk shows overtly to emphasize queer presences has decreased significantly. In fact, glbtq people have moved from talk-show audience members and participants to becoming hosts of their own shows.

Talking Queerly

Following the meteoric rise in the popularity of such shows as *The Jerry Springer Show* and *The Rikki Lake Show*, which debuted in 1993, network television executives began creating talk shows for numerous celebrities and television personalities. Tempestt Bledsoe, who played Vanessa Huxtable on the hit NBC comedy *The Cosby Show*, and Danny Bonaduce, former kid star on the 1970s sitcom *The Partridge Family*, hosted two such shows.

Amid this spate of celebrities were two notable gay personalities, Jim J. Bullock, who rose to fame as Monroe Ficus on ABC's *Too Close For Comfort* (1980–1985), and Charles Perez, who coanchored the entertainment news show *American Journal* from 1993 to 1998. In addition, a newer celebrity, drag star RuPaul, debuted a talk show in the late 1990s.

Perez's show, which aired from 1994 to 1996, was known mostly for its catchy theme song, "You Got It Goin' On." His show was indistinguishable from those of Springer and Lake and featured the same variety of dysfunctional heterosexuals and raucous queer characters, such as, for example, Consuela Cosmetica, a black drag-queen dominatrix.

Bullock's show, however, was particularly notable for its flamboyantly out host, as well as his choice for cohost, Tammy Faye Messner, former wife of televangelist Jim Bakker and former cohost of the *PTL Club*. The *Jim J. and Tammy Faye Show* had a short, four-month run in 1996, but it differed from other talk shows, relying on light, noncontroversial topics and a relentlessly happy atmosphere. Tammy Faye left the show after three months, citing health reasons, and the show was canceled soon afterward.

Also in 1996, an equally out and proud show debuted on the cable network VH1. *The RuPaul Show*, which featured the fierce drag diva RuPaul, premiered on October 12, 1996, and welcomed, during its two-year run, an eclectic mix of guests, including cross-dressing basketball star Dennis Rodman and lesbian country singer k.d. lang.

The show highlighted RuPaul's strong sense of camp, biting humor, and open expressions of his sexual orientation, but a 1998 episode entitled "The Family Show" was especially memorable. It contained touching footage of his family's reunion, as well as compassionate interviews with his three sisters.

Later the same year, the episode was nominated for a GLAAD (Gay and Lesbian Alliance Against Defamation) Media Award in the Outstanding TV Talk category. Despite this nomination, however, VH1 opted not to renew the show for its next season, and it left the air in September 1998.

Less Talk

The cancellations of the shows hosted by Perez, Bullock, and RuPaul were part of a concerted decision by network executives to clear the airwaves of so much talk. From a mid-1990s high of over thirty talk shows, the number has dwindled to fewer than ten major venues.

Even so, in 2000 controversial radio host Dr. Laura Schlessinger attempted to cross over into television. Schlessinger, whose moralistic and judgmental rhetoric angered many people, especially gay men and lesbians (whom she labeled "biological errors"), appeared briefly on the Paramount network.

However, due in no small part to furious protests and boycott threats from the glbtq and women's communities, over ninety-five advertisers withdrew their sponsorships from the show, and Paramount's affiliate stations either canceled the show outright or relegated it to late-night slots until the plug was finally pulled.

Oprah, Rosie, and Ellen

Television, it seems, has come full circle. Since 1998, Oprah Winfrey has been actively participating in an effort to clean up daytime talk shows. Her show now focuses on healing relationships, promoting books, making over wardrobes, and a strange, almost New Age mantra called "finding your spirit." Her core audience has also changed, and is now composed primarily of white heterosexual housewives.

Another show that renewed interest in conversation and variety is *The Rosie O'Donnell Show*, which aired from 1996 until 2002. O'Donnell's infectious humor, exhaustive knowledge of celebrity and showbiz trivia, and likability made her show a runaway success and reemphasized the clean side of television. At the same time, her role as an icon among lesbians and her status as the single mother of an adopted child made her show especially popular in the glbtq community.

Although O'Donnell was frequently criticized by gay and lesbian activists for failing to acknowledge her

homosexuality publicly, she refused to act until she was ready. In March 2002, in a widely hyped appearance on ABC's *Primetime Thursday,* she told Diane Sawyer, "I don't think America knows what a gay parent looks like: I am a gay parent."

While some critics have speculated that her decision to come out was predicated on her prior decision to leave her show and on the promotion of her autobiography *Find Me* (2002), her own explanation is that she needed a political reason to motivate her to come out publicly, and she found it in the discrimination against gay men and lesbians in the adoption policies of many states, especially Florida.

O'Donnell helped rehabilitate the talk show as a respectable form of entertainment. For her efforts, she won a total of ten Emmys in six years.

In 2003, comedian Ellen DeGeneres, who came out in a 1997 episode of her sitcom *Ellen,* debuted in a syndicated talk show. Eschewing controversial issues, including her lesbianism, and relying largely on her charm and comic riffs, DeGeneres scored a somewhat surprising hit. The show features a mix of celebrity interviews, musical performances, "real people" segments, and audience participation games, as well as DeGeneres's monologues. Having earned critical praise and solid ratings, the show was also honored with a daytime Emmy Award as Outstanding Talk Show in its first season.

Future Talk

Somewhat surprisingly, even the remaining trash television shows have begun to de-emphasize what Gamson, quoting former television producer Martin Calder, terms anything that looks "unclean." Although this attribute was applied initially to gay people, lower-class black people, drag queens, and risqué dressers, shows such as *The Rikki Lake Show, The Jenny Jones Show*, and *The Jerry Springer Show* no longer apply it to gay men and lesbians. They still strive to include lower-class blacks, drag queens, and especially risqué dressers. But middle-class gay people, *per se*, are now considered too normal, or boring, to qualify as trash television material.

Gay and lesbian couples are more likely be seen on HGTV home renovation and decorating shows than on trash television these days.

—Nathan G. Tipton

BIBLIOGRAPHY

Berkman, Meredith. "Daytime Talk Shows: Fake Guests Common in Battle for Ratings." *New York Post,* December 4, 1995.

———. "Liars Send in Clowns for Sicko Circuses." *New York Post,* December 4, 1995.

Birmingham, Elizabeth. "Fearing the Freak: How Talk TV Articulates Women and Class." *Journal of Popular Film and Television* 28.3 (2000): 133–139.

Dahir, Mubarak. "Homosexual Panicking." *Advocate*, June 22, 1999, 27.

Gamson, Joshua. *Freaks Talk Back: Tabloid Talk Shows and Sexual Nonconformity.* Chicago: University of Chicago Press, 1998.

_____. "Why They Love Jerry Springer." *Tikkun* 13.6 (1998): 25–28.

Kurtz, Howard. *Hot Air: All Talk, All the Time.* New York: Random House, 1996.

SEE ALSO

American Television: Situation Comedies; American Television: Drama; O'Donnell, Rosie; RuPaul (RuPaul Andre Charles)

Anderson, Lindsay (1923–1994)

FILM AND STAGE DIRECTOR LINDSAY GORDON ANDERSON was a foundational figure in the Free Cinema movement of the 1950s, a group of British filmmakers who created low-scale, realist works that focused on the ordinary or the socially marginalized, particularly the working class and the younger generation. A leader among such peers as Karel Reisz, Tony Richardson, Gavin Lambert, and John Schlesinger, Anderson was influential in shaping what now might well be considered the golden age of British cinema in the 1960s.

Ironically, as a result of his independence and idealism, he directed relatively few major films, and both his professional and personal lives were affected by the repression and sublimation of his homosexuality.

Anderson was born April 17, 1923, in Bangalore, India, where his father was a captain in the British Army. His family sent him to Cheltenham, an English private school, where he met his lifelong friend and colleague, Gavin Lambert, who, like Anderson, was not only gay but would also enjoy a significant directorial career.

Subsequently, Anderson attended Oxford University, where he specialized in Classics and later cofounded the film journal *Sequence* with Lambert. In his essays and reviews in *Sequence* and other journals, Anderson took aim at the conventions of contemporary British cinema, which tended to avoid controversy and favored the lives and loves of the upper middle class as its subject matter.

Anderson's first films were short semidocumentary studies, looking at the everyday activities of the lower classes. Yet while Anderson had paved the way for feature films about the lives of working-class individuals, such as those that Richardson, Reisz, and Schlesinger directed throughout the early 1960s, he left filmmaking in 1957, when he became a director at the Royal Court Theatre, London.

In this capacity Anderson directed many major theatrical works, including the 1975 revival of Joe Orton's *What the Butler Saw*, the first unexpurgated performance of the play. It was not until 1963 that he made his first feature film, *This Sporting Life*, which, in detailing the career of a young coal miner turned professional footballer, seemed to follow rather than lead then current trends. As such, it was not a commercial success, yet it is significant inasmuch as its depiction of the frustration and the emotional and physical violence that characterize the lives of ostensibly heterosexual working-class men has an inescapable homoerotic undercurrent, as seen in the film's nude bathing scenes.

Many of these themes, although in a very different context, recur in Anderson's best known film, *If...* (1968). Set in a British private school—indeed, filmed at Cheltenham—the film explores the social fascism that is inculcated in such privileged institutions and ends with student rebels machine-gunning a school assembly. It is also noteworthy for its frank representation of homosexual relationships among the schoolboys.

Although *If...* was well-received as a cinematic political statement in the zeitgeist of the late 1960s, Anderson's subsequent films, though often equally daring, fared less well. *O Lucky Man!* (1973), the second of a trilogy featuring the character Mick Travis, the protagonist of *If...* (played by Malcolm McDowell), is a rambling three-hour satire in the mode of Voltaire's *Candide* on the evils of military-industrial capitalism and scientific experimentation. Ambitious and idealistic, the film was nonetheless a commercial failure, and, as a result, Anderson had few offers or financial backers for subsequent film projects. The third film of the trilogy, the cult classic *Britannia Hospital* (1982), is a satire on the British national health service.

During the 1970s and 1980s, Anderson continued to direct for the stage and directed a number of television plays, as well as some rather uncharacteristic features, including *The Whales of August* (1987), starring Lillian Gish and Bette Davis as aged siblings, and *Glory! Glory!* (1989), a satire on televangelism. He also directed *Wham! in China: Foreign Skies* (1986), a documentary of George Michael's pop group on tour.

Anderson died on August 30, 1994, of a heart attack, while in southern France.

Despite Anderson's daring as a director, his recently published letters and Lambert's biography show a tormented man who struggled with his own sexuality. He tended to fall in love with his leading men, including Richard Harris, Albert Finney, and Malcolm McDowell, all of whom were heterosexual, married, and unattainable. His closest associates have speculated that his life was, for the most part, a celibate one. His films, in which homoerotic elements are often presented in a violent or disturbing manner, became the outlet for the desires he could not express in life.

—*Patricia Juliana Smith*

BIBLIOGRAPHY

Anderson, Lindsay. *The Letters of Lindsay Anderson.* London: Faber and Faber, 2000.

——. *Never Apologise: The Collected Writings of Lindsay Anderson.* Paul Ryan, ed. London: Plexus, 2000.

Hedling, Erik. *Lindsay Anderson: Maverick Film Maker.* New York: Continuum, 1998.

Lambert, Gavin. *Mainly About Lindsay Anderson.* London: Faber and Faber, 2000.

SEE ALSO

Film Directors; Richardson, Tony; Schlesinger, John

Anger, Kenneth   (b. 1927)

ONE OF AMERICA'S FIRST OPENLY GAY FILMMAKERS, and certainly the first whose work addressed homosexuality in an undisguised, self-implicating manner, Kenneth Anger occupies an important place in the history of experimental filmmaking. His role in rendering gay culture visible within American cinema, commercial or otherwise, is impossible to overestimate.

He was born Kenneth Anglemyer on February 3, 1927, in Santa Monica, California, but as a youngster renamed himself as part of his aggressive self-fashioning. A child actor, he was exposed to cinematic artifice early in his life and gained a precocious familiarity with films by masters such as Sergei Eisenstein. This exposure and familiarity informed the production values and narrative complexity of the short films Anger made as a teenager.

In 1947, Anger gained instant notoriety with *Fireworks*, a homoerotic nightmare/reverie in which a muscle-bound sailor enjoys posing for the protagonist's (Anger's) delectation, but then, with four others, bashes the youth in a public restroom. Despite the horrific scenario, the ending suggests redemption, with milky fluid spattering Anger's body, a sympathetic sailor's crotch spewing white sparks from a Roman candle, and Anger resurrected, wearing a flaming Christmas-tree headdress.

Encapsulated thus, *Fireworks* is deprived of its visual subtleties, irony, and sophisticated editing, which were precisely the qualities that exonerated it in a 1959 obscenity trial before California's Supreme Court after years of censorship and controversy, sometimes even when shown in European avant-garde film festivals. Thereafter, the artistic merits of gay-themed films were invoked with increasing success at censorship trials.

Some early Anger works never made it to the controversial screening stage because negatives were confiscated and destroyed by self-policing labs to which he had sent film for processing. Conversely, other viewers were overly appreciative of Anger's eroticism, pirating and showing his films in nightclubs during an era when gay porn was largely unavailable.

Similarly, the pervasiveness of iconic gay imagery in Anger's work, such as the leather-clad bikers of *Scorpio Rising* (1963), often caused his films to be grossly oversimplified as depictions of homosexual "pathology," rather than understood as critiques of American mass culture, particularly as it was propagated by Hollywood movies and the rock-and-roll music that Anger used for his soundtracks in pioneering ways, critically anticipating the music video genre.

In unfinished film projects such as *Puce Moment* (1949), with its close-up sequence of women's gowns, and *Kustom Kar Kommandos* (1965), in which a youth caresses a hot rod with a powder puff, Anger inventories American culture's most fetishized objects, evoking a profoundly camp sensibility. Elsewhere, in *Eaux d'artifice* (1953), whatever gay content does exist—Anger cites Ronald Firbank's novel *Valmouth* as inspiration and has likened the fountain imagery to sexual watersports—is subordinate to the film's elegant visual abstractions.

Although *Fireworks* and *Scorpio Rising* had earned Anger a reputation as an underground gay filmmaker, through the late 1960s and 1970s his films expressed less specifically gay content. His longtime fascination with the writings of occultist Aleister Crowley, which had imparted a dark, ritualistic atmosphere to even his earliest films, propelled works such as *Invocation of My Demon Brother* (1969) and *Lucifer Rising* (1973). Collaborative projects with Mick Jagger and Led Zeppelin's Jimmy Page recalled Anger's earlier professional engagements with Jean Cocteau, Anaïs Nin, and other iconoclasts, but the results fell short of Anger's expectations and, indeed, abilities.

Through the 1980s, Anger became known to a broader public through the film adaptation of his lurid book *Hollywood Babylon* (1958), which chronicled scandals of the film industry. *Hollywood Babylon* is, in essence, a counteraccusation of indecency and intemperance against America's self-righteous film establishment, an institution that at midcentury was so fearful of scandal that only underground filmmakers risked depicting overtly sexual content and exploring radical cinematic forms.

—*Mark Allen Svede*

BIBLIOGRAPHY

Anger, Kenneth. *Hollywood Babylon.* 1958. San Francisco: Straight Arrow Books, 1975. Reprint, New York: Dell, 1981.

Hunter, Jack. *Moonchild: The Films of Kenneth Anger.* London: Creation, 2002.

Landis, Bill. *Anger: The Unauthorized Biography of Kenneth Anger.* New York: HarperCollins, 1995.

Pilling, Jayne, and Michael O'Pray, eds. *Into the Pleasure Dome: The Films of Kenneth Anger.* London: British Film Institute, 1989.

Suárez, Juan Antonio. *Bike Boys, Drag Queens, and Superstars: Avant-Garde, Mass Culture, and Gay Identities in the 1960s Underground Cinema.* Bloomington, Ind.: Indiana University Press, 1996.

SEE ALSO

Film; Film Directors; New Queer Cinema; Pornographic Film and Video: Gay Male; Almodóvar, Pedro; Cocteau, Jean; Eisenstein, Sergei Mikhailovich; Grinbergs, Andris

Araki, Gregg   (b. 1959)

GREGG ARAKI'S FILMS ARE DIRECT RESPONSES TO THE "institutionalized homophobia" of media, politicians, and cultural watchdogs. The poster boy of radical and militant queer cinema, Araki disdains the ghettoizing label "gay filmmaker" and denies being part of the New Queer Cinema.

Frequently accused of displaying negative images of homosexuals, Araki has no tolerance for insular lesbian and gay organizations, and refuses to be a propagandist for any gay agenda. Aggressively skirting labels and appropriation by others, Araki's polemical, queer films explore polymorphous perversity, amorphous and pansexuality, omnisexual behavior, AIDS, and the modern *ménage à trois.*

Born to Japanese-American parents in Los Angeles in 1959, Araki grew up in Santa Barbara. After graduating from the University of California, Santa Barbara, with a B.A. in film history and criticism in 1982, Araki completed an M.F.A. in film production at the University of Southern California. Studying film history, he developed a love for screwball comedies and their irrational, subversive narratives, as well as for road movies and French New Wave filmmaker Jean-Luc Godard, who regularly broke filmic codes.

Scripting, photographing, editing, and producing his first four films, Araki polished the art of being a guerrilla filmmaker: someone who freely and spontaneously films anywhere and anytime with rudimentary equipment. He constantly dodged Los Angeles police in the streets for failing to have a shooting permit.

During this period, punk and post-punk music was as important to Araki's films as was his growing up gay in Los Angeles. He embraced the spirit of punk rock's intensity, anarchy, and anger, its unrefined confrontational style, and hyperexaggerated performances.

Araki's early films are crude in production values, and contentious. As the filmmaker explained to his friend Craig Lee, they attack Hollywood's conservative ideology as a "stagnant cesspool of conformity."

Made in 1989, *The Long Weekend (O' Despair),* "a minimalist gay/bisexual post punk antithesis to the smug complacency of regressive Hollywood tripe like *The Big Chill* (1983)," depicts the futile attempts of three couples to disentangle their lives. Their polymorphous sexuality becomes the source of confusion, distress, uncertainty, and depression. The gay press did not greet the film warmly.

With *The Living End* (1991), subtitled "An Irresponsible Film," critics associated Araki with the New Queer Cinema because its release coincided with other alternative gay films. In *The Living End,* two HIV-positive men, one antisocial and on the brink of lashing out at the world and the other a reserved film critic, fall in love and go on the run after accidentally killing a policeman. Referred to as the gay *Thelma and Louise* (1991), the film depicts how these reckless and irresponsible men clash with a homophobic society and with each other. Araki made *The Living End* in opposition to what he considered the sentimental "positive gay imagery" of *Longtime Companion* (1990).

After reading about the high rate of teenage suicide, and intrigued by the intensity of teen life, Araki began a "teen apocalypse trilogy," beginning with *Totally F***ed Up* (1993), subtitled "Another Homo Movie," followed by *The Doom Generation* (1994), and concluding with *Nowhere* (1997). The films focus on teenagers struggling with identity, sexuality, doubt, bitterness, and social torment in an irrational world.

Critics called the trilogy nihilistic, but the films are deeply romantic, and the characters desperately believe in ideal love. But, in their naïveté, the characters are blind to the ways in which an inhospitable world shatters romance. In all three films, Araki saturates images with bright red, orange, and green light, heightening romanticism while conveying a surreal environment. The trilogy reveals Araki's fascination with the oppressiveness of popular culture.

Central to Araki's queer aesthetic are extreme and unpredictable shifts in relationships and moods, from comic to tragic, sensitive to torturous. In *The Doom Generation,* subtitled "A Heterosexual Movie" and an attempt at a "purely queer" film that is sexually appealing to straights and gays alike, exaggerated, comic-book violence distances viewers from a vicious society until realistic and horrifically violent acts end the film. Critics walked out of screenings, and audiences, not prepared for the ending, left in shock.

The queerest event in Araki's career intertwined film and real life. While filming *Nowhere,* Araki's "*Beverly Hills 90210* set in hell," he became romantically involved with one of his actresses, Kathleen Robinson, who played Claire on the television series. *Variety* announced that the relationship had "tongues wagging," and another headline read "Gay filmmaker falls for 90210 babe."

The relationship led to a film Araki wrote for Robinson, *Splendor* (1999), an optimistic and glamorous screwball comedy with queer undertones that aims for a wider audience while remaining on Hollywood's fringe.

In summer 2000, Araki completed a pilot episode for the series *This is How the World Ends*, for MTV. Describing it as "Twin Peaks for the MTV generation," Araki was pleased that a truly radical program might enter millions of homes. MTV referred to it as "Dawson's Creek on acid" and announced that the series, from "one-time homosexual" Araki, would debut in fall 2000. It has yet to be shown. Before MTV silently abandoned the series, Araki explained why it would never air: "If we ever did manage to get the show on the air, it would change the face of broadcast TV."

After two successful screenings at the Venice Film Festival and London Film Festival in fall 2004, *Mysterious Skin* (2004), based on Scott Heim's novel of the same title, was finally released in the U.S. in spring 2005. In the film, Araki uses the "normal" setting of Hutchinson, Kansas, to enter the "dark and dangerous world" of adolescent sexuality, wherein a baseball coach's sexual abuse of two eight-year-old team members sparks two different journeys through late adolescence, and two radically different outcomes. One boy's embrace of the coach's advances calls into question the accepted "evil" image of the pedophile in a disturbing manner; viewers are confronted with a pedophile who elicits contradictory and unsettling emotional responses.

Araki's next project, *crEEEEps*, is set in Malibu Beach and combines two genres present in his early films, the horror film and the teenage sex comedy.

—*Richard C. Bartone*

BIBLIOGRAPHY

Bowen, Peter. "Designed for Living." *Filmmaker* 7.4 (Summer 1999): 28–31.

Chang, Chris. "Absorbing Alternative." *Film Comment* 30.5 (September/October 1994): 47–48, 50, 53.

Cole, C. Bard. "Out on the Lam." *New York Native*, August 17, 1992.

Gever, M., J. Greyson, and P. Parmar, eds. *Queer Looks: Perspectives on Lesbian and Gay Film and Video*. New York: Routledge, 1993.

Lee, Craig. "Introducing Gregg Araki." *L.A. Style* (August 1989).

Wu, Harmony H. "Queering L.A.: Gregg Araki's Homo-pomo Cinema City." *Spectator* 18.1 (1997): 58–69.

SEE ALSO

Film; Film Directors; Screenwriters; New Queer Cinema; Film Festivals

Arzner, Dorothy   *(1900?–1979)*

ALTHOUGH NOT THE FIRST WOMAN TO DIRECT FILMS in Hollywood, Dorothy Arzner was the only woman director to work through the turbulent, richly productive 1930s and 1940s—the period crucial to the development of classical Hollywood cinema.

Arzner had been familiar with the film industry almost her entire life. Although she was born in San Francisco, perhaps on January 3, 1900, or perhaps as early as 1897, she grew up around the filmmakers and actors who frequented her father's Hollywood restaurant. After dropping out of the University of Southern California, where she had intended to become a doctor, Arzner interviewed with William De Mille (of the Famous Players–Lasky Corporation, later to be Paramount Studios) and accepted her first film job as a script typist. She soon moved on to cutting and editing, eventually editing fifty-two pictures as chief editor for RealArt, a subsidiary of Paramount.

Arzner negotiated her directorial debut at Paramount with *Fashions for Women* in 1927. Between 1927 and 1933, she directed eleven films for Paramount; in the ten years between 1933 and when she left the Hollywood film industry in 1943, Arzner directed another six films as a freelancer with RKO, United Artists, MGM, and Columbia.

During this time, Arzner received a substantial amount of media attention as a "woman director" in the popular press; and as a woman, her work and her career were constantly scrutinized. For all this, however, Arzner remained enigmatic, even provocatively so: Observers commented on the juxtaposition of her petite figure and her "mannish" dress; journalists reassured readers that this woman gave her orders on the set with a soft and "feminine" voice; and publicity photos regularly romanced her relationship with her female stars, who included such actresses as Clara Bow, Claudette Colbert, Rosalind Russell, Katharine Hepburn, and Joan Crawford.

Arzner's lesbianism seems to have been well known within the Hollywood community, though little attention was paid to it publicly. She lived openly with her companion, Marion Morgan, a choreographer and dancer, from 1930 until Morgan's death in 1971. The prominence of dance in several of Arzner's films may reflect Morgan's influence.

As with the films of all directors who worked within the creative constraints imposed by the economic and ideological demands of the early studio system, Arzner's films must be read cautiously for signs of her personal politics. Nevertheless, her films are, predominantly, films that convey the varieties of women's experiences and desires, and the tenacity of women's relationships with other women, often within the intersections of gender and social class.

Arzner's films consistently depict controversial topics: extramarital sex and pregnancy (*Working Girls*, 1931; *Christopher Strong*, 1933), cross-class relationships (*The Bride Wore Red*, 1937), prostitution or erotic display (*Nana*, 1934; *Dance, Girl, Dance*, 1940). Some viewers have detected a playful homoeroticism in the schoolgirl comedy *The Wild Party* (1929).

Even those films that appear most "conventional" succeed in critiquing the actual conventions they participate in; for instance, in *Craig's Wife* (1936), the very character of Harriet Craig (Rosalind Russell) offers a compelling indictment of the institution of marriage and the social and economic dependency that described the lot of many wives at the time.

Similarly, in an important and much-cited scene, Arzner exposes and deflates the power of the "gaze" (understood both in terms of gender—namely, male—and social class) that underpins most classical American cinema: In *Dance, Girl, Dance*, Judy (Maureen O'Hara), a ballet dancer forced by poverty to dance in vaudeville, confronts her audience and, in a role reversal that anticipates much later feminist criticism and feminist filmmaking,

tells them exactly how she and the other dancers on the stage see them.

Arzner left Hollywood in 1943 to recover from an illness, and she never returned. Coincidentally, post–World War II Hollywood experienced a radical movement toward conservative "family values" quite incompatible with Arzner's general themes and interests, and her work seems to have fallen out of favor.

After her Hollywood career, Arzner directed training films for the Women's Army Corps, taught in the film program at UCLA (1959–1963), and was honored by the Director's Guild of America in 1975. She died on October 1, 1979.

As a woman "pioneer" in the film industry, and as a lesbian, Arzner has attracted considerable attention recently. She has been recognized for her innovations in using sound; and her films, though many are still hard to find outside of archives, have seen a renewed interest both academically and popularly.   —*Jacqueline Jenkins*

BIBLIOGRAPHY

Cook, Pam. "Approaching the Work of Dorothy Arzner." *The Work of Dorothy Arzner: Towards a Feminist Cinema*. Claire Johnston, ed. London: British Film Institute, 1975. 9–18.

Johnston, Claire. "Dorothy Arzner: Critical Strategies." *The Work of Dorothy Arzner: Towards a Feminist Cinema*. Claire Johnston, ed. London: British Film Institute, 1975. 1–8.

Mayne, Judith. *Directed by Dorothy Arzner*. Bloomington, Ind.: Indiana University Press, 1994.

_____. *The Woman at the Keyhole: Feminism and Woman's Cinema*. Bloomington, Ind.: Indiana University Press, 1990.

Peary, Gerald, and Karyn Kay. "Interview with Dorothy Arzner." *The Work of Dorothy Arzner: Towards a Feminist Cinema*. Claire Johnston, ed. London: British Film Institute, 1975. 19–29.

SEE ALSO

Film; Film Directors; Screenwriters; Film Actors: Lesbian

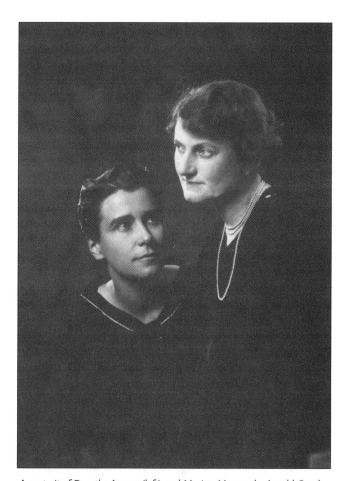

A portrait of Dorothy Arzner (left) and Marion Morgan by Arnold Genthe.

Asian Film

WITH THE PROLIFERATION OF INTERNATIONAL FILM festivals and a growing dissatisfaction with Hollywood hegemony, coinciding with film renaissances in Hong Kong, Taiwan, China, and Korea, Asian films have recently enjoyed an unprecedented popularity with English-language audiences. This popularity has allowed Western audiences a glimpse of Asian gay and lesbian identities through high-profile queer films such as Nakajima Takehiro's *Okoge* (1992) and Wong Kar-wai's *Happy Together* (1997), not to mention a constant stream of gender ambiguities in Japanese animation and Hong Kong martial arts fantasies.

Yet while many of the queer Asian films we see in the West have come from Japan and Hong Kong—probably because these are the most cosmopolitan film industries in Asia—queer films have both struggled and succeeded in countries throughout Asia, countries whose distinct cultures and histories inform their queer images.

We should, however, always keep in mind that many of the most noted Asian queer films, such as Chen Kaige's *Farewell My Concubine* (1993), Deepa Mehta's *Fire* (1996), and Zhang Yuan's *East Palace, West Palace* (1996), were made by professedly heterosexual directors and are films that arguably use homosexuality not as a subject matter in itself, but as an allegorical tool to critique political oppressions.

Mainland China and Taiwan

Although images of strong, masculinized women were an integral part of mainland Chinese propaganda films and revolutionary operas in the 1950s and 1960s, these images trapped women within a masculinist idea of gender, and pathologized any hints of lesbianism. Explicit homosexuality had, of course, been suppressed in a communist China where homosexuality was demonized as a sign of decadence, either Western or dynastic.

Mainland China's first "gay" film was director Chen Kaige's highly publicized Chinese opera tale *Farewell My Concubine* (1993), a somewhat whitewashed version of Lillian Lee's source novel. Although the director himself admitted that *Farewell* was basically a mainstream pageant that used homosexuality as a commercial selling point, the film is actually frustratingly shy about its gayness.

The film was banned nonetheless, a fate that also awaited China's first modern-day gay film, Zhang Yuan's *East Palace, West Palace* (1996), a bleak story of homoerotic tension between a gay prisoner and his interrogator that serves as a metaphor for the master/slave dichotomy that underpins politically repressive regimes. But more recently, China has witnessed a mild trend of gay and lesbian comedies such as Liu Bingjian's *Men and Women* (1999) and Li Yu's *Fish and Elephant* (2001), possibly pointing to a tentative liberalization of gay and lesbian subjects.

Only in the past fifteen or so years have Taiwanese films explicitly explored queer themes, and then it has been in singular or auteurist films, as Taiwan's film industry is, at the risk of oversimplification, neither populist nor large enough to support the kind of generic gender play that informs Hong Kong cinema. Seven years before the international distribution of Ang Lee's *The Wedding Banquet* (1993) allowed Westerners a glimpse of transnational gay Taiwanese identity, Yu Kan-ping directed *The Outcasts* (1986), the first gay film to receive approval from the Taiwanese government.

Taiwan has also delivered some very sensitive lesbian melodramas: Huang Yu-shan's *The Twin Bracelets* (1990) tells the rural love story of two young women who must choose between succumbing to patriarchal oppression and pursuing forbidden desires, and Cheng Sheng-fu's *The Silent Thrush* (1992) presents a classical Chinese opera setting as the backdrop to lesbian romance.

It is Tsai Ming-liang, however, who has emerged as Taiwan's foremost exponent of queer cinema. Both his juvenile delinquency tale *Rebels of the Neon God* (1992) and his minimalist character piece *Vive L'Amour* (1994) are shot through with (male) homoerotic undercurrents; and *The River* (1997) provides a devastating critique of sexual and familial alienation, presenting a modern family so distant that father and son unwittingly sleep with one another when one night the closeted father goes cruising in a darkened bathhouse.

Gay themes have also found a place in cosmopolitan Taiwanese films such as Wang Tsai-sheng's *A Cha-Cha for the Fugitive* (1997) and Edward Yang's transnationally themed *Mahjong* (1996), whose central setting of a gay bar suggests that an inclusion of gay identities (albeit stereotypical ones) is necessary in a consideration of East–West desires.

South Korea

South Korean films have often suffered from a stifling legacy of imported, family-centered Confucianism. If the controversy surrounding Jang Sun-Woo's *Lies* (1999) is any example, Korean cinema is still coming to terms with heterosexual erotica, so homosexual portrayals remain very controversial. Nevertheless, there are a few films that queer Korean audiences have claimed for themselves.

Ha Kil-jong's *The Pollen of Flowers* (1972), for example, is recognized as a subtle variation on Pasolini's *Teorema* (1968). Kim Su-hyeong's *Ascetic: Woman and Woman* (1976) is considered Korea's first lesbian film. It is a tragic protofeminist drama about two troubled women who erotically bond when one of them is abused by her husband.

In the 1990s, Park Jae-ho's *Broken Branches* (1995) emerged as a landmark in Korean cinema, an intergenerational gay romance, with moderately revealing sex scenes, whose intergenerational relationship becomes a metaphor for a new Korea reconciling its tenuous relationship with its conservative elders.

In 1997, the Seoul Queer Film and Video Festival was both founded and quickly banned by the government, attracting worldwide attention. Reinstated the following year with some success, it provides an overdue forum for queer films in Korea. However, most of the festival's films are not actually Korean. Moreover, the spotlighted feature of the proposed 1997 fest was in fact Wong Kar-wai's Hong Kong import *Happy Together*

(1997). Meanwhile, the most recent development in indigenous queer film has been Kim Tae-yong and Min Kyu-dong's commercially successful adolescent lesbian ghost story *Memento Mori* (1999).

The Philippines and Thailand

Unlike Confucianist China and Korea, many Southeast Asian cultures have more open traditions of alternative sexuality. However, it should be noted that the sexual "openness" the West often perceives in Thailand and the Philippines is often based on prostitutional economies and class exploitation.

The most internationally recognized director of Philippine films, the late Lino Brocka, was also the one most associated with gay films. Brocka's *Manila in the Claws of Light* (1975) tells of a poor fisherman who turns to male prostitution in the big city, and *My Mother, My Father* (1978) is concerned with a transvestite father toiling under the class stratifications of the Marcos regime. The most influential gay Philippine film is certainly Brocka's *Macho Dancer* (1988), an engagingly lurid exploration of Manila's male sex trade that combines equal elements of neorealism, soft pornography, and Philippine melodrama.

Brocka's associate, Mel Chionglo (who scripted Brocka's 1979 *Mother, Sister, Daughter*) later turned the "macho dancer" melodrama into its own veritable subgenre with *Midnight Dancers* (1994) and *Burlesk King* (1999).

In contrast to Chionglo's glossy films, which tend to romanticize the sex trade while simultaneously critiquing the poverty that produces it, independent director Nick Deocampo's lower-budgeted *Oliver* (1983), *Children of the Regime* (1985), and *Revolutions Happen Like Refrains in a Song* (1987) take more critical looks at the socioeconomic links between male prostitution and class exploitation during and immediately after the Marcos era.

In Thailand, a gay melodramatic aesthetic, perhaps comparable to that of the Philippines, informs M. L. Bhandevanop Devakul's *I Am a Man* (1986), sort of a Thai *Boys in the Band*, as well as Pisan Akarasainee's *The Last Song* (1986) and *Anguished Love* (1987), a two-part series about the loves and losses among a star-crossed intersection of gays, lesbians, transvestites, and, yes, heterosexuals.

Recently, Youngyooth Thongkonthun's comedy *Satree Lex* (U.S. title: *Iron Ladies*, 1999), based on the remarkable true story of a champion Thai volleyball team composed of gay men and transsexuals, proved something of a breakthrough in Thai cinema, becoming one of the biggest box office hits in Thai history.

Nevertheless, the film's popularity in Thailand may be attributed to the camp spectacle of its subject matter, as Thailand's kathoey (transgender) population, though

far more visible than transsexuals in the West, is still marginalized and objectified. We might compare Thongkonthun's treatment of the subject with that of gay Hong Kong director Manshi Yonfan in his Singaporean film *Bugis Street* (1995), whose steamy images of transgendered desire make no concessions to straight audiences.

India

While openly politicized homosexuality in India is a recent, Westernized phenomenon, popular Indian cinema has long offered glimpses of alternative sexualities, though sometimes not in the most positive terms.

We might go back as far as Fearless Nadia (real name: Mary Evans), the exotic, mannish Australian actress who starred in Homi Wadia's *Hunterwali* (1935) and other Hindi films as a kind of whip-wielding, "Perils of Pauline"-style heroine, and whose campy, gender-bending career is explored in Riyad Wadia's documentary *Fearless: The Hunterwali Story* (1993).

In the 1970s, the male buddy films of Hindi superstar Amitabh Bachchan, such as Ramesh Sippy's landmark *Sholay* (1975) and Raj Khosla's *Dostana* (1981), often featured homoerotic undercurrents that eclipse those of Hollywood's male buddy films. *Sholay* is, in fact, known for song sequences that valorize male platonic love.

Bollywood cinema is, however, also known for its caricatures of gay men and lesbians, and there are countless films featuring swishy men, such as the effeminate biker who lusts after the macho hero of Vikram Bhatt's *Ghulam* (1998), or sexless butch women, such as the cruel prison warden who punishes her lesbian charges in Jabbar Patel's *Subhah* (1981).

Hijras (transsexuals, eunuchs, or gender-ambiguous persons) and transvestites are also a fixture of Hindi cinema, yet usually as objects of derisive comedy or disgust, as in Rahul Rawail's *Mast Kalandar* (1991), Mahesh Bhatt's *Sadak* (1991), or Darmesh Darshan's popular *Raja Hindustani* (1996). While a film such as Mani Ratnam's *Bombay* (1995) may briefly provide a sympathetic hijra, the continuing persecution of hijra communities remains a critical social problem throughout India.

In the 1990s, a number of independent, liberal, English-language queer Indian films emerged to challenge conventional Bollywood morality, the best-known of which is Deepa Mehta's Canadian-produced *Fire* (1996). The feminist lesbianism of the film provoked outrage among the Hindu patriarchy and fundamentalists; and the film lived up to its name when arson and bombings rocked Indian theaters that dared show it.

Fire was immediately preceded, however, by Riyad Wadia's *BOMgaY* (1996), a short experimental film based on the verse of gay Indian poet Raj Rao, which celebrates gay Indian life while critiquing the government's homophobic antisodomy statutes. Although *BOMgaY* (which was shot on video) did not receive any public screenings, news of its existence spread quickly through the Indian press, and became an immediate topic of controversy.

Recently, feature-length films such as Kaizad Gustad's *Bombay Boys* (1998) and Dev Benegal's *Split Wide Open* (1999) have continued to address the politics of Indian gay identity. Admittedly, however, these films are considered semicommercial in India and are not aimed at a populist Hindi demographic.

Bombay Boys, the story of three overseas, Anglicized Indians who come to Bombay in search of their political, familial, and sexual identities, particularly draws connections between transnational identity and a burgeoning Indian gayness. This may be a sign that, as Asian films are increasingly products of transnational distribution, the politics and sexualities they engage may necessarily and inevitably become caught between imported ideas of Western queerness and the struggle to maintain an Eastern, autonomous self-identity.   —*Andrew Grossman*

BIBLIOGRAPHY

Berry, Chris. *A Bit on the Side: East-West Topographies of Desire.* Sydney: EM Press, 1994.

Grossman, Andrew, ed. *Queer Asian Cinema: Shadows in the Shade.* Binghamton, N.Y.: Harrington Park Press, 2000.

Kwan, Stanley. *Yang and Yin: Gender in Chinese Cinema.* Hong Kong: Media Asia, 1996.

Wadia, Riyad Vinci, dir. *Fearless: The Hunterwali Story.* Documentary film. Bombay/New York: Wadia Movietone, 1993.

Yang, Mayfair Mei-hui. *Spaces of Their Own: Women's Public Sphere in Transnational China.* Minneapolis: University of Minnesota Press, 1999.

SEE ALSO

Hong Kong Film; Japanese Film; Pasolini, Pier Paolo

Asquith, Anthony   *(1902–1968)*

DISCREET AND *REFINED* ARE ADJECTIVES USUALLY applied to director Anthony Asquith's films, which, for an international cinemagoing public, continue to represent a certain quintessential "Britishness."

While his works focus on the psychological dilemmas of the upper class into which he was born, Asquith was nevertheless a pioneer in securing union benefits for the working-class men and women who perform the necessary if unglamorous jobs of the film industry. His characteristic discretion and refinement, moreover, were not merely a facet of his art, but rather a highly developed way of life for the gay son of a famous politician in a society in which homosexual acts were criminal.

Anthony Asquith was born in London on November 9, 1902. His parents were Herbert Asquith (later Earl of Oxford and Asquith), who was British Prime Minister from 1909 to 1916, and the witty Margot Tennant Asquith, a highly visible figure in London literary and social circles. The gay eccentric Stephen Tennant was a cousin, and contemporary actress Helena Bonham Carter is his great-niece. Small, effeminate, and hook-nosed, Asquith was nicknamed "Puffin" (or "Puff") as a child, because he reminded his mother of a bird of that species. The name remained with him for life.

Asquith was educated at Balliol College, Oxford, where he was very much an aesthete and where he first became interested in film. In 1925, after graduating, he became a founding member of the Oxford Film Society and traveled to the United States to learn cinematic techniques from the Hollywood studios. His social connections gave him a rapid start in the fledgling British film industry; he codirected his first film, *Shooting Stars* (1927), at twenty-five.

Asquith's early films, however, did not bring him success, as they were deemed too "arty" for the public's taste. His commercial breakthrough came with *Pygmalion* (codirected with Leslie Howard, 1938), an adaptation of George Bernard Shaw's play. Soon thereafter, he embarked on a professional partnership with gay playwright Terence Rattigan, whose drawing-room dramas were then much in vogue.

Their collaboration began with an adaptation of Rattigan's hit comedy *French without Tears* (1939), and reached its high point with *The Winslow Boy* (1948) and *The Browning Version* (1951), the latter of which is memorable for Michael Redgrave's compelling portrayal of a teacher who has failed personally and professionally.

Other Asquith-Rattigan films include *Quiet Wedding* (1940), *Uncensored* (1942), *Way to the Stars* (1945), *While the Sun Shines* (1947), *The Final Test* (1953), *The V.I.P.s* (1963), and *The Yellow Rolls-Royce* (1965). In addition, Asquith also directed notable adaptations of Oscar Wilde's *The Importance of Being Earnest* (1952) and Shaw's *The Doctor's Dilemma* (1959) and *The Millionairess* (1960); war films such as *We Dive at Dawn* (1943) and *Carrington, V.C.* (1954); and psychological dramas such as *Libel* (1959).

Although his films are almost exclusively concerned with heterosexual subjects, some critics, particularly Stephen Bourne, argue that they are permeated with a gay sensibility.

Despite his privileged background, Asquith was a modest and unassuming man who was deeply concerned for those less powerful. For three decades he headed the British film technicians union and fought for workers' rights and government subsidies to the film industry. While many simply assumed his homosexuality, he was quite repressed in his personal life and apparently sublimated his desires in his films.

Anthony Asquith died in London after a long battle with cancer, on February 20, 1968. —*Patricia Juliana Smith*

BIBLIOGRAPHY

Bourne, Stephen. *Brief Encounters: Lesbians and Gays in British Cinema 1930–1971*. London: Cassell, 1996.

Minney, R. J. *The Films of Anthony Asquith*. South Brunswick, UK: A. S. Barnes, 1976.

_____. *"Puffin" Asquith: A Biography of the Hon. Anthony Asquith, Aesthete, Aristocrat, Prime Minister's Son and Film Maker*. London: Frewin, 1973.

Noble, Peter. *Anthony Asquith*. London: British Film Institute, 1958.

SEE ALSO

Film; European Film

Australian Film

OVER THE LAST DECADE THERE HAVE BEEN A NUMBER of Australian films that have, either overtly or implicitly, been informed by lesbian, gay, bisexual, transsexual, and queer themes. However, this vibrant, sometimes controversial contemporary queer flowering—now recognized by many critics as an integral part of Australian national cinema—must be placed in the context of a film industry that, prior to the 1970s, was characterized by a combination of social conservatism and strictly codified censorship.

The Early Years

Despite, or perhaps because of, its repression, early Australian cinema did yield some of the queer traces identified by Vito Russo in *The Celluloid Closet*, although the relative paucity of local film output resulted in fewer examples than the Hollywood product. For example, in *Dad and Dave Come to Town* (1938)—part of K. G. Hall's nationally beloved country bumpkin "Dad and Dave" series—the Rudd family meet Entwistle, a limp-wristed shop floorwalker who, despite his effeminate demeanor, becomes a family confidant, and appears again in *Dad Rudd MP* (1940).

Cross-dressing—specifically female to male—appeared via the masculine attire of the pioneer or squatter girl, producing some interesting ambiguities in films such as *Jewelled Nights* (1925), *Lovers and Luggers* (1937), *The Squatter's Daughter* (1933), and *Bitter Springs* (1950).

Ironically, however, the most notable gender bender appeared in a classic Australian war film—Charles Chauvel's *Forty Thousand Horsemen* (1941), a celebra-tion of the heroic masculinity of the Australian soldier that features a plot development involving a beautiful female French spy disguised as an Arab boy. Needless to say, all of these queer traces were strictly subtextual, and sealed with satisfactory heterosexual resolutions.

The 1970s and 1980s

In the 1970s, a growing drive for cultural self-definition, along with increased government funding, resulted in a greater quantity and quality of Australian films. This combined with the loosening of severe censorship laws to facilitate the exploration of "adult" themes.

For example, Bruce Beresford's *The Adventures of Barry McKenzie* (1972), a crude yet funny "innocent abroad" tale, exposes naive hick Bazza and Auntie (later Dame) Edna Everage to various sexual perversities, among them lesbianism and homosexuality, on their visit to the United Kingdom.

Meanwhile, the arrival of the permissive society in Australia was celebrated in *Felicity* (1978) and *The Guide to Australian Love and Sex* (1978), forgettable sex romps with sophisticated pretensions, which nevertheless extend some tolerance to same-sex desire.

More challenging (and perhaps surprisingly so), *Number 96* (1974), a movie version of a popular television nighttime soap, featured both camp stereotype Dudley ("ever so nice") Butterfield and "average guy/gay" Don Finlayson, a lawyer who, surprisingly, is the film's ethical center.

Serious films of the period saw only tentative, sometimes troublesome, explorations of queer themes. While Fred Schepisi's *The Chant of Jimmy Blacksmith* (1978) and George Miller's *Mad Max II* (1981) include demonizing caricatures of the predatory older male, Canadian director Ted Kotcheff's still controversial *Wake in Fright* (1971) offers a more complex account of Australian masculinity through an uncompromising study of the victimization—and eventual rape—of a "sissy" schoolteacher by the macho menfolk of a country town.

In Schepisi's visually stunning *The Devil's Playground* (1976), set in a repressive Catholic seminary in 1950s Australia, it is unclear whether adolescent homosexual experimentation is the object of repression or the (regrettable) product of it.

In *Lonely Hearts* (1982), by avant-garde director Paul Cox, a sympathetically portrayed gay male friend plays a key role in facilitating the heterosexual romance plot. Cox's explorations of troubled, off-center heterosexuality might well fit him in the category of "queer," though traces of lesbianism in his *Man of Flowers* (1983) might, for some, seem little more than standard voyeuristic fare in a study of male (hetero) sexual obsession.

Little represented in the period, lesbian desire does, nevertheless, play a crucial if seemingly tangential role in two important historical dramas, both set in girls' schools. Traces of lesbian eroticism underpin Peter Weir's haunting *Picnic at Hanging Rock* (1975), while Bruce Beresford's *The Getting of Wisdom* (1977) gives greater specificity to the teenage protagonist's sapphic crush than Henry Handel Richardson's turn-of-the-century novel.

The 1970s also saw the beginnings of a lesbian tradition in independent, experimental film. Often informed by feminist debates and academic gender theories, it includes fiction shorts such as Megan McMurchy's *Apartments* (1977) and Ann Turner's *Flesh on Glass* (1981), Digby Duncan's documentary *Witches, Dykes, and Poofters* (1979), and Leone Knight's confrontational, queer-theory-inflected *In Loving Memory* (1992) and *The Father Is Nothing* (1992).

The 1990s and After

The explosion of queer Australian films in the 1990s was, arguably, heralded by the stunning success of Baz Luhrman's *Strictly Ballroom* (1992). The romance plot may be straight but the film is saturated with camp and kitsch, and is a forerunner of Luhrmann's later international extravaganzas, *William Shakespeare's Romeo + Juliet* (1996) and *Moulin Rouge* (2001).

Ann Turner's feature-length *Dallas Doll* (1992), starring American comedienne Sandra Bernhard as a bisexual adventuress let loose on an "ordinary" Australian family, was a patchy yet intriguing venture that failed to find mainstream cinema release.

In 1994, however, three seminal films, all comedies, and all with serious thematic underpinnings, were released to critical acclaim and commercial success: P. J. Hogan's *Muriel's Wedding* (1994), with its friendship between two young women on the loose in Sydney, saturated in camp and grounded in an (unrealized) lesbian subtext; Stephan Elliott's exuberant *Priscilla, Queen of the Desert* (1994), the story of three Sydney drag queens (one transsexual, one homosexual, and one bisexual) who embark on a bus journey to Ayers Rock, scandalizing the local yokels on the way; and Geoff Burton and Kevin Dowling's *The Sum of Us* (1994), starring Russell Crowe as a working-class gay plumber, living with his sympathetic straight father.

The comic vein continued with Emma-Kate Croghan's *Love and Other Catastrophes* (1996), a witty take on the screwball genre focusing on the romantic misadventures of five young students in Melbourne, two of whom "just happen" to be lesbians.

Yet toward the end of the 1990s a more serious tone began to emerge. Lawrence Johnson's *Life* (1996)—acclaimed by critics but too confrontational to attract the crossover success of *Priscilla*—offered a searing, timely study of relationships between men in the HIV division of a state prison.

Ana Kokkinos's *Only the Brave* (1994), a sometimes scrappy, yet engaging, short film about the lesbian awakening of a working class Greek-Australian girl, paved the way for Kokkinos to direct and cowrite *Head On* (1998), a technically impressive adaptation of Christos Tsoilkas's grunge novel *Loaded*, featuring a striking performance by Alex Dimitriadis as the antihero Ari.

Novel-to-film adaptations have also provided the impetus for the work of Samantha Lang, who, with Kokkinos, heads the vanguard of younger queer-focused directors. *The Well* (1997), a visually stunning version of Elizabeth Jolley's story of closeted lesbian obsession, stumbles a little, perhaps due to uncertainty about the veiled homophobic strains of the original, but *The Monkey's Mask* (2000) works creditably to capture some of the intelligence and eroticism of Dorothy Porter's complex verse detective novel, eliciting powerful performances from Suzie Porter and Kelly McGillis.

Conclusion

Australia's diverse and distinctive contribution to queer film has secured increasing international recognition. While the halcyon highs of 1994 have yet to be matched, the tradition is, it is hoped, sufficiently solid to withstand the strands of social conservatism and fiscal restraint that mark Australian life in the new millennium.

—*Deborah Hunn*

BIBLIOGRAPHY

Bertrand, Ina. *Film Censorship in Australia*. Brisbane: University of Queensland Press, 1981.

Hunn, Deborah. "'It's Not That I Can't Decide, I Don't like Definitions': Queer in Australia in Christos Tsiolkas' *Loaded* and Ana Kokkinos' *Head On*." *Territories of Desire in Queer Culture: Refiguring Contemporary Boundaries*. David Alderson and Linda Anderson, eds. Manchester, UK: Manchester University Press, 2000. 112–129.

McFarlane, Brian, Geoff Mayer, and Ina Bertrand, eds. *The Oxford Companion to Australian Film*. Oxford: Oxford University Press, 1999.

Murray, Scott. *Australian Film 1978–1992*. Melbourne: Oxford University Press, 1993.

_____, ed. *Australian Cinema*. St. Leonards, NSW: Allen and Unwin, 1994.

O'Regan, Tom. *Australian National Cinema*. London and New York: Routledge, 1996.

Rayner, Jonathan. *Contemporary Australian Cinema: An Introduction*. Manchester, UK: Manchester University Press, 2000.

Robinson, Jocelyn, and Beverly Zalock. *Girls' Own Stories: Australian and New Zealand Women's Film*. London: Scarlet Press, 1997.

Sabine, James, ed. *A Century of Australian Cinema*. Port Melbourne: William Heinemann Australia, 1995.

Willett, Graham. "Minorities Can Win: The Gay Movement, the Left and the Transformation of Australian Society." *Overland* 149 (1997): 64–68.

SEE ALSO

Australian Television; Film; Transsexuality in Film; Transvestism in Film; Bernhard, Sandra

Australian Television

DESPITE SOME IMPORTANT BREAKTHROUGHS IN THE depiction of gay men and lesbians in the past, Australian television today lacks any regular and open discussion of queer issues and lives.

Australian television launched the careers of Nicole Kidman, Kylie Minogue, Guy Pearce, Paul Hogan, and Skippy the Kangaroo. One of its five networks led the world in producing a type of sexy, outrageous serial drama that spawned a cycle of soap opera that has beguiled audiences in Australia and in many other parts of the world for over thirty years. Certainly cult television would be the poorer without dramas like *Sons and Daughters* (with the infamous Pat the Rat), *Prisoner—Cell Block H* (featuring the dyke-you-love-to-hate), and *Return to Eden* (heroine escapes jaws of crocodile—just—and takes on new body, face, identity).

The combination of geographical isolation, an unpredictable climate, and hatred of pretension and authoritarianism has found its way into Australia's television programming. This was the country that produced the world's first positive gay character on television (*Number 96*, 1972–1977). And the world's first bisexuals, male and female (*Number 96*, *The Box*). And the world's first gay man to parent a young boy far more lovingly and effectively than the boy's own biological parents (*Players to the Gallery*, 1980).

Despite its small population (under 20 million), Australia has been able to maintain five television networks, three entirely commercial, one partly so, and the fifth—approximating to Britain's British Broadcasting Corporation—valiantly surviving on government subsidy alone. One of the quintet, SBS (Special Broadcasting Service), created in 1980, is the most successful and highly regarded multicultural service in the world.

The inclusion of "Australian content" in drama, documentaries, comedy, and other types of programming is a cornerstone that, though significantly eroded since the glory days of the 1960s and 1970s, is still in place.

Early Days

Gay men and lesbians, certainly on a superficial reading of the near half-century of Australian small-screen entertainment, have played an integral part in the mix. During the very first hour of transmission, in September 1956, urbane queer artist Jeffery Smart, standing in front of a studio fireplace, expatiated on painting in the children's series, *The Argonauts' Club*.

Smart was very much outside the stereotype of the hard-drinking, sun-browned, fair dinkum Aussie bloke, known as an "ocker," prepared to do and die for his "mates." Although less durable as the 1960s opened up Australia to more diverse influences, the ocker, with his sometimes unstable and dangerous mix of good humor and misogyny, was the predominant image of the Aussie male.

With this strain of homoemotionalism came a degree of sexual activity, none of which was ever fully reflected in Australian film or television. During the successive conservative governments of Robert Menzies, a lid was kept on the country's sexual tensions and injustices through a combination of legal sanctions, religious puritanism, and sometimes draconian censorship.

The 1970s

The mold was broken, or appeared to be, with the noisy arrival of a late-night soap called *Number 96* in 1972. Nudity, both male and female, sexual high jinks, and increasingly outrageous plotlines (including "The Knicker-Snipper") were *de rigueur*.

From the very first episode, *Number 96* was labeled immoral trash, pornography, designed to corrupt the nation. Heedless of these admonitions, the Australian public could not get enough of the very full lives of this group of people living in a Sydney apartment block.

One of its most popular residents was the quietly spoken, intelligent, handsome young lawyer Don Finlayson (played by Joe Hasham), who, it soon became clear, was gay, living with a lover, and inescapably good, kind, and decent: a pillar of the community. Not quite a fair dinkum Aussie bloke, but close.

Don was later joined by a more flouncing gay man, who, in a manner typical of a series vowed and determined to upset viewers' rigid expectations, began an affair with a woman.

Number 96 begat *The Box*, even sexier and set in a television station. It displayed a bisexual woman kissing an underage teenage girl. The same show also rang changes on the portrayal of the effeminate gay man: flapping wrists and camp patter but consistently presented as a competent professional and well respected. The actor playing this role, Paul Karo, won the Most Popular TV Actor award of 1975.

"Real" homosexuals began to appear occasionally on television after the advent of *Number 96*. On a segment of the Australian Broadcasting Corporation's groundbreaking *Chequerboard* series (1972), one man actually kissed his lover on-screen. The day after transmission, the man was dismissed from his administrative job with one of the Sydney churches.

The mid-1970s, with Australia spreading its wings under the radical government of Gough Whitlam before he was summarily dismissed by the Queen of Great Britain's representative, were a high-water mark for the regular airing of gay lives.

However, as well as the euphoria induced by fine-upstanding-if-rather-dull Don and his various lovers, boyfriends, and one-night stands, there was the occasional recognition that there was another, less accepting, Australia. In one edition of the ABC's current-affairs program *The Monday Conference* (1976), human excrement was thrown at a gay rights activist who was being interviewed before a generally fair-minded audience in the mining area of Mt. Isa in Queensland.

Lesbians remained relatively invisible, with a couple of exceptions. There was a wicked lesbian in a late-1970s serial called *Skyways*. She had her comeuppance in the shower: stabbed forty-seven times.

Much more to the lesbian community's liking—and to that of a cult television audience all over the world—was *Prisoner*, also known as *Prisoner—Cell Block H* (1979–1987). Set in a women's prison, the series sought to tease out all possible emotional and sexual *frissons* involving inmates and staff—women characters tough and tender, cynical and naive in profusion. Queening it over all was a sadistic lesbian warder nicknamed "The Freak": growly of voice, beady of eye, and thoroughly convincing in Maggie Kirkpatrick's imposing black-gloved hands.

Public broadcasting was far less committed to lesbian and gay stories. Apart from occasional episodes in short-run drama series, the only thing the ABC could offer that was remotely challenging was a miniseries called *Players to the Gallery* (1980). A story seen from three different viewpoints, one gay, it bravely focused on the plight of a political activist whose own personal life is totally taken up with his landlady and her young son. A custody case hinges on possible corruption of the child by the tenant, who is presented throughout as just the sort of mother/father society should be encouraging to parent its children.

The 1980s and 1990s
In the 1980s and 1990s, financial constraints, the need for overseas sales, and coproduction money seemed to force Australian television away from the relative radicalism of the 1970s. The portrayal of gay men and, apart from *Prisoner*, lesbians virtually ceased for fifteen years.

Making the greatest impact during this period were occasional documentaries, such as *Something to Sing About* (the Sydney Gay and Lesbian Choir) and *Positive Art* (HIV/AIDS and its impact on gay culture), and, notably, a 1991 interview with conductor Stuart Challender in which he revealed he was dying of AIDS.

Fictional representations were mainly medical, consisting of a few episodes of *A Country Practice* and *G.P.*, issue-based, and well researched. Their intention was missionary and awareness-raising.

Both series were much loved by middle Australia. *G.P.* courted and received some adverse criticism when, in 1994, its makers included a young gay doctor, played by Damian Rice, among its regulars. Even this mutedly negative reaction seemed to sap the producers' resolve, so the character never developed to anything like his full dramatic potential.

Although the high-definition bravado of the 1970s seemed a far distant memory, a cannonball hit the Australian viewing public full in the face in the mid-1990s in the form of "edited highlights" of Sydney's Gay and Lesbian Mardi Gras.

Initially—and bravely, in the teeth of much church and state opposition—this event was brought into the homes of mythical average Australians, including not a few diehard ocker homophobes, by the ABC, who cited its long-held commitment to showing all aspects of the country's human condition.

Taken over a few years later by commercial Channel Ten, the Mardi Gras seems to have become an annual fixture. However, it is seen by not a few people as presenting lesbians and gays as a freak show, light years away from the integration and honesty of *Number 96*'s Don and his day-to-day world.

The political message of Mardi Gras can be discerned beneath all the glitz and surging flesh and pulsating techno. Just.

Current Conditions
What is glaringly obvious in the Australian television landscape of today is the complete lack of any regular and open discussion of lesbian and gay issues and lives; and very little dramatization of same. Recent soaps featuring gays and lesbians in prominent roles were poorly promoted at home and failed to "sell" overseas. There is a total absence of a *Queer As Folk* or a *Tales of the City* made in Australia about queer contemporary or past Australian culture.

Openly queer figures such as sportsman Ian Roberts, television medical guru Dr. Kerryn Phelps, and comedian and pundit Julie McCrossin do pop up quite frequently on the screen, respected and liked by the television public, gay and straight.

These are the exceptions, a fact made quite clear by the extraordinary if not always positive impact of "gay Johnnie," one of the sequestered dozen in Australia's version of the reality television phenomenon *Big Brother* (2001).

Seen initially by some as a "backstabber," Johnnie was gradually rehabilitated until he was regarded as a role model, not only for gays but also for some of his young male "housemates." Much hugging, kissing, and crying ensued both during and after the incarceration.

It remains to be seen whether Johnnie's impression on average Australians, especially those under twenty, will be lasting. What was made obvious, through comments in the gay press and elsewhere, was the absence of a broad band of gays on Australian television. The turning point, Don in *Number 96* thirty years before, had failed to turn.

There is hope, however, that the turn will be made. *The Secret Life of Us* (2001–2004), an award-winning drama revolving around the lives of the residents of an apart ment block in an urban suburb of Melbourne, did have gay, lesbian, and bisexual characters, including Australia's first non-Anglo lesbian in the character of Chloe.

—Keith G. Howes

Bibliography

Howes, Keith. "Gays of Our Lives: 30 Years of Gay Australian TV." *OutRage* (Melbourne) 177 (February 1998): 38–49.

See also

Australian Film; British Television; American Television: Situation Comedies; American Television: Drama

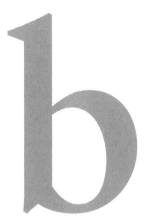

Bankhead, Tallulah   *(1903?–1968)*

TALLULAH BANKHEAD IS TODAY REMEMBERED MOSTLY as an irreverent wit and volcanic life force rather than as an actress. She was, however, a significant artist, originating two of twentieth-century American drama's most substantial female characters: Regina Giddens in Lillian Hellman's *The Little Foxes* (1939) and Sabrina in Thornton Wilder's *The Skin of Our Teeth* (1943).

Born in Huntsville, Alabama, on January 31, 1903 (or perhaps 1901), into a prominent political family, Tallulah was the daughter of a Speaker of the U.S. House of Representatives and the granddaughter and niece of U.S. Senators. Her career began when she won *Picture-Play* magazine's national talent search at the age of fifteen. Her prize, a three-week studio contract, brought her east. The promised silent screen career fizzled, but she was to have remarkable theatrical successes, both in London and in New York.

In the 1930s and early 1940s, Tallulah attempted a movie career, but with little success. However, her impact on the Hollywood community was considerable. She rented the palatial home of silent-movie star William Haines and hosted parties whose regular guests included Ethel Barrymore, Marlene Dietrich, and George Cukor.

Her drug-taking, her scatological language, and her voracious sexual appetite were widely reported. Her sexual liaisons allegedly included Dietrich and Greta Garbo. Summing up the breadth of her indulgences, Tallulah said,

"My daddy warned me about men and booze but he didn't say a word about women and cocaine!"

Unable to transfer stage success to cinema, Tallulah saw many of her most significant roles performed on-screen by Bette Davis, who starred in the film versions of *Dark Victory* (1935) and *The Little Foxes* (1941), for which she received Academy Award nominations. Davis won an Academy Award for another Bankhead-originated role in *Jezebel* (1938).

Eventually Tallulah played a part worthy of her talents in Alfred Hitchcock's *Lifeboat* (1943). Although the New York Society of Film Critics voted her Best Actress for her performance in *Lifeboat*, the Academy Awards overlooked her.

Disheartened, Tallulah left Hollywood in 1944, embarking on a legendary revival of Noël Coward's *Private Lives*, which would occupy her for the next six years.

Tallulah turned to radio in 1950 with *The Big Show*. The ninety-minute variety program was a final attempt by NBC to attract dwindling radio dollars from burgeoning television markets. NBC invested an unprecedented $50,000 per program.

As Mistress of Ceremonies, Tallulah was not only "Mistress" but also often the object of the show's humor, which centered on her drinking, advancing age, androgynous voice, and diminishing sexual appeal. A critical and commercial success, the program became a Sunday evening ritual in millions of homes.

The Big Show began an unintended transformation of Tallulah's career: She became a professional parody of herself. Ironically, that caricature is what resonates in gay mythology: the wisecracking, decadent, ambisexual, and larger-than-life diva.

Indeed, she profited from her persona, in lectures, personal appearances, and a best-selling autobiography, *Tallulah* (1952). She even played Las Vegas for a then astounding $20,000 per week.

However, the price of Tallulah's self-parody revealed itself in a fabled 1956 New York revival of Tennessee Williams's *A Streetcar Named Desire*. Despite her gallant and purportedly engrossing portrayal of Blanche DuBois, her legions of gay admirers would not surrender to her efforts and laughed inappropriately throughout the performances. She was humiliated.

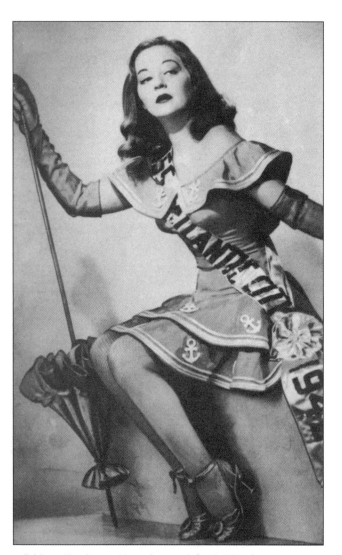

Tallulah Bankhead in a publicity photograph for *The Skin of Our Teeth* (1942).

Although continuing to work in the theater, she would never again attempt parts beyond her natural range.

In 1963, she flirted with brilliance in Williams's *The Milk Train Doesn't Stop Here Anymore*. Unfortunately, addled from thirty years of cigarettes, bourbon, and opiates, she was unable to memorize her lines. The play closed on Broadway after five performances.

Encumbered by emphysema, Tallulah took refuge in her New York townhouse. She ventured out professionally twice more. She played a fanatical harridan in the 1965 pseudo-Gothic horror film *Die! Die! My Darling!* And, in 1967, she portrayed a camp villainess, the Black Widow, on the popular television series *Batman*.

Tallulah Bankhead's death on December 12, 1968, warranted a photograph and two-column obituary on the front page of the *New York Times*.   —Benjamin Trimmier

BIBLIOGRAPHY

Bret, David. *Tallulah Bankhead: A Scandalous Life*. New York: Robson Books/Parkwest, 1996.

Gill, Brendan. *Tallulah*. New York: Holt, Rinehart and Winston, 1972.

Israel, Lee. *Miss Tallulah Bankhead*. New York: G. P. Putnam's Sons, 1972.

SEE ALSO

Film Actors: Lesbian; Cukor, George; Dietrich, Marlene; Garbo, Greta; Haines, William "Billy"

Barker, Clive   (b. 1952)

CLIVE BARKER IS PERHAPS BEST KNOWN AS THE WRITER and director of the modern classic horror film *Hellraiser* (1987), which spawned multiple sequels, and as the executive producer of Bill Condon's Oscar-winning film *Gods and Monsters* (1999), based on the Christopher Bram novel *Father of Frankenstein* (1995), about gay film director James Whale. However, Barker is also a prolific fiction writer, actor, playwright, painter, and illustrator, as well as a developer of comic books and computer games.

Barker's work often features gay, straight, and lesbian characters. While Barker commands a particularly loyal gay reading audience, to date he has had little success in placing positive gay characters into the world of his horror films.

Born in Liverpool, England, on October 5, 1952, the son of an Italian mother and Irish father, Barker moved to London at the age of twenty-one. He became the founder, playwright, and director of a small theater group there.

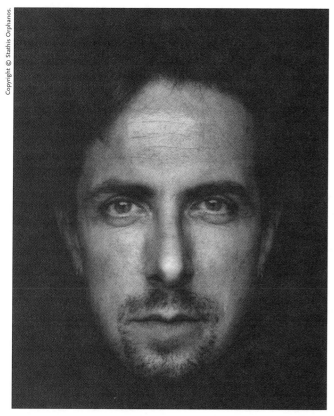

A portrait of Clive Barker by Stathis Orphanos.

When not working at the theater, Barker began writing short horror stories. These stories were eventually published as a three-volume set entitled *The Books of Blood* (1984 and 1985), which brought him international fame at the age of thirty-two and inspired Stephen King to declare him "the future of horror."

The success of Barker's stories enabled him to begin writing and directing horror films. He debuted as a director in 1987 with *Hellraiser*, which was based on one of his novellas and featured a character popularly known as "Pinhead"—a needle-pierced demon. Barker went on to produce three sequels, *Hellbound: Hellraiser II* (1988); *Hellraiser III: Hell on Earth* (1992); and *Bloodline: Hellraiser IV* (1996).

He also produced the horror film *Candyman* (1992) and its sequel, *Candyman II: Farewell to the Flesh* (1995). Other, somewhat less successful films Barker worked on include *Rawhead Rex* (1986), *Nightbreed* (1990), and *Lord of Illusions* (1995).

He has produced several made-for-television movies, some of which have been based on his stories, and has written others.

Barker is also the author of over a dozen novels. His early works in the genres of horror and suspense include such titles as *Weaveworld* (1987), *Cabal* (1989), and *Imajica* (1991). More recently, Barker has moved toward writing fantasy fiction, such as *Abarat* (2002).

In 1992, he wrote and illustrated *The Thief of Always*. Although marketed as a fable for all ages, *Thief* is really a children's book. Its hero is ten years old and the story, about the boy's visit to a land where each season passes in one day, is conveyed in simpler prose than that of Barker's adult books.

His later novels *Sacrament* (1996) and *Galilee* (1998) consider issues closer to Barker's life—gay sexuality, love, and the purpose of art.

Coldheart Canyon, published in 2001, distills motifs from nearly all of Barker's earlier writings. The novel's sophisticated merging of the fantastic and the real, as well as its central device—a room of painted tiles that come alive, luring mortals into the hell they depict—echo themes explored by Barker in his works of the late 1980s and early 1990s, books that sealed Barker's reputation as a writer of remarkable imagination.

Barker has also been the creative force behind a series of comic books published by Marvel Comics. His dark fantasy comics include *Razorline*, *Ectokid*, *Saint Sinner*, and *Hokum & Hex*, all of which debuted in 1993.

Barker currently resides in Los Angles, with his lover, the photographer David Armstrong.   —*Craig Kaczorowski*

BIBLIOGRAPHY

Lemon, Stephen. "King of Pain." *Salon*, February 4, 2000.
    www.salon.com/people/feature/2000/02/04/barker/index.html

Zaleski, Jeff. "The Relaunch of Clive Barker." *Publishers Weekly, Supplement*, October 1, 2001, S1.

Visions, The Official Clive Barker Web Site.
    www.clivebarker.com/html/visions/visions.html

SEE ALSO

Film; Horror Films; Screenwriters; Condon, William "Bill"; Whale, James

Bartel, Paul   *(1938–2000)*

FILMMAKER PAUL BARTEL'S CAREER IS IN MANY RESPECTS typical of the modern independent auteur. His filmography as a director is slight (ten features and a couple of television shows between 1969 and 1993). He tended to work when and where he could, with very low budgets, in disreputable genres, often writing and acting in his films and in those of others and calling on friends such as actress Mary Woronov to bring what star power they could to his work.

That Bartel was openly gay was not the issue in the independent film world that it would have been in mainstream film, which has so much more invested culturally and economically in the heterosexuality of its interpreters.

In a 1998 interview in the *Advocate*, Bartel said "I go to commercial Hollywood films and often think how glad I am that I didn't pursue a career in that kind of filmmaking"—a statement that may say as much about the opportunities available to openly queer filmmakers in Hollywood during his heyday as about where his own interests lay.

Born in Brooklyn on August 6, 1938, Bartel was the classic future filmmaker, creating marionette shows at the age of five, discovering movies and directors as a teenager, and by sixteen shooting his own animated shorts.

Early on, he evinced a talent for obtaining resources for little or no money—persuading his father to buy him a 16 mm camera and conning a high school teacher into excusing him from a semester to work on an elaborate animated project (a 3,000-cel undertaking that Bartel convinced the whole class to work on). This talent would serve him well throughout a flashy but far from lucrative career outside the mainstream.

After high school, Bartel worked in the Army Signal Corps Pictorial Center in Queens as a script clerk and assistant director on training films and documentaries. Fluent in French and Italian, he studied theater and film at UCLA and won a Fulbright scholarship that brought him to work at Rome's Cinecittà Studios.

In the early 1960s, Bartel moved to New York City, where he met future collaborator Mary Woronov and by the end of the decade had made his first feature, *The Secret Cinema* (1969). *The Secret Cinema* is a black-comic tale of a woman whose fear that her life is being filmed for the entertainment of her friends turns out to be true. The film presaged the sardonic tone of most of his later work, though he would mostly abandon *The Secret Cinema*'s experimental aspects in favor of linear narratives with perverse touches.

Three years later, the director made *Private Parts* (1972), another black comedy whose title was sometimes printed as *Private Arts* or *Private Party* by skittish newspapers. *Private Parts* introduces a typical Bartel tableau: a depraved San Francisco hotel riddled with leather queens, transvestites, runaways, and other social deviates, all treated as amusing denizens of the demimonde.

Bartel's career was kick-started the following year by his association with exploitation maestro Roger Corman, for whom he made *Death Race 2000* (1973). Bartel's vision of a future world in which drivers get points for running down pedestrians became a cult favorite and triggered a sequel, *Cannonball* (1976).

Six years later came *Eating Raoul*, the 1982 film that remains, to most Bartel watchers, his best. This edgy comedy features Paul and Mary Bland (played by Bartel and Mary Woronov), a nerdish, sex-hating couple who realize their dream of opening a restaurant by murdering and robbing swingers.

Eating Raoul's satirical take on marriage, adultery, cannibalism, the cult of "good taste," entrepreneurship, and swinging won it more critical and commercial success than any of his other films. It was chosen for such prestigious venues as Cannes and the New York Film Festival.

Eating Raoul did not catapult Bartel out of the minor leagues, however, perhaps because he had no more interest in the mainstream than the mainstream had in him. He made a few more films, some of them, such as *The Longshot* (1986) and his last effort, *Shelf Life* (1993), barely released.

Fans of Divine gave *Lust in the Dust* (1985), a comic Western promoted as a kind of queer *Blazing Saddles*, a modicum of notoriety. In addition, Bartel gained some cachet from *Scenes from the Class Struggle in Beverly Hills* (1989), where he had a larger (but not *large*) budget and better-known actors such as Jacqueline Bisset. The film was not successful, but it was hailed in some quarters for its caustic humor, political savvy, and casual introduction of a heated sex scene between Robert Beltran and Ray Sharkey.

Bartel's ultimate importance may lie less in his directorial efforts, which are variable in quality, than in his unwavering presence as an inspiring figure in the independent film world, particularly to queer filmmakers, an image reinforced by his genial, bearlike demeanor and eagerness to help struggling young auteurs.

He probably survived as much through his acting in both mainstream and independent films—*Heart Like a Wheel*, *National Lampoon's European Vacation*, *Rock and Roll High School*, *Basquiat*, and *Billy's Hollywood Screen Kiss* are among his seventy-seven acting credits—as through his own films.

Bartel died on May 13, 2000, of a heart attack, two weeks after undergoing surgery for liver cancer. At the time of his death, he was preparing a sequel to *Eating Raoul*, set twenty years after the original.

—*Gary Morris*

BIBLIOGRAPHY

Duralde, Alonzo. "End of the Reel," *Advocate*, July 4, 2000, 53.

Murray, Raymond. *Images in the Dark: An Encyclopedia of Gay and Lesbian Film and Video*. New York: Plume, 1996.

O'Haver, Tommy. "Two of a Kind." *Advocate*, July 21, 1998, 69.

SEE ALSO

Film; Film Directors; Divine (Harris Glenn Milstead)

Bernhard, Sandra   (b. 1955)

SHARP-TONGUED COMEDIAN, WRITER, SINGER, AND actor Sandra Bernhard is known almost as well for her amorphous sexuality as for her cynical wit.

Over the past three decades, the prolific entertainer has toured extensively on and off Broadway with her one-woman stage shows, appeared on numerous television programs and in movies (including films made of her live shows), written three books, and recorded several albums.

She has also been forthright regarding both her sexual orientation—perhaps best described as "pansexual"—and progressive political stance in countless interviews, speaking about her ex-girlfriends and her support of women's rights with equal candor.

Bernhard was born on June 6, 1955. She was raised Jewish alongside three older brothers in Flint, Michigan. Her artist mother and doctor father moved the family to Arizona when Bernhard was in high school.

At the age of nineteen, Bernhard relocated to Hollywood, where she worked as a manicurist and took acting classes before she began landing gigs at Los Angeles comedy clubs. Developing her distinctively acerbic style

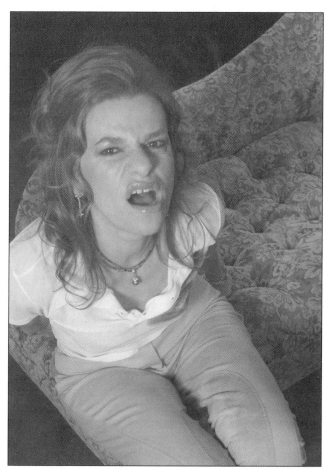

A portrait of Sandra Bernhard by Richard Mitchell.

of stand-up, Bernhard became popular locally, which led to her national television debut in 1977 on Richard Pryor's short-lived variety show.

Bernhard went on to appear in her first film, entitled *Shogun Assassin*, in 1980. But the movie that established her reputation as an actor came a few years later when she appeared opposite Robert De Niro and Jerry Lewis in Martin Scorsese's satire *The King of Comedy* (1983). Numerous bit parts in 1980s movies such as John Byrum's *The Whoopee Boys* (1986) and Genevieve Robert's *Casual Sex* (1988) followed.

In 1985, Bernhard toured with her first solo show, entitled *I'm Your Woman*, and she also released her first album, of the same name, that year. Her 1988 show *Without You I'm Nothing* was recorded and received a Grammy nomination for Best Comedy in 1991.

It was around this time, in the early 1990s, that Bernhard became closely linked with Madonna, and for some time the two maintained a widely publicized, erotically charged friendship that led to much public speculation about both being lesbians.

To this day, in fact, Bernhard is described interchangeably as bisexual and as lesbian, and she herself has claimed at different times that she is gay; that she does not understand labels; and that she simply does not gravitate toward a particular sexual preference.

Whatever her sexual identification, her visibility in queer culture is widespread. She appeared on the television show *Roseanne* in a lesbian role throughout the 1990s, steadily attracts lesbian audiences, and openly discusses the five-year relationship she had with model Patricia Velazquez.

In 1998, Bernhard was very busy: She launched her show *I'm Still Here...Dammit* (which became notorious for the fact that she wore a see-through dress on stage while very pregnant); she gave birth to daughter Cicely on July 4th; and she published her third autobiographical book, *May I Kiss You on the Lips, Miss Sandra?* Her film roles were also plentiful that year and included parts in Pat Proft's *Wrongfully Accused* and Daphna Edwards's *Exposé*.

Bernhard continues to expand her horizons, speaking frequently in interviews about her ongoing, intensive study of Kabbalah (Jewish mysticism) and promoting her latest show, entitled *The Love Machine*, in which she is accompanied by a five-piece rock band.

Her recent television appearances include spots on *Will and Grace*, *VIP*, and *Ally McBeal*. August 2001 heralded the debut of her talk show, *The Sandra Bernhard Experience*, on cable channel A&E; unfortunately, it aired for only one week before it was pulled because of poor ratings. In summer 2004, it was announced that Bernhard would join the cast of Showtime's *The L Word*, a dramatic series about a group of Los Angeles lesbians, during its second season, in 2005.   —*Teresa Theophano*

BIBLIOGRAPHY

Bernhard, Sandra. *Confessions of a Pretty Lady.* New York: Harper & Row, 1988.

Biography, Internet Movie Database (IMDb): http://us.imdb.com/Name?Bernhard,+Sandra

Biography, PlanetOut: http://www.planetout.com/pno/entertainment/ starstruck/feature/splash.html?sernum=169

O'Neill, Tom. "One Hot Mama." *OUT,* November 1998, 68.

http://sandrabernhard.com

Bisexuality in Film

THE HISTORY OF GAY MEN AND LESBIANS IN FILM IS well documented, but bisexuality, in both characters and performers, has been less examined. While some historians and filmmakers take the approach that bisexuality is a mediated and therefore acceptable representation of homosexuality, others vilify the bisexual as either a traitor to the gay world or a maniacally homicidal or suicidal deviant torn between two worlds.

The first documented appearances of bisexual characters in motion pictures are *A Florida Enchantment* (1914), an American film by Sidney Drew, and *Zapatas Bande*, a German film from the same year. These early silent films were not burdened by overt censorship, and filmmakers were free to represent sexuality in their characters' lives within the constraints of the mores of the period.

Still, characters' sexuality was more often implied than definitively stated. Depictions of homosexuality and bisexuality were often cloaked in religious themes in order to evade local censors, who frequently edited films before they were screened.

The Hays Code

Around 1915, Hollywood invented itself as the film capital of the world, and along with this new industry came widespread notoriety for rampant debauchery—especially drug use and promiscuous sex—among its employees, especially performers.

Eventually deciding the industry needed to regulate itself before external censors did, a group of filmmakers and producers hired Will H. Hays, former Postmaster General, to draft a series of guidelines that by 1934 had become the Motion Picture Production Code, or Hays Code, which banned any explicit representation of homosexuality or bisexuality in American films.

The words *gay, homosexual,* and *bisexual* could not even be uttered, and virtually no bisexual characters appeared in American films during the 1930s and 1940s. The lack of representation of bisexuals in film may have been abetted by the popular belief that bisexuality did not actually exist. Eventually, however, bold filmmakers began to release their films without adhering to the Code, which led to its complete abandonment in the 1960s.

Formulaic Scenarios

The demise of the Hays Code did not immediately translate into positive representations of homosexuals and bisexuals. Instead, what emerged were a few formulaic scenarios in which bisexual characters in film were presented.

In one scenario, a married bisexual's past is revealed, or he or she strays with a same-sex partner. Adhering to this formula, *Making Love* (1982) was the first mainstream Hollywood film to address the bisexual male character openly and directly and without vilification. Husband Michael Ontkean leaves wife Kate Jackson—the former *Charlie's Angel* Sabrina (and lesbian icon)—for another man, played by Harry Hamlin. While the film was not a commercial success, it was a watershed event in Hollywood's depiction of the bisexual as an ordinary, complex human being.

In another film formula, a gay man or lesbian is left by a bisexual lover who pursues a heterosexual relationship. In 1968's box-office success *The Fox*, the bisexual female character Ellen ultimately chooses a man over her female lover, who, in turn, is killed by the male, Paul.

In *Personal Best* (1982), the Mariel Hemingway character is awakened to her sexuality by Patrice Donnelly, but eventually settles with her coach, Scott Glenn.

A twist on this theme is Kevin Smith's *Chasing Amy* (1994). The character Alyssa is an avowed lesbian until she falls in love with a man; she has a relationship with him, but eventually returns to lesbianism.

In the third and most frightening scenario, the bisexual character is a deviant who kills or is killed for his or her sexuality. In the aforementioned *The Fox*, the lesbian's death is rife with symbolism: She is killed by a tree falling between her legs.

In *Basic Instinct* (1982), a film boycotted by gay, lesbian, and bisexual groups for its perpetuation of the criminal homosexual, Sharon Stone portrays the murderous bisexual seductress Catherine Tramell. Her former lover, a bisexual woman, is at one point assumed to be the murderer but ends up murdered by a man, Michael Douglas, with whom they have both been involved.

The Bisexual as Betrayer

The bisexual character in film is frequently represented as lacking commitment, someone who ultimately betrays his or her partners, gay or straight, or even his or her community.

Hollywood heartthrob Robert Redford played the bisexual husband Wade in 1966's *Inside Daisy Clover*; at the star's request, Wade was changed from homosexual to bisexual so that Redford could "play him as a guy who bats ten ways—men, women, children, dogs, cats, anything—anything that salves his ego." Although his bisexuality is barely alluded to in the film, the actor's intent was to represent bisexuality as a selfish, amoral endeavor.

In John Schlesinger's 1971 film *Sunday, Bloody Sunday*, a gay man and heterosexual woman share a bisexual male partner who is regarded as freewheeling because he does not "choose" either homo- or heterosexuality.

Cabaret (1972), based on the John Kander-Fred Ebb musical and inspired by Christopher Isherwood's *Berlin Stories*, features a relationship between the bisexual character Baron Max and the more clearly homosexual Brian Roberts. Roberts eventually ends up alone.

Rose Troche's 1994 independent film *Go Fish*, arguably the most successful and mainstream lesbian film, includes an openly bisexual character, Daria, who sleeps with a man and then undergoes an imaginary inquisition from her lesbian friends who disapprove and want to vote her out of the sisterhood.

Sidney Lumet's *Dog Day Afternoon* (1975) is a notable exception to these themes. Based on real events, the film presents Al Pacino as Sonny, who is married with children, but who is in love with Leon, his pre-op transsexual lover, played by Chris Sarandon. Sonny robs a bank in order to pay for Leon's operation. It is an extraordinary circumstance presented without hysterics or pretense.

The same year, however, hysterics and pretense were celebrated in the campy cult classic *The Rocky Horror Picture Show*. Dr. Frank-N-Furter, portrayed by Tim Curry in transvestite drag, satisfies both Brad and Janet, the newlyweds played by Barry Bostwick and Susan Sarandon (former wife of Chris).

Recent Depictions

Despite some advances, Hollywood still regards depictions of bisexuality as taboo. *Henry and June* (1990), which includes a relationship between bisexual women, was the first film to earn the *NC-17* rating from the Motion Picture Association of America (MPAA).

On the other hand, *Wild Things* (1998), which also presents an explicit sexual relationship between the two female lead characters, as well as an implied one between the two male lead characters, did not receive such a rating; the film, however, merely exploits a heterosexual fantasy lesbianism that has little or nothing to do with an actual lesbian relationship.

A more serious recent depiction is in the Wachowski brothers' *Bound* (1996), in which Jennifer Tilly's mobmoll femme leaves her gangster man for a slightly butch Gina Gershon and never looks back.

Bisexual Performers

Rumors of bisexuality have persisted about many performers, from James Dean to Cary Grant to Tom Cruise, but only a few actors, such as Madonna, Joey Lauren Adams, Anne Heche, and Sandra Bernhard, have openly revealed their bisexual identities. It is no coincidence that the majority of these actors are women, for female bisexuality is still much more acceptable than male bisexuality, since it plays into a particular male heterosexual fantasy.

An especially interesting instance of bisexual infiltration is the Julia Roberts film *My Best Friend's Wedding* (1997), which opens with bisexual singer Ani DiFranco's tongue-in-cheek cover of Dusty Springfield's "Wishin' and Hopin'" played over the credits. The film also starred bisexual actor Rupert Everett, who stole the show as the predictably lovable, laughable gay sidekick to Roberts's lead.

Bisexuality in film, as separate from gay and lesbian representation, has emerged as a significant genre in its own right, even spawning a separate bisexual film festival in San Francisco.

—*Carla Williams*

Bibliography

Bryant, Wayne M. *Bisexual Characters in Film: From Anaïs to Zee.* New York: Harrington Park Press, 1997.

Dyer, Richard, ed. *Gays and Film.* London: British Film Institute, 1977.

Ehrenstein, David. *Open Secret: Gay Hollywood 1928–1998.* New York: William Morrow, 1998.

Hadleigh, Boze. *The Lavender Screen: The Gay and Lesbian Film, Their Makers, Characters, and Critics.* New York: Citadel Press, 1993.

Russo, Vito. *The Celluloid Closet: Homosexuality in the Movies.* Rev. ed. New York: Harper & Row, 1987.

See also

Film; Film Actors: Gay Male; Film Actors: Lesbian; Film Festivals; Bernhard, Sandra; Dean, James; Everett, Rupert; Grant, Cary

Bogarde, Sir Dirk   *(1921–1999)*

IN HER EULOGY FOR SIR DIRK BOGARDE, GLENDA Jackson called him Britain's "first home-grown film star." Often dubbed "the British Rock Hudson"—both for his matinee-idol good looks during the 1950s and his discreet homosexuality—his film career spanned five decades and seventy films.

He was born Derek Jules Gaspard Ulric Niven van den Bogaerde to a Dutch-born father (a London *Times* arts editor) and an English mother (a former actress) in Hampstead, London, on March 28, 1921. After an inauspicious film debut as an extra in the comedy *Come On George* (1939), his career was interrupted by military service in World War II, during which he was decorated for valor as a major in the Queen's Royal Regiment.

Bogarde resumed acting after the war. Noël Coward, an early admirer, encouraged him to pursue a stage career, but in 1947, when Stewart Granger dropped out as the romantic lead in *Esther Waters*, Bogarde assumed the role. As a result, he earned a long-term film contract with the Rank studios and subsequently ceased theatrical work.

During the 1950s, Bogarde starred in romantic comedies, war films, and crime thrillers. As he entered his forties, however, he assumed more serious dramatic roles, some of which touched upon homosexual themes, a particularly risky venture in the years before the partial decriminalization of male homosexuality with the 1967 Sexual Offences Act.

The first and most significant of these was in *Victim* (1961), in which he played a married lawyer who is blackmailed for a homosexual affair. Bogarde's moving portrayal of a sympathetic homosexual may have helped sway public opinion in the debate leading to decriminalization.

With this role also came the first of six nominations for the British Academy Award for Best Actor, an honor he won twice, for his performance as the sexually ambiguous valet in Joseph Losey's *The Servant* (1963) and for the romantic lead opposite Julie Christie in John Schlesinger's *Darling* (1965).

Bogarde's other significant films include *Song Without End* (1960); *Damn the Defiant!* (1962); *I Could Go On Singing* (1963), opposite Judy Garland; *Modesty Blaise* (1966); *Accident* (1967); and *Our Mother's House* (1967).

In the mid-1960s, Bogarde moved to Provence in the south of France, where he lived with his manager and longtime companion, Tony Forwood. Subsequently, Bogarde appeared mostly in European films, most notably as Aschenbach in Luchino Visconti's *Death in Venice* (1971), based on Thomas Mann's novella about a dying writer who becomes obsessed with a beautiful boy. Other late and daring films include Visconti's *The Damned* (1969), Liliana Cavani's *The Night Porter* (1974), and Rainer Werner Fassbinder's *Despair* (1978).

When Forwood became terminally ill in 1983, Bogarde returned to England with him and saw to his care until Forwood's death in 1988. During this time, Bogarde curtailed his acting and embarked on another career, that of writer. During the 1980s and 1990s, he published sixteen books, including seven volumes of autobiography and numerous novels.

While in his autobiographical works Bogarde carefully avoids direct discussion of homosexuality, he does discuss his relationship with his partner, particularly his care of him during the latter's long terminal illness.

Bogarde was knighted in 1992. He died of a heart attack in Chelsea, London, on May 8, 1999, after being incapacitated by a stroke in 1996.

For most of his life, Bogarde acknowledged his homosexuality only tacitly, though, as his obituary in the *Independent* notes, "the public understood he was essentially gay." One result of his discretion is that he was ridiculed in the 1980s by some members of a younger generation of gay men who came of age after decriminalization. His reticence about his personal life should not, however, obscure the fact of his courage in being the first actor to create a sympathetic gay character in British film.

—*Patricia Juliana Smith*

BIBLIOGRAPHY

Bogarde, Dirk. *Backcloth*. Harmondsworth: Penguin, 1987.

_____. *Cleared for Take Off*. Harmondsworth: Penguin, 1996.

_____. *For the Time Being*. Harmondsworth: Penguin, 1998.

_____. *Great Meadow*. Harmondsworth: Penguin, 1993.

_____. *An Orderly Man*. Harmondsworth: Penguin, 1992.

_____. *A Particular Friendship*. Harmondsworth: Penguin, 1990.

_____. *A Postilion Struck by Lightning*. Harmondsworth: Penguin, 1988.

_____. *A Short Walk from Harrods*. Harmondsworth: Penguin, 1994,

_____. *Snakes and Ladders*. Harmondsworth: Penguin, 1988.

Bourne, Stephen. *Brief Encounters: Lesbians and Gays in British Cinema 1930–1971*. London: Cassell, 1996.

Hinxman, Margaret, and Susan d'Arcy. *The Cinema of Dirk Bogarde*. South Brunswick: A. S. Barnes, 1975.

Medhurst, Andy. "Dirk Bogarde." *All Our Yesterdays: 90 Years of British Cinema*. Charles Barr, ed. London: British Film Institute, 1986.

Morley, Sheridan. *Dirk Bogarde: Rank Outsider*. London: Bloomsbury, 1996.

SEE ALSO

Film Actors: Gay Male; European Film; Film; Fassbinder, Rainer Werner; Garland, Judy; Hudson, Rock; Schlesinger, John; Visconti, Luchino

Borden, Lizzie   (b. 1958)

BISEXUAL FILMMAKER LIZZIE BORDEN GAINED FAME IN the mid-1980s among gay audiences and fans of independent movies for her visionary films about the unexplored politics of women's lives. A sharp observer of social realities, Borden brings a feminist perspective and a dynamic authenticity to her films that make them relevant long after their creation.

Borden was born on February 3, 1958, the daughter of a Detroit stockbroker. Her given name was Linda, which she retained until she was eleven years old and heard the children's rhyme about the famed ax murderer. Perhaps foretelling her iconoclastic tendencies as an artist, young Linda changed her name to Lizzie Borden.

She majored in art at Wellesley College before moving to New York City to become an artist and art critic. Attending a festival of Jean-Luc Godard films persuaded her to try her hand at filmmaking. She taught herself the skills she needed to make movies.

Although she made a black-and-white film called *Regrouping* in 1976, Borden first received public attention with the release of *Born in Flames* in 1983. A feminist science-fiction film, *Born in Flames* envisions a future ten years after a bloodless "Second American Revolution" has brought democratic socialism to the United States.

Though smarmy politicians and media spokespeople assure the audience that equality has been universally achieved, the hypocrisy of the new society is soon revealed. Backed by the beat of an energetic punk sound track, the film's heroines, mostly lesbians of color, rise up and form a women's army to fight against the oppression they still face in the new society.

Made in a documentary style, *Born in Flames* delivers its powerful political message with intensity and poetry, leaving audiences energized. After its successful premiere at the 1983 Berlin Film Festival, the film went on to win First Prize at the women's film festival in Sceaux, France.

Released on video in 1997, *Born in Flames* remains a lesbian feminist standard. When some feminists criticized the violence of Borden's solution in the film, Borden responded by saying, "I asked many, many women if they would ever use violence, and the answer was always no. How convenient for the government. I'm posing the question: What if we did?"

Borden followed *Born in Flames* with another faux documentary, this time portraying a day in the life of a New York call girl. *Working Girls*, released in 1986, follows the life of Molly, a lesbian photographer who works as an upscale prostitute to pay the bills. Neither romantic nor lurid, *Working Girls* presents prostitution mundanely, as a job, often boring and occasionally dangerous. Like *Born in Flames*, *Working Girls* is a feminist film with a lesbian heroine that attempts to tell some unpleasant truths about society.

After directing some episodes of the syndicated television horror show *Monsters* in the late 1980s, Borden went to Hollywood to make her next film. *Love Crimes* (1991) is a dark exploration of erotic fantasy and violent reality. It was not well received by either film critics or many of the feminist fans of Borden's earlier films. Borden herself was not happy with the film and felt the need to move out of Hollywood again to gain more control of her work.

In 1992, continuing her exploration of female sexuality, Borden directed two episodes of the series *Inside Out*, produced by Playboy Video; and in 1994 she directed a segment of the film *Erotique*, titled "Let's Talk About Sex," which explores the life of a Latina phone-sex worker.

—*Tina Gianoulis*

BIBLIOGRAPHY

Brownworth, Victoria A. "Working Girl: Movie Director Lizzie Borden." *Advocate*, August 23, 1994, 82.

Gleiberman, Owen. "Feminist Kink: Love Crimes." *Entertainment Weekly*, February 7, 1992, 40.

Mills, Nancy. "Director Lizzie Borden." *Premier*, May 1991, 46.

Pally, Marcia. "Working Girls." *Nation*, April 11, 1987, 482.

SEE ALSO

Film; Film Directors

British Television

TELEVISION HAS BEEN INADEQUATELY RENDERED AS part of gay and lesbian artistic and cultural history. Many important milestones continue to be dismissed or ignored by lesbian and gay academics and cultural commentators. Unlike the study of gay and lesbian cinema, the discussion of television is often predicated on ill-informed and historically naive viewpoints that would be unacceptable if applied to other art forms.

Early Television History

A large proportion of early television productions in Britain (1936–1960) no longer exist, and what remains is often imperfectly preserved on crude technology. However, this does not mean either that gay men and lesbians were not represented in the ebb and flow of programming during this time or that fugitive details of their existence are not available.

Until September 1955, there was only one channel: the license-funded, politically neutral British Broadcasting Corporation (BBC), or "Aunty" as she was affectionately or slightly known.

The BBC offered a relatively broad-based range of choices: While stuck in traditional, white, middle-class values, the Corporation employed enough oddballs and eccentrics to spice up the most conservative fare. Carrying on the quality-first philosophy of the Corporation's first director-general, John Reith, the BBC believed in diversity: of talent, culture, geography, and even—though this had to be masked—of sexuality.

In glorious fuzzy black and white, with frequent breaks in transmission and hilarious glitches because most of the shows went out live, British television provided a number of regular "queer" sightings in the 1950s: a mannish policewoman, based on a real lesbian police officer, and an intellectual tramp disowned by his family in the enormously popular bobby-on-the-beat drama series *Dixon of Dock Green*. The tramp, Duffy Clayton, was based on a gay man who was a mentor for the show's creator and principal writer, Ted Willis.

Real-life lesbian journalist Nancy Spain, with her close-cropped hair, cravat, and trousers, was often seen on the small screen, as was gruff and ungracious Gilbert Harding, with whom she was, for a time, "romantically linked."

A panelist on the quiz show *What's My Line?*, Harding specialized in rude outbursts to contestants who were not quick on the uptake or who were syntactically challenged. His zingers were the talk of the nation the next day. The first British small-screen superstar, his private life remained publicly asexual. Maybe a word to the wise was being sent when an aging character actress based her role of a querulous fairy godmother in a 1955 children's television play, *Pots of Money*, upon this titan of tactlessness.

Gilbert Harding's lifelong attraction to males was masked by the facade of the snapping bulldog, which prevented too many questions from being asked by a postwar British public that, anyway, was officially ignorant of homosexuality. Indeed, the very word could not be spoken, let alone its meaning discussed in a direct manner. Television, nevertheless, was awash with clipped male poodles and sturdy female stallions: British culture's acceptance of eccentricity was their protection and their potting mix.

Homosexuality Rises to the Surface

It was the very rigidity of British society, its cap-doffing deference to royals and aristocrats still in place despite two devastating world wars and the destruction of an empire, that eventually forced homosexuality to rise to the surface, making it a television staple without which no viewing week would be complete.

With the arrest in 1953 of the esteemed and recently knighted actor John Gielgud and a high-profile court case a year later involving a lord and a boy scout or two, the establishment of that interbred, intermarried coterie without which the status quo could not be maintained or even slightly adjusted, decided to act.

Suddenly, certain realities were faced. There were men who were attracted to other men. Their natures led them to be prey for blackmailers and the law courts. Some were imprisoned for loving. Some didn't get that far: They just killed themselves.

A committee, significantly, on homosexuality and prostitution, was set up under the chairmanship of John Wolfenden. The publication of his report, recommending

the partial decriminalization of male homosexuality in private, was the Open Sesame! for the discussion of homosexuality, male and female, as well as other unacceptable facts of intimate human contact.

The relatively new and untried commercial network, which took the form of regionally based companies under the overall banner of Independent Television (ITV), took Wolfenden's findings—which were finally published late in 1957—and presented dramatizations of Oscar Wilde's trials, as well as adaptations of stage plays such as *South*, in which television heartthrob Peter Wyngarde risked his reputation if not his career by playing an unmistakable, if repressed, homosexual.

The actor revealed many years later that the day after the play had aired in 1959 he was set upon by a group of elderly women on the top of a London bus. They attacked him with their handbags for daring to play a "queer" and in so doing to sully forever their image of him as a real man.

The BBC responded with some original plays and episodes of popular series, such as *Z Cars*, set in Liverpool. In *Summer, Autumn, Winter, Spring* (1961), the homo-emotional story of David and Jonathan was updated: Safely, the protagonists become brothers not friends, and one dies early in the piece. In John Hopkins's play *Horror of Darkness* (1965), a character played by Nicol Williamson tells another male, ostensibly straight, that he loves him. A few scenes later, however, the gay man slits his throat and dies. Offscreen.

Throughout the 1960s, both before the 1967 Act decriminalizing male homosexuality and immediately after, homosexuality was an inescapable topic of television drama and documentary. It was a surefire way to provoke the right-wing press to foaming fury if the depiction was in any way sympathetic or encouraging.

In tandem with the generally liberal viewpoints and relatively diverse characterizations were the endless comic queens with flapping wrists and piping voices, whose one-note, coy rapaciousness found its apogee in Clarence. Clarence's gushing come-on ("Hello, honky tonks!") to a straight man each week on *The Dick Emery Show* became a late-1960s national catchphrase and shorthand for queer-baiting until the following decade, when it was replaced by Larry Grayson's "What a gay day!" on *The Larry Grayson Show* and John Inman's "I'm free!" on *Are You Being Served?*

Homosexuality with a Political Edge

It was not until the advent of *Monty Python's Flying Circus* in 1969 that any kind of political edge was given to gay or camp humor. Owing something to BBC Radio's anarchic *The Goon Show* (1951–1960) and also to the virtually unrestrained camp of *Round the Horne* (1965–1969), with its two very "bold" gay characters, Julian and Sandy, Python put the boot into all kinds of establishment stupidity, including its hypocritical stance on homosexuality, no matter that it was now—in certain circumstances—legal.

One of the Python team, Graham Chapman, became the first popular entertainer to talk openly about his gayness, being interviewed with his lover in the inaugural edition of the fortnightly London newspaper *Gay News*.

Chapman would remain the exception for quite a few years, despite the inroads made by the U.S. import gay liberation. This wave of political consciousness manifested itself in various "access" slots. These featured gays and lesbians talking about their lives without the mediation of interviewers, biased editing, and shadowy lighting.

Mainstream television followed the gay liberation lead slowly and—doubtless because the dramatic possibilities of victimhood were being eroded by the philosophy of personal politics and coming out—reluctantly. Singer Tom Robinson's gay anthem "(Sing If You're) Glad to Be Gay" received its first public performance on a Sunday-afternoon show for teenagers in 1977; and a comedy series called *Agony* (1979–1981), inspired by the success of *Soap* in the United States, featured a very out and—in contrast to the other characters—very well-adjusted pair of gay men.

But the real breakthrough had occurred in 1975 with the broadcast, on commercial television (the BBC had turned down the project), of the biography of "effeminate homosexual" Quentin Crisp. This was victimhood with a gay-lib message: To your own self be true. The public response to *The Naked Civil Servant*, in the United Kingdom and in many other countries, was overwhelmingly positive.

The Naked Civil Servant earned awards for its star, John Hurt, and enduring fame on the talk show circuit for its subject, Quentin Crisp. Its prestige did not, however, lead to other productions in which an openly gay or lesbian person was the lead character, save for modestly produced "single plays" of which *Only Connect* (1979) remains the most provocative and compelling.

This short play by Noel Greig and Drew Griffiths, former members of the Gay Sweatshop Theatre Company, centers upon the brief encounter between a gay student researching early gay rights activist Edward Carpenter and an elderly man, once a bed partner of Carpenter, with whom the young man sleeps.

The 1980s and 1990s

Big budget miniseries in the 1980s such as *Brideshead Revisited* and *The Jewel in the Crown* did include homosexual characters—as adolescent crushes, aristocratic decadents, or pathological villains.

But the lives of gay people and the culture they were developing went largely unreported on mainstream television. Two series of the show *Gay Life*—"about homosexuals"—came and went, televised around midnight in the London area in 1980–1981, but it would be another eight years before television—in the shape of ITV's pioneering Channel 4—would open the airwaves to a series "by and for" gay men and lesbians: *Out on Tuesday*.

Two huge blockades obstructed the free flow of non-problematic representations and depictions in the 1980s. The advent of AIDS once again drove homosexuality back into its medical-psychiatric problem box. The hysterical climate engendered by the disease, and by increasing media-stoked fears about "recruitment" and "promotion," led to the enactment of legislation prohibiting local authorities from in any way positively promoting homosexuality in schools or other services. This outrage—known as Section 28—inspired a group of lesbians to invade the BBC's *Six O'Clock News* to protest: a most un-BBC thing to do.

Despite its being created by a gay man (Tony Warren, who based at least one of its beloved female characters on himself), Britain's most enduring and beloved drama series, the Manchester-located *Coronation Street*, has never had—and at time of this writing still does not have—a gay or lesbian resident or even a regular visitor.

The soaps that followed, notably Channel 4's *Brookside* and the BBC's *EastEnders*—both gutsy and relatively fearless—presented a gay couple apiece in the 1980s: not always to the liking of the gay community or to the rabidly homophobic tabloid press. Questions were even asked in parliament when *EastEnders*'s Colin kissed a male admirer for a few seconds.

Gay men were not easy for British television. Most soaps were scheduled during family viewing hours, thus ensuring that any display of physical affection came under strict scrutiny. Such restrictions on natural, spontaneous behavior rendered any true exploration of character and emotion virtually impossible.

Lesbians, on the other hand, were much more to 1990s television's liking, especially in the wake of the Madonna-led "lipstick lesbian" phenomenon. In addition to two well-received literary adaptations in 1990, *Oranges Are Not the Only Fruit* (based on the Jeannette Winterson novel) and *Portrait of a Marriage* (which includes the story of Vita Sackville-West and Violet Trefusis), female couples appeared on both *Brookside* and *EastEnders*.

The most durable lesbian has proved to be veterinarian Zoe Tate (played by Leah Bracknell) in *Emmerdale*. Bracknell first appeared in the role in 1993 and is still going strong, winning television audience awards for the character.

EastEnders tried again with gay men. Bisexual Tony Hills and his lover, Simon Raymond, debuted in 1996; the results were mixed and after a year or so they were written out.

With the relative easing of the AIDS epidemic in Britain, renewed pressure came from sections of the gay and lesbian community to depict homosexuals honestly. To fill the gap came a loud and proud late-night BBC series called *Gaytime TV*: commercially oriented, youthful, fast and flashy. The show was not to everybody's liking but it was sufficiently appealing to run for four summers.

The End of the Twentieth Century

By the end of the century, homosexuality was a staple in every British drama and comedy series. Every night, somebody or other was either saying they were gay or denying they were; pundits and politicians were for and against; the issue and a whole raft of subissues were on every discussion program or talk show. Achingly predictable, most of it and, ultimately, unenlightening because of the rigid parameters in which queer lives were set.

Like a comet roaring across a night sky came Channel 4's *Queer As Folk* (1999), a rambunctious comedy-drama set in Manchester's Gay Village. Unapologetic, taboo-tweaking, and unconcerned with presenting a good public face, its mainly gay characters played havoc with previously acceptable notions of "homosexual TV drama." Written by Russell T. Davies, it was the *Naked Civil Servant* of the late twentieth century, spawning a sequel and a successful U.S. version.

The New Century

With *Queer As Folk*, many gay men, though by no means all, felt that, at last, they had a television drama series designed for them: sexy, confrontational, and presenting complex moral issues in an entertaining way. To date, however, only one series peopled almost entirely by gays has subsequently surfaced: *Metrosexuality* (2001), also from Channel 4.

Nevertheless, *Queer As Folk*'s influence can be seen in the refreshing approach a series such as the revamped *Crossroads* (debuted 2001) has taken to its queer incumbents, who are involved in all aspects of the plotlines, not just those dealing with homosexuality.

With the new century, a strong gay and lesbian presence is making itself felt. Openly gay and lesbian people present a range of faces, voices, attitudes, and opinions. These include comics Julian Clary, Graham Norton, and Rhona Cameron; drag queen Lily Savage, aka Paul O'Grady; political analysts Matthew Parris and Bea Campbell; actors Sir Ian McKellen and Stephen Fry; and pop stars Elton John, George Michael, Boy George, and Stephen Gately.

In popular drama series, a gay or a lesbian regular character is almost essential for a good-conduct medal. In 2001, even the cop series *The Bill* began employing a gay police officer in its Sun Hill police station, sixteen years after the show began. *Coronation Street* is the only holdout: no gay or lesbian sightings in its forty-plus years

of existence. However, the series does feature a transgender (male-to-female) character, who was recently granted that ultimate soap-opera accolade: the big wedding.

Not just one but two gay men were included in the second British edition of the wildly successful reality TV show *Big Brother* (2001); one of them won the contest by a substantial margin. A lesbian had been one of the housemates in the first edition.

Conclusion

British television's nearly eighty-year history has, until only recently, marginalized lesbians and gay men as Them rather than Us. With the rise of niche television, a much more demanding gay and lesbian audience, and many more openly gay and lesbian people working in all aspects of television, the appetite for a more diversified and nuanced approach to all kinds of sexuality is surely about to be satisfied.

While, for some, British television has assiduously opened up dialogue and debate since the 1960s, for others the medium remains one-dimensional and sensationalist, with gay men and lesbians presented mainly as figures of fun, or mad, bad, and dangerous to know.

In truth, British television has consistently worked to broaden knowledge of the human condition. Many talented people, of all sexual hues, have labored—sometimes at considerable risk—to present a balanced view of a marginalized sexuality.

British television's contribution to gay culture still has not been properly researched or promoted, despite the best efforts of Keith Howes (whose thousand-page, three thousand-entry encyclopaedia of gay television and radio, *Broadcasting It*, was published in 1993) and of Stephen Bourne, who has presented gay and lesbian plays, variety shows, soap-opera tributes, and documentaries each July since 1992 at London's National Film Theatre.

Despite the teeming and relatively welcoming queer landscape at present on display on British television, the innate insularity and knee-jerk conservatism of the British Isles should never be underestimated. For more than a few diehard Little Englanders, queers remain resolutely mired in the mirthful piping of *Are You Being Served?* and in the dangerous depths of political agitation, as represented by the tireless gay activist Peter Tatchell on news flashes and discussion programs.

—*Keith G. Howes*

BIBLIOGRAPHY

Howes, Keith G. *Broadcasting It : An Encyclopaedia of Homosexuality on Film, Radio and TV in the UK, 1923–1993*. London: Cassell, 1993.

Sanderson, Terry. *Mediawatch*. London: Cassell, 1995.

SEE ALSO

American Television: Drama; Chapman, Graham; Crisp, Quentin; Fry, Stephen; Gielgud, Sir John; McKellen, Sir Ian

Broughton, James   *(1913–1999)*

EVERY MOVEMENT HAS ITS MUSES. JAMES BROUGHTON probably would have copped to being a muse, or perhaps more accurately, a smiling spirit guide to pleasurable realms beyond the norm.

It is less likely he would have considered himself a leader of any movement, despite the fact that he more or less created the West Coast experimental film scene with two short films, *The Potted Psalm* (1946) and *Mother's Day* (1948), and has been identified with the San Francisco Renaissance, the literary movement that included Kenneth Rexroth and Robert Duncan.

Broughton is simply too individual for categorization, even when the evidence for labeling him this or that is overwhelming. But the lure of labels is strong, so for the sake of shorthand, and with apologies to Broughton, let us call him poet, avant-garde film artist, and Dionysian gay sage.

Broughton was born in Modesto, California, on November 10, 1913, into a wealthy family. His father died when he was a child and he was sent to a military academy, from which he was later expelled for having an affair with another boy. He was educated at Stanford and the New School for Social Research.

In his memoir *Coming Unbuttoned* (1993), Broughton recounts his childhood, reflects on his work, and remarks on his love affairs with both men and women. Among his male lovers were gay activist Harry Hay and publisher Kermit Sheets.

In 1962, Broughton married Suzanna Hart. The couple were divorced in 1978. On Christmas Eve, 1976, Broughton celebrated his relationship with artist Joel Singer in a marriage ceremony. Eschewing the labels *homosexual, heterosexual,* and *bisexual,* the poet and filmmaker describes himself as a "pansexual androgyne."

Broughton's poems reflect the influence of Blake, Whitman, Duncan, and Ginsberg. Collected principally in two volumes, *A Long Undressing: Collected Poems: 1949–1969* (1971) and *Special Deliveries: New and Selected Poems* (1990), his poems are ecstatic and visionary celebrations of life's pleasures, characterized by simple diction and experimental form.

He also wrote a number of plays and memoirs, including *The Androgyne Journal* (1977), though he remains best known as a filmmaker.

Mother's Day is a comic antitribute to Mother that envisions Father as mostly a face in a frame, staring dourly, and the children as childlike adults, mindlessly engaging in such rituals as playing hopscotch and shooting squirt guns. Broughton's attack on the family is wrapped in Firbankian whimsy: "Mother was the loveliest woman in the world," reads a title in the film, "And Mother wanted everything to be lovely."

Mother's Day's more jarring images—ruined buildings, inscrutable characters—are less in evidence in his later films, which take the motif of the child-man (and child-woman) and expand it to rhapsodic effect.

Broughton was busy in the 1950s and 1960s writing poetry, but he returned to filmmaking in 1968 with the fanciful *The Bed*. The film's central image is arresting and hilariously absurd—an empty bed is traveling leisurely down a hill as if it were a car. Eventually it settles in a meadow and becomes the locus of all manner of strange scenarios and woodland trysts.

Characters—mostly naked—appear suddenly on its sheets. Broughton pops in as a kind of laughing Pan, sitting nude in a tree serenading a series of revelers. He ridicules conventional rituals when a woman arrives and officiously begins making up the bed. More typical, though, are the polymorphous pleasures of wriggling bodies apparently liberated by the bed.

Broughton brings nature in harmony with humanity in odd and intriguing ways, as when a woman in close-up encounters a spider and reaches out to kiss it. In another scene, a live lizard appears to slither out of a man's mouth.

Broughton's poetic skills are often highlighted in the films; such is the case in one of his boldest efforts, *Song*

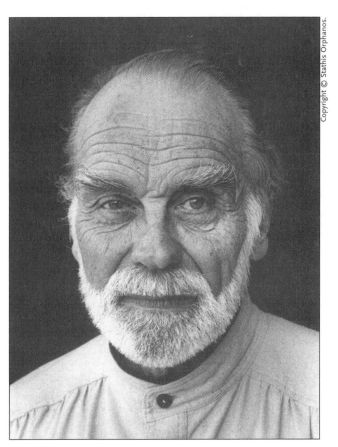

A portrait of James Broughton by Stathis Orphanos.

of the Godbody (1977). Here a male body—the film-maker's own, as it is featured in so much of his work—is shown in close-up, a kind of landscape of flesh that the camera lovingly surveys.

Broughton's beatific words accompany this exploration: "This is my body, which speaks for itself.... This is my body, which sings of itself." The comparisons to Whitman are inevitable, and Broughton could certainly lay claim to being Whitman's heir, celebrating the male body and male bonding unabashedly, and going further than Whitman in ways made possible in part by Broughton's appearance in the world decades later. What Whitman said, Broughton can say and show.

The Gardener of Eden (1981) is a brief document of his honeymoon with his lover and frequent collaborator, Joel Singer. The film was shot in Sri Lanka, and is typical in its treatment of the transporting beauty of nature and its positioning of the person as a fundamental part of it.

Two years later, in 1983, he made the masterful *Devotions*, also with Singer. Set in San Francisco and featuring a shimmering gamelan orchestra background, the film imagines an ecstatic world in which men are freed from tired, joyless convention. Broughton again appears as the sweet seer, playing a pipe, seducing his players into scintillating tableaux of union. His mostly naked men spend their time in loving embrace, washing each other, caressing, kissing.

Broughton's wit is never far away from his erotic celebrations: In one scene, two men kiss on a rooftop, then slowly don nuns' habits and saunter away in the fading day. Later, a pair of leather queens whip up a soufflé. Without being the least bit polemical, this graceful film, like all his work, shows the sweet rewards that come from living authentically and, above all, joyfully.

Broughton died of heart failure on May 17, 1999, in Port Townsend, Washington, in the arms of his lover, Joel Singer, and in the company of two close friends. He was eighty-five.

—*Gary Morris*

Bibliography

Broughton, James. *Ecstasies.* Mill Valley, Calif.: Syzygy Press, 1983.

———. *Coming Unbuttoned: A Memoir.* San Francisco: City Lights Books, 1993.

Elder, R. Bruce. *A Body of Vision: Representations of the Body in Recent Film and Poetry.* Waterloo, Ont.: Wilfrid Laurier University Press, 1998.

Sheehy, T. "Celebration; Four Films by James Broughton." *Film Quarterly* 29.4 (Summer 1976): 2–14.

Sitney, P. Adams. *Visionary Film.* New York: Oxford University Press, 1973.

See also

Film

Burr, Raymond   (1917–1993)

For millions of television viewers worldwide, actor Raymond Burr will always be identified with Perry Mason, the character he played in a long-running courtroom drama series, but in his career, which spanned five decades, he played a variety of roles in radio, television, and film and on the stage. He was also an avid breeder of orchids and the owner of a winery.

Quite apart from his importance as an accomplished actor, however, Burr has a particular significance in glbtq history for his response to the pressure he faced as a gay actor in a homophobic culture. It is clear that he felt the need to hide his homosexuality by carefully constructing (if not inventing out of whole cloth) a biography in which he seemed to conform to the heterocentric norms of the 1950s, when he rose to prominence as an actor.

Raymond William Stacy Burr was born in New Westminster, British Columbia, on May 21, 1917. When he was six, his parents, William Burr, a hardware dealer, and Minerva Smith Burr, a pianist and music teacher, divorced, and the boy and his mother moved to Vallejo, California, where his maternal grandfather owned a hotel.

Burr was sent to the nearby San Rafael Military Academy but, with the onset of the Great Depression, dropped out at the age of thirteen to help support the family. In the ensuing years he had various jobs, working on a sheep and cattle ranch, at a U.S. Forest Service weather station, and in China, as well as doing surveying and sales work.

At the age of twelve, Burr also began doing occasional acting jobs. He appeared on the stage in Canada, England, and Australia and also sang at a nightclub in Paris. He eventually worked on Broadway, appearing in *Crazy with the Heat* in 1941 and *The Duke in Darkness* in 1944.

After service in the navy, Burr headed for Hollywood and soon won his first film role in Mervyn LeRoy's *Without Reservations* (1946). The intense and physically imposing Burr was often cast as a villainous or intimidating character. Notable in his early work were his performances as a district attorney in George Stevens's *A Place in the Sun* (1951) and as the murderer in Alfred Hitchcock's *Rear Window* (1954).

In the course of his career, Burr had significant roles in over sixty cinematically released films and almost forty made-for-television movies. His work included dramas, Westerns, monster movies, and even comedies, such as Ken Finkleman's *Airplane II: The Sequel* (1982).

In 1955, Burr was asked to audition for the part of district attorney Hamilton Burger in a planned television series based on the Perry Mason mystery novels of Erle Stanley Gardner. Burr insisted on trying out for the title

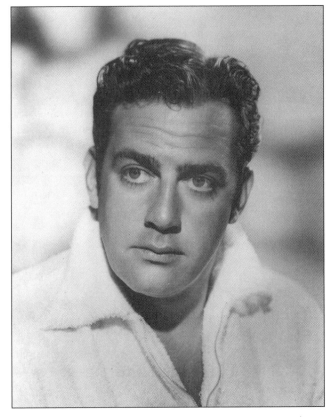

Raymond Burr.

role as well. Impressed by Burr's performance, Gardner chose him to play the lead.

Perry Mason ran from 1957 until 1966. Burr won two Emmy Awards (1959 and 1961) for his work on the popular series, and he became one of the highest-paid actors in television at the time. Burr returned to the role of the clever defense attorney in 1985, making over two dozen *Perry Mason* movies for television in the next eight years.

Burr starred in two other television series, the hit *Ironside* (1967–1975) and the flop *Kingston: Confidential* (1977), and appeared in several miniseries.

When it came to his private life, Burr has been described as "the most secretive of men." Reference sources state that he was married three times and had a son, but it is unclear how much of this information is true.

According to various accounts, Burr's first wife was Annette Sutherland, an English actress whom he married in 1941 and who supposedly died in the same plane crash as actor Leslie Howard when, on June 1, 1943, during World War II, the aircraft, en route from Lisbon to London, was shot down by the Germans.

At the very least, the story about Sutherland's death is a fabrication. There were only three adult females on the list of passengers and crew of Howard's ill-fated flight, and Annette Sutherland (or Burr) was not among them.

Burr's second marriage, which can be documented, was in 1947, to Isabella Ward. The union was annulled after a few months.

The name of Burr's third wife is given as Laura Andrina Morgan, who allegedly married Burr in 1953 and died of cancer in 1955.

The putative son of Burr and Sutherland, Michael Evan Burr, is said to have died of leukemia at the age of ten in 1953. In a rare public comment on his personal life, Burr claimed to have taken time off and traveled around the United States with his son in the last year of the boy's life.

Reports from Burr's closest associates cast doubt on the account. John Strauss, his publicist since 1953, said that Burr "never mentioned any wives or a son" and that he was in fact working steadily during the time when he claimed to have been on the road with his son. In addition, Burr's sister, Geraldine Fuller, said that neither she nor her mother ever saw Burr's son. None of Burr's longtime friends seems to have met any of his wives.

Despite the suspicious biography and occasional efforts to portray Burr as romantically linked to various actresses, including Natalie Wood, industry insiders were aware of his homosexuality. In 1961, Hedda Hopper, gossip columnist and mother of William Hopper, a costar on *Perry Mason*, wrote to tell Burr that she had received a compromising letter about him but said that she would not divulge the information, promising to "stand up and swear anything" for him.

In 1963, Burr and his partner, Robert Benevides, an actor whom he had met on the *Perry Mason* set, bought Naitaumba, an island in Fiji. There they pursued their shared interest in breeding orchids, a hobby that they turned into a successful business, Sea God Nurseries.

They also ran a cattle ranch and worked to improve the lives of the 150 residents of the island, building houses, a church, and a school. Burr sponsored the publication of the first dictionary of the Fiji language and also provided money to send the island's youngsters to school, a practice that he continued even after he and Benevides sold the island in 1983.

By 1980, Burr and Benevides had moved their orchid business to a farm in the Sonoma Valley of California. In the early 1980s, Burr donated two greenhouses and a portion of the orchid collection to the California State Polytechnic University at Pomona.

In the decade that followed, he and Benevides donated thousands more plants, and in 1992 they gave the university a collection of art and antique furniture valued in excess of $1.1 million. Other gifts made by Burr and Benevides include theater and law school scholarships.

In the 1980s, Burr and Benevides became interested in grape-growing and wine production. Vines were planted on their Northern California farm in 1986, and their first vintage was produced in 1990.

At the same time, both men were involved in the making of *Perry Mason* television movies, Burr as the star and Benevides as a producer. By the early 1990s, however, Burr was in failing health due to cancer. In August 1993, he completed his last film, *Perry Mason: The Case of the Killer Kiss*, after which he retired to the farm, where he died on September 12, 1993.

Although Burr had not wanted it, Benevides decided to name their business the Raymond Burr Vineyards as a tribute to his partner of thirty-five years.

—*Linda Rapp*

BIBLIOGRAPHY

Bergan, Ronald. "Bruising Baddie to Invincible Goodie." *Guardian* (London), September 14, 1993.

Biemiller, Lawrence. "From the Greenhouses of Cal Poly Pomona, Blooms of Rare Breeding." *The Chronicle of Higher Education* (March 23, 2001): A56.

Bounds, J. Dennis. "Burr, Raymond." *Encyclopedia of Television.* Horace Newcomb, ed. Chicago and London: Fitzroy Dearborn Publishers, 1997. 1:260–262.

"Burr, Raymond (William Stacy)." *Current Biography 1961.* Charles Moritz, ed. New York: H. W. Wilson Company, 1961. 88–90.

"The Defense Rests." *People,* September 27, 1993, 40.

Grimes, William. "Raymond Burr, Actor, 76, Dies." *New York Times,* September 14, 1993.

Hodges, Ann. "Defense Rests." *Houston Chronicle,* October 22, 1993.

Mann, William J. *Behind the Screen: How Gays and Lesbians Shaped Hollywood 1910–1969.* New York: Viking, 2001.

"No Trace Is Found of Howard's Plane." *New York Times,* June 4, 1943.

"Raymond Burr." *Daily Telegraph,* September 14, 1993.

Raymond Burr Vineyards website: www.raymondburrvineyards.com

SEE ALSO

Film; Film Actors: Gay Male

Butler, Dan   (b. 1954)

BEST KNOWN FOR HIS PORTRAYAL OF "BULLDOG" Briscoe, a lecherous heterosexual sports reporter on the television comedy *Frasier*, Dan Butler not only came out as a gay man, but also authored and starred in the gay-themed play *The Only Worse Thing You Could Have Told Me.*

Dan Butler's roots are in the American Midwest. Born on December 2, 1954, in Huntington, Indiana, he grew up in the nearby city of Fort Wayne. He showed an early

interest in acting, gathering neighborhood children to put on "little vaudevilles."

In high school, Butler pursued his penchant for the stage, winning leading roles in student plays. He also excelled in sports and was elected class president.

Upon graduating in 1973, he enrolled at Purdue University and then transferred to San Jose State University, but dropped out to study acting at the American Conservatory Theater in San Francisco from 1976 to 1978.

Although he had had girlfriends, Butler realized that he had always been attracted to men. His first gay romance, however, only came in 1977. He confided the news to his sister, Pam Conrad, announcing on the first page of a letter that he was in love and writing on the top of the second page, "And his name is Tommy." Although she and their mother, who subsequently happened upon the letter, were surprised by the revelation, both women were quick to accept Butler's sexual orientation.

Butler's father, on the other hand, did not take the news well at first. Although he eventually came to accept his son's sexuality, his initial reaction was one of anger. Even ten years later, when their relationship had improved, he said of the moment that Butler had revealed his sexual orientation, "The only worse thing that you could have told me is that you were dead"—a line that Butler would take for the title of his play.

Butler moved to New York in 1980 to pursue a career on the stage. Over the next decade he appeared in a number of plays, including Terrence McNally's *The Lisbon Traviata*. After a successful New York run in 1989 and 1990, the show moved to Los Angeles, where Butler performed in 1990 and 1991.

In the meanwhile, he had begun performing in films. He debuted in *Manhunter* (1986, directed by Michael Mann). His numerous movie credits include Norman René's *Longtime Companion* (1989) and Jonathan Demme's *Silence of the Lambs* (1991).

Butler also pursued opportunities in television. He landed a recurring role on the situation comedy *Roseanne* (1991–1992) and made guest appearances on many others, but he is best known for the character that he played on *Frasier* (1993–2004)—a libidinous heterosexual sports reporter named Bob "Bulldog" Briscoe.

It was during the run of *Frasier* that Butler came out publicly as a gay man. He did so in unusually dramatic fashion—starring in his own one-man play, *The Only Worse Thing You Could Have Told Me.* The show earned rave reviews when it opened in Los Angeles in 1994, and the accolades continued to pour in when Butler took it to New York the following year.

The semiautobiographical play presents a series of fourteen vignettes of different characters, all of them gay except for a macho jock whose best friend has just come out to him. The characters present a wide range of situations and experiences. Among them are an ACT UP demonstrator, an opera queen, an AIDS worker who falls in love with a dying patient, a man about to attend his high school class reunion, and an angry closeted man.

New York Times critic Ben Brantley described *The Only Worse Thing* as a "beautifully executed show" and "a remarkably clear-eyed and human portrait of the existential questions of gay identity that is more than the sum of its parts."

Butler incorporated a very personal element into the play, a taped conversation with his mother about why she had not revealed his homosexuality to his stepfather.

Butler did not, however, want to focus narrowly on his own experience. "There are so many different camps about what being gay means. The danger comes when each one is so rigid that it sees itself as the true picture," he commented.

Butler compared doing the play to working as a trapeze artist without a net. He feels that the experience made him stronger and more confident both personally and professionally.

Butler has become an active proponent of glbtq rights. In 1995, he and Candace Gingrich served as spokespersons for the National Coming Out Day Project. Butler appeared in public service announcements that included the gently humorous statement, "I'm not a straight man, but I play one on television."

Butler was among the public figures to speak out in 2000 against California's Proposition 22 (also known as the Knight Initiative), which sought to define marriage as a union between a man and a woman.

Butler has participated in fundraisers for AIDS charities, among them one in his native state of Indiana in 2002 that brought in a record amount of money for the event. He has also done volunteer service, including working as a counselor on the Trevor Helpline, a telephone resource for gay youth in crisis or considering suicide.

Butler has been in a stable relationship with acting teacher Richard Waterhouse since the mid-1990s. Although they had known each other before, they cemented their relationship soon after Waterhouse lost a former lover to AIDS. At first, they felt guilty for falling in love so soon after a bereavement, and Waterhouse asked Butler to "slow down" a little. He did, and the two have been together ever since.

Butler and Waterhouse were married—albeit without the sanction of the State of California—in a private ceremony in March 1999, on their fifth anniversary together. The families of both men were in attendance.

By making a public declaration of his homosexuality in mid-career, Butler showed courage. He realized that doing so might adversely affect his career, but he bravely took the chance. Happily, his career has not suffered, and he continues to appear in a variety of projects in film, television, and theater.   —*Linda Rapp*

BIBLIOGRAPHY

Brantley, Ben. "Familiar Attitudes on Gay Life Paint a Clear-Eyed Portrait." *New York Times*, April 3, 1995.

Epstein, Jeffrey. "Acting Independently: Frasier's Dan Butler Takes Center Stage with a Return to His First Love, Theater." *Advocate*, November 23, 1999, 73.

Guthmann, Edward. "Things Only Getting Better for Dan Butler; 'Frasier' Actor Is Out of the Closet and Proud of One-man Show." *San Francisco Chronicle*, September 15, 1996.

Holden, Stephen. "Two Solo Performers Embrace Multitudes." *New York Times*, June 18, 1995.

Israel, Betsy. "Bulldog Barks." *People*, April 24, 1995, 55.

Jones, Anderson. "Dan Butler and Richard Waterhouse." *Men Together: Portraits of Love, Commitment, and Life.* Essays by Anderson Jones; photographs by David Fields. Philadelphia: Running Press, 1997. 110–113.

SEE ALSO

Film Actors: Gay Male; American Television: Situation Comedies

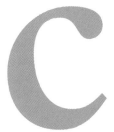

Cadinot, Jean-Daniel (b. 1944)

JEAN-DANIEL CADINOT, FRENCH PORNOGRAPHER *EXTRAordinaire*, has attracted an international following for his audacious films, which manage to be both unusually artistic and enormously arousing.

Cadinot was born in 1944 in Paris, at the foot of Montmartre in the Batignoles Quarter. His parents were tailors who custom-fit clothes. In reference to his parent's occupation, Cadinot notes the irony that whereas they clothed men, he has earned a reputation for undressing them.

Cadinot realized he was gay at the age of twelve, but he did not delve into gay erotica until 1972. Prior to that, in the early 1960s, he studied at the École des Arts et Métiers and at the National School of Photography. He then began his professional career at Valois Studios, where he directed mainstream films for French-speaking audiences.

Cadinot's professional coming-out as a gay photographer began in 1972, when he created nude photographs of gay author Yves Navarre and popular singers Patrick Juvet and Pascal Auriat. These photographs, which circulated only among a small, appreciative coterie, did not receive widespread notice.

In the early 1970s, Cadinot continued his mainstream career, but took ever more photographs of nude men, gradually earning a reputation as a skilled still photographer. By 1978, when he turned to filmmaking, he had published seventeen photo albums, which had sold more than 170,000 copies.

In 1978, Cadinot established his own production company, French Art, and issued his first 16 mm film, *Tendres adolescents*.

Cadinot explains his embrace of filmmaking as an expression of gay activism: "The still photo became too limiting. I quickly reached its boundaries and I had a desire for action and movement," he remarks. "I wanted to go further, to tell our collective stories as gay men. Video enabled me to do just that. I have to say that when I'm shooting photos I prefer to work as an artist and make artistic photos because otherwise it's not long before it gets pornographic and I don't like that. In that sense there was a progressive evolution towards films in order for me to tell stories about men. In a way it was my first gay activism to illustrate our sexual stories."

While Cadinot dislikes the term *pornography* because of its pejorative connotations, he has no apologies for the depictions of sexual action that animate his films. This action is often raw and even brutal, but sometimes tender and sweet.

Cadinot's films are plot-driven, usually featuring interesting and strong narratives. They also usually involve a journey, either literally, as in *Sex Bazaar* (1982) and *Sex Oasis* (1984), which feature young Frenchmen in North Africa; or figuratively, as in *Tough and Tender* (1989), which chronicles the search for love in a boys' reformatory. In *Sex Drive* (1985), the journey is imaginary. There, the protagonist is supposedly running away from home, but in the end it turns out to be a dream. Of course, all the journeys are picaresque; they, quite naturally, involve many adventures, especially of the sexual kind.

Another characteristic of Cadinot's films is that they feature young men in their late teens or early twenties. They are not the pumped-up, well-endowed, hot-waxed men who now dominate American pornography, however. Although they often interact with older and larger men, frequently of non-European background, the protagonists tend to be youthful and nonmuscular, and they tend to be more sexually versatile than actors in American pornography, who are often limited to top or bottom roles.

Regarding his young actors Cadinot has this to say: "To me they represent the freshness and innocence of youth. They are provocative: a 20-year-old is more subversive than a 30-year-old; there is not yet the weight of socialization and education on his shoulders; he is not yet molded into society. I like the freshness but also the intelligence of these guys. I do not choose Apollo-type men with big penises. I want men that could be your average next door neighbors, fresh, natural, without any complexes regarding their sexuality or their sexual tastes."

In devising his sex scenes, Cadinot states: "I write a scenario that fits the young guys. This is the essence of my films. The performers do not portray things that are imposed on them by me, but things they like to do themselves. These 'puppies' kiss each other with real passion, with real lust. It is emotions that make my particular style. I tell a story. I don't do things that are 'robotical' like we often tend to see in the porn industry, my scenarios are based on the actors' tastes."

Although Cadinot says that he tailors his films to his actors, he also, rather paradoxically, insists that his films are autobiographical, which may account for their intensely personal quality. He says that his works constitute a saga "that traces my life from the age of twelve when I became aware of my homosexuality, with all of the problems of

religion and existentialism." While the films are not literally autobiographical, they are informed by events in the director's life.

For example, Cadinot did not spend time in a reformatory, the setting of *Tough and Tender,* yet the film nevertheless derives from his own experience: "It is a transposition of my vacations as an adolescent in religious camps," he explains. "The universe was, for me, similar (like a concentration camp, and the product of hierarchy among the teenagers). The same with the time I spent in the Boy Scouts."

The time Cadinot spent in the Boy Scouts is used to good effect in *Hot on the Trail* (1984), a film that is notable for its fetishization not only of youth and genitalia, but also of underwear, especially jockey-style briefs.

To date Cadinot has made sixty films, usually limiting himself to directing no more than four a year. In 1992, he bought and restored a farm, which he now utilizes as his studio. "It is very satisfying to have this studio now," he has commented, "to live with the actors for many days, to discuss with them and understand their personalities, which helps me to develop scenes. Here, there is space for more than a dozen people and each youth can do whatever pleases him, whether it is staying with the group and having fun or having some privacy."

Cadinot's films have earned an international audience and numerous accolades. In 1997, Cadinot was honored with a Venus Award as Best Director at the International Erotic Film Awards in Berlin, the first time the organization recognized gay erotic films. More recently, Cadinot won an AVN award, the adult Oscars, awarded in Los Angeles, for his entire body of work, and another Venus for *C'est La Vie* (2001). He has completed his autobiography, *Premier,* but has yet to find an American publisher for it.

—*George Koschel*

BIBLIOGRAPHY

Gardiner, Stephen "Outspoken: Bad Puppies-The films of JD Cadinot." www.outuk.com/index.html

Koschel, George. E-mail interview with Jean-Daniel Cadinot. Linda Rapp, trans. October 2002.

Sibalis, Michael. "Cadinot, Jean-Daniel." *Who's Who in Contemporary Gay and Lesbian History: From World War II to the Present Day.* Robert Aldrich and Garry Wotherspoon, eds. London and New York: Routledge, 2001. 69–70.

www.cadinot-films-france.com

SEE ALSO

Pornographic Film and Video: Gay Male

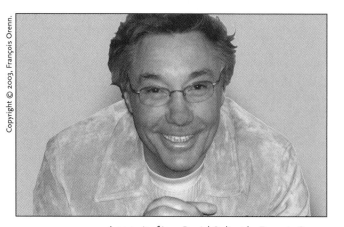

A portrait of Jean-Daniel Cadinot by François Orenn.

Callow, Simon (b. 1949)

VERSATILE BRITISH ACTOR SIMON CALLOW HAS PLAYED a wide variety of roles on the stage, in movies, and on television. He has also directed the film *The Ballad of the Sad Café* (1991) and numerous theater productions, including *Carmen Jones* (1991), for which he won an Olivier Award for Best Director of a Musical.

Callow was born on June 15, 1949, in South London. His parents separated when he was a child and he was educated at a variety of schools, including private schools in England and secondary schools in Zambia and South Africa.

Callow's fascination with the theater began when, at the age of seven, he heard a radio performance of *Macbeth*. As a student at the London Oratory Grammar School, he founded the Literary and Debating Society so that he and his schoolmates could read plays.

After leaving school, Callow wrote to Laurence Olivier, telling him of his interest in the theater and his willingness to work at the National Theatre "in however humble a capacity." His first job was humble indeed—he worked in the box office and the mailroom.

Deciding that he needed a university education, Callow went to Queen's University in Belfast. There he joined the Drama Society and played Trigorin in Chekhov's *The Seagull*.

More inclined to the stage than to academia, Callow soon left the university and returned to London, where he was accepted as a student at the Drama Centre. Even before leaving drama school, he got a role in C. P. Taylor's *Schippel*. The play, first produced at a fringe theater, eventually moved to the West End, where it was very well received.

In 1975, Callow played the lead in the Gay Sweatshop's production of Martin Sherman's *Passing By*. He was impressed by the text, which presented "self-accepting, unagonised, uncaricatured gay people."

Performing in this "quiet and funny play" was an important professional experience for Callow, who felt a particular synergy with his audiences. His and their reaction to the play led him to reflect on the relationship of the actor himself to his character.

When playing a gay role, Callow said, he was "able to go deeper and wider" into the part even in a play such as *Kiss of the Spider Woman*, in which his character "had very little to do with [him] personally, very little to do with the kind of gay man that [he was]." Among the gay roles for which Callow is particularly well known is Gareth in Mike Newell's film *Four Weddings and a Funeral* (1994).

Callow has appeared in more than twenty plays and as many films. His work first came to general public attention in 1979, when he starred as Mozart in the stage version of Peter Shaffer's *Amadeus*. In 1984, he played impresario Emanuel Schikaneder in Milos Forman's film of the same work.

Callow's first classical role was as the title character in Shakespeare's *Titus Andronicus* in 1978. He also appeared in *As You Like It* in 1979 and in Sir John Vanbrugh's Restoration comedy *The Relapse* in 1983.

Callow's movie roles have allowed him to demonstrate his versatility as an actor. He earned considerable praise for his work in a string of Merchant-Ivory films, *A Room With a View* (1984), *Maurice* (1986), *Mr. and Mrs. Bridge* (1991), *Howards End* (1992), and *Jefferson in Paris* (1994).

His remarkably wide-ranging film credits also include the Master of Revels in John Madden's *Shakespeare in Love* (1998), the voice of the Grasshopper in Henry Selick's animated film *James and the Giant Peach* (1996), and a pompous official in a Jean-Claude Van Damme movie, *Street Fighter* (1994). Other recent credits include appearances in Stephen Fry's *Bright Young Things* (2003), based on Evelyn Waugh's novel *Vile Bodies*, in Mike Nichols's television miniseries of Tony Kushner's *Angels in America* (2003), and in Joel Schumacher's movie of Andrew Lloyd Webber's *The Phantom of the Opera* (2004).

In addition to his acting, Callow has directed over two dozen plays in England and on Broadway. He also directed a radio play, *Tomorrow Week*, in 1999.

An excellent writer as well as an unusually thoughtful actor, Callow has written a number of books on acting and the theater as well as biographies of Orson Welles and Charles Laughton. The Laughton biography is particularly interesting as an analysis of the acting style and development of one great gay character actor by another. Callow also writes weekly columns that appear in several English newspapers.

Fluent in French, Callow has translated works by Cocteau, Kundera, and Prévert.

Callow has been involved romantically with a number of partners, including the late Turkish-Egyptian filmmaker Aziz Yehia and designer Christopher Woods. He recently described his current relationship as a happy one and described his partner as "very determined and exploratory and intellectual."

In 1991, when actor Ian McKellen was attacked by filmmaker Derek Jarman for accepting a knighthood from the homophobic Thatcher government, Callow, along with such other gay and lesbian artists as Nancy Diuguid, Stephen Fry, Bryony Lavery, John Schlesinger, and Antony Sher, came to McKellen's defense.

In 1999, Callow was named a Commander of the British Empire (CBE) in recognition of his richly varied career and achievements.

—*Linda Rapp*

BIBLIOGRAPHY

Callow, Simon. *Acting in Restoration Comedy.* New York: Applause Theatre Books, 1991.

_____. *Being an Actor.* London: Methuen, 1984.

_____. *Charles Laughton: A Difficult Actor.* London: Methuen, 1987.

_____. *Love Is Where It Falls.* London: Nick Hern Books, 1999.

_____. *The National: The Theatre and Its Work 1963–1997.* London: Nick Hern Books, 1997.

_____. *Orson Welles: The Road to Xanadu.* London: Jonathan Cape, 1995.

_____. *Oscar Wilde and His Circle.* London: National Portrait Gallery Publications, 2000.

_____. *Shooting the Actor or The Choreography of Confusion.* London: Nick Hern Books, 1990.

Durrant, Sabine. "The Business of Feeling." *Guardian,* February 15, 1999.

Fitzwilliams, Richard, ed. "Callow, Simon Philip Hugh." *International Who's Who 2002.* London: Europa Publications, 2001. 244–245.

Jourdan, Thea. "Nothing Callow in His Art." *Scotsman,* September 19, 2001.

Tweedie, Neil, and Jessica Callan. "Queen's Birthday Honors." *Daily Telegraph* (London), June 12, 1999.

Zucker, Carole. "Simon Callow." *In the Company of Actors: Reflections on the Craft of Acting.* New York: Theatre Arts Books/Routledge, 1999. 30–46.

SEE ALSO

Film Actors: Gay Male; Cocteau, Jean; Fry, Stephen; Laughton, Charles; McKellen, Sir Ian; Ivory, James, and Ismail Merchant; Schlesinger, John

Canadian Television

THE PORTRAYAL OF GAY, LESBIAN, BISEXUAL, TRANS-gendered, and queer people in English Canadian television programming has been sporadic. There have been several significant appearances of glbtq characters on the CBC (Canadian Broadcasting Corporation), Canada's national public broadcasting system.

The recent advent of PrideVision, a digital cable television network with a mandate to air glbtq Canadian content, will certainly lead to an increase not only in the presence of gay men and lesbians on television, but also in the number of shows developed for a glbtq audience.

Canadian Broadcasting Corporation

Perhaps because it is a public broadcaster with a mandate to inform and enlighten as well as entertain, CBC has aired more television programs with glbtq content than Canada's other national network, CTV.

CBC's *Degrassi Jr. High* (1987–1989), part of the youth-centered Degrassi series, dealt with abortion, single parenthood, sex, death, racism, AIDS, feminism, and gay issues as situations that the characters had to work through within the serialized narrative structures, while avoiding the "topic of the week" feel that is endemic to the genre. One episode, for example, featured the pre-adolescent character Caitlin discussing lesbianism with her English teacher, Miss Avery.

A spin-off of the Degrassi series, *Liberty Street* (CBC, 1995–1996), featured Billy Merasty as Nathan Jones, a gay Native North American ex–bicycle courier. The producers of *Liberty Street* went on to create *Riverdale* (CBC, 1997–2000), with gay character George Patillo.

In early 2003, CBC announced that gay playwright Michel Tremblay will write Quebec's first television show to feature an ongoing gay relationship, *Le Coeur Découvert.*

Comedy

In the 1990s, CBC's Ivan Fecan programmed an hour of adult comedy that preceded Canada's national newscast each Thursday.

Gay and lesbian characters, content, and liberation politics were also contained in the satire of sketch comedy series *CODCO* (1987–1994, starring Tommy Sexton, Greg Malone, Cathy Jones, Mary Walsh, Andy Jones) and *Kids in the Hall* (1989–1995, starring David Foley, Bruce McCulloch, Kevin McDonald, Mark McKinney, and Scott Thompson).

All five members of *CODCO* frequently cross-dressed and traversed gender. Their pointed satire took aim at regional differences, national assumptions, and gay codes. The show had a recurring "Queen's Counselors" sketch about two fey, gay Newfoundland lawyers.

The more outrageous *Kids in the Hall* had a penchant for drag, gender-bending, and pro-homo skits, featuring nellie bon vivant Buddy Cole; the Sappho Sluggers (a lesbian softball team); Running Faggot—a new folk hero; and Dracula, a gay aesthete with a taste for rough trade. The show both satirized and celebrated glbtq culture, and ended up developing a loyal cult following.

Under the rubric of comedy, a number of special presentations of lesbian comedian Elvira Kurt and gay comedian Gavin Crawford (who also created *The Gavin Crawford Show* for the Comedy Network in 2000) were produced and aired on Canadian television in the 1990s.

Documentaries and Reality Television

Canada has a strong history of documentary filmmaking, and since 1992 the National Film Board (NFB) has produced seventeen glbtq-themed films. Several have aired on Canadian television: David Adkin's *Out: Stories of Lesbian and Gay Youth* (1993) and Aerlyn Weissman and Lynne Fernie's *Forbidden Love: The Unashamed Stories of Lesbian Lives* (1992) are but two award-winning examples.

The Life Network's "reality" television program,

U8TV: The Lofters (debuted 2001) follows the lives of eight young adults living together in a loft. The first season featured Mathieu Chantelois and his boyfriend Marcello and bisexual Valery Gagne. Chantelois now hosts the Internet television show *So Gay TV*, which has also been adopted by the new PrideVision TV network.

Public Access Television

Public access channels in Canada's larger urban centers have also created programming for the glbtq community. *Cable 10%* (1995–2000, renamed *10%-Qtv* in 1997) premiered on Rogers Community Television in Toronto and aired for six seasons in southern and eastern Ontario. Produced entirely by volunteers, *Cable 10%* lacked the production values of network television, but did chronicle queer love, families, and communities, exploring issues of diversity, religion, politics, arts, and culture.

Similarly, Vancouver's *Outlook TV* now offers glbtq current-affairs television programming produced entirely by volunteers on Shaw Cable 4 (British Columbia).

Toronto's CHUM (City TV) presented *QT-Queer Television* (1998–1999), a weekly program about gay, lesbian, and trans cultures. Hosted and produced by Irshad Manji, *QT* grew directly out of the success of *Q-Files*, also hosted by Manji and broadcast on Toronto's Cable Pulse 24. *QT* was concurrently broadcast on the Internet in fully streamed video via www.planetout.com. Although the television program lasted for only two seasons, the episodes are still available online.

QT's emergence paralleled the increasing visibility of the gay and lesbian (especially gay male) market as a significant demographic. Since 1992, the glbtq community has become increasingly desirable to marketers because research demonstrated that they had disposable income, were trendsetting consumers, and were more likely to try new products than the rest of the population.

Niche programming and television networks devoted to the glbtq community have developed in Canada, as they have in the United States.

PrideVision TV

PrideVision TV was launched on September 7, 2001, and is touted as the world's first gay, lesbian, bisexual, and transgender television network to broadcast twenty-four hours a day, seven days a week. The network is licensed by the Canadian Radio Television and Telecommunications Commission (CRTC) to provide television service targeted to the gay, lesbian, bisexual, and transgender community.

The network is guaranteed distribution through cable and direct-to-home satellite companies that provide digital television services in Canada. As many as 2.5 million households are expected to have access to digital channels in Canada, though the number who have subscribed to PrideVision is still unknown.

PrideVision TV offers a range of programming, dealing with subjects ranging from current affairs, documentaries, health and fitness, lifestyle, and finance to relationships, music, cooking, and travel. Entertainment programming includes popular movies and comedies from around the world, Canadian drama, arts programming, biographies, and variety shows.

Among the offerings of PrideVision TV is *Shout!* (debuted 2001), a weekly current-affairs program dealing with the ongoing concerns of the glbtq community. Indeed, PrideVision TV opened its studio in the heart of Toronto's "gay ghetto" to promote the network and facilitate audience interaction on *Shout!*

PrideVision has also developed a travel show titled *Bump!* (debuted 2001). Its two hosts travel the world in search of fascinating glbtq human-interest stories. *Bump!* presents a new location each week, delving into the local social scene.

Another new program, *The UnderCovers* (debuted 2001), offers live phone-in sex advice. It takes viewer emails and phone calls from the glbtq community. PrideVision also airs popular glbtq dramas and comedies, such as *Gimme Gimme Gimme*, *Undressed*, *So Graham Norton*, and *Metrosexuality*.

Although an emerging network, PrideVision's mandate to air Canadian content should give cause for optimism to Canadian gay, lesbian, bisexual, and transgendered filmmakers, producers, directors, and performers.

—Jennifer Burwell

BIBLIOGRAPHY

Attallah, Paul. "Kids in the Hall." *Encyclopedia of Television*. Museum of Broadcast Communication website. www.museum.tv/archives/etv/index.html

Bednarski, P. J. "What? No gay channel?" *Broadcasting & Cable*, June 25, 2001, 17.

CBC Mandate: http://cbc.radio-canada.ca/htmen/1_2.htm

Knoebel, John. "Nontraditional Affluent Consumers." *American Demographics* 14.11 (November 1992): S10(2).

Kryhul, Angela. "PrideVision's Tough Sell: The New Gay and Lesbian-themed Channel Faces Special Challenges Getting onto Media Plans." *Marketing*, October 15, 2001, 21.

Nicks, Joan. "CODCO." *Encyclopedia of Television*. Museum of Broadcast Communication website. www.museum.tv/archives/etv/index.html

———. "Degrassi." *Encyclopedia of Television*. Museum of Broadcast Communication website. www.museum.tv/archives/etv/index.html

Shecter-Barbara. "CRTC Slaps Shaw over PrideVision Discrimination: Gay-themed TV Channel." *National Post*, September 29, 2001, 1.

Wyatt, David. "Gay/Lesbian/Bisexual Television Characters." http://home.cc.umanitoba.ca/~wyatt/tv-characters.html

SEE ALSO

American Television: Situation Comedies; Documentary Film; Fernie, Lynne

Carné, Marcel   (1906–1996)

THE MASTER OF POETIC REALISM, MARCEL CARNÉ WAS a prodigy who created some of the defining films of French cinema from 1936 until 1945, including the Dadaist comedy-thriller *Drôle de drame* (1937; American title: *Bizarre Bizarre)*, the fatalistic melodrama *Le quai des brumes* (1938; American title: *Port of Shadows*), the intricate, flashback-structured tragedy *Le jour se lève* (1939), the medieval allegory *Les Visiteurs du soir* (1942), and his masterpiece, the magnificent theatrical epic *Les Enfants du paradis* (1945; American title: *Children of Paradise*).

Working with a powerful team of collaborators (the poet Jacques Prévert as scenarist, the designer Alexandre Trauner, the composers Maurice Jaubert and Joseph Kosma, the editor Henri Rust, the cinematographer Roger Hubert), Carné provided the French cinema with some of its most emblematic images, including Michèle Morgan with trench coat and beret walking through the fog in *Port of Shadows*, Jean Gabin waiting for the police alone in his attic room in *Le jour se lève*, and the mime sequences, with Jean-Louis Barrault's lovesick Baptiste pining for Arletty's statuesque Garance, in *Children of Paradise*.

Carné's poetic realism consists of a meticulously recreated studio environment in which every element of lighting, decor, and design could be utilized to maximum expressivity.

After World War II, there was a dispersal of his collaborative team. Carné himself would remain a master craftsman as a director, but his insistence on themes of fatalism and doomed romance did not have the same urgency.

Still, *Juliette ou la Clef des songes* (1951) had atmospheric design and a wonderful performance by Gerard Philipe, and *Thérèse Raquin* (1953) proved to be a vigorous updating of Zola's novel, with exceptional performances by Simone Signoret and Raf Vallone.

Carné's last feature film, *Le Merveilleuse visite* (1974), about a beautiful young man who turns out to be an angel visiting Earth, is an allegory in which male beauty is used as an indicator of innocence.

A man noted for his generosity and sensitivity, in his private life Carné tended to place personal relationships above political considerations: On the sets of *Les Visiteurs du soir* and *Children of Paradise*, there were artists who would later be tried for collaborating with the Nazis, as well as artists who were members of the Underground resistance and Jews in hiding who were given shelter.

During the 1970s, however, Carné issued several statements to the press indicating that he wished the openness of the post-Stonewall era had been available to him earlier in his career. Although he regretted that he had not infused his work with a political consciousness, he believed that his partiality to themes of impossible romance derived from his acute awareness of the societal oppression of homosexuals.

He was an outspoken champion of filmmakers such as Pier Paolo Pasolini and Rainer Werner Fassbinder, who politicized questions of gender and sexual orientation.

Although his career was uneven, Carné will be remembered for the masterful films that began his career: *Jenny* (1936), *Drôle de drame, Port of Shadows, Hôtel du Nord* (1939), and, above all, for *Children of Paradise*. The latter, indisputably one of the classics of French cinema, was voted one of the greatest films in French history by a poll of French film critics in 2000.

—*Daryl Chin*

BIBLIOGRAPHY

Armes, Roy. *French Cinema.* New York: Oxford University Press, 1985.

Carné, Marcel. *La Vie à belles dents: Mémoires.* Paris: L'Archipel, 1996.

———. *La Vie à belles dents: Souvenirs.* Paris: J.-P. Ollivier, 1975.

Turk, Edward Baron. *Child of Paradise: Marcel Carné and the Golden Age of French Cinema.* Cambridge, Mass.: Harvard University Press, 1989.

SEE ALSO

European Film; Film Directors; Fassbinder, Rainer Werner; Pasolini, Pier Paolo

Chamberlain, Richard   (b. 1935)

AMERICAN ACTOR RICHARD CHAMBERLAIN BUILT A career in television, film, and theater playing romantic heterosexual roles. Deeply closeted for most of his life, he at last publicly acknowledged his homosexuality in his 2003 memoir *Shattered Love*.

Chamberlain, born in Los Angeles on March 31, 1935, grew up in Beverly Hills, but, he says, on "the wrong side of the now-vanished streetcar tracks" in a city whose name is synonymous with affluence. Although the Chamberlains were not rich, they were reasonably comfortable financially.

Emotional comfort was a far rarer commodity in the household. Chamberlain's father was an alcoholic who terrorized his wife and two sons with psychological rather than physical violence. In his memoir Chamberlain describes consistent feelings of inadequacy and failure to live up to his father's expectations.

Chamberlain entered Pomona College in 1952. He intended to major in art, but soon began appearing in the drama program's plays, enjoying enough success that he decided to pursue an acting career after graduating.

His plans were briefly interrupted when he was drafted and served two years in the army. Upon his return to civilian life, he enrolled in acting classes, in one of which he met a young man who became his first love. Because of the homophobia prevalent in the late 1950s, the pair were careful to keep the year-long affair "as secret as possible."

Chamberlain made his movie debut in the forgettable *The Secret of the Purple Reef* (1960, directed by William Witney), and filmed a pilot for a proposed television series that never materialized. Shortly thereafter, however, he won the title role in the NBC drama *Dr. Kildare*, which began its immensely successful five-year run in 1961 and established the handsome Chamberlain as a romantic leading man, the object of desire of both men and women.

When *Dr. Kildare* ended, Chamberlain declined offers of other television series to work in theater and film. This led him to England, where he lived for four and a half years. A highlight of his British sojourn was the opportunity to play Hamlet at the Birmingham Repertory Theatre in 1968.

Chamberlain's movie career includes an eclectic mix of projects. His roles in Bryan Forbes's *The Madwoman of Chaillot* (1969) and Ken Russell's *The Music Lovers*

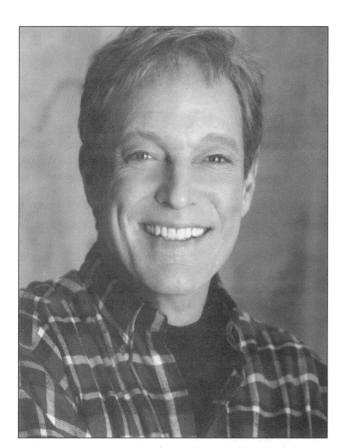

A portrait of Richard Chamberlain by Greg Gorman.

(1971), in which he played Pyotr Ilich Tchaikovsky, are generally considered among his best, earning critical accolades. He also appeared in Irwin Allen's disaster films *The Towering Inferno* (1974) and *The Swarm* (1978) and Richard Lester's *The Three Musketeers* (1974), among others.

In the late 1970s and 1980s, Chamberlain reigned on television as "the king of the miniseries," starring in *Centennial* (1978, based on the novel by James Michener and directed by Harry Falk, Paul Krasny, Bernard McEveety, and Virgil Vogel), *Shōgun* (1980, based on James Clavell's novel and directed by Jerry London), and the phenomenally successful adaptation of Colleen McCullough's *The Thorn Birds* (1983, directed by Stan Margulies).

Around 110 million television viewers watched the tale of Father Ralph de Bricassart's doomed love for Meggie, an Australian sheep rancher, putting *The Thorn Birds* among the highest-rated miniseries in the history of television. The miniseries also solidified Chamberlain's status as mysterious heartthrob to legions of female fans.

When cable television began drawing an ever increasing share of the audience, the major networks moved away from producing costly miniseries. Chamberlain returned to the theater, where he undertook such mature roles as Henry Higgins in a 1994 Broadway revival of Lerner and Loewe's *My Fair Lady* and Baron von Trapp in a national tour of Rodgers and Hammerstein's *The Sound of Music* in 1999.

When Chamberlain publicly acknowledged that he is gay in his 2003 memoir *Shattered Love*, the news came as a shock to virtually no one. That he chose at the age of sixty-eight finally to speak of his sexuality was considerably more surprising.

Although the tabloids had outed him in the early 1990s, and his homosexuality was an open secret in much of the theatrical and television community as well as the subject of gossip in the gay male community, throughout his career he had refused to comment on the topic because of, he stated later, his "own self-rejection" as a gay man. He also feared that coming out might jeopardize his job prospects, certainly a valid concern when he was starting out in the early 1960s. Even today many gay male actors wonder if they can be accepted in romantic heterosexual roles if they are openly gay.

When Chamberlain finally revealed "the worst kept secret in Hollywood," however, he found his fans "supportive, …positive, and friendly."

In his memoir Chamberlain writes of his search for inner peace and of his relationship with producer-director Martin Rabbett, his partner since the mid-1970s. For the past decade, the couple has made their home in Hawaii, where Rabbett grew up.

The two have worked together on various professional projects over the years. One of the most recent was a July 2003 production of Timothy Findley's *The Stillborn Lover* at the Berkshire Repertory Theater in Stockbridge, Massachusetts. Rabbett directed the play, in which Chamberlain starred as an ambassador who reveals to his family that he is gay. Critic Malcolm Johnson observed that Chamberlain brought "a deep reserve and quiet dignity" to the role, perhaps reflecting both his many years of reticence and his newfound self-acceptance.   —*Linda Rapp*

BIBLIOGRAPHY

Bernstein, Fred A. "A Night Out with Richard Chamberlain; A Couple Makes a Debut." *New York Times,* July 13, 2003.

Chamberlain, Richard. *Shattered Love: A Memoir.* New York: ReganBooks, 2003.

Guthmann, Edward. "The Doctor Is Out; New Memoir, New Honesty from TV's 'Dr. Kildare.'" *San Francisco Chronicle,* June 18, 2003.

Johnson, Malcolm. "Bold 'Stillborn Lover' a Play of Timely Ideas." *Hartford Courant,* July 12, 2003.

Levine, Bettijane. "Richard, Reconciled; In His New Book, Leading Man Chamberlain Reveals He Is Gay, and It's Liberated Him." *Los Angeles Times,* June 13, 2003.

SEE ALSO

Film Actors: Gay Male

Chapman, Graham   (1941–1989)

COMIC ACTOR AND WRITER GRAHAM CHAPMAN, a member of Britain's madcap Monty Python troupe, was in the vanguard of actors to come out publicly as gay.

Chapman's first entrance was dramatic: An air raid was in progress when he was born on January 8, 1941, in Leicester, England.

Because his father served in the police force, the family moved quite often as he was posted to a succession of different towns. Chapman's favorite place growing up was Melton Mowbray, a town in Leicestershire famous for its pork pies, where he participated actively in the school theater program.

After graduation from Melton Mowbray Grammar School, Chapman entered Emmanuel College, Cambridge, in 1959, following his older brother into the study of medicine.

In his second year at Cambridge, Chapman auditioned successfully for the prestigious Footlights acting troupe, as did first-year student John Cleese, with whom he soon began writing sketches. Eric Idle joined the group the following year.

After graduating from Cambridge in 1962, Chapman pursued his medical studies at St. Bartholomew's Hospital, a teaching institution in London. Later that year, the annual Footlights show, originally called *A Clump of Plinths* but subsequently retitled *Cambridge Circus,* came to play in London's West End. When a cast member dropped out, Chapman replaced him, and he began juggling his medical training and his acting.

The well-received show was slated for a tour in New Zealand. Chapman decided to interrupt his medical course and sign on after he had occasion, as secretary of the students' union, to lunch with Queen Elizabeth, the Queen Mother, who told him that New Zealand was "a beautiful place" and "you must go."

After the tour Chapman resumed his medical studies and eventually qualified as a physician, but he also began performing in cabaret shows and writing sketches and dialogue for a number of television programs, including for Footlights alumnus David Frost's satirical *The Frost Report.* Also writing for the Frost show were Michael Palin, Terry Jones, and Eric Idle. Soon, together with John Cleese and Terry Gilliam, they formed the troupe that launched *Monty Python's Flying Circus* on the BBC.

The show first appeared in England in October 1969 and continued in first runs until 1974. A few years after its British debut, the program aired on American PBS stations. It quickly became a favorite, especially among college-age viewers. The zany sketches featured both amusing and irreverent—and often ludicrous—dialogue and broad physical humor. The actors appeared in a variety of costumes, frequently in drag.

Some of the Python skits, especially those written by Chapman, were gay or gay-inflected in theme. Perhaps the most famous of these is "The Mouse Problem," a sketch involving men who dress in mouse costumes and secretly engage in cheese-tasting parties. The skit is in effect a parable about the secretive lives led by British homosexuals in the years after decriminalization of homosexuality, but before social acceptance was widespread.

Some of the sketches that Chapman wrote with John Cleese, such as "The Ministry of Silly Walks" and "Dead Parrot," are now considered classics of British comedy.

Although his comic imagination was in many ways the most surreal and subversive of the Pythons, Chapman often played figures of authority and the "straight man" in situations that sometimes revealed the looniness that could lurk behind a buttoned-down upper-class British exterior.

The Python troupe wrote and appeared together in several films, beginning with Ian McNaughton's *And Now for Something Completely Different* (1971), the title of which is a catchphrase from the television show. The movie, which comprised remade sketches from the series, did not do well in the United States, where the Pythons were as yet unknown.

Their second feature, *Monty Python and the Holy Grail* (directed by Jones and Gilliam, 1975), received a more enthusiastic reaction from their growing number of American fans. Chapman's portrayal of King Arthur in the medieval spoof garnered him enthusiastic notice.

He played the title role in the third Python movie, *Life of Brian* (directed by Jones, 1979). The film drew criticism from some conservative groups that viewed it as sacrilegious, but audiences were appreciative. Indeed, the publicity generated by the fulminations of religious groups against the film is probably what made it so successful at the box office, despite its being banned in many jurisdictions. Many consider Chapman's turn as Brian of Nazareth, a man mistaken for the Messiah, as his finest work.

Chapman also appeared in the final Python film, Jones's *The Meaning of Life* (1983).

In addition to their collaborative work, the Pythons undertook independent projects. Chapman's included cowriting and starring in the pirate spoof *Yellowbeard* (directed by Mel Damski, 1983), which was not a commercial success.

He continued writing scripts. Among these were some that he coauthored in 1988 with his lover, David Sherlock, for a comedy/fantasy television series entitled *Jake's Journey*, loosely based on Mark Twain's *A Connecticut Yankee in King Arthur's Court*, in which Chapman would have starred. The project was never realized.

In 1980, Chapman published a memoir, *A Liar's Autobiography, Volume VI*, which mixes truth and fiction. Along with fantasy passages are serious discussions of his medical studies, his involvement with Monty Python, his battles with alcohol, and his homosexuality.

Chapman, who was twenty-five before he realized that he was homosexual, was among the first British entertainers to come out as openly gay, which he did in 1969, soon before the launching of *Monty Python's Flying Circus*. His openness provoked some hostility from television viewers and critics.

Chapman met his life partner, Sherlock, in 1966 in Ibiza, where the latter was hoping to rekindle a "holiday romance" from the previous year. That plan fizzled, but he and Chapman fell in love and remained together for the next twenty-four years.

Chapman became, in his own words, "an early campaigner for gay liberation." In 1972, he cofounded the publication *Gay News*, to which he lent his financial support. The inaugural issues of *Gay News*, England's first national gay-liberation newspaper, featured an interview with Chapman and Sherlock.

In the early 1970s, Chapman and Sherlock adopted John Tomiczek, a teenage runaway from a large family. Tomiczek, who recognized Chapman from his television acting work, approached him; and Chapman, realizing that the youth was running a fever, provided for his medical treatment and returned him to his home in Liverpool.

When Tomiczek ran away again, his father eventually surrendered custody of him, and he joined Chapman and Sherlock's household. The couple agreed to adopt him on condition that he finish school. Tomiczek eventually became Chapman's manager. He died of a heart attack in 1992.

Chapman faced medical challenges of his own. He suffered from alcoholism for several years, but gave up drinking during the filming of *Monty Python and the Holy Grail*, when he realized that the situation had gotten out of hand. In 1977, he entered a hospital to undergo a recovery process and thereafter completely abstained from alcohol.

Chapman was unable to overcome cancer, however. Diagnosed with a malignant tumor on his tonsil in November 1988, he underwent an operation, but the disease had spread to other parts of his body, including his spine. Despite further surgery and radiation therapy, he died on October 4, 1989. Sherlock was at his bedside at the end, and the couple's last words to each other were affirmations of their love.

Chapman's death came the day before the twentieth anniversary of the first broadcast of *Monty Python's Flying Circus*. Only a month earlier, he had been able to take a limited part in the troupe's special anniversary program, *Parrot Sketch Not Included*, which aired later that year.

Susan Schindehette has called Chapman "the most doggedly different member of his era's most unpredictable comedy troupe." A BBC biographical sketch describes him as "the only genuine anarchist within Python, and the most subversive element in a group of subversive elements," adding that "it was his unique outlook on life that coloured some of Python's most surreal, most bizarre and, most importantly, funniest moments."   —*Linda Rapp*

BIBLIOGRAPHY

Chapman, Graham, John Cleese, Terry Gilliam, Eric Idle, Terry Jones, and Michael Palin with Bob McCabe. *The Pythons Autobiography by the Pythons*. New York: St. Martin's Press, 2003.

"Graham Chapman—Comedy Writer and Actor." www.bbc.co.uk/dna/h2g2/alabaster/A687954

Morgan, David. *Monty Python Speaks*. New York: Avon Books, 1999.

Perry, George. *Life of Python*. Boston: Little, Brown and Company, 1983.

Schindehette, Susan. "Mourning Monty Python Lays to Rest Silly, Brave, Unique Graham Chapman." *People*, October 30, 1989, 52.

Yoakum, Jim. "Graham Chapman's Journey." *Rolling Stone*, November 17, 1988, 47.

SEE ALSO

British Television; Screenwriters

Cheung, Leslie   (1956–2003)

Leslie Cheung first gained legions of fans in Asia as a pop singer. He went on to a successful career as an actor, appearing in sixty films, including the award-winning *Farewell My Concubine* (1993). Androgynously handsome, he sometimes played sexually ambiguous characters, as well as romantic leads in both gay- and heterosexually-themed films.

Leslie Cheung, born Cheung Kwok-wing on September 12, 1956, was the tenth and youngest child of a Hong Kong tailor whose clients included Alfred Hitchcock and William Holden.

At the age of twelve, Cheung was sent to boarding school in England. There he adopted the English name Leslie, in part because he admired Leslie Howard in *Gone with the Wind*, but also because the name is "very unisex."

Cheung studied textiles at Leeds University, but when he returned to Hong Kong, he did not go into his father's profession. He entered a music talent contest on a Hong Kong television station and took second prize with his rendition of Don McLean's "American Pie."

His appearance in the contest led to acting roles in soap operas and drama series, and also launched his singing career. His first album, *The Wind Blows On* (1981), was a best seller in Asia and established him as a rising star in the "Cantopop" style. He would eventually make over twenty albums in Cantonese and Mandarin.

Quickly gaining an enthusiastic fan following, Cheung played concerts in packed theaters, auditoriums, and stadiums. Although never as well known in North America, Cheung drew full houses for his concerts at Caesars Palace in Las Vegas in 2000, for which tickets cost as much as $238.

Beginning in the late 1970s, Cheung also pursued a movie career. His first film was the soft-porn *Erotic Dream of the Red Chamber* (1978).

In his next film, Patrick Tam's *Nomad* (1982), Cheung played a young man fixated on his mother. The initial version included a scene in which Cheung's character, clad only in underwear, fondled himself while talking on the telephone with his mother. Hong Kong censors objected, and the scene had to be reshot with Cheung in trousers.

Cheung had a featured role as a rookie policeman in John Woo's 1986 crime thriller *A Better Tomorrow*, one of the films that established the Hong Kong action genre. He also appeared in the movie's two sequels (1987 and 1989).

In 1989, Cheung was one of the stars of Stanley Kwan's *Rouge*, a stylish drama in which he played a young man who falls in love with a courtesan who is dressed as a man when he first encounters her. The young man reneges on a suicide pact with his sweetheart, whose ghost returns to visit him fifty years later.

Cheung also starred in Wong Kar-Wai's *Days of Being Wild* (1990), this time as a callous, womanizing playboy, a role that earned him the Best Actor Prize at the Hong Kong Film Awards.

Shortly after this success, Cheung announced his retirement from his singing career and moved to Vancouver, British Columbia, for a period.

The actor next went to China to make Chen Kaige's *Farewell My Concubine* (1993). The film won the Palme d'Or at the Cannes Film Festival and was nominated for an Academy Award for Best Foreign Film, but was banned in China because of its homosexual theme.

In *Farewell My Concubine*, Cheung played a young actor at the Peking Opera who specializes in women's roles. This was in accordance with the Opera's tradition that all characters, male and female, be portrayed by men. In preparation for his role, Cheung spent months studying the conventional movements and gestures used by the Opera's actors for such parts. He also learned the dialect of Beijing for the film.

Cheung's character in *Farewell My Concubine* is a boy who is made to chant "I am by nature a girl, not a boy" to prepare him for a career impersonating women. The youth is befriended by one of the Opera's leading men, of whom he becomes enamored. Critic Jay Carr called Cheung's performance the "most affecting and unceasingly fascinating" of the film.

Cheung next appeared in Peter Chan's gender-bending comedy *He's a Woman, She's a Man* (1995), playing a man who falls in love with a woman disguised as a man.

In Chen Kaige's *Temptress Moon* (1996), Cheung starred as an unsympathetic heterosexual character, a manipulative, blackmailing gigolo. Although the film was considered somewhat flawed, critic Stephen Holden described Cheung's performance as "arresting."

Cheung played one of a pair of gay lovers in Wong Kar-Wai's *Happy Together* (1997), an ironically titled piece because the couple, who make a trip to Argentina to rekindle their relationship, fail to find their longed-for happiness.

Cheung's personal situation was more fortunate. After making *Happy Together*, he came out publicly and acknowledged his lover, Tong Hock Tak, a banker. Speculation about Cheung's sexual orientation had been rife for some years, but he had always dodged questions, fearing that revealing his relationship might be deleterious to Tong's career. By this time, however, Cheung's fortune—skillfully managed by Tong—had grown to the point that Tong was able to retire from his job.

Still, coming out was not without risk for Cheung, since very few star Asian entertainers are openly gay. In Cheung's case, as the journalist Ronald Bergan reported, "the move did nothing to diminish his following; it only increased it."

In the late 1990s, Cheung resumed his singing career. His comeback album, *Legend* (1997), was a great success, and several more best sellers followed. He returned to the concert stage as well, and in 2000 played a year-long "Passion" tour, described by Allan Hunter as "noted for the kind of spectacular costume changes and flamboyant attitude that would have made Liberace seem self-effacing." His onstage wardrobe featured eight outfits by Jean-Paul Gaultier, including a white tuxedo with angel wings, gold hot pants, and a "naughty skirt."

In reviving his singing career Cheung made music videos, one of which featured a *pas de deux* with a Japanese male ballet dancer so sexy that it was banned by Hong Kong's top channel, TVB.

In his last film, Law Chi-Leung's *Inner Senses* (2002), Cheung played a psychiatrist tempted by evil spirits to kill himself.

Thus, fans who heard of Cheung's suicide on April 1, 2003, hoped at first that the story might be a macabre April Fool's Day joke. But soon they learned that Cheung had indeed taken his own life by jumping from a twenty-fourth-floor balcony at Hong Kong's Mandarin Oriental Hotel.

Cheung had long suffered from depression and reportedly had tried to commit suicide the previous year by taking an overdose of sleeping pills. He left a note in which he thanked Tong, his family, and his friends, but concluded poignantly, "I have not done one single bad thing in my life. Why is it like that?"

Disconsolate fans quickly created a shrine at the spot of Cheung's death. Their memorial offerings of flowers, notes, personal mementos, and photographs covered half a block. Admirers of all ages joined in paying tribute to the popular artist.

—*Linda Rapp*

Bibliography

Bergan, Ronald. "Leslie Cheung: Asian Actor and Pop Star Famed for His Androgynous Performances on Stage and Screen." *Guardian* (London), April 5, 2003.

Carr, Jay. "'Farewell My Concubine' Holds an Unflattering Mirror to China." *Boston Globe*, October 29, 1993.

Corliss, Richard, and Stephen Short. "Forever Leslie." *Time* (International Edition), May 7, 2001, 44.

Goodman, Peter S. "Farewell to a Troubled Star and a City's High Times." *Washington Post*, April 5, 2003.

Hartl, John. "'Farewell My Concubine' Latest Film to Explore World of Sexual Ambiguity—a First for China." *Seattle Times*, October 24, 1993.

Holden, Stephen. "A 'Gone with the Wind' in China, without War." *New York Times*, October 5, 1996.

Hunter, Allan. "Leslie Cheung." *Scotsman*, April 3, 2003.

Mizui, Yoko. "Gender Bender from H.K." *Daily Yomiuri*, November 30, 1995.

Rayns, Tony. "Leslie Cheung; Pop singer and star of 'Farewell My Concubine.'" *Independent* (London), April 3, 2003.

Stuart, Jan. "Happy Together." *Advocate*, November 11, 1997, 67.

See also

Hong Kong Film; Film Actors: Gay Male; Liberace

Cho, Margaret   (b. 1968)

"COMEDY WAS ALL I EVER WANTED," MARGARET CHO declares in her memoir *I'm the One That I Want* (2001). "When I began, I don't think anyone believed I would go anywhere." But the bisexual actress turned stand-up comedian has become one of the most prominent Asian Americans in show business and in glbtq culture.

Born to Korean immigrant parents on December 5, 1968, in San Francisco, Moran "Margaret" Cho draws from her bicultural experience as Korean American as well as from everyday queer culture to forge her seductive style, which is enticing and amusing and never fails to surprise.

Her humor is a distinctively witty and candid kind of truth telling. It is funny, yet it is also enlightening; it teaches even as it amuses.

For Cho, comedy offers the occasion for good laughs while it also allows her the freedom to contest, reverse, and play with stereotypes. It also helps her make sense of her sexual, racial, and ethnic differences, which she says often come in direct conflict with her self-identified Americanness—an identity that is often denied her because of the shape of her face and character of her eyes.

Comedy thus helps Cho deal with the pain of racism and discrimination, as it also helped her deal with drug addiction, a false haven that eased her pain temporarily but almost destroyed her life.

Cho inherited her comedic gift from her father, who writes joke books in Korean—though Cho admits she is often unaffected by Korean jokes and by written Korean because of her American upbringing. She describes Korean script, for example, as "looking like a bunch of sticks" on the page.

Cho draws from her experience as an assimilated daughter of more traditional parents to educate Americans about generational cleavages among grandparents, parents, and teenagers—prominent themes in Asian American literature and an arresting focus in her own book.

Cho emphasizes that she eats with a fork and not with chopsticks. Her point is that being Korean does not necessitate using chopsticks any more than eating tortillas and tacos indicates that one is Latina.

Hence, when Cho performed before an appreciative crowd at Carnegie Hall, she joked about being the first Korean American to set foot on the stage "without a violin."

Yet Cho has not always enjoyed stardom and prestigious venues. Indeed, she has had to deal with the cold fact that roles for Asian Americans are limited. She has had to fight to overcome stereotypical casting, a problem that people of color often face.

Cho's penchant for comedy commenced in San Francisco, when she entered the McAteer High School of the Performing Arts, aspiring to be an actress. Her first professional performance was at a comedy club, where she appeared as part of the Batwing Lubricant, her high school improv collective. Upon graduation in 1988, Cho studied theater at San Francisco State University, but soon left to pursue her real passion, stand-up comedy.

Cho perfected her talent at the Rose & Thistle, a stand-up comedy club above a bookstore her parents ran in San Francisco. Then she won a comedy contest whose first prize was opening for Jerry Seinfeld.

She soon took her show across the country. She appeared at malls, colleges, theaters, and comedy clubs. She became especially popular on the college circuit, performing hundreds of concerts. This trajectory led to her "discovery," with showcase clips of her act on A&E, Fox television, MTV, and VH1, and to performance stints on *The Montel Williams Show* and *Star Search International*, where she represented Korea (despite being an American citizen).

In 1994, Cho burst into the big time with the ABC sitcom *All-American Girl*, the first comedy show about an Asian American family. Although it was supposedly based on her life and on her stand-up comedy show, the producers attempted to remake her to fit their stereotypical expectations.

In many ways, the show was a disaster, both professionally and personally, but it brought her to national attention and it provided fodder for her comic mill.

Asked by the producers of *All-American Girl* to lose weight, Cho dropped forty pounds in two weeks before filming the debut episode. The night after filming was completed, her kidneys collapsed. She was also coached to become more "Asian" in the same fashion that she was showcased as "foreign" and asked to be more "Chinese" by the talent coordinator of *Star Search International*.

These attempts to make her fit within preconceived categories have fueled her protests against demands for ethnic stereotypes and against arbitrary standards of beauty and body image.

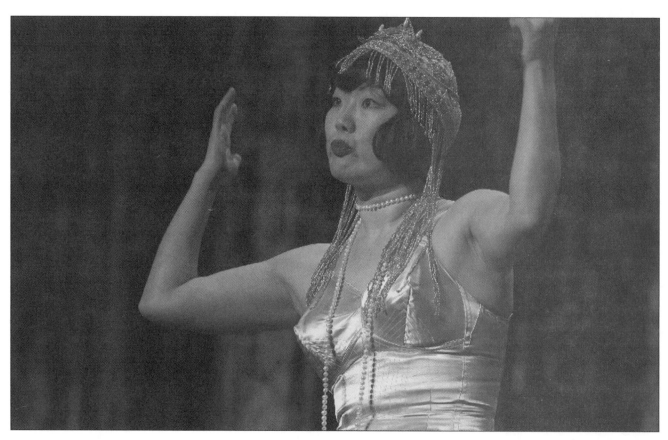

Margaret Cho. Photograph by Phil Nee.

After the cancellation of *All-American Girl*, Cho was almost destroyed by a bout of alcohol abuse and drug addiction. But she resumed her stand-up comedy career and appeared in several films, the most notable of which was Randall Kleiser's poignant *It's My Party* (1996), where she plays the best friend of a gay architect suffering from AIDS.

Frustrated by the paucity of good film and stage roles being offered her, Cho wrote her own one-woman show and scored a triumph. *I'm the One That I Want* (1999) addresses critical issues of race, gender, sexuality, AIDS, and drug and alcohol addiction even as it showcases her comedy. The show toured the country, attracting a diverse audience. It was subsequently released as an independent film.

Notorious C.H.O. (2002), her second one-woman show, has also been successful both in the theater and onscreen. Somewhat edgier and raunchier than her previous show, *Notorious C.H.O.* puts a distinctively female spin on machismo.

In 2003, Cho embarked on her third sold-out national tour, *Revolution*. The CD of *Revolution*, released in the fall of 2003, was nominated for a Grammy for best comedy album of the year. The concert film *Revolution* premiered on Sundance Channel in June 2004 and was released on DVD in August.

Cho's most topical work to date is her show *State of Emergency* (2004), designed to motivate people to vote in the 2004 presidential election.

Cho is the proud recipient of the first Golden Gate Award, given by the Gay and Lesbian Alliance Against Defamation (GLAAD), a distinction she shares with Elton John and Elizabeth Taylor. The citation recognizes her as "an entertainment pioneer who has made a significant difference in promoting equal rights for all, regardless of sexual orientation or gender identity."

—*Miguel A. Segovia*

BIBLIOGRAPHY

Cho, Margaret. *I'm the One That I Want*. New York: Ballantine Books, 2001.

Gan, Geraldine. *Lives of Notable Asian Americans: Arts, Entertainment, Sports*. New York: Chelsea House Publishers, 1995. 103–112.

www.margaretcho.com

SEE ALSO

American Television: Situation Comedies; Film Actors: Lesbian; Wong, B. D.

Clift, Montgomery   *(1920–1966)*

BROODING AND INTENSE, MONTGOMERY CLIFT WAS ONE of a group of young actors in the 1950s who personified the emotionally repressed loss of innocence of the post–World War II generation. A dedicated actor who exhausted himself both emotionally and physically with the depth of his characterizations, Clift was also an isolated and tortured, closeted gay man who used drugs and alcohol to escape his pain.

Although he was both friend and inspiration to the likes of Marlon Brando and James Dean, Clift felt his own acting achievements were undervalued, and he died as bitter and broken as the characters he played in many of his films.

Clift was born into privilege in Omaha, Nebraska, on October 17, 1920, the son of a wealthy stockbroker. His father spent most of his time working in New York, leaving Clift, his twin sister Roberta, and his older brother Brooks in the care of their high-strung mother.

An upper-class childhood filled with lengthy trips to Europe and the Bahamas ended suddenly with the stock market crash of 1929, and the family moved to a small house in Sarasota, Florida. There Clift discovered the theater in a local teen acting club.

Clift's mother encouraged her son's acting ambitions, and when the family moved back to New York in 1935

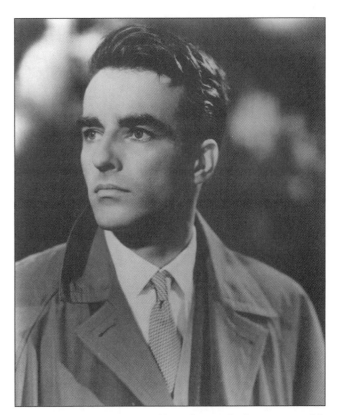

A Columbia Pictures publicity photograph of Montgomery Clift.

he auditioned and was cast in a Broadway production, *Fly Away Home*. His 1938 performance in the male lead in *Dame Nature* established Clift's acting career. He was seventeen years old.

Clift's success on Broadway continued, and he soon found himself courted by Hollywood film executives. He rejected a number of scripts before finally making a memorable film debut in Howard Hawks's 1948 film *Red River*. He followed that with a critical success in Fred Zinneman's *The Search* (1948), which earned him the first of four Academy Award nominations.

Clift continued to make successful films and developed friendships in Hollywood, the closest of which was with actress Elizabeth Taylor. Taylor and Clift were both passionate and vulnerable people who felt a bond immediately. They worked together on several films, beginning with George Stevens's *A Place in the Sun* in 1951, and remained friends until the end of his life.

Clift had always had relationships with men, but he dated Taylor and other women to conceal his homosexuality. In the early 1950s, he turned down a role in Alfred Hitchcock's *Rope*, based on the infamous Leopold and Loeb gay murder case, probably because it might have led to speculation about Clift's own life.

Although at the beginning of his career he drank only moderately and conducted his private life discreetly, by the mid-1950s he was using alcohol and drugs excessively and spending wild nights cruising.

In 1954, Clift rented a house in the gay resort of Ogunquit, Maine, and spent the summer picking up men on the beach for S/M parties. The studios did their best to keep Clift's exploits out of the press, but rumors about his lifestyle abounded.

On May 12, 1956, after leaving a party at Taylor's house in Beverly Hills, Clift drove his car into a telephone pole. The crash caused scarring and partial paralysis of his face, which would affect his appearance for the rest of his life. Although he continued to act, and gave some of his most memorable performances after the accident (in, for example, Stanley Kramer's *Judgment at Nuremberg* and John Huston's *The Misfits*, both in 1961), both his expressive acting and his personal life were never the same.

In his final years, Clift plunged more deeply into drug and alcohol abuse and wild sexual behavior. He began to be considered unreliable by studio bosses. Sadly, by the time his companion, Lorenzo James, found him dead of a heart attack at their home, on July 23, 1966, he was virtually unemployable.
                                                                    —*Tina Gianoulis*

BIBLIOGRAPHY

Finch, Stephen. "The Montgomery Clift Shrine: A Celebration of a Great Movie Star." www.montyclift.com/shrine/

Hoskyns, Barney. *Montgomery Clift, Beautiful Loser*. New York: Grove/Atlantic, 1992.

Kalfatovic, Mary C. *Montgomery Clift*. Westport, Conn.: Greenwood, 1994.

LaGuardia, Robert. *Monty: A Biography of Montgomery Clift*. New York: Arbor House, 1977.

Purtell, Tim. "No Place in the Sun." *Entertainment Weekly*, July 23, 1993, 76.

SEE ALSO

Film; Film Actors: Gay Male; Dean, James

Cocteau, Jean   (1889–1963)

A PROLIFIC POET, ARTIST, PLAYWRIGHT, ACTOR, AND filmmaker, Jean Cocteau published his first poems in his early twenties. He established his reputation, as both respected artist and popular Parisian man-about-town, with the success of several ballet scenarios and plays that he wrote in his late twenties. But today he is best remembered as one of France's most important filmmakers.

Born into a middle-class family on July 5, 1889, Cocteau was orphaned at age ten, when his father died. After the death of a classmate whom he idolized, and whose memory haunted him for the rest of his life, Cocteau ran away from Paris to Marseille, where he lived among sailors and prostitutes, before returning to Paris, where he quickly became established as a promising young poet. He soon became associated with Sergei Diaghilev and the Ballets Russes, for whom he wrote scenarios for several ballets, including *Parade* (1917), with sets by Picasso and music by Satie.

Although his formal schooling was ragged, Cocteau educated himself through his wide reading and extensive travel. In the early 1920s, Cocteau's lover, novelist Raymond Radiguet, died of typhoid fever; the despondent Cocteau, reportedly to escape the pain of this loss, soon after began using opium.

In 1930, the poet broached filmmaking, which critics often cite as the medium best suited for his artistic expression. For instance, in *Le sang d'un poète* (*Blood of a Poet*, 1930), a stylized, homoerotic short feature about the arduousness of poetic creation, characters come to life out of Cocteau's own characteristic drawings—bold, simple strokes, accentuated eyes, minimalist outlines and profiles, and erotic, surrealistic portraits—which dominate the sets.

In his later films, Cocteau includes portions of his poetry written in his distinctive handwriting, samples of his drawings and paintings, narration in his own voice, and even himself in pivotal roles.

Frequently marked by whimsical special effects and exotic landscapes, Cocteau's films—at times adaptations

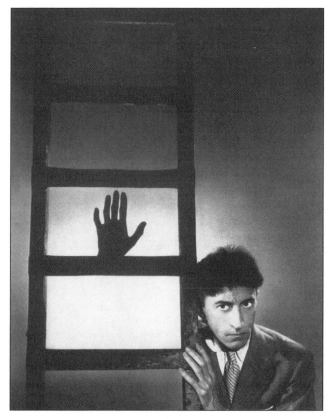

A photograph of Jean Cocteau by George Platt Lynes.

of his own literary works, such as *L'aigle à deux têtes* (1947) and *Orphée* (1950)—contain themes and symbols common to the entirety of the artist's oeuvre, such as narcissism, the Orpheus myth, poetic creation, mirrors and other passages to secret worlds, fairy tales, flowers, and beautiful people in iconographic settings.

In 1937, Cocteau met Jean Marais, the most famous of his lovers, and helped make his talented, handsome, and athletic protégé into one of France's most beloved cinema stars. Among the notable films that Cocteau made with Marais are such classics as *La belle et la bête* (*Beauty and the Beast*, 1946) and *Orphée*.

Cocteau's cinema demonstrates the artist's mastery of spectacular imagery. His cinepoems do not rely on a large studio system or fixed, narrative structures, but on his independent vision and experimentation.

Homoeroticism pervades Cocteau's films, especially through the featuring of attractive men and the suggestive depictions of their relationships. For instance, at the beginning of *Orphée*, Cocteau frames the Orphée and Cégeste characters (played by Marais and Edouard Dermit, Cocteau's last protégé and official heir) under a threshold as the two exchange a lingering gaze before crossing paths. Then, as the film progresses, Orphée becomes obsessed with listening to Cégeste's voice over a mysterious radio.

With Marais, Cocteau contributed to the rebirth of the French cinema industry during and after World War II. At the same time, the artist endured criticism, usually unfair and homophobic in nature, for not taking a more active stance in the French Resistance. Although Cocteau encouraged artists to speak out against unjust political domination, he himself was disadvantaged by the open secrets of his opium use and homosexuality, which made him particularly vulnerable to attack by the right-wing Vichy government.

During the Nazi Occupation, Cocteau's plays were interrupted or banned outright, and Cocteau himself experienced physical violence and homophobic insults. Despite such difficulties, Cocteau wrote, made films, traveled, and attracted famous friends, patrons, and protégés during this period and throughout the rest of his life.

Cocteau received numerous awards and honors, including election to the prestigious Académie Française. The artist died while recovering from a heart attack, on October 11, 1963, one hour after learning of singer Édith Piaf's death. Cocteau continues to this day as one of France's most famous, and most adored, cultural icons.

—*David Aldstadt*

BIBLIOGRAPHY

Anderson, Alexandra, and Carol Saltrus, eds. *Jean Cocteau and the French Scene.* New York: Abbeville, 1984.

Cocteau, Jean. *Cocteau on the Film: Conversations with Jean Cocteau Recorded by André Fraigneau.* Trans. Vera Traill. New York: Dover, 1972.

Evans, Arthur. *Jean Cocteau and His Films of Orphic Identity.* Philadelphia: Art Alliance Press, 1977.

Steegmuller, Francis. *Cocteau.* Boston: Little Brown and Company, 1970.

Touzot, Jean. *Jean Cocteau.* Lyon: La Manufacture, 1989.

SEE ALSO

European Film; Film Directors; Set and Costume Design; Anger, Kenneth; Marais, Jean

Collard, Cyril (1957–1993)

FRENCH WRITER, FILMMAKER, AND ACTOR CYRIL Collard was among the first artists in France to announce publicly his HIV-positive status. Along with writers Vincent Borel and Guillaume Dustan, he became a key figure in the struggle to revise attitudes toward AIDS in art. Principally known for his highly controversial autobiographical novel and subsequent film *Les nuits fauves* (*Savage Nights*), Collard also garnered a great deal of critical acclaim in France and England for his unapologetic portrayals of both bisexuality and HIV.

Collard came from a liberal, bourgeois family and received a Catholic education in Versailles. Aside from his decision to drop out of the University of Lille, where he had been pursuing a science degree, his youth was lived relatively predictably.

He traveled extensively with his father, and it was a father–son trip to Puerto Rico for the Pan American Games in 1979 that truly awakened Collard's artistic potential as well as his burgeoning sexuality. Collard stayed on to write in Puerto Rico after his father's departure, and there he began to realize fully his bisexuality—a theme he would address in most of his later works.

Upon his return to Paris, Collard began work in the film world. Claude Davy, who served as mentor to Collard, introduced him to directors Maurice Pialat and René Allio, and Collard acted as assistant director and actor in À nos amours, a 1983 film by Pialat. From there, Collard went on to direct his first short film, an exploration of violence, race, and passions entitled Alger la blanche. Also a musician, Collard created the score for his television film Taggers in 1986, a work that explored the world of young graffiti artists.

Condamné amour, the first of Collard's two autobiographical novels, appeared in 1987. Reflecting his knowledge of his HIV-positive status, the novel explores a young man's physical and spiritual crisis when confronted with an unnamed "divine virus."

Two years later, Collard published Les nuits fauves. (The English translation, Savage Nights, was published in 1994.) The main themes of Les nuits fauves are bisexuality and the search for meaning in contemporary life in the shadow of AIDS. Because of its unsentimental—even defiant—portrayal of sexuality and AIDS, it has been immensely influential on French representations of the disease.

Collard himself wrote and starred in the film based on Les nuits fauves. In the movie, Collard plays the lead role of Jean, a self-absorbed thirty-year-old filmmaker. Jean, whose male-oriented sexuality shifts when he meets Laura, a seventeen-year-old actress, is HIV-positive but refuses to change his risky habits. He becomes involved with Laura—neglecting to mention his illness despite having unprotected sex with her—while sleeping with a boy named Samy throughout the relationship.

The film demonstrates a remarkable honesty and grit in its lack of sentimentality toward the less-than-heroic character of Jean, as well as toward AIDS itself. The controversy sparked by the book and film was only magnified by the fact that the woman on whom Laura was based contracted HIV herself and later died of AIDS-related illnesses.

Savage Nights was, alas, not only Collard's first full-length film but also his last. It won four Césars—the prestigious French equivalent of the Oscars—in 1992, including Best Film, Best First Film, Best Editing, and Best Female Newcomer (for Romane Bohringer as Laura). The awards were announced a mere seventy-two hours after Collard's death at age thirty-five, from HIV-related complications, on March 5, 1993.

The following year, Flammarion published a collection of Collard's poems, entitled L'animal.   —Teresa Theophano

BIBLIOGRAPHY

Bülow, Louis. "Cyril Collard—Savage Nights..." www.auschwitz.dk/Collard.htm

Collard, Cyril. Savage Nights. Woodstock, N.Y.: Overlook Press, 1994.

Robinson, Christopher. "Collard, Cyril." Who's Who in Contemporary Gay and Lesbian History: From World War II to the Present Day. Robert Aldrich and Garry Wotherspoon, eds. London: Routledge, 2001. 87–88.

SEE ALSO

Film; Film Directors

Condon, William "Bill"   (b. 1955)

BILL CONDON HAS EARNED CRITICAL ACCLAIM FOR directing and writing the films Gods and Monsters, about openly gay director James Whale, and Kinsey, on the life of the famed sex researcher. Among Condon's other writing credits is the Academy Award–nominated script for the movie musical Chicago.

William Condon was born October 22, 1955, into an Irish Catholic family in Queens, New York. He attended Regis High School, an all-male Jesuit institution in Manhattan. As he remarked in an interview, he found high school "liberating" since "the priests were much more radical than you could ever hope to be," especially in actively opposing the war in Vietnam.

In his sophomore year of high school Condon began his first serious romance, a two-year relationship with a young man in the class ahead of his. Condon's parents eventually learned of the love affair and spoke about it at first, but subsequently "it was never talked about," Condon recalled.

Condon earned a bachelor's degree in philosophy from Columbia University. Following his graduation in 1976, he moved to Los Angeles, planning to establish residency and then pursue film studies at UCLA.

In the interim, Condon began freelancing as a writer. One of his articles in the movie periodical Millimeter caught the eye of British producer Michael Laughlin, who hired him to write scripts for two horror films, Strange Behavior (1981) and Strange Invaders (1983), both of which Laughlin directed. Although Strange Behavior was set in Illinois, it was filmed in New Zealand, so all the Americans on hand were pressed into service for bit parts. Thus, Condon made his screen debut as the first victim of a mad doctor. He has since appeared occasionally in other movies.

Condon continued in the horror genre, revising a screenplay originally titled *The Louisiana Swamp Murders* into a movie called *Sister, Sister* that he directed in 1987. The film flopped, putting Condon into what he described as "film director's jail"—making movies, including crime thrillers such as *Murder 101* (1991), for cable television, some of which he produced as well as wrote and directed.

After several such efforts he returned to the big screen with the 1994 film *Candyman: Farewell to the Flesh*, which was based on a short story by Clive Barker, whom he met during the shooting of the movie in New Orleans.

Making *Candyman* was a turning point in Condon's career. He learned about financing independent films, and the contacts that he made helped him secure the movie rights to Christopher Bram's novel *Father of Frankenstein*, about director James Whale. Barker agreed to serve as executive producer of the film, which was realized as *Gods and Monsters* in 1998.

Bringing the project to fruition was a considerable challenge. Condon was disappointed that although the distinguished actor Sir Ian McKellen was slated to play Whale, even production companies that had previously backed films with gay themes showed little interest in funding *Gods and Monsters*. Eventually a small company, Lion's Gate, provided a $3 million budget—modest by Hollywood standards—and the film was shot in a mere four weeks. The demanding schedule was necessary because of McKellen's pending commitment to appear at the National Theatre in London.

McKellen, then fifty-nine, was at first reluctant to play the septuagenarian Whale, since he had recently accepted another role as an older man and was afraid of becoming typecast. Condon allayed his fears by pointing out that he would also be playing Whale in his forties in flashback scenes. Upon seeing a picture of the fortysomething Whale, McKellen declared him "rather dishy," and the die was cast.

Other actors in the film include sweet-natured hunk Brendan Fraser, somewhat miscast as the young gardener who Whale hopes will assist him in committing suicide, Lolita Davidovich as the gardener's girlfriend, and Lynn Redgrave as Whale's devoted Hungarian housekeeper, who fears that "Mister Jimmy" will go to hell because he is gay.

Gods and Monsters opened to enthusiastic critical response, winning numerous awards at film festivals. When the Academy Awards for the year were given out, McKellen's extraordinary performance was overlooked, but Condon's script earned him an Oscar for Best Adapted Screenplay.

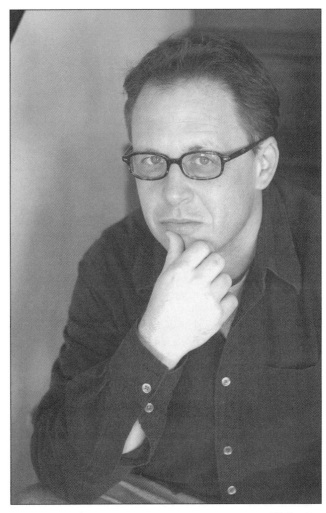

Bill Condon.

Condon received a second Academy Award nomination for the superb script that translated the cynical Kander and Ebb musical hit *Chicago* from the stage to the screen. Rob Marshall directed the movie version in 2002.

Acclaimed as the best movie musical in years, *Chicago* is actually the product of the collaboration of several out gay men, including—in addition to Condon and Marshall—executive producers Neil Meron and Craig Zadan. Winner of the Academy Award for Best Motion Picture of the year, it may have done more than any other recent film to resurrect the musical as a viable film genre.

Condon's most recent project is *Kinsey* (2004), a film biography of the legendary sex researcher Alfred Kinsey, which he both wrote and directed. Featuring brilliant performances by Liam Neeson as Kinsey and Laura Linney as Kinsey's wife, Clara Bracken MacMillen, the film explores the contradictions of the scientist's complex personality and recreates the conditions under which he conducted his pioneering research.

A crucial element of *Kinsey* is its depiction of the sexual relationship between Kinsey and his younger associate Clyde Martin (Peter Sarsgaard), who also had an affair with Kinsey's wife. As he began his film, Condon said, he was skeptical about the concept of bisexuality and "less comfortable with the idea than [he] knew [he] was." In the course of making the film, however, he came to understand Kinsey as "really someone who moved on that scale"—a reference to the measurement that Kinsey devised to describe human sexual behavior, with 0 denoting exclusively heterosexual activity and 6 exclusively homosexual.

Condon said in a 2004 interview in the *Advocate*, "It was very important for me as a gay filmmaker that *Kinsey* not be a movie that could be typed exclusively as a gay film." He stated that he sees Kinsey as "truly one of the fathers of the gay movement," but added, "Because Kinsey didn't believe in labels and because he spoke to everybody, I didn't want it to dominate."

What does dominate in *Kinsey* are the ideas that every individual's sexuality is different, that diversity is valuable, and that tolerance in sexual matters is an enormous virtue. Thus, it is entirely appropriate that a movie telling the story of the man who pioneered in collecting other people's sexual histories be structured as Kinsey's own sexual history, and that that history be presented in as nonjudgmental a way as Kinsey presented the histories of his subjects.

Condon saw a parallel between Kinsey and Whale, in that for each man there was a "deep connection between his personal life and the work for which he's famous." Moreover, he felt "a certain personal connection" with Kinsey, "having grown up in an Irish Catholic household with a father who was very kind but also very skittish about any mention of sex."

Indeed, one of the real virtues of *Kinsey* is that it recognizes the enormous contribution the sex researcher made by helping dispel some of America's widespread ignorance and skittishness about sex, including male homosexuality in particular and female sexuality in general. Among the consequences of his work was to question the notion of "normality" in sexual behavior and to reassure sexual minorities that they were not alone.

Precisely because he told the truth about the disparity between Americans' actual sexual behavior and the rigid social and legal codes intended to regulate it, Kinsey exposed the national hypocrisy in regard to sex and helped liberate individuals from the tyranny of convention. His role as liberator is touchingly dramatized in the movie by a scene between the ill scientist and a lesbian (portrayed by Lynn Redgrave) who thanks him for having made her life altogether better. For being a liberator, however, Kinsey paid a heavy price.

As the film documents, after the publication of Kinsey's landmark books on male and female sexual behavior, he was vilified by political and religious leaders, who in effect hounded him to his death. Even today religious and social conservatives continue to defame the man and his research, accusing him of everything from condoning pedophilia to practicing "junk science" (an epithet far more applicable to their own pseudoscientific approaches than to Kinsey). Luckily, their homophobic campaign to boycott Condon's film is likely to garner greater publicity for it and increase attendance, which may in turn lead to greater appreciation for Kinsey and his remarkable achievement.

Condon lives in Los Angeles with his life partner, who is a screenwriter and director. The couple have been together since the mid-1990s.

In addition to writing and directing, Condon is on the board of IFP/Los Angeles, an association for independent filmmakers, and is also a founding member of the Independent Writers Steering Committee of the Writers Guild of America.

Since he has made films about Whale and Kinsey, Condon has found himself described as a "homosexual activist," a designation with which he is not entirely comfortable. "I'm proud to wear those stripes," he says, adding, "I just haven't done enough to earn them."

—Linda Rapp
—Claude Summers

BIBLIOGRAPHY

Arnold, Gary. "From Monster to Godlike Films?; The Low-Budget Adventures of a Director." *Washington Times*, November 22, 1998.

Hartl, John. "'Monsters' Brings Unlikely Success to Indie Director." *Seattle Times*, November 15, 1998.

Rosen, Steven. "'Gods' Gives Filmmaker His Just Due; 'Best Picture' Designation Puts Light on an Unknown." *Seattle Times*, December 13, 1998.

Steele, Bruce C. "Bill & Al's Excellent Adventure." *Advocate*, November 23, 2004, 70.

Vargas, Jose Antonio. "Naked Contradictions; 'Kinsey' Creator Analyzes the Famed Sex Researcher." *Washington Post*, November 20, 2004.

SEE ALSO

Film Directors; Screenwriters; Barker, Clive; McKellen, Sir Ian; Whale, James

Crisp, Quentin   (1908–1999)

ACTOR, WRITER, PERFORMANCE ARTIST, AND WIT Quentin Crisp described himself as "one of the stately homos of England" and "not merely a self-confessed homosexual, but a self-evident one." He became a celebrity in England as a result of his extraordinary autobiography, *The Naked Civil Servant* (1968), and a celebrity in the United States when its dramatization as a television movie starring John Hurt was broadcast in New York in 1976.

Crisp was born Denis Charles Pratt on December 25, 1908, the youngest of four children of a solicitor and a nursery governess. He was educated at a minor public school in Staffordshire and then took art courses at Battersea Polytechnic and High Whitcomb.

As a young man in London, he supported himself in a variety of ways, including designing book covers, freelancing as a commercial artist, and occasionally working as a prostitute and a tap-dancing teacher. During World War II, exempt from military service because of his open homosexuality, he was employed by a government-funded art school as a nude model. Hence he became a "naked civil servant," as he entitled his autobiography.

Because his homosexuality was so self-evident, as epitomized by his effeminacy, hennaed hair, long fingernails, and makeup, Crisp not only became a London "character" in the 1930s and 1940s, but frequently aroused the anger of total strangers, who sometimes attacked him physically, beating and spitting upon him, simply for being who he was.

In this sense, his crusade of making visible the existence of effeminate homosexual men certainly succeeded, though at a high cost in self-esteem and safety.

Published in 1968, only one year after the Sexual Offences Act partially decriminalized male homosexual acts in private in Great Britain, *The Naked Civil Servant* made Crisp famous (or, as he would say, notorious) in England.

Perhaps the first modern, unapologetic, noneuphemistic, uncoded account of the life of a living homosexual, *The Naked Civil Servant* presented Crisp's flamboyant (but self-denigrating) personality, and his arch—sometimes sardonic—observations about English society and conventions, straightforwardly yet wittily and unsentimentally.

Its success was greatly multiplied when it was made into a television movie in 1975, featuring a dazzling performance by John Hurt in the title role.

The Naked Civil Servant vividly documents the indignities and absurdities to which a certain kind of homosexual was subject in pre–gay liberation Britain. It also, however, partakes of many of the same homophobic attitudes that contributed to the persecution of homosexuals.

Although he thought that by wearing cosmetics he "managed to shift homosexuality from being a burden to being a cause," Crisp clearly also himself thought of homosexuality as unnatural, and he internalized many of the most damaging stereotypes about homosexuals, including the notion that homosexuals are mentally ill and inevitably frustrated in their search for love.

While Crisp can hardly be seen as particularly enlightened about homosexuality, he deserves enormous credit for his courage. His refusal to be cowed into the closet and his insistence on his right to live as he chose were significant acts of defiance for which he paid a heavy price.

In the autumn of 1977, Crisp traveled to New York for the first time. Long an admirer of Americans, whom he found to be more generous of spirit and open than his fellow Britons, he determined to live in the city, where the broadcast of *The Naked Civil Servant* the previous year had made him well known in gay circles.

In 1980, at the age of seventy-two, he emigrated to the United States, with the intention of beginning his life anew. He moved into a room on East 3rd Street on Manhattan's Lower East Side and obtained "Resident Alien" status. He always felt grateful to America for the kindness and tolerance that he found there.

In Crisp's American years, he became a fixture on the New York gay scene, as a writer, performance artist, and wit. Even before moving to New York, he had created a one-man show in which he talked about style with only a bentwood chair and a hat stand as props.

For the rest of his life, he would periodically revive (and update) this show. Full of bons mots and witty observations about style (or its absence), the show proved very popular and Crisp often toured with it around the country.

In the 1980s, Crisp also became a film critic and columnist. He wrote film criticism for *Christopher Street* and a column for the *New York Native*. He was to collect many of the columns written for the *Native* in *Resident Alien: The New York Diaries* (1997), a work in which he manages to be both charming and iconoclastic.

Other books from his later years include *How to Have a Life-Style* (1975), *How to Become a Virgin* (1981), and *Manners from Heaven* (1985).

As a writer, and as a persona, Crisp managed to be at once witty and generous. His books are funny, but they are also often penetrating. He himself was unfailingly gracious, but often also relentless in exposing the absurdities and injustices of English and American social mores.

If *The Naked Civil Servant* chronicles the mistreatment and pain (both borne with a stiff upper lip) of his youth in England, his later books stress the contentment he found in America, where life is presented as a comedy of manners.

Crisp also gained fame in his old age as an actor. He appeared as himself in a number of documentary films, including *Resident Alien* (1991), *Naked in New York* (1994), and *The Celluloid Closet* (1995), and in small parts in commercial films, such as *Philadelphia* (1993) and *To Wong Foo, Thanks for Everything, Julie Newmar* (1995).

Perhaps his most interesting performance was as Queen Elizabeth I in *Orlando* (1993), Sally Potter's film based on Virginia Woolf's novel. He also starred opposite Lea DeLaria in Sara Moore's farcical *Homo Heights* (1997).

Crisp's life not only inspired several documentary films, but it was also the subject of a skillfully constructed play. Crisp gave playwright Tim Fountain permission to turn his diaries into a dramatic monologue entitled *Resident Alien*. Performed with style and subtlety by transvestite actor Bette Bourne, a veteran of drag shows, the play enjoyed successful runs on both sides of the Atlantic in 1999 and 2000.

Crisp died in Manchester, England on November 21, 1999, at the age of 90. He suffered a heart attack while on tour with his one-man show, *An Audience with Quentin Crisp*.

Although he lived in notoriously squalid conditions (his theory being that housework was entirely useless: "After the first four years the dirt doesn't get any worse," he quipped), Crisp left an estate valued in excess of $600,000. But his greatest legacy was his example of courage.

Despite the contradictions of his life, particularly the fact that he refused to campaign for homosexual equality and failed to grasp the seriousness of the AIDS epidemic, by the end of his life he had become a beloved figure in glbtq culture.

                                              —*Claude J. Summers*

BIBLIOGRAPHY

Bailey, Paul, ed. *The Stately Homo: A Celebration of the Life of Quentin Crisp.* London: Bantam, 2000.

Robinson, Paul. *Gay Lives: Homosexual Autobiography from John Addington Symonds to Paul Monette.* Chicago: University of Chicago Press, 1999.

www.quentincrisp.com

SEE ALSO

British Television; Film Actors: Gay Male

Crowley, Mart   (b. 1935)

PLAYWRIGHT MART CROWLEY SAW HIS FIRST PLAY, *The Boys in the Band*, become a huge off-Broadway hit that was later adapted as a motion picture. Although a groundbreaking representation of gay men, *The Boys in the Band* is now considered somewhat controversial, partly for the attitudes of the characters and partly for its now anachronistic setting in the age before AIDS.

Crowley is a son of the South. Born in Vicksburg, Mississippi, on August 21, 1935, he used his familiarity with the culture and his personal experience to inform his writing.

Crowley's childhood was not a happy one. His father, a tavernkeeper, was an alcoholic, and his mother, who was addicted to both drugs and alcohol, eventually had to spend considerable time in mental institutions. For a respite from his miserable home life, the young Crowley frequented the local movie theater.

After graduating from a Catholic boys' high school in Vicksburg, Crowley enrolled at Catholic University in Washington, D.C. When he received his degree in theater in 1957, he went to New York, where he became a production assistant to director Elia Kazan on the film *Splendor in the Grass*.

Crowley became friends with the film's star, Natalie Wood, who encouraged him to go to Hollywood to pursue a career in screenwriting.

Crowley succeeded in writing a script that was slated for production, but the project was canceled at the last moment. Other disappointments followed. Crowley wrote the pilot episode for a television series that was to star Bette Davis, but the show was never produced. Next, he got a screenwriting job at Paramount, but was soon fired.

After these setbacks, Crowley wrote a play about a group of gay men while house-sitting for a friend. A friend brought the work to the attention of producer Richard Barr, who ran the Playwrights' Unit with Edward Albee. They agreed to put it on in a workshop in January 1968, and Crowley burst onto the literary scene with his best-known work, *The Boys in the Band*. It opened off-Broadway in April and ran for over a thousand performances. The play was made into a film directed by William Friedkin in 1970.

The Boys in the Band is a groundbreaking work that uses both humor and melodrama to offer a look at the lives of a group of openly gay men. Queer audiences welcomed it when it appeared, but over the years it became controversial. Objections centered on traits of various characters that critics felt perpetuated negative stereotypes—self-loathing, flamboyance, and promiscuity. Rather than offering an upbeat, positive look at the gay subculture, it presented a depressing snapshot of individuals tormented by internalized homophobia.

Set at a birthday party in New York, *The Boys in the Band* introduced audiences to a number of gay men with different attitudes and backgrounds. The birthday celebrant is Jewish, one of the guests African American. Another guest is thoroughly campy and brings a hustler dressed as a cowboy as a birthday gift. The guests also include a couple, one of whom is a divorced father of three. The pair, though committed to each other, are arguing over whether their relationship needs to be exclusive.

At the center of the piece is the host, Michael, the character with whom Crowley most strongly identifies. The cynical and pessimistic Michael has been the focus of many who became detractors of the play in later years. His most famous line, "You show me a happy homosexual, and I'll show you a gay corpse," has often been quoted to indicate the character's self-loathing, and sometimes to indict Crowley for his negative depiction of the period's gay subculture.

Crowley, however, has strongly defended his play, calling it a period piece—from an era before both Stonewall and the AIDS epidemic. He stated in 1996 that the play's "self-deprecating humor was born out of a low self-esteem, if you will; from a sense of what the times told you about yourself." He said that he understood "the need for positive images" and pointed out that "the lovers in the play, Hank and Larry, make a most positive statement about commitment to each other" at the end of the piece. He also called the "flaming and incendiary" character Emory "very positive" because "he never hides who he is, and that's a very brave thing to do."

Certainly, it is true that even today it is difficult for glbtq people to grow up in America without internalizing the homophobic attitudes of the larger society. That would have been even more true for the characters in Crowley's play, most of whom grew up in the 1950s, a decade in which homosexuals were routinely abused and their self-esteem systematically attacked.

Rather than being dismissed for presenting a politically incorrect view of gay men, *The Boys in the Band* should be respected for calling attention to the destructive effects of the pervasive societal homophobia with which gay people in the period before Stonewall had to cope.

Crowley's next play, *Remote Asylum*, was produced in 1970. The comedy received unfavorable notices and quickly closed.

His third play, *A Breeze from the Gulf*, which is based on his memories of growing up in Mississippi, enjoyed a much warmer critical reception but did not find an audience. It had only a six-week run off-Broadway in 1973.

During the 1970s, Crowley lived off his money from *The Boys in the Band*. He stated in 1996 that he "was just running around the world, drinking too much" at the time, and so his funds were dwindling by the end of the decade.

In 1979, Crowley's friend Natalie Wood and her husband, Robert Wagner, helped Crowley get a job as head writer for the television show in which they starred, *Hart to Hart*. When the producer abruptly quit, Crowley replaced him and remained in that post until 1983.

Crowley then returned to work as a screenwriter. "I have original movie scripts in the files of every major studio in Hollywood," he declared in 1993. Although he was successful in selling them, none has ever been produced. He has, however, written some television screenplays that have been produced, including an adaptation of James Kirkwood's *There Must Be a Pony* (1986).

Crowley's next stage play, *Avec Schmaltz* (1984) was written for the Williamstown Theater Festival in Massachusetts. It has not been produced since.

His next play, For *Reasons That Remain Unclear* (1993) deals with the theme of sexual abuse of a student by a Catholic priest. Crowley has stated that the story is a fictionalized version of his own experience. The play was first presented at the Olney Theatre in Maryland. It was optioned for a year, but the production was soon abandoned. The play has since been performed in several regional theaters.

The Boys in the Band was revived in New York in 1996 to mostly favorable reviews and had a respectable run. By the time of the revival Crowley had already let it be known that he was planning a sequel. It was not until 2002, however, that *The Men from the Boys* premiered in San Francisco.

The setting for the sequel is the same New York City apartment that was the site of the birthday party in *The Boys in the Band*. This time it is the venue for a wake for Larry, who has died of pancreatic cancer. Seven of the nine original characters return, and three younger ones have been added.

While reviewers generally found the play entertaining and pointed to some wickedly witty lines by Crowley, they were somewhat disappointed by the lack of evolution of the characters. Critic Dennis Harvey commented

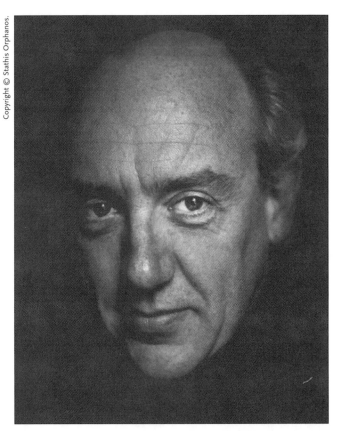

A portrait of Mart Crowley by Stathis Orphanos.

that they "end up defined mostly by the degree to which they've resisted 35 years of social and potential personal change."

While Crowley has never been able to recapture the success and acclaim that he had with his debut play, he deserves honor for having blazed the trail for subsequent gay-themed theater with *The Boys in the Band*.

—*Linda Rapp*

BIBLIOGRAPHY

Bilowit, Ira J. "Mart Crowley on 'The Boys in the Band': From Author's Anguish to NYC Revival." *Back Stage*, June 14, 1996, 17.

Dodds, Richard. "'The Boys' Are Back." *New Orleans Times-Picayune*, July 20, 1996.

Harvey, Dennis. "The Men from the Boys." *Variety*, November 25, 2002, 32.

Richards, David. "Bringing Back 'The Boys'; Will N.Y. Warm to Crowley's Play?" *Washington Post*, June 16, 1996.

Rickard, John. "The Boys in the Band, 30 Years Later." *The Gay & Lesbian Review Worldwide*, March 2001, 9.

Roca, Octavio. "'Boys' to 'Men'; Mart Crowley's Latest Play Takes 'Boys in the Band' through the Past 30 Years." *San Francisco Chronicle*, October 26, 2002.

SEE ALSO

Screenwriters; Film Sissies

Cukor, George   (1899–1983)

GEORGE CUKOR, THE PREEMINENT "WOMAN'S DIRECTOR" and gay auteur of Hollywood's classical era, was born on July 7, 1899, in New York. Cukor evinced an early interest in the theater, becoming a stage manager for a stock company and then on Broadway while still in his teens (1919–1924). From there he graduated to being a stage director of some renown, working with top female stars of the period, including Jeanne Eagels and Ethel Barrymore, from 1925 to 1929.

In 1929, Cukor was part of the wave of Broadway talent that migrated to Hollywood, where he worked as a dialogue coach on other people's films before codirecting one of his own, *Grumpy*, in 1930. Following two more codirecting efforts (with Cukor working with the actors and dialogue and more experienced directors handling the action), he made his first film, *Tarnished Lady* (1931), with Tallulah Bankhead. By 1933, with *Dinner at Eight* and *Little Women*, he was firmly established as a major talent.

Throughout his long career, he worked on prestigious, often stage-derived, productions with the most important stars of the day.

Cukor was responsible for many of the most popular and critically praised films of Hollywood's golden age, including *Camille* (1935), *The Women* (1939), *The Philadelphia Story* (1940), *Born Yesterday* (1950), *A Star Is Born* (1954), and *My Fair Lady* (1964). So skilled was he with actors, but particularly female stars, that he became typed as a "woman's director," a provocative phrase that also spoke obliquely of Cukor's homosexuality.

Many female stars adored Cukor, whom they eagerly sought to work with and counted as a friend. Joan Crawford, for example, who gave her best performances under his demanding eye, insisted on working with him as often as possible. They responded not only to his oft-remarked personal charisma and wit, but also to his ability repeatedly to elicit Oscar-winning performances from them.

However, the director's reputation as a "woman's director" (and homosexual) may have got him kicked off the set of *Gone with the Wind* (1939), when star Clark Gable allegedly said, "I won't be directed by a fairy." (Another version of this story has Gable's refusal to work with Cukor motivated by his belief that the director knew of the actor's own earlier same-sex escapades.) Typical of the loyalty Cukor could generate, however, was Vivien Leigh's continuing to be coached by him despite the objections of Gable and Victor Fleming, who replaced him as director.

Cukor always denied the "charge" of being a "woman's director." He correctly pointed out that in spite of his legendary collaborations with such talents as Crawford, Jean Harlow, Katharine Hepburn, Judy Garland, and Judy Holliday, more men than women had won Oscars for their work in his films.

Cukor's private life was well known within the limits of Hollywood. His Sunday-afternoon pool parties are legendary in queer circles, having been described at lurid length in recent Cukor biographies and published remarks by some of the attendees, such as novelist John Rechy.

These events were studies in egalitarianism, with Cukor and his sophisticated friends socializing with their boyfriends, who were often hustlers, rough trade, would-be actors, or ambitious artists and writers who saw these parties as entrée to the high life.

Cukor's personal reputation has suffered somewhat from these accounts, with Rechy (quoted in David Ehrenstein's *Open Secret*), for example, portraying the "gentleman director" as a catty, sometimes cruel queen who was as gifted at separating his private and public personas as he was at making films.

Not surprising for a semicloseted gay artist in Hollywood, one of Cukor's constant themes as a director was how to reconcile a schizoid existence, particularly that of an outsider or artist figure constantly at war with his or her own demons and the limits imposed by

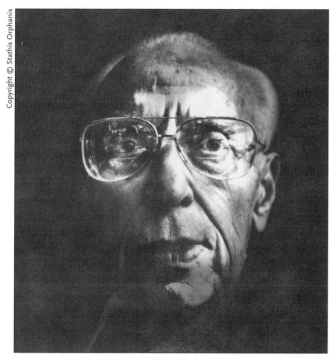

A portrait of George Cukor by Stathis Orphanis.

relationships and humdrum reality. Sometimes this conflict ends in a break with reality, as in *A Double Life* (1948), where the Ronald Colman character is eventually driven to madness while playing Othello.

In other cases, there is a merging of two artistic temperaments that, for Cukor, represents a transcendent state. This happens tellingly in, for example, *Holiday* (1938), where free spirit Johnny Case (Cary Grant) rejects his rich, stuffy fiancée in favor of her spinster sister (Katharine Hepburn), who turns out to be a dreamer like himself.

In spite of his devotion to the dream and the dreamer, Cukor was realist enough to know that such liaisons are rare and fleeting. In *A Star Is Born*, the relationship of two larger-than-life actors—here played by James Mason and Judy Garland, in her best performance—begins in triumph but ends in abuse and finally suicide.

Cukor's reputation as the pioneer maker of divas does not take into account his brilliance in exploring the artistic temperament and the struggle for self-expression in subtle variations throughout his career. Moreover, this reputation fails to acknowledge the grittiness of his 1950s films, which despite strong performances by actresses cannot be consigned to the ghetto of the "woman's picture."

Particularly in his collaborations with Garson Kanin and Ruth Gordon, such as *The Marrying Kind* (1952), shot on location, there is an almost neorealist feeling in the unflinching treatment of the sometimes squalid reality of people's daily lives.

Cukor died on January 24, 1983, two years after directing his last film, *Rich and Famous*. This film, which revisits Cukor's theme of the artistic temperament at odds with society and itself, was an update of the Bette Davis–Miriam Hopkins vehicle *Old Acquaintance* (1943). As such, it is a suitable coda for the career of one of America's great gay artists in or out of cinema.

—*Gary Morris*

BIBLIOGRAPHY

Ehrenstein, David. *Open Secret.* New York: Harper Perennial Library, 2000.

Hadleigh, Boze. *Conversations with My Elders.* New York: St. Martin's Press, 1986.

Lambert, Gavin. *On Cukor.* New York: Rizzoli, 2000.

Levy, Emanuel. *George Cukor: Master of Elegance: Hollywood's Legendary Director and His Stars.* New York: William Morrow, 1994.

McGilligan, Patrick. *George Cukor, a Double Life: A Biography of the Gentleman Director.* New York: Harper Perennial, 1992.

SEE ALSO

Film; Film Directors; Set and Costume Design; Transvestism in Film; Bankhead, Tallulah; Garland, Judy; Goulding, Edmund; Grant, Cary; Haines, William "Billy"

Cumming, Alan   (b. 1965)

Versatile actor Alan Cumming has performed a wide variety of roles on stage, screen, and television. He has earned numerous awards for his acting and also for his support of glbtq causes.

The younger son of a forester and a homemaker, Alan Cumming was born on January 27, 1965, in Aberfeldy, Perthshire, Scotland. He spent his first year in the neighboring town of Dunkeld, where his father worked on a large estate. The family then moved to Fassfern on the west coast of the country, and three years later settled on the east coast, on another estate near Carnoustie.

As a child growing up on an isolated estate, he lacked playmates—his only sibling was six years older than he—and so he amused himself by acting out stories of his own invention. His cast, he recalled, consisted of "me and my dog. And imaginary others."

After graduating from Carnoustie High School, Cumming worked for a year at a publishing company in Dundee, initially in the fiction department and then interviewing bands for a pop culture magazine called *TOPS*.

Cumming then enrolled in the Royal Scottish Academy of Music and Drama in Glasgow. While attending the academy, Cumming met and married fellow student Hilary Lyon.

After graduating in 1985, Cumming and a friend, Forbes Masson, developed a stand-up comedy act that proved extremely popular. Following this success, Cumming starred in a BBC sitcom, *The High Life*, which he also cowrote.

Cumming's first love was the stage, however, and he and Lyon won the lead roles in a very well-received production of *Hamlet* in London in 1993. Cumming was nominated for the Richard Burton Award at the Shakespeare Globe Awards and received the Martini Rossi TMA Award for his work.

Cumming and Lyon appeared destined to become a theatrical star couple, but it was not to be. Near the end of the run of *Hamlet*, Cumming suffered from panic attacks and depressive episodes that led to a nervous breakdown. The marriage disintegrated, and the couple divorced.

Thereafter, Cumming was involved in several gay relationships, but while filming *Circle of Friends* (1995, directed by Pat O'Connor) he fell in love with actress Saffron Burrows. The two became engaged but broke up before there was a wedding.

Since then, Cumming has had a number of romantic relationships, mainly with men, but he has not yet found a life partner.

Cumming is reluctant to put a label on his sexual orientation. In a 1999 article in the *Advocate*, he said, "I'm not going to say I'm one thing when I'm not just so I can fit into people's notions of how things are. I think people deny themselves by putting themselves into categories."

As an actor, Cumming has certainly defied categorization. In his work on stage, in films, and on television, he has played roles in productions that range from the plays of Shakespeare to the animated adventures of Garfield the cat. He has already appeared in over fifty movies, with more in production.

Cumming's first film role was in the little-noticed *Prague* (1992, directed by Ian Sellers), in which he plays a young Scot who has returned to his ancestral home, Prague, in search of film that depicts his grandparents being taken away by the Nazis in World War II. The 1995 James Bond film *Goldeneye* (directed by Martin Campbell), in which he plays a computer programmer, brought him to public attention, and he went on to more prominent roles in *Circle of Friends* and *Emma* (1996, directed by Douglas McGrath). As the egregious Reverend Elton in *Emma* and the slimy Sean Walsh in *Circle of Friends*, Cumming brings unexpected humanity to unappealing characters.

Before becoming a film actor, he had already won acclaim for his stage work in London's West End. He was nominated for a Laurence Olivier Award as Most Promising Newcomer for his performance in Manfred Karge's *The Conquest of the South Pole* in 1989. He received an Olivier Award for his work in Dario Fo's *Accidental Death of an Anarchist* in 1990 and was nominated for another in 1992 for David Hirson's *La Bête*. The following year, he gave his award-winning performance as Hamlet.

While *Hamlet* was still in production, Cumming began rehearsals for a London revival of *Cabaret* (book by Joe Masteroff, based on Isherwood's Berlin stories; music by John Kander, lyrics by Fred Ebb). In a 1987 production, he had played a minor role. But in the 1993–1994 West End production, he had a leading role as the Emcee and earned another Olivier Award nomination for Best Actor in a Musical.

Cumming reprised his role as the Emcee in *Cabaret* on Broadway in 1998–1999. The New York production was a smash hit, and Cumming earned numerous honors for his performance, including the Tony, Drama Desk, Outer Critics Circle, Theatre World, and New York Public Advocate's Awards.

Cumming's success in *Cabaret* led to the opportunity to star in a New York production of Noël Coward's *Design for Living*, a play that he had long wanted to do. Critic Elysa Gardner praised Cumming's 2001 performance, writing that he "imbues Otto with a delightful mix of impishness and innocence."

The following year, also in New York, he appeared in *Elle*, a short play by Jean Genet. The work had never been performed in English, and so Cumming wrote an adaptation based on a translation by Terri Gordon.

The simple premise of the play is that a young photographer is trying to take a perfect picture of the pope for worldwide distribution. As *New York Times* critic Ben Brantley noted, however, " 'Elle' is a dense, ornately verbal meditation on the tyranny of fame and manufactured images of glamour and authority."

The French feminine pronoun *elle* actually refers to the pope, since his title, *Sa Sainteté* ("His Holiness"), is a feminine noun; thus, the pope is called "she."

Cumming gave a flamboyant performance as the pontiff. Brantley described his entrance as one "which for audacity and spectacle is unlikely to be topped...even by touring rock stars," with its special effects and Cumming's designer dress "that makes the most lavish Oscar-night gowns look modest." The reviewer went on to say that Cumming brought "miraculous new variety to the premise of the actor as war-weary whore that he perfected in 'Cabaret.' "

In addition to his work on stage, Cumming has appeared in dozens of films, in which he has shown remarkable versatility as an actor. His movies include light-hearted fare such as the three *Spy Kids* films (2001, 2002, and 2003, all directed by Robert Rodriguez) and the animated feature *Garfield* (2004, directed by Peter Hewitt), for which he did voice-overs. He has also appeared in adaptations of the works of Shakespeare—*Titus* (1999, directed by Julie Taymor); Charles Dickens—*Nicholas Nickleby* (2002, directed by Douglas McGrath); and Patricia Highsmith—*Ripley Under Ground* (2005, directed by Roger Spottiswoode).

With Jennifer Jason Leigh, who played Sally Bowles to his Emcee in the New York production of *Cabaret*, Cumming has cowritten and codirected a film, *The Anniversary Party* (2001). The two costarred with a cast that included Gwyneth Paltrow (with whom Cumming had worked in *Emma*), Phoebe Cates, and John C. Reilly. The low-budget film, which was shot on digital video in only nineteen days, was not a great commercial success but received favorable reviews. Critic Eric Harrison called it a "nicely acted and appealing drama" with "sterling performances" from the "marvelous cast."

Among Cumming's recent film projects are Lorena Machado's *Bam Bam and Celeste* (scheduled for release in 2005), which will star Margaret Cho, and Sara Sugarman's *Coming Out* (planned for release in 2006), in which Cumming will play a gay cabaret performer who takes charge of a hapless Welsh rugby team after the death of his father, its coach.

Cumming is the author of a novel, *Tommy's Tale* (2002), about a bisexual man who, as he approaches his thirtieth birthday, is both enjoying a freewheeling party scene and yearning for a more settled life as a father. The book received polite but unenthusiastic reviews.

In February 2005, Cumming introduced Cumming The Fragrance, which is called "beyond gender." *Cosmetics International Cosmetic Products Report* states that the "fusion of basic, masculine notes with adventurous ones... makes it original." A line of other body-care products is planned.

While pursuing his many projects, Cumming has still found time to work for worthy causes. He serves on the Board of Directors of Broadway Cares/Equity Fights AIDS and has taken part in many events on behalf of the organization. He is also a member of the Board of Advocates of the Planned Parenthood Federation of America, the Ambassadors Committee of Free Arts for Abused Children NYC, and the Honorary Advisory Board of Living Beyond Belief, an organization that encourages New York City high school students to become active in the fight against AIDS.

In addition, he participates in numerous events for Bailey House, a New York organization that provides housing and other important services to people with HIV/AIDS. He has also done a comedy benefit for Beverly Hills's Trevor Project, whose goal is to promote tolerance for glbtq teens and whose national Trevor Helpline (866-4-U-TREVOR) provides around-the-clock suicide prevention services. He also served as the Celebrity Grand Marshal of the 2004 San Francisco LGBT Pride Parade.

Despite all these efforts, Cumming said that he "felt such a fraud for being publicly lauded" for his charity work. He therefore decided to take part in a project of the American Foundation for AIDS Research's TREAT Asia program by going on an eight-day fundraising walk on the Great Wall of China. The twenty-five walkers raised more than $275,000 and also learned about the cultural issues that complicate combating the disease in China.

In a 2001 interview, Cumming stated, "I get bored quite easily. I like to do different things. I'd be horrified to think I was going to be doing the same thing all the time." With his many projects, both professional and charitable, it seems unlikely that he will fall prey to ennui any time soon.

—*Linda Rapp*

BIBLIOGRAPHY

Brantley, Ben. "Cutting Down Icons to Clay Feet." *New York Times,* July 25, 2002.

"Conquering Mountains: Out Actor Alan Cumming Tells Us What It's Like to Hike the World's Most Momentous Monument—All in the Name of Charity." *Advocate,* March 1, 2005, 38.

De Bertodano, Helena. "The Sting in 'Tommy's Tale.'" *Sunday Telegraph* (London), March 30, 2003.

"Following the February Launch of Cumming The Fragrance, Scottish Star of 'X-Men,' Alan Cumming Is Preparing for the Roll-out of a Body Care Line." *Cosmetics International Cosmetic Reports* (April 2005): 13.

Gardner, Elysa. "'Design for Living' Still Delivers Sexy Shocks." *USA Today,* March 15, 2001.

Harrison, Eric. "'Anniversary Party' Lets Fine Cast Shine." *Houston Chronicle,* June 22, 2001.

McQuaid, Peter. "The Artful Swinger." *Advocate,* September 28, 1999, 59.

Painter Young, Jamie. "Don't Fence Him In." *Back Stage West,* June 14, 2001, 5.

Walsh, John. "The Flying Scotsman." *Independent* (London), April 28, 2003.

www.alancumming.com

SEE ALSO

Film Actors: Gay Male; British Television; Cho, Margaret

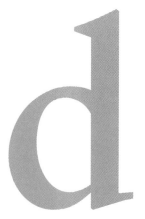

Davies, Terence (b. 1945)

BRITISH FILMMAKER TERENCE DAVIES CREATES AESTHET-ically compelling films that offer honest and complex psychological portraits of gay adults and youths.

Davies was born on November 10, 1945, into a working-class Catholic family in Liverpool, the youngest of ten children. At fifteen, he began work as a bookkeeper, a profession he continued for the next twelve years. This background provides the subject matter for much of Davies's work, which is to a large degree autobiographical.

In 1972, Davies won a place at Coventry Drama school, where he wrote the screenplay for his first short film, *Children* (1976), the first part of what is known as the Terence Davies Trilogy. The remaining two parts of the trilogy are *Madonna and Child* (1980), made while Davies attended the National Film School, and *Death and Transfiguration* (1983), which was funded by the British Film Institute and the Greater London Arts Council.

In 1984, Davies published a novel, *Hallelujah Now*, which, like the short films, similarly takes the form of a trilogy concerned with sexual and religious guilt. Both the films and the novel document, in a fragmentary and elliptical way, the life of a working-class gay man from childhood to death.

Davies's first feature film, *Distant Voices, Still Lives* (1988), was highly acclaimed, winning the International Critics' Prize at Cannes and awards at sixteen other film festivals, including Locarno and Toronto. This film, along with his next feature, *The Long Day Closes* (1992), is set in the Liverpool of Davies's childhood. The first film explores in two parts a working-class family dominated by a tyrannical father; the second film is focused more closely on the relationship between the youngest son in a family and his mother.

Both films are highly formalist attempts to convey the structure of memory. They are characterized by loose (virtually absent) narratives, associative editing, and long takes that attempt to bring out the extraordinary in the mundane. In one celebrated and exquisitely beautiful example of the latter technique, the camera focuses on a faded carpet for a number of minutes as sunlight slowly moves across it.

Music, in this case the popular music of the 1950s, plays a prominent role in all of Davies's films, often providing what would otherwise be conveyed through dialogue or narrative. This reliance on music may be the product of Davies's fascination with the Hollywood musical.

Distant Voices, Still Lives and *The Long Day Closes* act as something of a corrective to the British kitchen-sink dramas of the 1950s and 1960s, which portrayed working-class life in gritty black and white, typically showing it to be nasty, brutish, and short. While Davies does not romanticize this life, he does attempt to show, along with the privations, the beauty and the culture of the British working-class community.

The Neon Bible (1995), set in the American South in the 1940s, is an adaptation of the novel by John Kennedy Toole. In it, a sensitive youth remembers his childhood, which is populated by a domineering father, a withdrawn mother, and a glamorous former nightclub singer, Aunt Mae. While this is Davies's first nonautobiographical film, it does exhibit many of his usual interests—for example, mimicking the structure of memory and using songs as structuring or bridging devices.

Davies's most recent film is an adaptation of Edith Wharton's novel *The House of Mirth* (2000). Another film, *Sunset Song,* based on the novel by Scottish author Lewis Grassic Gibbon, was in production in 2005 but not yet released.

In spite of his relatively small canon, Davies is highly regarded among critics and other filmmakers for his artistry. Davies's representations of gay adults and alienated youths do not conform to the school of positive stereotypes. Indeed, they are often infused with great sadness. Yet these aesthetically compelling films offer uncompromisingly honest cinematic visions.   —*Jim Ellis*

BIBLIOGRAPHY

Cousins, Mark. "Interview with Terence Davies." *Projections 6: Filmmakers on Film-making.* John Boorman and Walter Donohoe, eds. London: Faber and Faber, 1996. 173–184.

Davies, Terence. *Hallelujah Now.* London: Brilliance Books, 1984.

———. *A Modest Pageant.* Six screenplays. London: Faber and Faber, 1988.

Dixon, Wheeler Winston. "The Long Day Closes: An Interview with Terence Davies." *Re-Viewing British Cinema, 1900–1992.* Wheeler Winston Dixon, ed. Albany: State University of New York, 1994. 249–259.

Eley, Geoff, "The Family is a Dangerous Place: Memory, Gender, and the Image of the Working Class." *Revisioning History: Film and the Construction of a New Past.* Robert A. Rosenstone, ed. Princeton, N.J.: Princeton University Press, 1995. 17–43.

Hunt, Martin. "The Poetry of the Ordinary: Terence Davies and the Social Art Film." *Screen* 40.1 (1999): 1–16.

Williams, Tony. "The Masochistic Fix: Gender Oppression in the Films of Terence Davies." *Fires Were Started: British Cinema and Thatcherism.* Lester Friedman, ed. Minneapolis: University of Minnesota Press, 1993. 237–254.

SEE ALSO

Film; Film Directors; Screenwriters

Davis, Brad   *(1949–1991)*

BOYISHLY HANDSOME BRAD DAVIS ROSE TO FAME FOR his starring role in *Midnight Express* (1978). The homoerotic shower scene in that movie, along with Davis's performance as a gay sailor in Rainer Werner

Fassbinder's *Querelle* (1983) and other homosexual roles, made him a gay film icon. After his death, newspaper reports described him as "the first heterosexual actor to die of AIDS," but his bisexuality was well known to people in the entertainment industry.

Robert Creel Davis was born in Tallahassee, Florida, on November 6, 1949. Known in his youth as Bobby, he changed his name to Brad in 1973 because there was already a Bobby Davis listed with Actors Equity.

In Davis's earliest years, his family enjoyed a relatively affluent life. His father, Eugene Davis, was a successful dentist; however, as he took to drink, his practice declined. His alcoholism became a serious problem, and in the late 1950s he injured a patient on whom he was working while drunk.

After the incident, Dr. Davis moved his family to Titusville, Florida, in hopes of making a fresh start. Although he gave up drinking, he was never able to achieve prosperity again. His wife, Anne Creel Davis, took the reversal of fortune badly, sinking into a severe depression.

Acting was young Brad Davis's lifelong ambition. After winning a music talent contest at the age of seventeen, he worked at Theatre Atlanta. Later, he attended the American Academy of Dramatic Arts and studied acting at the American Place Theater in New York.

After appearing in several off-Broadway productions, he won a regular part on a television soap opera, *How to Survive a Marriage*, in 1974. He came to greater public attention in 1976 with a major role in the television movie *Sybil*, directed by Daniel Petrie; and the following year he appeared in the highly acclaimed miniseries *Roots*, directed by Marvin J. Chomsky and John Erman.

Davis's cinematic breakthrough came in 1978 when he starred as imprisoned drug smuggler Billy Hayes in Alan Parker's *Midnight Express*. His performance earned him a Golden Globe Award as best new actor, but other important roles were not immediately forthcoming. His next film, Rob Cohen's *A Small Circle of Friends* (1980), was not a success, and his role in Hugh Hudson's 1981 hit *Chariots of Fire* was a relatively minor one.

In 1983, Davis took a professional risk by accepting the title role as a gay sailor in *Querelle*, Rainer Werner Fassbinder's screen adaptation of a novel by Jean Genet. Associates in the entertainment industry warned Davis that taking this part, especially after performances in other gay-themed theatrical works such as Larry Kramer's *Sissies' Scrapbook* (1973) and Joe Orton's *Entertaining Mr. Sloane* (1981), would be detrimental to his career. Nevertheless, Davis chose to work with Fassbinder on what would turn out to be the director's last film. Unfortunately, *Querelle* was a commercial failure and generally not well received by critics.

In 1985, Davis won critical acclaim for his portrayal of the lover of a man dying of AIDS in Larry Kramer's play *The Normal Heart*. Still, his film career foundered. The only other movie in which he starred was Percy Adlon's 1989 comedy *Rosalie Goes Shopping*.

Davis continued to find work in foreign films and on television, including the title role in Marvin J. Chomsky's 1985 miniseries *Robert Kennedy & His Times*, but he never realized his full potential as a film actor. Homophobia in Hollywood is one likely cause of this, but the problem was exacerbated by Davis's reputation for erratic behavior—mostly off the set—caused by alcohol and drug use.

Davis, a longtime alcohol abuser who had begun using cocaine while filming *Midnight Express*, joined Alcoholics Anonymous in 1981 and eventually became sober; but during the period of his substance abuse he was involved in a number of incidents of unruly conduct, some of which led to arrests.

In 1985, Davis learned that he was HIV-positive. Fearing that he would be unemployable if word of his condition became known, he shared the information only with his wife, Susan Bluestein Davis, whom he had married in 1976, and a few close friends. He received medical treatment from a doctor who came to his home; and later, when he required hospital stays, he checked in late at night and used his given name, Robert Davis.

The treatments were unsuccessful, and, according to Robert Pela, Davis ended his life by committing an assisted suicide at his home in Studio City, California, on September 8, 1991.

In his final months, Davis had been working on a proposal for a book about his struggle with AIDS. In 1997, his widow published a biography, *After Midnight: The Life and Death of Brad Davis*. In it, she echoed the description of her husband that had appeared in newspaper articles about him, "the first heterosexual actor to die of AIDS." She expressed the belief that he must have contracted the disease through his drug abuse, though she also stated that he had an aversion to needles and had consumed cocaine by snorting it or rubbing it on his gums.

Bluestein Davis acknowledged that, in his early years in New York, her late husband had "hustled" in Times Square and had lived with a transvestite, but she insisted that he was heterosexual. However, this assertion is contradicted by other sources.

Davis's friend the gay writer and AIDS activist Rodger McFarlane stated that Davis "never [said] he wasn't gay when someone asked." The late actor Timothy Patrick Murphy spoke of having had an affair with Davis in the mid-1980s. And in an interview that appears in Boze

Hadleigh's book *Hollywood Gays*, Davis himself acknowledged having had sex with men. When asked if he considered himself bisexual, he replied, "Didn't someone once say that everyone's bisexual, deep down?" —*Linda Rapp*

BIBLIOGRAPHY

"Davis, Brad." *The Hollywood Who's Who.* Robyn Karney, ed. New York: Continuum, 1993. 113–114.

Davis, Susan Bluestein, with Hilary de Vries. *After Midnight: The Life and Death of Brad Davis.* New York: Pocket Books, 1997.

Hadleigh, Boze. *Hollywood Gays.* New York: Barricade Books, 1996.

Pela, Robert L. "Our Man Brad." *Advocate*, July 8, 1997, 36.

Zonana, Victor F. "Profile in Courage, Anger." *Los Angeles Times*, September 11, 1991.

SEE ALSO

Film Actors: Gay Male; Fassbinder, Rainer Werner

Dean, James (1931–1955)

ALTHOUGH HE SPENT ONLY TWO YEARS IN HOLLYWOOD before his untimely death, James Dean became an enduring icon of American film, one whose brooding nonconformity helped challenge rigid notions of masculinity.

James Byron Dean was born on February 8, 1931, in Marion, Indiana. His mother, Mildred, died when he was nine, and Winton, his father, sent him to live with his grandparents. A talented youth who won high school dramatic competitions while attending Fairmount High School, Dean led a life of longing caused by the early death of his mother.

A star basketball player in high school, Dean lost his front teeth in a trapeze accident and had to wear false ones for the rest of his life. Despite this misfortune, and his terrible eyesight, he excelled in acting, and his brooding good looks promised success as a movie star. He soon left Indiana for Hollywood, where he struggled to land a few theater roles and bit parts in films.

In 1951, he took the advice of actor and teacher James Whitmore and traveled to New York. Although admitted to Lee Strasburg's Actors Studio, Dean rarely attended classes at the prestigious acting school. Nevertheless, he immersed himself in the techniques of method acting. Hence, as an actor, he is often compared with such other young method actors of the period as Montgomery Clift and Marlon Brando.

In New York, Dean found work in television commercials, which in turn led to stage jobs. In 1952, he was cast in N. Richard Nash's *See the Jaguar*, a play that ran only five days on Broadway. Brief as it was, however, Dean's exposure in *See the Jaguar* garnered him opportunities as a television actor and a role on Broadway as an Arab boy who seduces a male British tourist in the stage production of André Gide's *The Immoralist* (1954).

Despite his success in *The Immoralist*, Dean quit the show only three weeks after its opening in order to fly to Hollywood to begin filming *East of Eden* (1955). On the set of *East of Eden*, Dean had disagreements with director Elia Kazan, but he delivered an unusually mature and affecting performance as Cal, the young protagonist of the sprawling family drama based on John Steinbeck's novel.

Off camera, Dean studied dance with Eartha Kitt and painted erotic pictures of bullfighters. He had several torrid romances with actresses and, according to some biographers, with men as well. Among the men cited as having had affairs with Dean are actors Clifton Webb, Bill Bast, and Jack Simmons, as well as producer Rogers Brackett.

Dean's engagement to actress Pier Angeli temporarily quieted rumors of his bisexuality, despite his having been widely quoted as saying, when pressed about his orientation, that he "wouldn't go through life with one hand tied behind [his] back." Angeli's abrupt breaking off of the engagement and her subsequent marriage to singer Vic Damone left Dean alone and the subject of further speculation.

Dean hurled himself into his work on director Nicholas Ray's *Rebel Without a Cause* (1955)—the film, released soon after his death, that would establish him as an enduring Hollywood star. A classic film about teenage alienation and angst, it features prominently a gay subtext embodied in the relationship between the characters portrayed by Dean and Sal Mineo.

In its honesty and tenderness, the relationship between these characters, coded though it is, has touched several generations of gay youth. As Jim Stark, who lovingly accepts and protects Mineo's adoring Plato, Dean conveyed a new, nonconformist masculinity that boldly challenged the rigid gender-role expectations of 1950s America.

After completing *Rebel Without a Cause*, Dean began working on director George Eastman's epic *Giant* (1956), based on the Edna Ferber novel. In this film, Dean's transformation from farmhand to oil baron is astonishing. On set, tempers flared between Dean and his then closeted costar Rock Hudson, according to accounts by Dean's friend and costar Elizabeth Taylor.

Soon after finishing all his scenes for *Giant*, on September 30, 1955, Dean, a race car enthusiast, went for a drive with his mechanic, Rolf Weutherich, in his prize Porsche Silver Spyder. The drive proved fatal. Dean's vehicle collided with another on a rural road near Paso Robles, California, and the actor was nearly decapitated. His untimely death, just as he was on the verge of a major acting career, catapulted him to fame and helped make both *Rebel Without a Cause* and *Giant* box office hits.

Film studios were deluged with thousands of fan letters to the actor, who had spent less than two years in Hollywood. An obsessive cultlike following soon developed, and Dean's image, usually in a black T-shirt and with a cigarette dangling from his mouth, quickly became one of the most recognizable symbols of 1950s youth culture.

Numerous films, plays, documentaries, photographs, artworks, and advertising images attempt to capture the spirit of Dean's allure, but the actor's charisma continues to be vital, at least in part because he is shrouded in mystery. The image of Dean in the *Rebel* red windbreaker remains an icon of twentieth-century pop culture.

—*Jim Provenzano*

Bibliography

Alexander, Paul. *Boulevard of Broken Dreams: The Life, Times, and Legend of James Dean.* New York: Viking, 1997.

Dalton, David. *James Dean: American Icon.* New York: St. Martin's, 1984.

Grant, Neil. *James Dean: In His Own Words.* London: Michelin House, 1991.

Holley, Val. *James Dean: The Biography.* New York: St. Martin's Griffin, 1995.

Martinetti, Robert. *The James Dean Story.* New York: Pinnacle, 1975.

Spoto, Donald. *Rebel: The Life and Legend of James Dean.* New York: HarperCollins, 1996.

See also

Film; Film Actors: Gay Male; Bisexuality in Film; Clift, Montgomery; Hudson, Rock; Mineo, Sal; Webb, Clifton

DeGeneres, Ellen   (b. 1958)

Comic Ellen DeGeneres's act is characterized by slapstick zaniness, split-second timing, and rambling monologues delivered with a hapless charm that invites audience identification. But no matter how great her contribution to the world of comedy, DeGeneres will probably be best remembered as the first lesbian to star as a lesbian on her own network television series.

Born on January 26, 1958, into a middle-class family in Metairie, Louisiana, DeGeneres grew up riding her bicycle through the streets of New Orleans, a city that prides itself on a diverse and quirky population. Although the family moved to Texas for several years, DeGeneres, after dropping out of college in the mid-1970s, returned to New Orleans to follow her own unconventional path.

She worked a series of jobs, from oyster shucker to housepainter, before stumbling into comedy. Her first stand-up act was performed at an informal show at a friend's party. DeGeneres came onstage with a burger and fries and proceeded to eat as she talked, forcing the audience to wait as she chewed between lines. In this first show, she not only entertained her friends, but she began to create the bumbling everywoman character who would later convulse audiences across the country.

DeGeneres began to perform stand-up in coffeehouses and comedy clubs in New Orleans, and then around the country as she developed her act. In 1982, she won a cable television contest for "Funniest Person in America," and soon she had her own cable specials and guest spots on shows such as *The Tonight Show* and *Arsenio Hall*. In the early 1990s, she made the most of supporting roles in the short-lived ABC sitcom *Laurie Hill* and the Fox network's *Open House*. She also won the American Comedy Award for Best Female Standup.

In 1994, ABC offered DeGeneres her own sitcom, a *Seinfeld/Friends* clone, titled *These Friends of Mine*. The show was fairly successful, and the next season the network changed the title to *Ellen*.

DeGeneres had realized that she was a lesbian while still a teenager, and by the time she was in her twenties she was living a fully, if closeted, lesbian life. As her career and her public recognition grew, so did the chasm between her public and private lives. As her sitcom approached its third season, DeGeneres made the decision not only to come out as a lesbian performer, but also to bring out the other Ellen, her sitcom alter ego.

The decision would have a huge impact on DeGeneres's life and career, and also on anyone exposed to the barrage of media coverage. The coming-out of the actress and her character led to an international discussion of the presence of gay men and lesbians in prime-time television.

On April 30, 1997, Ellen Morgan, heroine of *Ellen*, came out as a lesbian in a highly touted hour-long special episode. The show was one of the highest-rated television shows ever, attracting 36.2 million viewers and winning an Emmy Award for writing. DeGeneres's success was short-lived, however. ABC canceled *Ellen* at the end of the season, citing the poor quality of the show and declining ratings.

An angry and disappointed DeGeneres blamed lack of network support for her show's failure. She felt especially betrayed by a parental advisory warning that the network placed on shows with gay content.

The coming-out episode of *Ellen* received intense scrutiny from both gay and mainstream press. Conservatives were, predictably, horrified; and, while many gays have hailed DeGeneres as a courageous pioneer, others have criticized her for not being political or radical enough. The media blitz surrounding her coming-out affected DeGeneres's family as well. Her mother supported her by becoming an outspoken advocate of gay rights.

Shortly after the coming-out episode, DeGeneres became romantically involved with (previously heterosexual) actress Anne Heche. Their relationship was constantly monitored by the press, which criticized them for such blatancy as public displays of affection at a White House function. Heche and DeGeneres dissolved their relationship at the end of 1999.

DeGeneres continues to work on network television. She had a recurrent role in the 1998 season of *Mad About You*, and she starred in another sitcom for CBS in 2001–2002. She has also appeared on cable (in Part 3 of HBO's *If These Walls Could Talk*) and in feature films (*EdTV* and *Goodbye Lover* in 1999). She has also gone back on the road as a stand-up comic, which resulted in another HBO comedy special.

In 2003, DeGeneres began hosting a syndicated talk show. Offering a mix of celebrity interviews, musical performances, "real people" segments, and audience participation games, as well as a daily monologue by DeGeneres, the show has earned critical praise and solid ratings. In 2004, it won a daytime Emmy Award for Outstanding Talk Show.

Thus, despite the failure of her sitcoms, the future for Ellen DeGeneres seems bright. Rather than harming her career, her highly publicized coming-out seems only to have increased her celebrity.

After the very public dissolution of her relationship with Heche, DeGeneres embarked on a much less publicized relationship with photographer Alexandra Hedison, with whom she was together for almost four years. Ironically, soon after the December 2004 publication of an *Advocate* cover story on DeGeneres that featured photographs by Hedison, the two decided to end their relationship.

—*Tina Gianoulis*

BIBLIOGRAPHY

DeGeneres, Betty. *Love, Ellen: A Mother/Daughter Journey.* New York: Rob Weisbach Books, 1999.

Flint, Joe. "As Gay As It Gets? Prime-time Crusader Ellen DeGeneres Led TV Into a New Era. But at What Cost to her Show—And to Her?" *Entertainment Weekly*, May 8, 1998, 26.

Stockwell, Anne. "A Day in the Year of Ellen." Photos by Alexandra Hedison. *Advocate*, January 18, 2005, 44.

Tracy, Kathleen. *Ellen: The Real Story of Ellen DeGeneres.* Secaucus, N.J.: Carol Publishing Group, 1999.

Wieder, Judy. "Ellen: Born Again." *Advocate*, March 14, 2000, 28.

SEE ALSO

American Television: Situation Comedies; American Television: Talk Shows; American Television: News; Film Actors: Lesbian

Dietrich, Marlene   *(1901–1992)*

PROBABLY NO ONE, GAY OR STRAIGHT, OF ANY GENDER, could tear her or his eyes from the sight of Marlene Dietrich, leaning back with lewd abandon, grasping a shapely gartered leg as she growls out her signature song, "Falling in Love Again." That song, and the role of Lola Lola, the sizzling slut with a heart of ice, brought Dietrich to international stardom in Josef von Sternberg's landmark 1930 film, *Der blaue Engel (The Blue Angel)*.

Born Maria Magdalene von Losch on December 27, 1901, to a bourgeois family in Berlin, Dietrich had been a promising student of the violin until a hand injury forced her to give up playing. In 1924, she married Rudolf Sieber, a film director who introduced her to acting; but it was Josef von Sternberg who would be the most powerful influence on her career.

In *Der blaue Engel,* von Sternberg created a powerful allegory of German society and spirit in the aftermath of World War I. Within this allegory, Dietrich's character symbolized a harsh and unfeeling decadence that threatened both to captivate and to destroy what was good and innocent in German culture.

Although Dietrich had had several previous film roles, her portrayal of Lola Lola crystallized her stage persona forever. While that persona would be softened and glamorized for her American films, for the rest of her career Marlene Dietrich would be the dangerously sexy femme fatale with the cool and sardonic exterior.

In the early 1930s, both von Sternberg and Dietrich left Germany and its rising Nazi party to settle in the United States. Dietrich soon became a deliciously controversial figure in American cinema. Although she remained married to Rudolf Sieber, the relationship was what would later be called an "open marriage." They remained close, but did not live together, and both had other relationships, often publicly.

Dietrich always retained her Continental sophistication, and she scandalized society almost as much by wearing trousers in public as by her numerous love affairs with both men and women. In the 1930 film *Morocco,* audiences were shocked and titillated when Dietrich's character, a nightclub singer in glamorous top-hat-and-tails drag, finishes a number by kissing a female audience member on the lips.

According to Marjorie Rosen, the actress once said, "In Europe it doesn't matter if you're a man or a woman. We make love with anyone we find attractive." Rumors of her numerous affairs with such celebrities as Frank Sinatra, John Kennedy, Edith Piaf, and writer Mercedes de Acosta only added to the Dietrich mystique.

Dietrich became an American citizen in 1937. During World War II, she denounced the German government and, at some risk, entertained Allied troops abroad. After the war, she followed a successful film career with an equally successful cabaret act. Her cool, knowing, self-mocking persona appealed to both gay men and lesbians, who composed a significant portion of her nightclub audiences.

In some ways, however, the actress felt trapped by her own glamorous image; and, as she grew older, she became obsessed with concealing her changing body.

In 1975, the last of several onstage falls resulted in a broken leg, and Dietrich finally retired from performing altogether. She moved to Paris and lived the rest of her life in semiseclusion, surrounded by mementos of her career and her romantic exploits.

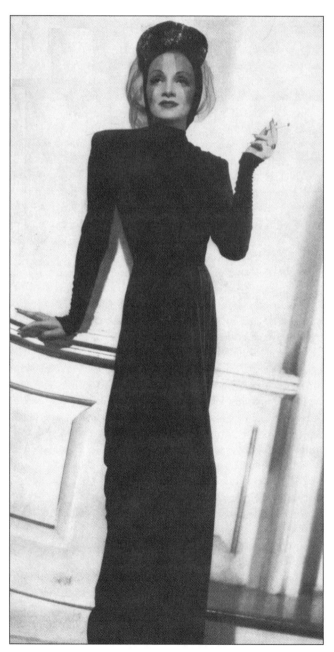

Marlene Dietrich.

Dietrich died in Paris on May 6, 1992. At her request, she was buried beside her mother in Berlin. She was welcomed back to the city of her birth by the tributes of her friends and fans, and over the protests of neo-Nazi groups and others who considered her support for the Allied cause in World War II treasonous.   —*Tina Gianoulis*

BIBLIOGRAPHY

Dietrich, Marlene. *Marlene*. Salvator Attanasio, trans. New York: Grove Press, 1989.

Riva, Maria. *Marlene Dietrich: By her Daughter, Maria Riva*. New York: Knopf, 1993.

Rosen Marjorie. "A Legend's Last Years: To the Very End, Marlene Dietrich Lived Out Her Life a Daring Original." *People*, June 1, 1992, 42.

Schickel, Richard. "The Secret in her Soul." *Time*, May 18, 1992, 72.

Spoto, Donald, *Blue Angel: The Life of Marlene Dietrich*. New York: Doubleday, 1992.

SEE ALSO

Film Actors: Lesbian; Transvestism in Film; Set and Costume Design; Bankhead, Tallulah; Fassbinder, Rainer Werner; Garbo, Greta

Divine (Harris Glenn Milstead)   *(1945–1988)*

A VERSATILE CHARACTER ACTOR, NIGHTCLUB SINGER, AND international cult star who generally performed his stage show and movie roles in drag, Divine first became famous through his appearances in John Waters's films of the late 1960s and early 1970s.

Born Harris Glenn Milstead on October 19, 1945, in Towson, Maryland, the future actor grew up in Baltimore suburbs. His parents, Bernard and Diana Francis Milstead, were generous and indulgent, perhaps because Harris was picked on at school for being plump and effeminate. When he was twelve, the family moved to Lutherville, another Baltimore suburb. The family lived just six houses from a boy Harris's age named John Waters.

Waters, who became a neighborhood friend, was responsible both for creating Milstead's stage name, supposedly a religious reference, and for crafting a host of outrageous roles for him.

Two scenes in particular from Waters's films contributed to Divine's cult status. In *Pink Flamingos* (1972), Divine eats real dog feces so that her character can prove she is "the filthiest person alive." In *Female Trouble* (1975), the Divine character Dawn Davenport gets sexually attacked by dirty-old-man Earl, also played by Divine (with help from a body double for certain shots).

Other films in which Divine appears include *Polyester* (1981) and *Hairspray* (1988), directed by Waters; *Lust in the Dust* (1984), directed by Paul Bartel; and *Trouble in Mind* (1985), directed by Alan Rudolph.

After beginning in films, Divine gained celebrity in the mid-1970s by performing campy stage plays and disco acts in San Francisco. In the late 1970s and early 1980s, Divine made films and performed in clubs around the world. He became famous in Australia, England, the Netherlands, and Israel, as well as in the United States.

Although Divine often had difficulty releasing records in the United States, his hits such as "Walk Like a Man" and "I'm So Beautiful," both released in 1985, became popular both at home and abroad. During the 1980s, Divine was a frequent guest on talk shows and cable television programs, and often appeared at celebrity events. But a life constantly on the road began to take its toll on the performer.

Professionally, Divine yearned for greater Hollywood stardom and for recognition of his talent, both in and out of drag, as a character actor. In his personal life, Divine faced worry over his romantic involvements, increasing weight, and financial difficulties.

In 1988, when Waters cast him in *Hairspray* as a leading lady—in addition to a cameo as a male character—Divine's personal and professional situations began to improve. With the film's success came publicity and offers for more interesting roles, as well as the possibility of the stardom Divine desired. However, in a sad twist of fate, Milstead died in his sleep on March 7, 1988, soon after the film's opening, the victim of an enlarged heart.

Divine's appeal to audiences springs not only from his innate talent and likableness, but also from his willingness to do absolutely anything, no matter how bizarre or subversive, in his quest for fame.

As a film actor, Divine constructed serious characterizations even in roles that called for him to perform outlandish actions. On stage and in personal appearances, he exhibited the same measure of control and professionalism. He created a stage persona marked by raunchy humor and sarcastic exchanges with audience members; but he could also moderate this persona by projecting a more subdued appearance and a calm, avuncular demeanor.

Today, with recent video releases and television airings of his films, Divine's wild looks, expressive gestures, strong delivery, and undeniable talent continue to attract new fans.   —*David Aldstadt*

BIBLIOGRAPHY

Bernard, Jay. *Not Simply Divine*. New York: Simon & Schuster, 1993.

Waters, John. *Shock Value*. New York: Thunder's Mouth, 1981.

SEE ALSO

Film; Transvestism in Film; Bartel, Paul; Fierstein, Harvey; Waters, John

Documentary Film

THE QUEER COMMUNITY HAS AGGRESSIVELY USED DOC-umentary film to resurrect historical memory and to permit the marginalized to bear witness, as well as to build an image base that reflects our diversity and counters distorted and misleading representations.

The availability of relatively inexpensive, lightweight, and high-quality video equipment has contributed to these efforts, as queer documentarians have challenged the conventional forms and aesthetic principles of a long documentary tradition. Documentary entries at the major U.S. lesbian and gay film festivals have increased at a phenomenal pace over the last ten years.

The number and quality of documentaries being produced spawned the yearly QueerDOC Festival, which began in 1998 in England. Documentary film is an indispensable medium for glbtq people to reevaluate and reposition themselves in different contexts.

Direct Cinema and the Birth of Gay Documentaries

Lesbian and gay documentaries were unheard of until the release of Ken Robinson's *Some of Our Best Friends* in 1971. Robinson, a student at the University of Southern California, found activists willing to speak and, in most cases, be seen on camera (albeit sometimes in shadow), including gay protesters at a psychiatric convention, a man entrapped by vice-squad ploys, and representatives of a New York homophile group.

But it was not until 1977 that documentaries received wide attention and broad distribution. Arthur Bressan's *Gay U.S.A.* and Peter Adair's *Word Is Out: Stories of Some of Our Lives*, both from that year, have been praised as excellent examples of "direct cinema," a term used by documentarians since the early 1960s to indicate minimal intrusion by filmmakers in the interview process and on the narratives that unfold.

Gay U.S.A. took six people three years to make. The filmmakers chose twenty-six people as subjects after "pre-interviewing" 200 people across America. With one stationary camera directed at the interviewees, who never shift their positions, the film records narratives of self-discovery, of discrimination, of ways to cope in a homophobic society, and of living an open life. It is a startling document of national gay identity.

Word Is Out forged an even stronger sense of a national civil rights movement. The Mariposa Film Group sent film crews to six cities to capture Gay Pride marches and activities over one weekend. It is the first queer documentary to see politics as an integral part of queer celebration, and is a more far-reaching film than *Gay U.S.A.* in the number of people interviewed and the range of questions posed to them.

In the 1990s, documentaries such as Karen Kiss and

Paris Poirier's *The Pride Divide* (1997) and Lucy Winer and Karen Eaton's *Golden Threads* (1999) also communicated a collective sense of lesbian and gay identity, but with a more complicated visual style and dramatic structure. *The Pride Divide* contrasts the differences and conflicts between gay men and lesbians in their movement toward civil rights. Lesbians in *Golden Threads* celebrate their commonality at a retreat as the film reveals the difficulties they encountered defining their identity in the 1940s and 1950s.

Producing and Distributing Queer Documentaries

Most queer documentaries are independent productions. In the 1970s and 1980s, many documentarians undertook the time-consuming and arduous task of funding their own films. As queer documentaries started achieving visibility and acclaim, however, funding opportunities appeared from noncommercial outlets.

The Public Telecommunications Act of 1988 mandated that Congress allocate funds to PBS "for programming that involves creative risks and addresses the needs of under-served audiences." With these monies PBS set up the Independent Television Service, which funded in whole or part such important documentaries as Arthur Dong's *Coming Out Under Fire* (1995), Meema Spadola's *Our House: A Very Real Documentary about Kids of Gay and Lesbian Families* (1999), Debra Chasnoff's *It's Elementary: Talking About Gay Issues in School* (1996), *The Pride Divide* (1997), Tom Shepard's *Scout's Honor* (2000), *Golden Threads* (1999), Eric Slade's *Hope Along the Wind: The Life of Harry Hay* (2001), and two four-part series, *Positive: Life with HIV* (1995) and *The Question of Equality: Gay and Lesbian Struggle Since Stonewall* (1995).

ITS-funded films are usually shown first at film festivals and sometimes move to brief runs at art film houses before airing on PBS nationwide. Although ITS funds are vital to the continuing production of queer documentaries, they impose some restrictions. For example, most films produced by ITS must fit a sixty-minute time slot. This has not deterred filmmakers happy to advance beyond festival venues and reach a different and larger audience, but it has to some extent shaped the form of their work.

In Canada, the National Film Board has funded such important works as David Adkin's *Out: Stories of Lesbian and Gay Youth* (1994) and Aerlyn Weissman and Lynne Fernie's *Forbidden Love: The Unashamed Stories of Lesbian Lives* (1992). The sixty-minute time limit is rarely a prerequisite, as it is with PBS. The NFB also has a tough skin in deflecting attacks by politicians. It has been accused of making queer films that "attack the traditional family," but it has never backed down in funding documentaries or supporting their distribution on CBC.

PBS is much more susceptible to the outcries of politicians. The network frequently refuses to air documentaries, and sometimes individual affiliates refuse to broadcast films approved by the national network. For example, PBS executives refused to air Kelly Anderson and Tami Gold's *Out at Work* (1997), a documentary about workforce discrimination, ostensibly because the filmmakers received funds from labor unions, even though many PBS programs receive funds from corporations. Many PBS stations refused to air Marlon Riggs's *Tongues Untied* (1989), about homosexuality in the black community.

The Historical Compilation Documentary

One of the largest documentary genres, the historical compilation film, has permitted queer filmmakers to take control of how they are represented by resurrecting and reconfiguring history. Films such as Greta Schiller and Robert Rosenberg's *Before Stonewall: The Making of a Gay and Lesbian Community* (1986) and John Scagliotti, Janet Baus, and Dan Hunt's *After Stonewall* (1999) vitally document the strength of the queer community. These films permit glbtq people to make initial connections with their past or to rethink their relationship to past events and places.

Historical compilation documentaries comb numerous sources for actuality footage, sometimes referred to as archival footage, to reconstruct history. Actuality footage is film or video shot for another purpose and collected by researchers, as opposed to "originally shot" footage filmed by a documentary unit specifically for that project.

Actuality footage comes from individuals, local and national television news archives, newsreel archives, photographic still archives, public and private organizations, medical research institutions, glbtq community centers, and educational films. The unique characteristic of a compilation documentary is that it selects and assimilates footage from disparate sources to construct a vision of the past.

Most compilation documentaries rely to varying degrees on eyewitnesses to past events. Their testimony becomes a dialogue with and from the past. Eyewitnesses serve a pivotal role in making actuality footage come alive through historical memory. When directors Rob Epstein and Jeffrey Friedman located eyewitnesses for *Paragraph 175* (2000), an investigation of homosexuality in Hitler's Germany, the actuality footage, some never before seen and some familiar, took on new levels of meaning as a result of eyewitness testimony.

The content of compilation documentaries varies, including sweeping historical chronicles, biographical profiles, representations of one historical event, and portraits of places central to queer life. Documentarians mine the past to expand historical memory. Paris Poirier's

Last Call at Maud's (1993) and Peter L. Stein's *The Castro* (1997) both cover decades, but they configure the world from the perspective of a specific place and the people who populated those environments, providing history with a more personal narrative.

Queer compilations continue to find creative ways to express history. In Jeff Dupre's *Out of the Past* (1998), a seventeen-year-old student starting a Gay–Straight Alliance goes in search of queer history, only to discover that oppressive forces prevent student access to historical knowledge. In this film, a student unearthing knowledge of the past becomes the catalyst for sequences constructed with actuality footage.

The Biographical Compilation Documentary

In 1984, Robert Epstein and Richard Schmiechen's *The Times of Harvey Milk* won an Academy Award for Best Feature-Length Documentary, thus signaling a broader acceptance of queer narratives by the film community. This outstanding documentary also set a very high standard for biographical compilation films.

The Times of Harvey Milk made extensive use of actuality footage from news organizations to reconstruct Milk's life and his tragic death and the events that followed. But the film is most impressive in the way it strategically employs the testimony of five eyewitnesses, with different backgrounds and from different sections of society, to convince audiences that Harvey Milk was a leader of all the people of San Francisco.

Biographical compilations vary in their structure and the amount of actuality footage utilized, but all serve the crucial function of placing an individual in the historical record.

Other notable biographical compilations include Richard Schmiechen's *Our Minds: The Story of Dr. Evelyn Hooker* (1992), Jerry Aronson's *The Life and Times of Allen Ginsberg* (1993), Monte Bramer's *Paul Monette: The Brink of Summer's End* (1994), Ada Gay Griffin and Michelle Parkerson's *A Litany for Survival: The Life of Audre Lorde* (1996), and Susan Muska and Greta Olafsdottir's *The Brandon Teena Story* (1997). Slade's *Hope Along the Wind: The Life of Harry Hay* (2001) makes extensive use of actuality footage from disparate sources.

Interrogating the Image

Queer documentaries have rigorously interrogated fictional film images from mainstream British and American movies that claim to represent our lives and behavior. Interrogation reveals the nature and pattern of negative representations of glbtq people, and documents any shift toward positive portrayals.

The best-known documentary of this kind is Robert Epstein and Jeffrey Friedman's *The Celluloid Closet* (1995), based on the book of the same title by Vito Russo. The film is a historical overview of Hollywood's negative construction of homosexuality and the homosexual.

Andrea Weiss takes the same approach with mainstream British films in *A Bit of Scarlet* (1996). In *Dry Kisses Only* (1990), filmmakers Jane Cottis and Kaucyila Brooke add comedy to the deconstruction of classical Hollywood films by reediting scenes to bring out a lesbian subtext and satirizing the seriousness gay studies brings to interrogating the film image.

Homo Promo (1991), curated by Jenni Olson, investigates the ways Hollywood sold queer people to the general public in the period from 1956 to 1976. By editing together film trailers and promotional material that dealt with homosexuality and deviant sexual behavior, the film documents how Hollywood depicted the homosexual as self-hating, disturbed, and dangerous.

Documentarians have also dissected mainstream fictional films to steer viewers to queer subtexts and queer expressions in the behavior and speech of "straight" characters. These documentaries analyze for the queer community images that some lesbians and gay men have already appreciated and appropriated.

Mark Rappaport pioneered this approach in *Rock Hudson's Home Movies* (1994) and *The Silver Screen: Color Me Lavender* (1997). In the former film, Rappaport meticulously isolates and juxtaposes the words, phrases, and glances of Hudson that suggest that some of the characters he plays are queer and that Hudson himself is leading an illusionary life. One extensive section of *The Silver Screen* argues for a homosexual subtext in Walter Brennan's relationships with John Wayne and Gary Cooper in several Westerns.

Documenting AIDS

Documentaries played a central role in demystifying HIV/AIDS by presenting the faces and bodies of people with AIDS and letting them speak in their own voices. Peter Adair's *Absolutely Positive* (1991), Kermit Cole's *Living Proof: HIV and the Pursuit of Happiness* (1993), and Ellen Spiro and Marina Alvarez's *(In)visible Women* (1991) employ the techniques of direct cinema, letting narratives unfold with nominal editing and minimal questions by the interviewer.

The camera in Juan Botas and Lucas Platt's *One Foot on a Banana Peel, the Other Foot in the Grave* (1993) simply records a group of men in an intravenous medication room as they talk about surviving.

These AIDS documentaries present diverse voices, as people with AIDS discuss symptoms, medical treatments, and the ways they cope with the disease and a homophobic society. Another type of AIDS documentary, the memorial film, also tells individual stories. Robert Epstein and Jeffrey Friedman's *Common Threads:*

Stories from the Quilt (1990) is the best known of the memorial documentaries.

Documentaries such as Jay Corcoran's *Life and Death on the A-List* (1996) and Tom Joslin and Peter Friedman's *Silverlake Life: The View From Here* (1993) graphically depict HIV ravaging the body. In *Silverlake Life,* Tom Joslin and Mark Massi—both HIV positive—carry a video camera everywhere they go, unflinchingly chronicling each other's activities as AIDS racks their bodies. *Silverlake Life* is gut-wrenching as we watch intimate moments of suffering and the horrible conditions of death.

The unrelenting exposure of the victim speaking and the body displayed in AIDS documentaries led Derek Jarman to alter radically the representation of AIDS in his film *Blue* (1993). Blind during the production of *Blue,* Jarman mounts an auditory assault on the audience over a single solid-blue image for seventy-five minutes, privileging the vision of the mind's eye over sight. Jarman believed representational images distracted viewers from identifying on an experiential level with the conditions of living with AIDS.

Jarman's aural images condemn a homophobic British government and society, memorialize friends who have died, and depict a battle to save his sight. But the primary "content" of *Blue* is the series of poetic images that let Jarman's imagination, and the viewer's, transcend the limitations imposed by the representational visual image. With Jarman, the viewer also has lost sight, but not the vision of the mind.

Documentaries as the Battleground for Social and Political Change

Individuals representing national and local glbtq organizations are at the forefront of the fight against discrimination in all parts of society, but increasingly documentaries are taking center stage in clarifying and examining that struggle and in participating in the advancement of glbtq rights. These documentaries attempt to control and direct debate over civil rights and to respond to the discourses of heterosexism generated by homophobic groups.

Late in 1992, right-wing fundamentalist groups produced *The Gay Agenda: The Report,* which generalizes "the ills of gay life" that would infect a city or state following legislation giving "special rights" to glbtq people. In 1993, the Southern Baptist Convention produced *Gay Rights–Special Rights: Inside the Homosexual Agenda.*

Both films circulated in Oregon, where the Oregon Citizens Alliance was pushing for passage of antigay Ballot Measure 9, and in Colorado, where conservative groups were campaigning for Amendment 2, which would have prohibited discrimination claims based on sexual orientation.

Deborah Fort and Ann Skinner Jones made *The Great Divide* in 1993 in response to these films, and Heather

McDonald produced *Ballot Measure 9* in 1994 partly in response to *The Gay Agenda* but also to expose the tactics of hate and violence by conservative forces in Oregon. With these two films, these documentarians became activists resisting antigay initiatives.

The battle among documentaries occurred again in 1999 after Debra Chasnoff's *It's Elementary: Talking about Gay Issues in School* (1996) aired on many PBS stations and Meema Spadola's *Our House: A Very Real Documentary about Kids of Gay and Lesbian Parents* (1999) began to circulate in schools.

In direct response to PBS's airing of *It's Elementary*, the American Family Association quickly made *Suffer the Children: Answering the Homosexual Agenda in Public Schools* (1999), which even lifted scenes from *It's Elementary* to argue that children were being indoctrinated by homosexuals. The AFA succeeded in getting some PBS stations to air the film, but Fort, Jones, and McDonald responded with efforts to screen their films in schools.

The recent release of Tom Shepard's *Scout's Honor* (2000), chronicling thirteen-year-old scout Steven Cozza's nationwide campaign against discrimination by the Boy Scouts, is evidence that documentarians will continue to participate in the national debates on glbtq rights.

Activist Organizations and Activism

Although the label *activism* can apply to the function of many glbtq documentaries, a distinct subgenre of films depict activist organizations. Janet Baus and Su Friedrich's *The Lesbian Avengers Eat Fire Too* (1993) chronicles the first year of the Lesbian Avengers; Rosa von Praunheim's *The Transexual Menace* (1996) depicts the activism of the organization of the same name; and Sandra Elgear, Robyn Hutt, and David Meieran's *Voices from the Front* (1991) and Rosa von Praunheim's *Positive* (1990) and *Silence = Death* (1990) examine strategies of AIDS activists and ACT UP.

Portraits of activists and activist organizations have the potential to galvanize glbtq people, increase participation in organizations, and make a lasting impression in the fight for a specific cause.

Robert Hilferty's *Stop the Church* (1990), a documentary showing members of ACT UP demonstrating against New York's Cardinal O'Connor by entering St. Patrick's Cathedral and lying down until removed by the police, is a disturbing film about the disruptive power of activism. Perhaps not surprisingly, PBS refused to air the documentary.

Documentaries can also be tools for individual activism, as Tim Kirkman proves in *Dear Jesse* (1997), a long letter to Senator Jesse Helms interspersed with images that depict his hatred and interviews with people on the street about their attitudes toward Helms.

Lyrical Form in Autobiographical Documentaries

Sadie Benning, Barbara Hammer, and Su Friedrich, three of the most successful and popular experimental filmmakers, have sought innovative ways of seeing themselves as lesbians. They create images that reflect their visions of the world. Their work has expanded the notion of what constitutes a documentary. All three filmmakers claim the right to define lesbianism as an individual construction.

Most of Sadie Benning's short and personal documentaries were filmed in her bedroom and incorporate numerous television images. In *Me and Rubyfruit* (1989), *Jollies* (1990), and *Girlpower* (1992), Benning constantly seeks to define her sexual identity within a fiercely homophobic society that has produced narrow and negative images of women and lesbians.

Barbara Hammer's experimental documentaries *Women I Love* (1979), *Multiple Orgasm* (1976), and *Double Strength* (1976) are highly autobiographical, employing abstract images to investigate the filmmaker's sexuality and relationships with other women.

In the hour-long *Tender Fictions* (1995), Hammer sketches a complex personal and cultural autobiography from the events surrounding her life, including footage from Shirley Temple movies, the AFL/CIO faculty strike at San Francisco State College, the San Diego Women's Music Festival, and the "Take Back the Night" march in San Francisco.

Su Friedrich's film *Rules of the Road* (1993) is both oblique and engaging. Featuring images of Friedrich's car traveling along roads, with minimal narration, the film traces the growth and deterioration of a long-term relationship.

The Documentarian as Auteur

Several queer filmmakers working in the documentary form have produced distinctive and unified bodies of work that set them apart from other documentarians. Three such filmmakers are Marlon Riggs, Stuart Marshall, and Arthur Dong.

The six films directed by Marlon Riggs—*Ethnic Notions* (1987), *Tongues Untied* (1989), *Affirmation* (1990), *Anthem* (1990), *Color Adjustments* (1992), *No Regrets* (1992), and *Black is...Black Ain't* (1994)—center on issues of representation. They explore the ways in which mass-media institutions control images of African Americans, and they investigate the complexities of black gay identity.

Stuart Marshall's four films—*Bright Eyes* (1986), *Desire: Sexuality in Germany 1910–1945* (1989), *Comrades in Arms* (1990), and *Over Our Dead Bodies* (1991)—are unique in their broad conceptualization of issues. They are also remarkable for their ability to connect different perspectives within a single film. Marshall's *Bright Eyes* was the first feature-length documentary about AIDS.

Critics praise Arthur Dong for his extensive and shrewd historical and cultural analysis, and for the intensity that he brings to such subjects as men murdering gays (*Licensed to Kill*, 1997), gays and lesbians in the army during World War II (*Coming Out Under Fire*, 1994), queer rights (*The Question of Equality: Out Rage '69*, 1995), and gender-bending entertainment in a Chinese nightclub of the 1930s and 1940s (*Forbidden City*, 1989).

Boundless Paths of Inquiry

Queer documentarians have also rigorously pursued difficult, hidden, and taboo topics that would have been inconceivable a decade ago. For example, Alexandra Shiva, Sean MacDonald, and Michelle Gucovsky's *Bombay Eunuch* (2001) looks at the *hijras* of India, transvestites and transgendered people who are both revered and feared for their power. Kate Davis's *Southern Comfort* tells the story of Robert Eads, a male-to-female transsexual hillbilly in conservative rural America who, after a diagnosis of uterine cancer, is shunned by medical communities.

Over a period of five years, filmmaker Sandi DuBowski earned the trust of gay and lesbian Orthodox Jews in order to tell their story in *Trembling Before G-d* (2001). The film presents an intricate narrative of fear and self-hatred in the quest to reconcile religion and sexual identity.

Greta Schiller's *The Man Who Drove With Mandela* (1999) traces the life of Cecil Williams, a gay American theater director and activist against the racist government of South Africa, who through a startling series of events was in the car with Nelson Mandala as Mandela returned to South Africa.

By pursuing such unusual yet fascinating narratives, documentarians are revising history and changing public perceptions of the queer community.

Recent Trends in Queer Documentary

All of the documentary forms noted above have been used recently by filmmakers grappling with contemporary topics and debates. The very diversity of the topics and debates addressed by queer documentarians is evidence of the diverse interests of the glbtq community and of the centrality of our issues in the national dialogue about civil rights and equality.

For example, recent biographical documentaries have focused a lens on a wide range of queer issues by exploring the lives of both well-known and relatively unknown people. Examining the accomplishments and heritages of individuals has facilitated the exploration of issues ranging from the intolerance of organized religion to the unconventional expression of gay painters and fashion designers.

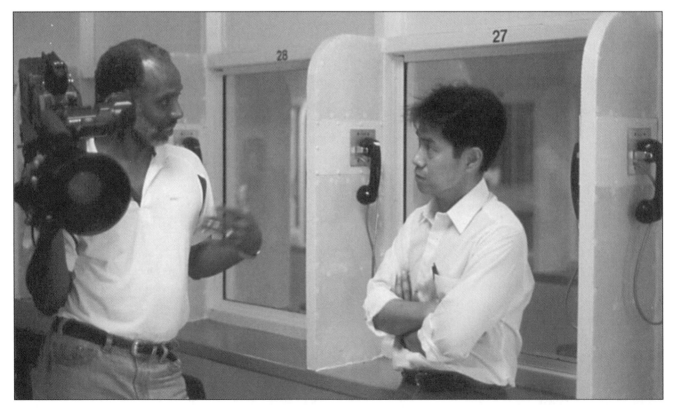

Director of cinematograhy Robert Shepard (left) and filmmaker Arthur Dong on location for *Licensed to Kill* at Robertson Correctional Unit, Abilene, Texas, in 1996.
Photograph by Angie Rosga.

These documentaries include Charles Atlas's *The Legend of Leigh Bowery* (2003); Carole Bonstein's *A Swiss Rebel: Annemarie Schwarzenbach 1908–1942*, produced in 2000 but receiving new exposure at recent film festivals; ; Matt Sneddon's *The Truth or Consequences of Delmas Howe* (2004); and Fenton Bailey and Randy Barbato's *Hidden Führer: Debating the Enigma of Hitler's Sexuality* (2004).

Two biographical documentaries, Nancy D. Kates and Bennett Singer's *Brother Outsider: The Life of Bayard Rustin* (2002), and Joan Elizabeth Biren's *No Secret Anymore: The Times of Del Martin and Phyllis Lyon* (2003), contribute to queer history by illuminating the individual's role in sweeping historical change.

Brother Outsider: The Life of Bayard Rustin (2002) relies on archival footage to trace the civil rights movement in the 1960s, and document racism and homophobia in the United States. Rustin, the organizing figure behind the 1963 March on Washington, lived with the possibility that exposure of his homosexuality could harm the momentum of the movement. When the homophobia of his allies and enemies generated public scrutiny, Rustin detached himself from the central figures of the movement but remained an outspoken activist on many civil rights issues. A wealth of archival footage of Rustin provides an insightful personal profile within the sweep of history.

No Secret Anymore: The Times of Del Martin and Phyllis Lyon (2003) covers fifty years in the history of lesbian and gay civil rights. Filmmaker Joan Biren started making the film in 1999, and it premiered on the fiftieth anniversary of the partnership of Del Martin and Phylis Lyon, activists who were at the forefront of the struggle for glbtq equality. Through documenting their lives, director Biren assembles a dynamic history of lesbian rights in the United States and the growth of the glbtq community.

Established documentary filmmakers have also contributed to the recent national debate on topics central to lesbian and gay rights. Arthur Dong's *Family Fundamentals* (2002) poses the question: What happens when parents believe that their own kids represent the very element that will lead to the destruction of the human race? Dong attempts to understand the vehement reactions of religious families to their college-age children's homosexuality.

Since 2001, more than twenty-five documentaries have examined gay marriage from different perspectives. Jim de Sève's *Tying the Knot* (2003) ambitiously depicts the political and social forces arrayed against gay marriage, as well as the struggles of lesbian and gay couples in different states with different laws and differing public opinion. It reveals the complexity of a national battle often simplified by other documentaries. Abigail Honor's *Saints and Sinners* (2004) depicts the struggle of a gay male couple to receive the Holy Sacrament of Marriage in the Roman Catholic Church.

Canadian filmmaker Alexis Fosse Mackintosh's *Let No One Put Asunder* (2004) depicts the obstacles to marriage faced by three Canadian same-sex couples in the context of a national political debate in which a major figure in the Conservative Party supported a legislative ban on gay marriage.

Several recent documentaries on AIDS examine its global impact. For example, Rory Kennedy's *Pandemic: Facing AIDS* (2003) chronicles the devastation wrought by AIDS in countries such as Uganda and Thailand. But Louise H. Jogarth shocked the American gay community with *The Gift* (2003), about the efforts of some HIV-negative men to become infected with the disease.

Judy Wilder and Laura Barton's *The Dildo Diaries* (2003) examines the Texas Penal Code (which makes owing six or more dildos a felony) and its effects on the adult sex toy industry. Through probing and sometimes hilarious interviews with legislators, porn stars, sex shop owners, and others, the film honors the dildo's fight for legitimacy and underscores the danger of antisodomy laws, while exposing the absurdity of the actions of the Texas legislature.

Other topics that documentary filmmakers have investigated since 2002 include the history of the women's music movement, in Dee Mosbacher's *Radical Harmonies* (2002); the persecution of gay men and lesbians in the less-developed world, in Janet Baus and Dan Hunt's *Dangerous Living: Coming Out in the Developing World* (2003); the impact of the "first all-lesbian" punk band, in Tracy Flannigan's *Rise Above: The Tribe 8 Documentary* (2003); and the problems and contentments of rural gay life, in Tom Murray's *Farm Family: In Search of Gay Life in Rural America* (2003).

The stakes are high for queer documentary filmmakers: the preservation of our history. They have responded to political change and shifting public opinion in a manner that admirably represents the various positions of the queer community.

—*Richard C. Bartone*

BIBLIOGRAPHY

Bad Object-Choices, ed. *How Do I Look: Queer Film and Video*. Seattle: Bay Press, 1991.

Dyer, Richard. *Now You See It: Studies on Lesbian and Gay Film*. London: Routledge, 1990.

Gever, Martha, John Greyson, and Pratibha Parmar, eds. *Queer Looks: Perspectives on Lesbian and Gay Film and Video*. London: Routledge, 1993.

Holmlund, Chris, and Cynthia Fuchs, eds. *Between the Sheets, In the Streets: Queer, Lesbian, Gay Documentary*. Minneapolis: University of Minnesota Press, 1997.

Juhasz, Alexandra. *AIDS TV: Identity, Community, and Alternative Video*. Durham, N.C.: Duke University Press, 1995.

Dong, Arthur   (b. 1953)

THE DOCUMENTARIES OF FILMMAKER ARTHUR DONG, including several works that examine the roots of antigay attitudes in American culture and society, are distinguished by their humanity and complexity. This gay Asian American director's subtle, open-ended approach deepens understanding by encouraging viewers to situate themselves in relation to the issues, including homophobia and racism, that he explores in such films as *Coming Out Under Fire*, *Licensed to Kill*, and *Family Fundamentals*. Dong's movies amount to a particularly thoughtful form of activism.

Coming Out Under Fire, completed in 1994, is based on Allan Bérubé's well-received nonfiction book of the same title. It comments on the development (and the stupidity) of the "Don't Ask, Don't Tell" policy of the U.S. military by focusing on a group of gay and lesbian veterans of World War II. Speaking candidly for the camera, these men and women tell what it was like to hide their sexuality while in uniform during wartime. A former marine who entertained fellow service members by performing in drag says, "That was why we were marines—to make other marines laugh." His powerfully ambivalent comment is characteristic of the film as a whole.

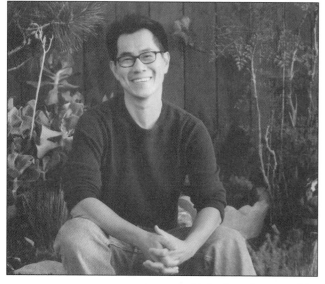

A portrait of Arthur Dong by Amy Rachlin.

Licensed to Kill, televised by the PBS network in 1998, is Dong's harrowing look at antigay violence. For this film, he went to prisons around the country and interviewed killers of gay men, asking them directly, "Why did you do it?" Not surprisingly, their answers point to religious and political leaders whose antigay pronouncements seemingly gave them license for committing their crimes.

Dong, who survived a gay-bashing attack in 1977 by throwing himself against the front of a passing Volkswagen bus and holding on as it carried him up the street to safety, was castigated for giving killers a platform—after all, critics said, these men had already had their say. "Once the film got out," Dong said later, "I think I quelled those fears. People said, 'Why would you give them a forum?' My idea was that we need to learn from them if we're going to overcome the problem."

Family Fundamentals, released in 2002, focuses on three families in which fundamentalist Christian parents reject their gay son or daughter. "*Family Fundamentals* is a little tame," Dong acknowledged, "but I wanted to reach a certain audience. We need to speak their language to get the message across." In another interview, Dong said that the question boils down to: "Do you want to shout down the opposition or do you want to work with them? My film is trying to ask, 'Can't we work on this together?' "

These three films are available in a boxed set under the umbrella title *Stories from the War on Homosexuality*. In keeping with his grassroots philosophy, Dong distributes his own work through DeepFocus Productions, his company based in Los Angeles, where he lives with his partner of more than twenty-five years.

"Self-distribution is a big part of what I do," Dong has said. "I've been doing it since the early '80s, when that notion was kind of crazy. Now more and more people are doing it, and it's become easier with the Internet, which has changed the marketing of films for independents. They don't need to rely so much on the machine."

Arthur Dong was born the son of Chinese immigrants in 1953 in San Francisco, where he came out in 1969 and made his first film in a high school art class in 1970. Entitled *Public*, it was a five-minute animated short presenting a child's-eye view of the war in Vietnam and other issues.

Dong went on to study filmmaking at San Francisco State University and at the American Film Institute.

Sewing Woman, Dong's 1982 film focusing on his mother's experience as a Chinese immigrant making a new life in America, was nominated for an Academy Award. *Lotus* (1987) is a dramatic short condemning the binding of women's feet in China. *Forbidden City, U.S.A.* (1989) spotlights a San Francisco nightclub featuring Asian American performers that became an international tourist attraction during the 1930s and 1940s.

Another documentary directed by Dong, *Out Rage '69* (1995), was the first of four episodes in the PBS series, *The Question of Equality*, a history of the gay rights movement. Typically for this filmmaker, it asked difficult questions, focusing on racism, sexism, and class prejudice *within* the movement, and not just outside it.

Arthur Dong's work has won numerous honors and awards, including a George Foster Peabody Award, three Sundance Film Festival Awards, five Emmy nominations, and two GLAAD (Gay and Lesbian Alliance Against Defamation) Media Awards.

He is a member of the Board of Governors of the Academy of Motion Picture Arts and Sciences, representing the Documentary Branch. In that capacity as in his own distinguished work, he heightens awareness of (and appreciation for) the documentary form.

—*Greg Varner*

BIBLIOGRAPHY

Dong, Arthur. Biographical Statement. www.deepfocusproductions.com

Goldman, Walter. "The Ugliness at Work in Attacks on Homosexuals." *New York Times,* June 23, 1998.

Guthmann, Edward. "How Fundamentalists, Gays Sit at Same 'Family' Table; Arthur Dong Explores Conflicts in Latest Documentary." *San Francisco Chronicle,* October 9, 2002.

Herlinger, Chris. "At Home, Conflicts Over Homosexuality: Documentary Follows Gay Men, Lesbians From Conservative Christian Families." *Washington Post,* July 13, 2002.

King, Loren. "Reconciling Old-Time Religion and Gay Sexuality." *Boston Globe,* June 9, 2002.

Varner, Greg. "A Look at the Dark Side: Documentarian Arthur Dong Asks Killers of Gay Men Why They Did It." *Washington Blade,* June 12, 1998.

SEE ALSO

Documentary Film

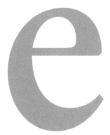

Edens, Roger
(1905–1970)

ROGER EDENS WAS A GIFTED COMPOSER AND ARRANGER who gave a new look to movie musicals through his work with the Arthur Freed unit at the MGM studios. He was mentor and friend to many in the entertainment industry, including Judy Garland.

Edens came from a large family in Hillsboro, Texas. The youngest of eight brothers, he was born Rollins Edens on November 9, 1905. Unlike his rambunctious siblings, Edens was of an artistic and studious nature. His parents, though not well off, managed to scrape together enough money to finance his education at the University of Texas.

Upon graduation, Edens found work playing piano on a cruise ship. A manager from New York heard him and helped him land a job with a jazz band. Edens, who always enjoyed a close relationship with his family, brought his widowed mother to stay with him on Long Island.

At this time, Edens changed his first name to Roger. The reasons for this are unclear, but William J. Mann suggests that it is "possible he considered 'Rollins' just too precious, too dandy, for the hard-drinking, woman-chasing world of orchestras and musicians."

Edens moved on to a job with the Red Nichols Orchestra, which played at the Alvin Theater on Broadway. In a dramatic turn of events, Edens was called from the orchestra pit to the stage when Ethel Merman's pianist suffered a heart attack before the second performance of George and Ira Gershwin's *Girl Crazy,* in 1932. Impressed by Edens's work, Merman employed him as her accompanist and arranger for her next show and for her nightclub act. When she headed for Hollywood, she brought along Edens to be music director for Roy Del Ruth's *Kid Millions* (1934), in which she would star.

Also moving to California was Edens's wife, the former Martha LaPrelle, whom he had dated in college. Their marriage was characterized by long periods apart, since her job as a buyer for a fashion house entailed extensive travel. According to Edens's nephew J. C. Edens, his aunt "never cared much for Hollywood." Even Edens's closest friends in California rarely saw her. The couple soon separated and eventually divorced.

Edens meanwhile had attracted the attention of MGM producer Arthur Freed when the latter heard him play at the audition of a singer. Freed was not much impressed by the singer but instantly recognized Edens's skill as a composer and arranger. He quickly hired him as a member of his creative staff.

The Arthur Freed unit was a team of talented composers, arrangers, lyricists, choreographers, and other artisans who set the standard for movie musicals during their golden age, from the late 1930s to the early 1960s. Because so many members were gay, the Freed unit was known in the industry as "Freed's Fairies."

Freed, who was not gay, never intended to create a team of gay artists, nor were all the members of the Arthur

Freed unit gay. But Freed wanted a first-rate team, and he hired without regard to sexual orientation. The many gifted and gay members of the team, in addition to Edens, include songwriters Cole Porter and Frederick Loewe, choreographers Robert Alton and Jack Cole, and directors Charles Walters and the closeted Vincente Minnelli.

Edens became the heart and soul of the Freed unit, and Freed had the utmost confidence in him. Production assistant Lela Simone stated that "Freed did not occupy himself with details because he had Roger and he knew that Roger was going to do the best job there is." Freed's reliance on Edens is reflected in his decision to elevate him to the rank of associate producer on a number of films, beginning with Minnelli's *Meet Me in St. Louis* (1944). It was extremely rare in Hollywood to move from a job as a musician to one in production.

Edens's first film with Freed was Victor Fleming's *Reckless* (1935), for which he was musical supervisor. During his career, Edens worked on over forty films as composer, musical director, producer, or a combination of these. His long list of credits includes Robert Z. Leonard's *The Great Ziegfeld* (1936), Fleming's *The Wizard of Oz* (1939), Busby Berkeley's *Babes in Arms* (1939), Minnelli's *Cabin in the Sky* (1943), Charles Walters's *Easter Parade* (1948), Gene Kelly and Stanley Donen's *Singin' in the Rain* (1952), and George Cukor's *A Star Is Born* (1954).

The Freed unit, with Edens at the helm, created a new kind of musical. Whereas previously musical movies had been essentially stories interrupted by the occasional song, Edens insisted that "songs in film musicals should be part of the script itself." In the Freed unit, songs fit seamlessly into the plot.

Hollywood honored Edens with three Academy Awards. His first, for *Easter Parade*, was followed in rapid succession by Oscars for Donen's *On the Town* (1949) and George Sidney's *Annie Get Your Gun* (1950).

Edens played an important part in the career of gay icon Judy Garland. The two met in 1935 when Edens was called in to replace Garland's father, Frank Gumm, an amateur pianist, at Garland's audition at MGM. Edens was quick to appreciate her talent and became not only her musical mentor but also a lifelong friend.

Edens wrote a song for Garland to sing at Clark Gable's birthday party in 1937. It not only delighted Gable but also favorably impressed the producer of Del Ruth's *Broadway Melody of 1938* (1937), who had Garland sing it in the film.

After working with Garland on a couple of other projects, Edens served as musical director for *The Wizard of Oz* and also as rehearsal pianist for Garland. Garland's daughter Lorna Luft credits Edens with teaching her mother to have the courage to show her vulnerability in her performances. "Without Roger," she commented, "we might never have had 'Over the Rainbow,' at least not the way we remember it."

Edens continued to contribute to Garland's professional success. He provided her "Born in a Trunk" number for *A Star Is Born*—uncredited, because he was under exclusive contract to MGM and the film was a Warner Brothers production.

Edens and Charles Walters were also indispensable in arranging Garland's triumphant 1951 vaudeville act at the RKO Palace Theatre, which won rave reviews from the critics.

Edens's professional star continued to rise. Freed chose him as producer of two movies, Donen's *Deep in My Heart* (1954), featuring the music of Sigmund Romberg, and *Funny Face* (1957).

By this time, the heyday of the movie musical was waning, and various members of the Freed unit had moved on. Edens worked on a few more films, notably Walters's *The Unsinkable Molly Brown* (1964) and Kelly's *Hello, Dolly!* (1969), but also pursued other opportunities. During the 1960s, he renewed his professional association with both Garland and Merman, penning material for their nightclub acts. He also coached Katharine Hepburn for her performance in Alan Jay Lerner and André Previn's stage musical *Coco* in 1969.

Edens succumbed to cancer on July 13, 1970, in Hollywood.

Edens's career is a stunning success story, the more remarkable because his achievements came in an era of widespread homophobia. Gay performers sometimes resorted to "lavender marriages" or invented fictitious wives to conceal their sexual orientation. Even working behind the scenes and in the congenial atmosphere of the Freed unit, Edens, according to Mann, kept a photo of his ex-wife on his desk for years though he was living openly with another man.

Mann also recounts a touching recollection of Frank Lysinger, an MGM messenger whom Edens had befriended around 1939. Edens often invited him to dinner along with Lena Horne and musical director Lennie Hayton—a gathering of two "officially unsanctioned" couples, since studio head Louis B. Mayer had forbidden Horne, an African American, and Hayton, who was white, to date each other. Edens, who championed Horne at the studio, also tried to bring happiness to her personal life.

This kindness and compassion were typical of Edens's character. His collaborator and longtime friend Kay Thompson described him as "a darling man," and Michael Morrison, another friend and the business partner of gay actor William Haines, commented that "all sorts of people were drawn to him."

Edens was a model of professional success and personal dignity.

—Linda Rapp

BIBLIOGRAPHY

Eder, Bruce. "Roger Edens."
http://movies2.nytimes.com/gst/movies/filmography.html?p_id
=88652&mod=bio

Fricke, John. *Judy Garland: The World's Greatest Entertainer.* New York:
Henry Holt and Company, 1992.

Kenrick, John. "Edens, Roger." www.musicals101.com/who2d.htm

Mann, William J. *Behind the Screen: How Gays and Lesbians Shaped
Hollywood, 1910–1969.* New York: Viking, 2001.

SEE ALSO

Cukor, George; Garland, Judy; Haines, William "Billy"; Minnelli, Vincente

Eisenstein, Sergei Mikhailovich   *(1898–1948)*

ONE OF THE GREATEST FILMMAKERS IN THE HISTORY OF cinema, Sergei Eisenstein was one of the first directors to take seriously the role of film editing as a means of narrative, a way of manipulating time and space by linking and juxtaposing images.

Eisenstein was born on January 23, 1898, in Riga, Latvia. He attended the science-oriented Realshule to prepare himself for engineering school, but he also performed in a children's theater troupe while a student. In 1915, he entered Petrograd's Institute of Civil Engineering, his father's alma mater. However, he evinced as much interest in art and theater as he did in engineering.

During the February 1917 Revolution, Eisenstein served in the volunteer militia and in the engineering corps of the Russian Army. In the spring of 1918, following the October Revolution of 1917, he joined the Red Army. His father, however, supported the White Russian Army and subsequently emigrated.

In 1920, Eisenstein entered the General Staff Academy in Moscow, where he joined the First Workers' Theater of Proletcult as a scenic and costume designer. He collaborated with several experimental theater groups.

Despite his success in the theater, Eisenstein eagerly embraced film as the artistic medium that could most effectively convey communist ideas and ideals. From the beginning of his career as a filmmaker, he took a theoretical approach. The idea of editing to create a truly cinematic language became codified as "montage."

This theoretical approach to the cinema can be found in Eisenstein's first feature film, *Strike* (1924). Although *Strike* is based on an agitprop theater piece, one would never know it, for the film became, in Eisenstein's fevered cinematic imagination, a torrent of visceral imagery, edited for maximum impact.

Strike's narrative is often obscured by the onslaught of imagery; nevertheless, the work remains one of the most startling debut films in the entire history of cinema, and might have attained legendary status were it not for the fact that Eisenstein's follow-up feature proved to be one of the most famous films ever made, the incendiary masterpiece *The Battleship Potemkin* (1925).

Potemkin's more linear narrative allowed the impacted editing and the rush of images to attain a greater emotional effect. Shot with the immediacy of a newsreel, this story of the naval revolt in Odessa in 1905 produced some of the most celebrated sequences in twentieth-century art: the Odessa Steps scene must be the single most quoted, imitated, and parodied sequence in movie history.

Eisenstein's triumph with *Potemkin* was instantaneous and worldwide. But political problems surfaced during the filming of his next epic, *October* (1928). In that film, begun in 1927 to celebrate the October Revolution of 1917, Eisenstein planned his most elaborate scenario, which was to display his theory of "dialectical montage" to maximum effect. By the time filming was completed, however, Stalin's cultural policies were firmly in effect, which wreaked havoc with the film's final cut and the content.

When *October* was finally shown in 1928, the battles with the cultural bureaucracy had been fought, and Eisenstein had lost. His next movie, *Old and New* (1929), his paean to collective farming, proved a more conventional propagandistic piece, but it too was subject to censorship.

Chafing under the constraints of Stalinism, Eisenstein accepted offers to work abroad, which led to unfulfilled projects in the United States and to the spectacular debacle of *Que Viva Mexico!* That film, never completed, was taken over by the producers and edited into three separate films: *A Time in the Sun, Thunder Over Mexico,* and *Death Day* (1935–1938).

Eisenstein returned to the Soviet Union in 1935, where he continued the spiral of falling out of and back into favor with the Stalinist regime. His remaining films—*Bezhin Meadow* (1937), *Alexander Nevsky* (1939), *Ivan the Terrible, Part I* (1942), *Ivan the Terrible, Part II: The Boyars' Plot* (1946), and the fragment of *Ivan the Terrible, Part III* (1947)—were marked with the tensions of the political turmoil in which Eisenstein was embroiled.

Eisenstein's personal life was also chaotic. He married twice in response to political pressure, but his marriages were never consummated. His unexpurgated diaries, recently published as *Immortal Memories*, are filled with accounts of his infatuations with many young men, including his assistant, Grigori Alexandrov.

Often, his infatuations (as in the case of Alexandrov) were with young heterosexual men, whom he would educate and assist in their careers. His drawings, recently exhibited during the centenary of his birth, include many illustrations of homosexual activity.

Despite his difficulties with censorship and other problems, Eisenstein created a remarkable legacy. His films reveal his continued commitment to experimentation in form. *Nevsky*, his first sound film, contains spectacular scenes, most notably the Battle on the Ice, as well as the incomparably thrilling film score by Sergei Prokofiev.

Ivan the Terrible, an intensely Expressionistic study of political power and corruption, with immense sets, voluminous costumes, and amazingly hyperbolic lighting, represents a contrast to this earlier work. It was not dynamically edited, but relied on extended long takes, in which dialogue, sound effects, and music were crucial. *Ivan the Terrible* pointed to new operatic possibilities in motion pictures.

In addition, *Nevsky* and *Ivan the Terrible* benefited from the charismatic performances of Nikolai Cherkassov, a "golden Adonis" on whom the director doted.

From *Strike* to *Ivan*, Eisenstein's career always excited controversy, but he remains one of the most important filmmakers in history, the exemplar of the true intellectual artist.

—*Daryl Chin*

BIBLIOGRAPHY

Bergen, Ronald. *Eisenstein: A Life in Conflict*. Boston: Little, Brown, 1997.

Eisenstein, Sergei M. *Beyond the Stars: The Memoirs of Sergei M. Eisenstein*. Richard Taylor, ed.; William Powell, trans. Calcutta: Seagull Books, 1995.

———. *Immortal Memories: An Autobiography*. Herbert Marshall, trans. Boston: Houghton Mifflin, 1983.

Montagu, Ivor. *With Eisenstein in Hollywood: A Chapter of Autobiography*. New York: International Publishers, 1969.

Seton, Marie. *Sergei M. Eisenstein: A Biography*. London: Dennis Dobson, 1978.

SEE ALSO

Film; Film Directors; Anger, Kenneth

Epperson, John   (b. 1955)

JOHN EPPERSON HAS HAD AN EXTREMELY SUCCESSFUL career performing as the glamorous and hilarious drag character Lypsinka. In addition, he has appeared, both in and out of character, in several plays and films.

Epperson was born on April 24, 1955, in Hazlehurst, Mississippi, not a particularly gay-friendly place to grow up. He said in a 2002 interview, "I was always like a changeling in my home...like an alien among them." He wondered why he was so fascinated by show business when no one else in his family was.

From an early age Epperson took lessons in classical piano, but he was also intrigued by popular music and culture. By the age of four, he was lip-synching to his father's records and soon gave dancing a try as well, mimicking Ann-Margret's moves in George Sidney's *Bye Bye Birdie* (1963).

School days were a trial for the boy seen as a "sissy," who was "teased, taunted, [and] physically threatened." He had to teach himself to be less effeminate in order to cope with his schoolmates' cruelty.

After high school, Epperson enrolled at Belhaven College, a small Presbyterian institution in Jackson, Mississippi. While there, he went to a gay bar—a "sawdust-on-the-floor-dump," as he recalled it—for the first time and saw drag performers doing lip-synching acts. He called the experience "totally frightening because I saw myself up on stage." He realized that drag performers might draw enthusiastic audiences but were also subject to ostracism. Not wishing the latter fate, he stopped going to gay bars for a year.

When Epperson graduated from Belhaven, he landed a job playing piano in Colorado, but in 1978 he moved to New York, where he became a rehearsal pianist for American Ballet Theater. In addition, despite his earlier misgivings, Epperson began doing drag performances at nightspots such as Club 57 and the Pyramid.

When Epperson went on tour with American Ballet Theater, he had the opportunity to see sophisticated drag acts in Europe. Modeling his performances on those, Epperson wrote and starred in two drag pieces—*Dial "M" for Model* (1987) and *Ballet of the Dolls* (1988), a send-up of Jacqueline Susann's *Valley of the Dolls*—before beginning to perform as Lypsinka.

In creating the Lypsinka character, he "chose a one-word name to show a sense of humor, but also as an homage to European models with one name." Epperson has said that Lypsinka owes much of her look to 1950s supermodel Dovima, and that stage actress Dolores Gray was also part of the "prototype for Lypsinka." Among others who influenced his work he cites Ann-Margret, Charles Pierce, and Charles Ludlam.

Lypsinka first met her public in late 1988, when Epperson's act was a late-night addition to the bill of Charles Busch's *Vampire Lesbians of Sodom* at the Provincetown Playhouse in New York. *I Could Go on Lip-Synching* is the story of Lypsinka's rise from modest beginnings in Louisiana to the status of diva.

The show, which soon moved to the Theater Off Park, was a resounding success, running for slightly over a year in New York. It then went to California, where the production was financed in part by Madonna.

Epperson quit his job with American Ballet Theater in 1991 in order to devote himself full-time to performing as Lypsinka. His repertoire includes *The Fabulous Lypsinka*

Show, Lypsinka! Now It Can Be Lip-Synched, Lypsinka! A Day in the Life, Lypsinka! As I Lay Lip-Synching, and *Lypsinka! The Boxed Set*. For the last, he won the Los Angeles Drama Critics' Circle Award for Best Sound Design, the L.A. Weekly Theatre Award for Best Solo Performance, and the Helen Hayes Award for Best Nonresident Production in 2003. He was also a nominee for Outstanding Lead Actor at the Hayes Awards.

The Lypsinka shows are technically complex, as Epperson weaves together scores of source materials to tell a story. Ringing telephones, bringing matters that demand immediate attention, are a staple of the act as Lypsinka expends extraordinary energy in coping with the exigencies of life. Scenery and lighting designer Mark T. Simpson calls Lypsinka "a 'schizophrenetic' character" whose "cueing requires rapid-fire color-wash changes and flashing strobes." He praises Epperson for his planning of the productions: "He's aware of everything. His attention to detail feeds the whole process. In a certain sense, if you can keep up with him, you can't go wrong."

Epperson's performances as Lypsinka can be enjoyed simply as comedic entertainment. Adelina Anthony calls him "a master of mad elegance, hilarious timing, and perfect physical expression." But there is more to a Lypsinka performance than light comedy. As Anthony also notes, Epperson's "gender-bending show is also a refreshing delight in the way he explores the dilemma of being pigeon-holed, stereotyped, and feared. His work is very pro-woman, pro-individual, and pro-dignity, without the political preaching."

Epperson has commented, "It's so easy to do misogynistic drag humor" and states that he has "deliberately tried to avoid that." He adds, "A lot of women, when they see the show, feel liberated and empowered."

Epperson rejects the term *drag queen* for himself and has stated that he does not enjoy much of the drag that is being done because "it is loud and tacky and trashy and has no sensibility or thought behind it." He intends his own work as "a commentary of performance in general and drag performance specifically." However outrageous Lypsinka may be, she is always at heart affectionate toward the women to whose work she performs.

In his cabaret act as Lypsinka, Epperson typically does not utter a sound. The entire shows are meticulously crafted from recordings of music and the spoken word, which Epperson interprets through expression and gesture. He has been praised for his ability to convey the wide array of emotions to which Lypsinka is subject as she works her way through the existential crises of her life.

Although Lypsinka does not speak in solo performances, she does when appearing on stage with other actors. The first such occasion came in 1998 in the show *Lypsinka Is Harriet Craig!*, a send-up of Vincent Sherman's 1950 film *Harriet Craig*, with Joan Crawford in the title role. The Lypsinka production costarred drag artist Varla Jean Merman (Jeffery Roberson) as Craig's much-put-upon cousin. Epperson has also been seen as Lypsinka on the big screen, in Barry Shils's *Wigstock: The Movie* (1995).

In his most recent performance as Lypsinka, in *The Passion of Crawford* (2005), Epperson recreates an interview that Crawford recorded late in her career. The work has been hailed as both richly comic and unexpectedly poignant.

Lypsinka has appeared in the George Michael music video "Too Funky" (1999), in several television specials, and in ads for companies such as the Gap and L.A. Eyewear. She has paraded down the runway of Thierry Mugler's fashion shows in Paris, Los Angeles, and Tokyo with other celebrities, including Sharon Stone, Julie Newmar, Jeff Stryker, and Ivana Trump.

Epperson has played drag roles as characters other than Lypsinka on both stage and screen. He earned plaudits as the wicked stepmother in New York City Opera's 2004 production of Richard Rodgers and Oscar Hammerstein's *Cinderella*. He portrayed a madam in Paul Schrader's 1994 HBO movie *Witch Hunt*, and he also plays a woman in Todd Stephens's *Another Gay Movie*, scheduled for release in 2005.

Epperson has played masculine roles as well, including a turn as RuPaul's boyfriend in Charles Winkler's 1996 film *Red Ribbon Blues*, which did not see theatrical release but has been shown on cable television. He appeared onstage at the New York International Fringe Festival in Patrick E. Horrigan's one-act drama *Messages for Gary*.

In 2004, Epperson launched a new cabaret piece, *Show Trash*, in which he plays piano and sings show tunes. Critic Peter Marks cited "eerie parallels between Superman and Lypsinka.... Each is an exaggerated version of a manly or feminine ideal. Both might view a red cape as a legitimate fashion statement...[but] both have mild-mannered alter egos." Marks praises Epperson for his voice—"strong and clear"—and his choice of selections—witty, soulful, honest, and showing, like his performances as Lypsinka, a sincere and caring appreciation of the material that he presents.

Epperson has also written a play, *My Deah*, his version of the Medea tale transplanted to Mississippi. It has been given several readings, including one at the Studio Theatre in Washington, D.C., in 2004 as a benefit for the Whitman-Walker Clinic, a glbtq health services provider.

Epperson does not see himself as a particularly political person. On the possibility of gay marriage, he commented in a 2002 interview, "I understand why people want the legal benefits of marriage. It just doesn't appeal to me to be married at all." A year later he called himself "too idiosyncratic for anybody to live with," adding that "traditionally most gay guys aren't interested in going with drag performers, because they just can't go there."

Epperson has stated on various occasions that, though the status of outsider can be difficult, he prefers individualism to assimilation. In a 2003 interview, he said, "When I see [gay] people who want to be assimilated into the mainstream, I can only say that if Tennessee Williams had wanted to be assimilated into the mainstream, he would never have written *Streetcar*. Being an outsider made him what he was."   —*Linda Rapp*

BIBLIOGRAPHY

Anthony, Adelina. Review of *Lypsinka! The Boxed Set*. *Back Stage West*, May 10, 2001, 15.

"As I Light Lypsinka." *Lighting Dimensions* (October 1, 2003): www.lightingdimensions.com/mag/lighting_light_lypsinka

Barnes, Michael. "Viva la Diva: Lypsinka Does It Her Way." *Austin American Statesman*, November 29, 2001.

Dullea, Georgia. "At Home with John Epperson: A Day in the Life of Lypsinka's Maid." *New York Times*, April 16, 1992.

LaSalle, Mick. "From the Lips of Lypsinka; Epperson Talks, in His Own Voice, about His New Show." *San Francisco Chronicle*, February 2, 1994.

Marks, Peter. "It's a Musical Life: Epperson Is Good 'Trash.'" *Washington Post*, June 16, 2004.

Padget, Jonathan. "Lypsinka Speaks!: Interview with John Epperson." *Metro Weekly* (Washington, D.C.), June 20, 2002. www.metroweekly.com/feature/?ak=12

Pela, Robert L. "Kind of a Drag: Lypsinka Is Much More Than a Drag Queen." *Phoenix New Times*, April 8, 2004.

Tallmer, Jerry. "Lypsinka Unplugged: John Epperson Works Hard to Remain on the Outside Looking in." *Gay City News* (New York), August 22, 2003. www.gaycitynews.com/gcn234/lypsinkaunplugged.html

www.lypsinka.com

SEE ALSO

RuPaul (RuPaul Andre Charles)

European Film

EUROPEAN FILMS HAVE BEEN GREATLY INFLUENTIAL IN shaping the history of queer cinema. In the first thirty years or so of cinema (roughly from the 1920s through the 1950s), European films, like their American counterparts, rarely included honest, nonjudgmental portrayals of gay and lesbian characters or dealt seriously with the theme of homosexuality.

However, as attitudes and ideas evolved in Europe throughout the 1960s and 1970s, the lives and culture of homosexual men and women became more visible, and film became more explicit about sexual behavior. Consequently, glbtq filmmakers across many European countries were able to bring their personal sensibilities to the screen, creating socially, as well as artistically, significant queer-themed films.

Although working across an array of styles and exploring a variety of subjects, glbtq European films exhibit several common themes, such as conflicts between classes and generations, the plight of the marginalized, and the yearning for love and freedom in a repressive society.

Early Gay and Lesbian European Films

The first known gay-themed film is Swedish director Mauritz Stiller's *Vingarne* (*The Wings*, 1916). Based on Herman Bang's novel *Mikael*, the film concerns a sculptor and his attraction to his young and handsome apprentice (who is primarily attracted to women). The younger man takes advantage of his patron at every opportunity, and their romance ends unhappily, with the older man dying of a broken heart.

The same material was used by German filmmaker Carl Theodor Dreyer in 1924, under the title *Mikaël*. As with the earlier Swedish film, the relationship between the two men is handled discreetly and conveyed mainly through glances and tone.

Another early gay-themed film is Richard Oswald's *Anders als die Andern* (*Different from the Others*, 1919), written by Oswald and Magnus Hirschfeld, the renowned German sexologist and founder of the Institute for Sexual Science in Berlin. Conrad Veidt stars as a musician blackmailed after making advances on a stranger at a men-only dance. The story is prefaced by a direct-to-camera monologue by Hirschfeld and ends with an explicit plea for the abolishment of Paragraph 175, the German law that punished homosexuality. The film was banned by the German government after a short commercial run.

In 1931, Leontine Sagan directed *Mädchen in Uniform* (*Girls in Uniform*), one of the earliest films with a strong lesbian undertone. Based on a play by the German writer Christa Winsloe, it tells the story of Manuela, an unhappy schoolgirl sent to a strict boarding school, who develops a romantic attraction to one of her teachers. When Manuela openly declares her love, the headmistress denounces such feelings as "sinful" and decides the student must be expelled. Faced with separation from her beloved, Manuela is driven to the point of suicide. Two endings were created for the film; in one, Manuela dies, but in the other she is saved by her classmates. The latter version was deemed objectionable by American censors; therefore, the more tragic ending, where the schoolgirl is irrevocably punished for her feelings, was the only version available in the United States for decades.

Cocteau and Genet

Other significant examples of early European gay cinema include the films of Jean Cocteau and Jean Genet's *Un chant d'amour*.

Jean Cocteau was one of the most versatile French artists of the twentieth century; in addition to being a director, he was a poet, novelist, painter, playwright, set designer, and actor. He was also openly homosexual; many of his films feature his lover of many years Jean Marais.

Cocteau's first film, *Le sang d'un poète* (*The Blood of a Poet*, 1930), explores the process of creating art through a series of dreamlike tableaux. Cocteau has stated that the film was an attempt to tell "where poems come from." He denied that the film contained any symbolism and instead called the movie "a realistic documentary of unreal happenings."

Cocteau wrote dialogue and adapted several stories for the screen over the next several years, but let fifteen years pass before writing and directing his second film, *La belle et la bête* (*Beauty and the Beast*, 1946). Using haunting images, and romantically elegant sets and costumes, Cocteau tells the story (based on the eighteenth-century fable by Madame Leprince de Beaumont) of a lonely and misunderstood Beast, played by Jean Marais, who falls in love with a beautiful young woman. *La belle et la bête* is, by general consensus, one of the most enchanting films ever made.

Cocteau and Marais subsequently collaborated on several more films, including *L'aigle à deux têtes* (*The Eagle Has Two Heads*, 1947) and *Les parents terribles* (*The Storm Within*, 1948). Perhaps the most significant of their collaborations is *Orphée* (*Orpheus*, 1949). Cocteau sets his retelling of the Greek myth of Orpheus in postwar Paris, and casts Marais as a poet who follows the spirit of his dead wife to the Underworld. Instead of rescuing his wife, however, he abandons her in his search for the treasures Death may hold. Self-consciously homoerotic, *Orphée* features striking and original imagery; the film became famous for its use of two leather-clad motorcyclists as the errand boys of Death.

Following the completion of *Orphée*, Cocteau made no films of his own for ten years; he blamed his withdrawal on the commercialism of the cinema and the dependence of filmmakers on financial backers. He did, however, contribute dialogue, narration, and occasionally full screenplays to the films of others. In 1960, Cocteau directed his last film, *Le testament d'Orphée* (*The Testament of Orpheus*), another retelling of the Orpheus legend, this time reinterpreted as the story of an eighteenth-century poet who time-travels in search of inspiration. Cocteau cast himself as the poet; the film also includes uncredited appearances by Pablo Picasso, Jean Marais, and Charles Aznavour, among others.

Another French artist who has had a significant influence on both queer and experimental cinema is Jean Genet. Although more widely known as a novelist and playwright, Genet also created *Un chant d'amour* (*A Song of Love*, 1950), one of the earliest and most remarkable attempts to portray homosexual passion onscreen.

Less than half an hour in length and silent, the film tells the story of three prisoners in solitary confinement and the prison's warden. Realistic scenes of the prisoners attempting to communicate their desires for one another (for example, two prisoners share a cigarette by blowing smoke back and forth through a hole in the wall) give way to fantasy images of same-sex lovemaking.

Since its first release, *Un chant d'amour* has been subject to censorship and banned in several countries on the ground of obscenity. The film is explicit in its portrayal of gay male desire, showing several scenes of masturbation and containing possibly the earliest images of erect penises seen in a legitimate, nonpornographic film.

Victim

Another landmark in the evolution of European gay and lesbian cinema occurred with the release of the British film *Victim* (1961). The film, directed by Basil Dearden, broke serious ground by addressing the adverse public perception of homosexuality in Britain. At the time, Britain had laws against homosexual activity, which left many gay men vulnerable to blackmail or exposure. *Victim* concerns a self-confessed, but nonpracticing, homosexual, portrayed by Dirk Bogarde, who risks his marriage and career to track down a ring of blackmailers preying on wealthy gay men. The film is reputedly the first in Britain to use the term *homosexual;* it was initially banned in the United States simply because the word was uttered in the movie.

Although perhaps timid in its treatment of homosexuality by today's standards, *Victim* is, nonetheless, a very courageous film. Made in the aftermath of 1957's Wolfenden Report, which recommended that homosexual behavior between consenting adults no longer be criminalized in England, the filmmakers consciously set out to change British law and the public's perceptions of homosexuality. Six years after the film's release, the Sexual Offences Act of 1967 finally decriminalized most homosexual behavior between consenting adults over the age of twenty-one in England and Wales.

As political and social changes gradually took place in Europe throughout the 1960s and 1970s, the portrayal of homosexual men and women onscreen became more acceptable, and brought several gay and lesbian directors and their queer-themed films to the forefront. Such directors include, among others, Italy's Luchino Visconti and Pier Paolo Pasolini, Germany's Rainer Werner Fassbinder and Rosa von Praunheim, Britain's Derek Jarman, and Spain's Pedro Almodóvar.

Visconti and Pasolini

Luchino Visconti is usually credited as one of the founders of Italian neorealism (along with Roberto Rossellini and Vittorio De Sica), with films notable for their use of non-professional actors and naturalistic settings. However, as his work progressed, Visconti's films became more stylized and, ultimately, more deeply personal. While Visconti was openly bisexual himself, his films have few explicitly gay characters, though there is often an undercurrent of homoeroticism.

Perhaps Visconti's most important contribution to gay cinema is *Morte a Venezia* (*Death in Venice*, 1971), an adaptation of Thomas Mann's classic homoerotic novella. The film tells the story of Aschenbach, a vain but aging composer, who travels to Venice to rest after a period of artistic and personal stress. A man obsessed with an ideal of beauty and perfection, Aschenbach becomes entranced with a beautiful young boy, Tadzio. Although only intending to stay at the Venetian resort for a short time, the composer invents reasons for prolonging his holiday, despite the threat of a deadly outbreak of cholera. Aschenbach lingers in the city and courts his own demise in his quest to understand the meaning of perfection.

Other notable films by Visconti include his first feature, *Ossessione* (1942), an unauthorized version of the James M. Cain novel *The Postman Always Rings Twice*. Visconti subtly portrays the friendship between the young drifter Gino and a street magician as a one-way gay romance. For example, in one scene, the two men are together in bed and the street magician strikes a match to survey Gino's handsome face as he sleeps.

Rocco e i suoi fratelli (*Rocco and His Brothers*, 1960) looks at southern Italian peasants who relocate to Milan in search of economic stability. The film includes a subplot involving a boxing promoter who pays young men for sex.

Il gattopardo (*The Leopard*, 1963), one of Visconti's most acclaimed films, chronicles the decline of the Sicilian aristocracy during the Risorgimento, the nineteenth-century movement that led to the unification of Italy, a subject close to Visconti's own family history.

Visconti explored the rise of Nazism in *La caduta degli dei* (*The Damned*, 1969), a portrait of the disintegration of a German industrialist family during the Third Reich. Homoeroticism is rampant in the film. Helmut Berger, as the German industrialist's grandson and successor, makes his first appearance in the film in full Marlene Dietrich drag; an explicit gay orgy precedes a scene depicting the Night of the Long Knives, June 30, 1934, when Hitler purged the party of his homosexual associate Ernst Röhm and some 300 other members of the "Brown Shirts." The stylized decadence depicted by Visconti was of such graphic intensity that the film was originally released in the United States with an X rating.

Ludwig (1972) is Visconti's film biography of the nineteenth-century homosexual "mad" King Ludwig II of Bavaria. The film includes a portrayal of the aging king's obsession with a handsome young actor and features an all-male orgy reminiscent of the one in *The Damned*. The 1974 film *Gruppo di famiglia in un interno* (*Conversation Piece*) is a culmination of the themes that run through most of Visconti's films: the disintegration of family, the decay of traditional values, and the obsessive pursuit of beauty.

Poet, painter, playwright, essayist, and novelist, Pier Paolo Pasolini is best known outside of Italy as a filmmaker. Indeed, Pasolini is considered one of the most significant directors to emerge in the second wave of Italian cinema in the 1960s. Although politically radical and openly gay, Pasolini infrequently addressed homosexuality in his films.

Pasolini's first film, *Accattone* (1961), adapted from his own novel *Una vita violenta* (*A Violent Life*), is a realistic depiction of the life of an *accattone*, or pimp, in Rome's petty-criminal underworld. The film's sympathetic attitudes toward its amoral characters caused an immediate uproar; Italian authorities originally sought to ban the film outright, but eventually allowed a release restricted to adults only.

His next film, *Mamma Roma* (1962), with Anna Magnani in the lead role, explores similar territory, and centers on a woman who is fatefully drawn back to her former life as a prostitute. This film, too, attracted official censure for "offending against the common sense of decency," but was finally released after lengthy legal proceedings.

Pasolini once again courted public outrage and legal battles with his third film, *La ricotta*. Pasolini was invited to contribute an episode to the 1963 compendium film titled *RoGoPaG* (named after the four contributing directors: Rossellini, Godard, Pasolini, and Gregoretti). In Pasolini's short film, a petty criminal finds work as an extra on a film about the life of Christ. When he is cast as one of the thieves crucified with Christ, he, ironically, suffers from a fatal case of indigestion and actually dies while on the cross. Italian authorities considered the film an "outrage against the established religion"; Pasolini was consequently tried for blasphemy and received a three-month suspended sentence. A significantly edited version of Pasolini's film was eventually allowed to be released.

It might have been suspected that his next feature film, *Il Vangelo secondo Matteo* (*The Gospel According to St. Matthew*, 1964), told in an almost documentary-like style, would again create outrage and receive censure. This time, however, the film was praised by Catholic organizations as one of the few honest portrayals of Christ onscreen, and was attacked instead by left-wing critics who accused it of pietism and hagiography. Despite all the controversy, or perhaps in part because of it, the film brought Pasolini his first international recognition.

Pasolini followed that film with *Uccellacci e uccellini* (*Hawks and Sparrows*, 1966), about the adventures of a father and son. (The son was played by Ninetto Davoli, Pasolini's onetime lover.) Pasolini next shifted his focus to the mythic past with *Edipo re* (*Oedipus Rex*, 1967).

Pasolini returned to a contemporary setting with *Teorema* (1968), one of his most controversial works. The story concerns a handsome, enigmatic stranger who insinuates himself into the home of a bourgeois Milanese family and proceeds to physically and emotionally seduce them all, including the father and the young son. Catholic authorities were outraged by the film and had it withdrawn and the director charged with obscenity. The charges were finally dismissed two years later, and the film was formally released in 1970.

In the early 1970s, Pasolini concentrated on lush, erotic adaptations of classical texts, which at the time he characterized as his most "nonpolitical" films. *Il Decameron* (*The Decameron*, 1971), *I racconti di Canterbury* (*The Canterbury Tales*, 1972), and *Il fiore delle mille e una notte* (*Arabian Nights*, 1974) provided Pasolini with his greatest commercial successes and broadest audiences. Later, Pasolini suggested these were instead his most "political" films; the politics being sexual in the eroticized male and female bodies celebrated onscreen.

Pasolini's final film is the intensely controversial *Salò o le 120 giornate di Sodoma* (*Salò, or The 120 Days of Sodom*, 1976), an uncompromising and explicit fusion of Mussolini's Fascist Italy with the philosophies of the Marquis de Sade. Scenes of rape, sodomy, coprophagia, sexual humiliation, and torture are repeatedly depicted. The film was released (and withdrawn on charges of obscenity) two weeks after Pasolini's death at the hands of a male prostitute. *Salò* was subsequently banned in Italy, and nearly everywhere else, for several years.

Fassbinder and the New German Cinema

One of the most remarkable phenomena of cinema was the brief but prolific career of German filmmaker Rainer Werner Fassbinder, who died at the age of thirty-six. Few directors in cinema history have matched his productivity. From 1966 to 1982, Fassbinder completed forty-four films for theatrical or television release. His prodigious output was matched by a wild, self-destructive nature that earned him a reputation as the *enfant terrible*, and central figure, of the New German Cinema. Openly gay (he declared his homosexuality to his father at age fifteen), Fassbinder nonetheless married twice; one of his wives acted in his films and the other served as his editor.

Fassbinder's films typically detail the hopeless yearning for love and freedom and the many ways in which society, and the individual, impedes it. Many of his films deal candidly with sexuality; homosexual themes often appear, either central or incidental to the films' plots.

Fassbinder achieved his first international success with *Die Bitteren Tränen der Petra von Kant* (*The Bitter Tears of Petra von Kant*, 1972), a highly stylized film that is both a tribute to and a deconstruction of Hollywood's "women's pictures" of the 1940s and 1950s. The story (adapted from Fassbinder's own play) concerns a lesbian love affair between a successful fashion designer and a young, working-class model, and its aftermath.

Working again in the genre of the Hollywood melodrama, *Faustrecht der Freiheit* (*Fox and His Friends*, 1975) focuses on a gay circus worker (played by Fassbinder himself) who wins a large fortune in a state lottery and is befriended and systematically exploited by a clique of younger, bourgeois gay men. Criticized by some gay and lesbian critics as being homophobic, Fassbinder insisted that his central focus was less on sexual behavior and more on the power relations among people sexually involved with one another, and on the intersections of age, beauty, and social class.

Fassbinder explored his own self-destructive tendencies in *Satansbraten* (*Satan's Brew*, 1976), about an artist named Kranz who is no longer able to create. The film features several sexually explicit scenes played for surreal comedy. In one scene, Kranz receives a public-restroom proposition from a male hustler who masturbates frankly for the camera throughout their conversation; in another, Kranz is beaten up by a pimp and discovers he enjoys the pain.

In einem Jahr mit 13 Monden (*In a Year of Thirteen Moons*, 1978) explores issues of sexual identity and the familiar Fassbinder theme of the "outsider among outsiders" in the story of Elvira, a male-to-female transsexual who, in the last few days before her suicide, decides to visit some of the important people and places in her life. In a virtuosic sequence, Elvira wanders through the slaughterhouse where she worked as Erwin, recounting her history amidst the carnage. Filmed in the aftermath of the suicide of Fassbinder's estranged lover, the work is an unrelenting, emotionally candid, and profoundly personal study of the human quest for love, approval, and acceptance.

Fassbinder's best-known homoerotic work is his final film, *Querelle* (1982), adapted from the Jean Genet novel *Querelle de Brest*. The film, a fetishized, flamboyant examination of the various forms of love and sexuality, concerns a young sailor (played by the American actor Brad Davis) discovering his homosexuality. In the first of several erotically charged scenes, Querelle purposely loses a bet and allows himself to be sodomized by the husband of the local brothel owner. To tell his story, Fassbinder utilized such archetypal gay imagery as leather-clad men and debauched sailors in white uniforms, and a self-consciously stylized landscape of phallic architecture.

Fassbinder died in 1982 from an overdose of sleeping pills and cocaine.

Another prolific filmmaker of the New German Cinema with a highly individualized style is Rosa von Praunheim (born Holger Mischwitzky). He chose the name Rosa as an allusion to the pink triangle (*rosa Winkel)* that homosexuals were forced to wear in the Nazi concentration camps.

Beginning his career in the late 1960s, von Praunheim developed a confrontational approach to filmmaking, offering little comfort to spectators and explicitly disavowing inspirational or optimistic treatments of gay life. He has been quoted as saying, "I don't want audiences at my movies to have a good time, I want them to be upset."

In 1971, von Praunheim gained notoriety, and created controversy, throughout Germany with his film *Nicht der Homosexuelle ist pervers, sondern die Situation, in der er lebt (It Is Not the Homosexual Who Is Perverse, but the Society in Which He Lives, 1971).* The appearance of this film has been cited as crucial to the founding of the new German gay rights movement. His film *Armee der Liebenden oder Revolte der Perversen (Army of Lovers or Revolution of the Perverts, 1979)* documents the American gay and lesbian rights movement from the 1950s to 1976.

With the black comedy *Ein Virus kennt keine Moral (A Virus Knows No Morals, 1985),* von Praunheim made one of the earliest feature films about AIDS. He subsequently directed a trilogy of films about AIDS and AIDS activism: *Positiv (Positive), Schweigen = Tod (Silence = Death),* and *Feuer unterm Arsch (Fire Under Your Ass),* all made in 1990.

In 1992, he directed the life story of the East German transvestite Charlotte von Mahlsdorf, *Ich bin meine eigene Frau (I Am My Own Woman),* employing both documentary footage and re-creations utilizing actors. *Vor Transsexuellen wird gewarnt (Transsexual Menace, 1996),* originally made for German television, documents the transgender community.

The gay sexologist Magnus Hirschfeld is the focus of *Der Einstein des Sex (The Einstein of Sex, 1999). Can I Be Your Bratwurst, Please?* (1999), a thirty-minute comedy, stars the gay pornography icon Jeff Stryker.

Frank Ripploh is another gay German filmmaker whose work has courted controversy. Ripploh achieved international art-house success with his first feature film, *Taxi zum Klo (Taxi to the Loo, 1981),* an explicit account of the director's own sexual escapades and fantasies. He returned to the same milieu several years later with *Taxi nach Kairo (Taxi to Cairo, 1987),* in which the main character's mother threatens to disinherit him if he does not settle down and marry. Ripploh died in 2002, at the age of fifty-two.

Director Wolfgang Peterson first gained recognition for his film *Die Konsequenz (The Consequence, 1977),* an understated and unsentimental coming-out story that he cowrote as well as directed. Peterson went on to earn international acclaim for *Das Boot (The Boat, 1981),* a wartime drama about a German submarine crew. He subsequently relocated to California, where he has since directed a number of mainstream Hollywood films.

German filmmaker Ulrike Ottinger has become a significant figure in lesbian cinema with her extravagant avant-garde fantasies. The attractions and desires of her female characters are never overtly presented, but are instead subtly encoded in the stylized *mise en scène* of her films.

Her first film, *Laokoon und Söhne (Laocoön and Sons, 1975),* stars Tabea Blumenschein, an underground film actress and Ottinger's lover at the time. Ottinger and Blumenschein collaborated again on *Madame X—eine absolute Herrscherin (Madame X: An Absolute Ruler, 1978),* a satiric and erotic fantasy, which has since reached cult status, about a group of women who join a female pirate on her sea voyages.

Ottinger has also directed several documentaries, primarily about marginalized cultures, such as *China. Die Künste—Der Alltag (China. The Arts—The Everyday, 1985),* about everyday life in the Sichuan and Yunnan provinces of China; *Taiga* (1992), concerning nomadic tribes in northern Mongolia; and *Exil Shanghai (Exile Shanghai, 1997),* the story of six exiled Jews in Shanghai who later settled in the United States.

Monika Treut has explored controversial social issues and celebrated transgressive sexuality in such films as *Verführung: Die grausame Frau (Seduction: The Cruel Woman, 1985),* about the psychological aspects of sadomasochism, and *Die Jungfrauenmaschine (Virgin Machine, 1988),* in which a female German journalist investigates the lesbian subcultures of San Francisco.

The compilation documentary *Female Misbehavior* (1992) is perhaps Treut's best-known work. "Bondage" (1983) examines the lesbian S/M and bondage scene; "Annie" (1989) showcases lesbian performance artist Annie Sprinkle; "Dr. Paglia" (1992) focuses on bisexual critic Camille Paglia; and "Max" (1992) documents the female-to-male transsexual journey of Max Velerio.

Derek Jarman and British Film

The British filmmaker Derek Jarman was a uniquely idiosyncratic artist known for his opulent imagery, social criticism, and bold explorations of homosexuality. He routinely revisited history from a gay perspective, and his work was influenced by such gay European filmmakers as Cocteau, Fassbinder, and Pasolini and the American underground director Kenneth Anger.

Sebastiane (1976), Jarman's debut feature film (co-directed by Paul Humfress), is an overtly homoerotic interpretation of the life and martyrdom of Saint Sebastian, with dialogue spoken entirely in Latin. The film opens with an extended scene set in a Roman orgy, where naked men covered in body paint dance while wearing comically exaggerated penises. The film's explicit content and groundbreaking full-frontal male nudity earned it an *X* rating when it was first released; the film went on to become a critical and commercial success.

Jarman followed that film with *Jubilee* (1977), a political fantasy in which Queen Elizabeth I time-travels to find England a wasteland of violence and anarchy, and *The Tempest* (1979), a visually lush reworking of Shakespeare's play. Jarman returned to Shakespeare for his next feature, *The Angelic Conversation* (1985), a unique, nonnarrative exploration of the underlying theme of homosexual desire in fourteen of Shakespeare's Sonnets.

Caravaggio (1986), which examines the art and sexuality of the late-Renaissance Italian painter, is perhaps Jarman's most popular work. Told in an intentionally anachronistic manner—motorcycles and jazz music are juxtaposed with richly rendered, painstaking recreations of Caravaggio's most famous works—the film emphasizes the artist's homosexual affairs with his models and the various scandals in which he was involved.

In 1991, Jarman created a film version of Christopher Marlowe's play *Edward II*. Although the film is relatively faithful to Marlowe's Elizabethan text, Jarman's direction turned the source material into a parable of homosexual martyrdom in the face of institutionalized homophobia, with direct references to the repressive nature of Thatcher-era British politics. Jarman augmented the film with graphic visualizations of homosexual love and sadomasochistic violence.

Other significant films by Jarman include *The Last of England* (1988), *War Requiem* (1989), *The Garden* (1990), *Wittgenstein* (1993), and his final work, *Blue* (1993), in which a densely interwoven soundtrack of voices, sound effects, and music is performed against a plain, unchanging, cobalt-blue screen to convey Jarman's experiences with AIDS.

Jarman died of an AIDS-related illness in 1994.

British filmmaker Terence Davies began his career with the short films *Children* (1976), *Madonna and Child* (1980), and *Death and Transfiguration* (1983). These intensely personal films chronicle the main character from childhood to death and examine how he copes with his working-class family, his religious upbringing, and his homosexuality. The three films were released together in 1984 under the title *The Terence Davies Trilogy*.

Davies's first feature film, the autobiographical *Distant Voices, Still Lives* (1988), paralleled the director's own harsh life in Liverpool during the 1940s and 1950s. The film won international acclaim for its structural innovations and lyrical imagery. Davies followed that film with *The Long Day Closes* (1992), a somewhat more uplifting look at a working-class Catholic childhood, again set in Liverpool.

Davies continued his career with nonautobiographical films, including *The Neon Bible* (1995), based on the novel of the same name by John Kennedy Toole, and *The House of Mirth* (2000), based on the novel by Edith Wharton.

Other notable glbtq-themed British films include the groundbreaking *A Taste of Honey* (1961), directed by Tony Richardson, about a young, unwed pregnant woman who befriends and sets up house with a gay art student. The film, based on the play by Shelagh Delaney, rendered one of the first sympathetic portrayals of a homosexual character in the history of cinema.

John Schlesinger's *Sunday Bloody Sunday* (1971) is the story of a young bisexual sculptor who divides his affections between a divorced woman and a well-to-do male doctor. *Maurice* (1987), created by the distinguished gay partnership of James Ivory (director) and Ismail Merchant (producer), and based on the posthumously published novel by E. M. Forster, concerns an upper-class man coming to terms with his homosexuality in Edwardian England.

Stephen Frears's early feature films *My Beautiful Laundrette* (1985), the story of a cross-race, cross-class, and same-sex relationship in London, and *Prick Up Your Ears* (1987), a study of gay British playwright Joe Orton, who was murdered at the height of his fame by his mentor and lover Kenneth Halliwell, are also noteworthy additions to the history of gay cinema.

Sally Potter's film *Orlando* (1992), based on the fanciful novel by Virginia Woolf, features a metaphoric transsexual character who is born a nobleman in the Elizabethan age and changes sex midway through his/her life. "Same person, no difference at all. Just a different sex," Orlando remarks, after falling asleep as a man and waking as a woman. Orlando is played throughout the film by actress Tilda Swinton; Queen Elizabeth I is portrayed by the openly gay writer and performance artist Quentin Crisp.

Further key British works include *Beautiful Thing* (1996), directed by Hettie MacDonald, a love story between two teenage boys in a London housing project, and Brian Gilbert's *Wilde* (1997), about the poet and playwright Oscar Wilde, with the openly gay actor Stephen Fry in the title role.

Pedro Almodóvar and Eloy de la Iglesia

Pedro Almodóvar is the most internationally acclaimed filmmaker to emerge from post-Franco Spain. He began his career making short films in the early 1970s. His earliest efforts became cult hits, but his third feature film, *Entre tinieblas* (*Dark Habits*, 1983), an offbeat comedy about a nightclub singer who seeks refuge in a convent of delinquent nuns (who indulge in such secular pleasures as hard-core drugs and soft-core porn), gained the director a wider audience.

Almodóvar's popularity increased with *¿Qué he hecho yo para merecer esto?!!* (*What Have I Done to Deserve This?*, 1984) and *Matador* (1986), which established the filmmaker's distinct style of combining elements of camp, comedy, melodrama, and sexual intrigue that often exceed the boundaries of socially acceptable norms.

Mujeres al borde de un ataque de nervios (*Women on the Verge of a Nervous Breakdown*, 1988), an elaborate farce deconstructing the clichés of female hysteria, became Almodóvar's first worldwide success. Throughout the 1990s, with such films as *¡Átame!* (*Tie Me Up! Tie Me Down!*, 1990), *Tacones lejanos* (*High Heels*, 1991), and *Kika* (1993), Almodóvar continued to craft brightly colored confections with tragicomic plots often focusing on death, violence, rape, and betrayal.

With the release of *Todo sobre mi madre* (*All About My Mother*, 1999), Almodóvar brought a greater refinement and emotional subtlety to his work. The film centers on a woman who, after the tragic death of her teenage son, journeys through Barcelona's underworld in search of the son's father, now a transsexual. Almodóvar followed with *Hable con ella* (*Talk to Her*, 2002), a complex tale of love, obsession, and loss; and *La mala educación* (*Bad Education*, 2004), an exploration of the effects of sexual abuse at a religious school on two friends.

Almodóvar's most significant gay-themed film, as well as his self-confessed most personal work, is *La ley del deseo* (*Law of Desire*, 1987). This intricately plotted film—part fantasy, part murder mystery, and part erotic comedy—centers on Pablo, a gay writer/director deeply in love with a young man, Juan, who will not respond to his affections. Under Almodóvar's direction, the film becomes both an appreciation of, and a satire on, the conventions of romantic love.

One of the earliest Spanish directors working within queer cinema is the Basque-born Eloy de la Iglesia. Outspokenly gay, de la Iglesia has stated that his films are about "the world of which the majority of filmmakers do not care to speak, the marginal world." His films often feature gay, or otherwise marginalized, characters. De la Iglesia has explained that he is a director who "always wants to make the films that are not supposed to be made," on subjects that "everyone else has agreed not to talk about." Despite censorship constraints and hostile reactions from Catholic leaders to many of his films, de la Iglesia has enjoyed commercial success as a director, especially in Spain.

De la Iglesia began his film career in 1966 with *Fantasia...3*, a collection of three short films based on children's stories by Hans Christian Andersen, L. Frank Baum, and the Grimm brothers. His first commercial achievement in his native country was *El techo de cristal* (*The Glass Ceiling*, 1971); two years later saw de la Iglesia's first international success with the release of *La semana del asesino* (*Week of the Killer* / *Cannibal Man*, 1974), a violent account of a young man who goes on a killing spree. The film also includes a gay character who is presented in an open, nonstereotypical, manner.

The death of dictator Francisco Franco in 1975 brought more latitude and a new openness for artists in Spain. As a result, de la Iglesia created *Los placeres ocultos* (*Hidden Pleasures*, 1977), the first gay film to be produced in Spain. The film concerns a closeted homosexual banker attracted to a poor, heterosexual young man. The banker brings the young man into his life, and though the attraction is one-way, the youth is accepting of the situation and even brings his girlfriend into the arrangement.

In 1979, de la Iglesia returned to a similar subject with *El Diputado* (*The Deputy* / *Confessions of a Congressman*), the story of a married gay congressman who risks his political career when he falls in love with a young man and attempts to integrate the man into his family life. The homosexual affair in this film, however, ends tragically.

De la Iglesia continued his career with such films as *El sacerdote* (*The Priest*, 1979), which was banned by the Catholic Church and heavily censored upon its initial release; *Colegas* (*Pals*, 1980); and *El pico* (*The Shoot*, 1983). After an absence of fifteen years, de la Iglesia returned with *Los novios búlgaros* (*Bulgarian Lovers*, 2003), a comedy of sexual obsession about a middle-aged gay lawyer who falls in love with a handsome young foreigner.

Other Notable European Films

Another notable filmmaker in European glbtq cinema is Belgian-born Chantal Akerman, whose works, typically filmed in a direct but distanced manner, address such themes as alienation, voyeurism, and marginalization. *Je, tu, il, elle* (1974) concerns a young woman's quest for sexual knowledge; in the final section of the film the young woman, played by Akerman herself, shows up at another woman's house, where they proceed to make love. *Jeanne Dielman, 23 Quai du Commerce, 1080 Bruxelles* (1976), perhaps Akerman's best-known film, focuses on a young middle-class widow whose life begins to unravel as she rigorously tries to maintain her role as housewife and mother while discreetly serving as a prostitute.

Italian director Ettore Scola's *Una giornata partico-lare* (*A Special Day*, 1977), starring Sophia Loren and Marcello Mastroianni, concerns a woman who befriends her homosexual neighbor on the eve of Hitler's 1938 visit to Fascist Italy.

The Danish films *Du er ikke alene* (*You Are Not Alone*, 1978), codirected by Ernst Johansen and Lasse Nielsen, and *Venner for altid* (*Friends Forever*, 1987), directed by Stefan Henszelman, both deal with the confusions of gay male teenagers coming to terms with their homosexuality.

Noteworthy French films include Jean Delannoy's *Les amitiés particulières* (*This Special Friendship*, 1964), which focuses on the youthful friendships, with homo-erotic overtones, among a group of boys in a strict French Roman Catholic boarding school in the 1930s. The popular farce *La cage aux folles* (1978), directed by Edouard Molinaro, is about a gay couple whose lives are turned upside down when the son of one of the men announces he is getting married.

Coup de foudre (*Entre Nous*, 1983), directed by Diane Kurys, concerns two women who meet in the aftermath of World War II and gradually form a deep bond that excludes their husbands and children. André Téchiné's *J'embrasse pas* (*I Don't Kiss*, 1991), focuses on a young man who leaves his home in the country to pursue an acting career in Paris but is eventually forced to prosti-tute himself to men, while *Les roseaux sauvages* (*Wild Reeds*, 1994), is a gracefully sensual coming-of-age story set in the early 1960s.

Les nuits fauves (*Savage Nights*, 1992), directed by Cyril Collard, concerns a promiscuous bisexual male (played by Collard himself) coping with the knowledge that he is HIV-positive; Collard died the following year of an AIDS-related illness. *Ma vie en rose* (1997), directed by Alain Berliner, is the tale of an eight-year-old boy who wants to live his life as a girl.

European glbtq cinema has a long and rich history. With the lessening of government and religious censor-ship and an increased public acceptance of sexual and gender nonconformity in the final decades of the twenti-eth century, queer filmmakers have created a number of artistically significant films that honestly explore glbtq issues.

—*Craig Kaczorowski*

BIBLIOGRAPHY

Bacon, Henry. *Visconti: Exploration of Beauty and Decay*. Cambridge: Cambridge University Press, 1998.

Baranski, Zygmunt, ed. *Pasolini Old and New: Surveys and Studies*. Dublin: Four Courts Press, 1999.

Dyer, Richard. *Now You See It: Studies on Lesbian and Gay Film*. New York: Routledge, 1990.

Gever, Martha, John Greyson, and Pratibha Parmar, eds. *Queer Looks: Perspectives on Lesbian and Gay Films and Video*. New York: Routledge, 1993.

Hanson, Ellis. *Outtakes: Essays on Queer Theory and Film*. Durham, N.C.: Duke University Press, 1999.

Kuzniar, Alice. *The Queer German Cinema*. Stanford, Calif.: Stanford University Press, 2000.

Lippard, Chris, ed. *By Angels Driven: The Films of Derek Jarman*. Westport, Conn.: Greenwood Press, 1996.

Murray, Raymond. *Images in the Dark: An Encyclopedia of Gay and Lesbian Film and Video*. Philadelphia: TLA Publications, 1994.

Sklar, Robert. *Film: An International History of the Medium*. New York: Harry N. Abrams, Inc., 1993.

Stack, Oswald. *Pasolini on Pasolini; Interviews with Oswald Stack*. Bloomington, Ind.: Indiana University Press, 1969.

Steegmuller, Francis. *Cocteau, a Biography*. Boston: D. R. Godine, 1986.

Vernon, Kathleen, and Barbara Morris, eds. *Post-Franco, Postmodern: The Films of Pedro Almodóvar*. Westport, Conn.: Greenwood Press, 1995.

Watson, Wallace Steadman. *Understanding Rainer Werner Fassbinder: Film as Private and Public Art*. Columbia, S.C.: University of South Carolina Press, 1996.

Weiss, Andrea. *Violets and Vampires: Lesbians in Film*. London: Penguin, 1993.

SEE ALSO

Film; Film Directors; Bisexuality in Film; Transsexuality in Film; Akerman, Chantal; Almodóvar, Pedro; Anger, Kenneth; Bogarde, Sir Dirk; Cocteau, Jean; Collard, Cyril; Crisp, Quentin; Davies, Terence; Davis, Brad; Dietrich, Marlene; Fassbinder, Rainer Werner; Fry, Stephen; Iglesia, Eloy de la; Ivory, James, and Ismail Merchant; Marais, Jean; Ottinger, Ulrike; Pasolini, Pier Paolo; Praunheim, Rosa von; Richardson, Tony; Schlesinger, John; Stiller, Mauritz; Treut, Monika; Visconti, Luchino

Everett, Rupert (b. 1959)

SINCE 1989, WHEN HE CAME OUT IN A PRESS INTERVIEW in Paris, Rupert Everett has defined and redefined himself for the mass media as a gay male actor, being notably open about his homosexuality. While Everett's career has led to heightened attention and debate regard-ing Hollywood's acceptance of openly gay movie stars, it has deflected attention from his own considerable accomplishments as a screen and stage actor.

After a stunning box-office and critical success in *My Best Friend's Wedding* (1997), Everett found it impossi-ble to control Hollywood's publicity machine and he was swamped with queries from entertainment maga-zines about his homosexuality. In response, he succeeded in shattering stereotypes and helped advance public dis-course about homosexuality, gay actors, and the film industry. Recently, however, he has charged that homo-phobia in the industry has cost him a number of roles.

Everett was born into an upper-class British family on May 29, 1959. His parents sent him at age seven to a prestigious Roman Catholic school, Ampleforth, in York. Everett has commented, "The most lasting effect of my childhood is the rejection I felt by my mother." Growing up away from home, he added, "calcifies your heart."

He became involved in theater at Ampleforth. Then, at age fifteen, he transferred to the Central School for Speech and Drama in London. Two years later, the intensely individualistic and rebellious young man was expelled on grounds of "insubordination." When accounts of this incident surfaced in 1990s news reports about Everett's moodiness and difficulties on film sets, Everett, admitting bouts of insecurity and lapses of confidence, finally told the press that "neurosis and insecurity can appear as arrogance."

Everett completed his theatrical education as a member of the Glasgow Citizens' Company, which he joined at the age of seventeen.

Everett's first major success came in a London production of Julian Mitchell's play *Another Country* (1982) and in the film adaptation directed by Marek Kanievska (1984). He played David Blakeley, a young, gay Soviet spy modeled on the life of Guy Burgess. He also earned acclaim in the British film *Dance with a Stranger* (1985), directed by Mike Newell.

Despite these successes, Everett was unable to break into Hollywood films during the 1980s. After a fruitless period of seeking work in Hollywood, he returned to Britain to concentrate on his stage career and also to pursue roles in European films. He appeared in nine films that went unnoticed in the United States.

Among his most memorable stage roles was that of Flora Goforth, a dying elderly woman frantically recalling her life, in Tennessee Williams's *The Milk Train Doesn't Stop Here Any More.* He also performed in productions of Shaw's *Heartbreak House,* Coward's *The Vortex* and *Private Lives,* and an adaptation of Wilde's *The Picture of Dorian Gray.*

Everett emerged as a film actor in the mid-1990s, first receiving attention for his performances in Nicholas Hytner's adaptation of Alan Bennett's *The Madness of King George* (1994) and Robert Altman's *Ready to Wear* (1994).

But P. J. Hogan's *My Best Friend's Wedding* (1997) shifted Everett onto the path from character actor to movie star. Favorable audience responses to Everett at test screenings of the unfinished movie led to shooting and adding seventeen minutes of onscreen time for the actor. Everett's character evolved from a friend of the character played by Julia Roberts to a closer, more appealing "gay confidant," with insight, charm, humor, and suavity, a distinctly different role from the gay comic sidekicks of earlier Hollywood films.

In John Schlesinger's *The Next Best Thing,* Everett attempted to focus attention on alternative families. He spent a year rewriting the original script, removing stereotypical elements. (In arbitration, Everett lost his demand for a scriptwriter credit.) In this film, he plays a gay man who fathers a child with the character played by costar Madonna, then has to fight for custody of the child when another man enters her life.

Everett believes that he was able to give the character he played greater depth as a result of his sexuality in real life. According to the actor, he and Madonna intentionally blurred the division between their characters and themselves to allow the public "real access to our lives."

Everett's openness as a gay actor, coupled with his success playing gay roles, led to a great deal of discussion about whether openly gay actors could be accepted as movie stars. More specifically, the question was raised whether Everett could be convincing in a heterosexual love scene.

Since Everett has managed not to be pigeonholed in upper-class British dramas, where his aloof, erudite, defiant, and privileged persona receives much praise, he probably can avoid being pigeonholed in gay roles. Among the upper-class British dramas in which he has appeared is Oliver Parker's film based on Oscar Wilde's *An Ideal Husband* (1999). He also plays Algernon Moncrieff in the same director's film version of *The Importance of Being Earnest* (2002).

In P. J. Hogan's *Unconditional Love* (2002), Everett plays a British valet, "a really bitter queen," searching for the murderer of his lover, a rock star, with the help of a woman (Kathy Bates) who fanatically adored the singer. Despite a stellar cast that includes Julie Andrews, Lynn Redgrave, Jonathan Pryce, and Dan Aykroyd, the film was never released theatrically, and premiered in 2003 on cable television.

Recently, Everett has reassessed the impact of coming out on his career. Although he does not regret coming out, he told television host Tina Brown that in Hollywood "Gay actors could only go a certain distance," and charged that his sexual preference cost him roles such as the lead in Chris and Paul Weitz's *About a Boy* (2002). He also told Brown that he was denied a role in *Basic Instinct 2: Risk Addiction* (2005) when an MGM executive told him he was "a pervert" and would "never be accepted by the American public in this role."

In 2004, Everett lashed out at the homophobia in Hollywood executive suites, lambasting Hollywood as "a trophy business," adding that "it's not a trophy thing to be gay." Although playwright and screenwriter Paul Rudnick has declared that Everett has "universal crush material," appealing to both men and women," the actor now feels that his openness has caused studio executives to stereotype him.

Perhaps not surprisingly, most of Everett's recent films have been produced outside the United States, in Britain, Germany, and even Russia. The most acclaimed of these recent roles is his flamboyant portrayal of Charles II in Richard Eyre's *Stage Beauty* (2004).

Everett is also a novelist. He published *Hello Darling, Are You Working?* in 1994 and *The Hairdressers of St. Tropez* in 1995.

—*Richard C. Bartone*

BIBLIOGRAPHY

Casillo, Charles. "Rupert Everett Close Up." *New York Native*, December 26, 1994, 18.

Goldstein, Patrick. "How One Actor Changed a Movie Before It Even Came Out." *Los Angeles Times*, June 6, 1994.

Karger, Dave. "The 'Best' Man." *Entertainment Weekly*, July 11, 1997, 30.

Miller, Mark. "Meet Rupert Everywhere." *Newsweek*, July 12, 1999, 64.

Patrick, John. "Rupert Everett: The Best Thing." *Encounter*, March 22, 2000, 6.

"Topic A with Tina Brown: Slutty Stepsister Gets Her Due." www.gawker.com (October 11, 2004).

Vilanch, Bruce. "Rupert Everett: Leading Man on the Rise." *Advocate*, January 20, 1998, 30.

SEE ALSO

Film Actors: Gay Male; Bisexuality in Film; Schlesinger, John

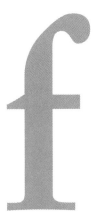

Fassbinder, Rainer Werner   *(1946–1982)*

DIRECTING OVER FORTY FILMS IN A SEVENTEEN-YEAR period, Rainer Werner Fassbinder was responsible for bringing the much-acclaimed New German Cinema of the 1960s and 1970s to the attention of international audiences. From early on, Fassbinder's ambitious, often audacious, films used the cinematic conventions of Hollywood to deliver the ideological arguments of the New Left.

Fassbinder simultaneously transformed the practice of political filmmaking and prompted critical reevaluation of certain underappreciated genres of American commercial cinema, such as the "women's picture" and domestic melodrama. His films not only articulated issues of gender and sexual relations, but also framed these issues within broader (and certainly no less problematic) social and political circumstances.

Homosexuality is an important presence in his work, but it most frequently is used to articulate or illuminate interpersonal themes and political issues.

Born in Bavaria on May 31, 1946 (or 1945), Fassbinder recalled spending his childhood in movie houses—five times a week, often three times a day. His parents divorced when he was five or six years old. Feeling abandoned by his father, he found comfort at the movies. The Allied military presence in post–World War II Germany assured his exposure to mainstream American film.

Fassbinder made his first films while in his early twenties: two short works starring his mother and his male lover. These productions foreshadowed a career in which the personal and the professional were often coextensive. Soon thereafter, when denied admission to Berlin's DFFA film school, Fassbinder turned to the theater. He joined an activist company in Munich, where he met key actors whom he would cast repeatedly in future projects, and where he became politically conscious.

The stage experience also compelled Fassbinder to hone his acting skills, and he went on to appear in many of his own films as well as those of numerous other directors. Until his untimely death from a drug and alcohol overdose on June 10, 1982, Fassbinder tirelessly produced work for stage, screen, television, and radio, his prodigious career sustained by state subsidies and bolstered by a flamboyant persona that sometimes generated more publicity than his art.

Homosexual themes featured in Fassbinder's films almost from the start, variously central or incidental to their plots, but always handled so that sexuality is just one factor within a complex of social forces buffeting his hapless characters.

Early works parody 1940s gangster films, foregrounding that genre's homoerotic motif of pivotal male friendships at odds with romantic male–female relationships. Fassbinder's international reputation was established with *The Bitter Tears of Petra von Kant* (1972), whose narrative centers on a female fashion designer's obsessive love for her model, a woman who, for a host of reasons besides sexual identity, is unwilling to submit to a suffocating lesbian relationship.

With *Fox and His Friends* (1975), Fassbinder directly addressed gay milieus in a story about an affable carny (played by himself) whose sudden wealth propels him into unfamiliar social territory, where a lover exploits and ruins him. Criticized for portraying clichés of gay culture, Fassbinder insisted that his satire focused attention on the class conflict he believed to be paramount. That is, the cause of the problems experienced by the characters is not their sexuality but their class differences and individual flaws.

Himself an exploitative personality who was later to feel responsible for driving his lover Armin Maier to suicide in 1978, Fassbinder acknowledged that his role as victim in *Fox and His Friends* reversed unflattering autobiographical parallels.

In a Year of Thirteen Moons (1978) explores complicated issues of sexual identity, as it recounts the final days of a male-to-female transsexual who is rejected by her lover after she has had surgery to please him. The protagonist is finally brutalized when a group of gay men discover she is not the homosexual transvestite they presumed. The film may reflect Fassbinder's pessimistic assessment of our ability to transcend our notion of binary gender roles.

Despite the violence and austerity of his work, Fassbinder also understood the campier pleasures inherent in cinema. Whether by showcasing a degraded movie-star protagonist (*Veronika Voss*, 1981), reprising Marlene Dietrich's iconic *Blue Angel* role in *Lola* (1981), or adapting Clare Booth Luce's *The Women* for German stage and television, Fassbinder reveals a camp sensibility.

In his final film, *Querelle* (1982), Fassbinder interpreted Jean Genet's controversial novel *Querelle de Brest*. In this work, Fassbinder refracted his exploration of cruel interpersonal rivalries through the brutish homoeroticism of sailors and leathermen.

Fassbinder died, perhaps a suicide, on June 10, 1982, of an overdose of sleeping pills and cocaine.

— *Mark Allen Svede*

BIBLIOGRAPHY

Appignanesi, Richard. *Fassbinder, Mishima, Pasolini*. London: Radius, 1989.

Braad Thomsen, Christian. *Fassbinder: The Life and Work of a Provocative Genius*. Trans. Martin Chalmers. London and Boston: Faber and Faber, 1997.

Elsaesser, Thomas. *Fassbinder's Germany: History, Identity, Subject*. Amsterdam: Amsterdam University Press, 1996.

Katz, Robert. *Love Is Colder Than Death: The Life and Times of Rainer Werner Fassbinder*. New York: Random House, 1987.

Schidor, Dieter. *Rainer Werner Fassbinder dreht "Querelle."* Munich: W. Heyne, 1982.

Watson, Wallace Steadman. *Understanding Rainer Werner Fassbinder: Film as Private and Public Art*. Columbia, S.C.: University of South Carolina Press, 1996.

SEE ALSO

Film; Film Directors; European Film; Transsexuality in Film; Transvestism in Film; New Queer Cinema; Bogarde, Sir Dirk; Carné, Marcel; Davis, Brad; Dietrich, Marlene

Fernie, Lynne   *(b. 1946)*

FILMMAKER, LYRICIST, AND EDITOR LYNNE FERNIE, A native of British Columbia, has had a varied career in the arts. Her principal work is the award-winning documentary *Forbidden Love: The Unashamed Stories of Lesbian Lives* (1992), which she codirected with Aerlyn Weissman.

As a young woman, Fernie moved to Toronto, where she became a member of LOOT (Lesbian Organization of Toronto), a lesbian feminist group in existence from 1976 to 1980.

In 1978, Fernie, along with other members of the Women's Writing Collective in Toronto, founded *Fireweed: A Feminist Quarterly of Writing, Politics, Art & Culture*. She coedited that journal's first lesbian issue (Issue 13) in 1983. Later, she worked as coeditor and then editor of *Parallelogramme*, a magazine of Canadian contemporary arts.

Fernie has been the lyricist for various Canadian recording artists, most notably the group The Parachute Club. She won gold records for her work on two of the group's albums and received a Juno award—the Canadian equivalent of a Grammy—for their single "Rise Up" (1983), which became an anthem of the Toronto gay community.

In 1989, Fernie was among a group of Canadian artists who founded the Inside Out Lesbian and Gay Film and Video Festival, held annually in Toronto.

Fernie directed a documentary, *Fiction and Other Truths: A Film about Jane Rule*, for which she won the Academy of Canadian Cinema and Television's Genie Award for short documentary in 1995. She also directed an educational video, *School's Out!* (1996), that places society's views toward homosexuality in a historical context and is intended for use in high schools to promote discussion of homophobia. In 1997, she directed another video for high school students, *Jane Rule...Writing*, in which the lesbian author discusses her writing process.

Fernie is best known as the codirector of *Forbidden Love: The Unashamed Stories of Lesbian Lives*, which won the Genie Award for feature-length documentary in 1993.

Forbidden Love was a product of Studio D of the National Film Board of Canada, the first publicly funded unit for women's films. In 1989, the executive director of Studio D, Rina Fraticelli, brought together Fernie and Aerlyn Weissman, a Vancouver filmmaker, to develop an ambitious project that would survey international lesbian history. Eventually, however, they decided to make a film with a very specific focus, the lesbian bar culture in major Canadian cities during the 1950s and 1960s.

Fernie and Weissman considered it essential to let the women of that milieu speak for themselves. For that reason they eschewed voice-over narration, opting instead for an interview format that allowed the women to tell their own stories of coming out and frequenting the bars, as well as what had happened to them in later years.

Weissman expressed their aim by saying, "Lynne and I felt quite strongly that it was important not to overlay the experiences of these women with a vocabulary of nineties feminist discourse. We really tried to structure the film in a way that would allow the women to speak for themselves, to give their experiences as they lived them, but to provide their contexts as well."

Nine women, ranging in age from approximately forty to eighty, described their experiences. They were a culturally diverse group, including a member of the Haida Nation from British Columbia, a black immigrant from Costa Rica, and a white woman who had been a middle-class Toronto housewife prior to coming out as a lesbian. Archival footage supplements these first-person accounts.

The period depicted in *Forbidden Love* was the heyday of lesbian pulp novels, paperback romances of a formulaic nature generally centered on college sorority members, dissatisfied housewives, or habituées of Greenwich Village bars. Ann Bannon, author of the extremely popular "Beebo Brinker" series of pulp novels, is among the women interviewed in the film.

Bannon's discussion of her experiences as a novelist and also a suburban wife and mother who explored the Greenwich Village lesbian bar scene helps tie together the recollections of the women and the fictional elements in *Forbidden Love*.

Departing from the standard documentary format, Fernie and Weissman interspersed a pulp-style love story with the reminiscences of the interviewees. Using the technique of freeze-frame and dissolve, the film moves from images of covers and illustrations in the style of pulp novels to the film-within-a-film.

The tale recounted in *Forbidden Love* is that of Laura, a country girl who moves to the big city, where, with some trepidation, she goes to a lesbian bar. There she meets and falls in love with Mitch.

The lesbian love affair brings fulfillment to Laura, and her story has a happy—even triumphant—ending. This is at odds with the typical dénouement of the pulp novels, which generally ended with the protagonist going mad or dying. (Bannon's novels were an exception to the pattern.)

It is also inconsistent with some of the stories of the interviewees, whose accounts include discussion of the difficulties and dangers that they faced in trying to create a public lesbian space in a homophobic society. Nevertheless, the women emerge as clever, witty, and courageous. Their stories of survival and endurance can be regarded as a triumph.

Forbidden Love garnered positive reviews in both the gay and mainstream press. In addition to the 1993 Genie, it won awards at the Durban International Film Festival and the International Women's Film Festival in France.

In 2003, Fernie completed *Apples and Oranges*, a short documentary/animation film for elementary-school-aged children that addresses issues of homophobia and bullying. Classroom discussions about these subjects are brought to life when two paintings made by children magically morph into animated stories based on characters the kids created.

In the first story, Anta, her two moms, and her all-girl band find a way to overcome a bully; in the second, a friendship between skateboarders Habib and Jeroux runs into homophobia when Jeroux reveals that he is gay. Produced and distributed by the National Film Board of Canada, the film has been screened at numerous festivals in Canada, the United States, and Europe, winning awards at many of them.

Fernie teaches film and video production at York University in Toronto, where she is also a programmer for the Hot Docs International Documentary Film Festival.

—*Linda Rapp*

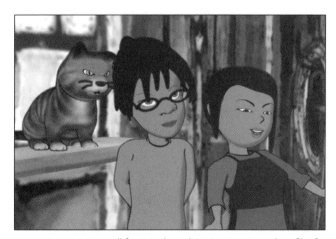

An animation still from *Apples and Oranges* (2003), a short film for children directed by Lynne Fernie and produced by Tamara Lynch.

BIBLIOGRAPHY

Anderson, Elizabeth. "Studio D's Imagined Community: From Development (1974) to Realignment." *Gendering the Nation: Canadian Women's Cinema.* Kay Armitage, Kass Banning, Brenda Longfellow, and Janine Marchessault, eds. Toronto: University of Toronto Press, 1999. 41–61.

FitzGerald, Maureen. "Fernie, Lynne." *Contemporary Gay and Lesbian History from World War II to the Present Day.* Robert Aldrich and Garry Wotherspoon, eds. London and New York: Routledge, 2001. 133.

Hankin, Kelly. " 'Wish We Didn't Have to Meet Secretly?': Negotiating Contemporary Space in the Lesbian-Bar Documentary." *Camera Obscura* 15.3 (2000): 34–69.

McKenty, Margaret. Review of "Forbidden Love." *Herizons* 7 (July 31, 1993): 41.

Rich, B. Ruby. "Making Love." *Village Voice,* August 17, 1993, 58.

Ross, Becki L. *The House That Jill Built: A Lesbian Nation in Formation.* Toronto: University of Toronto Press, 1995.

Tilchen, Maida. "Pre-Stonewall Lesbians Tell All." *Sojourner: The Women's Forum* 19.1 (1993): 33–34.

Wexler, Alice. Review of "Forbidden Love." *American Historical Review* 99.4 (1994): 1270–1272.

SEE ALSO

Documentary Film; Canadian Television

Fierstein, Harvey   (b. 1954)

Gravel-voiced actor Harvey Fierstein has had phenomenal success as both a performer and a playwright, earning many awards and accolades. He has also been recognized for his steadfast commitment to the cause of glbtq rights.

The younger of two sons of Jewish immigrants from Eastern Europe, Harvey Forbes Fierstein was born on June 6, 1954, in Brooklyn, New York. His parents and brother were extremely supportive of him when he came out to them at the age of thirteen.

The Fiersteins encouraged their sons to attend cultural events in New York City. Saturday matinees on Broadway were a favorite. Young Harvey Fierstein developed an act of his own, dressing in drag and belting out Ethel Merman songs. At sixteen, he began his career as a female impersonator at a gay club in Manhattan's East Village.

As a result of his club act, Fierstein was offered a role in a 1971 production of Andy Warhol's play *Pork* at the La MaMa Experimental Theater Club.

Fierstein continued to appear at La MaMa and other venues but also, having some aspirations to become a painter, enrolled at the Pratt Institute in Brooklyn. He received a B.F.A. degree from Pratt in 1973.

Rather than pursuing a career in painting, Fierstein turned to playwriting. Several of his early "raunchy chic" works were produced off-off-Broadway, and the New York Theater Ensemble staged his *Flatbush Tosca,* a drag interpretation of Puccini's opera, in 1975.

The following year, Fierstein became dangerously depressed after breaking up with a lover. His therapist recommended that he write about the experience, and the result was *The International Stud,* which was produced at the Theater for the New City in 1976 and at La MaMa in 1978, both times with Fierstein in the leading role of Arnold Beckoff, a gay man whose bisexual lover jilts him for a woman.

Critical reaction was not particularly enthusiastic, but Fierstein went on to write two more plays about Arnold, *Fugue in a Nursery* and *Widows and Children First!* Both premiered at La MaMa in 1979, with Fierstein again playing the lead. *Fugue in a Nursery* subsequently moved to an off-Broadway venue.

Backed by The Glines, a nonprofit corporation devoted to sponsoring gay-themed cultural works, Fierstein crafted the three Arnold plays into a single show, entitled *Torch Song Trilogy,* which was first presented off-off-Broadway at the Richard Allen Center in 1981.

Critic Mel Gussow of the *New York Times* had dismissed *The International Stud* as "a sincere but sentimentalized view of a transvestite in extremis," but he joined the chorus of praise for *Torch Song Trilogy.* He wrote that "Arnold's story becomes richer as it unfolds," and of Fierstein's performance he stated that his "self-incarnation is an act of compelling virtuosity." He also noted Fierstein's distinctive "throaty Tallulah voice and manner."

Torch Song Trilogy won the Obie Award for Best Play and the Oppenheimer Playwriting Award in 1982. The accolades and the awards continued when it moved to Broadway, where it played to sold-out houses and garnered a Drama Desk Award and a Tony Award. Fierstein also won the Theatre World Award as outstanding new performer, the Drama Desk Award for outstanding actor, and the Tony for best leading actor in a play in 1983.

While Fierstein was appearing in *Torch Song Trilogy,* producer Alan Carr offered him the opportunity to write the book for a projected musical version of *La Cage aux Folles,* a play—originally in French—by Jean Poiret. As he had in *Torch Song Trilogy,* Fierstein sought to make respect, both for oneself and for others, central to the story.

As a drag artist, Fierstein felt a strong responsibility to craft the role of Albin, the drag queen character in *La Cage aux Folles,* to show that he was fully human and worthy of respect. In a 1983 interview, Fierstein cited the indignities that he had seen people endure—"gay bars being raided by the police, drag queens being beaten in cells." He also recalled arriving at the theater to see "fifty drag queens dancing their hearts out" at an audition for the show on the morning he learned the news of Tennessee Williams's death and was mourning both the loss of the great playwright and the pain that Williams had suffered in his life. The poignant moment only increased Fierstein's desire and resolve to promote dignity and acceptance of all people, especially the marginalized.

With a great score by Jerry Herman, *La Cage aux Folles* was a smash hit on Broadway and won numerous honors, including the 1983 Tony Award for best book.

Fierstein's next three plays, *Spookhouse* (1984), *Safe Sex*, another trilogy of one-acts (1987), and *Forget Him* (1988), met with considerably less success at the box office, though some critics found parts of *Safe Sex* to be some of his best work. Fierstein also wrote the book for the musical flop *Legs Diamond* (1988). The show, which starred Peter Allen, was a disaster that has achieved a kind of legendary status in Broadway lore.

In the mid-1980s, Fierstein began his career in movies, some cinematic and others for television. His early projects include the narration of Rob Epstein and Richard Schmiechen's *The Times of Harvey Milk* (1984) and an acting role in Sidney Lumet's *Garbo Talks* (1984).

Fierstein revised the script of *Torch Song Trilogy* to bring the story to the big screen. Producers expressed reservations, saying that the play had become a "period piece" since it is set in the 1970s, before the AIDS crisis became acute. They also felt that a more prominent actor—either Dustin Hoffman or Richard Dreyfuss—should play the lead role. However, both Hoffman and Dreyfuss, having seen Fierstein onstage as Arnold, told him that they believed he was the best choice for the part.

The independent production company New Line Cinema made the 1987 film, starring Fierstein and directed by Paul Bogart. The movie was enthusiastically received. Critic Brian D. Johnson called it "a funny, poignant, and surprisingly wholesome tale of romantic love and old-fashioned family values," and David Ansen pronounced Fierstein's "generous, overspilling performance…a marvel."

Fierstein became a commentator for the television series *In the Life* in 1992. He also continued acting in a wide variety of films, including Chris Columbus's *Mrs. Doubtfire* (1993), Woody Allen's *Bullets over Broadway* (1994), Rob Epstein's *The Celluloid Closet* (1995), in which he appeared as himself, Roland Emmerich's *Independence Day* (1996), and Emily Squires's *Elmo Saves Christmas* (1996). As a favor to his friend the director John Nicollela, he played a pirate villain in *Kull the Conqueror* (1997). Critic Rafer Guzman, though commenting that "the acting in *Kull*…leaves a lot to be desired," singled out Fierstein's performance as "the most delightful surprise in the film."

Fierstein also made guest appearances on numerous television shows, including *Miami Vice* (1986), *The Simpsons* (1990), *Murder, She Wrote* (1992), and *Ellen* (1998). His 1992 turn in the *Cheers* episode "Rebecca's Lover…Not" won him an Emmy nomination.

In 1998, Fierstein voiced a character in the animated Disney feature *Mulan* (directed by Tony Bancroft), a story loosely based on the ancient Chinese tale of a girl who disguised herself as a boy so that her family could comply with an imperial decree that every household must supply one soldier to the army. Before accepting the part, Fierstein verified that the majority of the cast was Asian so that he would not be "tak[ing] work away from an Asian actor."

One of Fierstein's many works on the theme of respect for all was the 1999 television movie *The Sissy Duckling* (directed by Anthony Bell). The project, for which Fierstein wrote the script and voiced the title character (Melissa Etheridge voiced his mother), won a Humanitas Prize in 2000. His adaptation of the story as a children's book (2002) was warmly received and sold extremely well.

Another of Fierstein's television projects was the movie *Common Ground* (directed by Donna Deitch, 2000), made for the Showtime cable network. Fierstein, Paula Vogel, and Terrence McNally each wrote a piece for the trilogy. The film, set in a fictional small town in Connecticut, looks at the lives of gay men and lesbians in the 1950s, the 1970s, and at the turn of the twenty-first century. Fierstein's contribution, "Andy & Amos," in which he also acted, concerns the issue of gay marriage.

After a lengthy absence, Fierstein made a triumphant return to Broadway in the runaway hit musical *Hairspray* (2002), an adaptation of John Waters's 1988 film. The highly regarded team of Marc Shaiman and Scott Wittman wrote the music, and Mark O'Donnell and Thomas Meehan supplied the book.

Fierstein made his Broadway musical debut in a dress, as Edna Turnblad, the role played by the legendary drag performer Divine in the Waters film. Fierstein was thrilled to get the part and declared that he would "always be grateful, because for this brief, shining moment, I am Ethel Merman, starring in a musical."

Fierstein made the most of the opportunity and won a Tony Award. He became the first man to earn a Best Actor prize for playing a woman and only the second person to win Tony Awards in four different categories. (Tommy Tune was the first.) Among other honors, he also garnered a Drama Desk Award for best lead actor in a musical.

After 711 performances as Edna, Fierstein left the show to continue his movie career. His recent projects include two Danny DeVito films, *Death to Smoochy* (2002) and *Duplex* (2003), and the Craig B. Highberger documentary *Superstar in a Housedress* (2004), about Jackie Curtis, a flamboyant drag performer in the late 1960s and 1970s. Fierstein has also toured with his club act, "This Is Not Going to Be Pretty." In 2005, he returned to Broadway as Tevye in a revival of the Jerry Bock–Sheldon Harnick musical *Fiddler on the Roof*.

On the occasion of his final performance in *Hairspray*, Fierstein auctioned off two tickets to benefit the New York City Gay & Lesbian Anti-Violence Project. He has long been a vocal and outspoken champion of glbtq rights. He has pressed for AIDS research and also for education about safe sex. He has contributed his time and effort to a number of organizations, including the Services Legal Defense Fund, a group that assists gay men and lesbians in the military.

In an eloquent speech in 1998, Fierstein decried the homophobia that had led to the vicious murder of gay college student Matthew Shepard. He called upon glbtq people to be visible and active—to speak out, to vote, and to boycott—and work toward an end to bigotry.

Fierstein created a stir in 2003 when he appeared in the Macy's Thanksgiving Day Parade as Edna Turnblad dressed as Mrs. Santa Claus. Prior to the event he had written an op-ed piece for the *New York Times* questioning whether a figure as beloved as Santa would continue to enjoy respect as a partner in a same-sex couple, and used the example to advocate for gay marriage.

Fierstein has vigorously encouraged all glbtq people to come out publicly but disagrees with the tactic of outing. He believes that the decision to come out is a personal one, and he also feels that people dragged from the closet make poor representatives of the community.

Fierstein is conscious of his own opportunities and responsibilities as a prominent gay man. He turned down the part of a child-eating clown in *Stephen King's It* (directed by Tommy Lee Wallace, 1990) lest he provide fuel for people who unjustly portray gay men as preying on children. He has consistently tried to write and perform roles that affirm personal dignity and encourage people to take pride in who they are and respect others who may be different.

For that, Harvey Fierstein may take pride in himself.

—*Linda Rapp*

BIBLIOGRAPHY

Ansen, David. "In Search of Mr. Right." *Newsweek*, January 2, 1989, 58.

Bennetts, Leslie. "Harvey Fierstein's Long Journey to the Tony and Beyond." *New York Times*, June 26, 1983.

Campbell, Scottie. "Color Me Harvey." *Watermark*, May 25, 2000. www.gayday.com/news/2000/watermark_000525b.asp

Cuthbert, David. "Harvey's Hairy Hit." *New Orleans Times-Picayune*, February 23, 2003.

"Fierstein, Harvey." *Current Biography Yearbook*. Charles Moritz, ed. New York: H. W. Wilson Company, 1984. 122–126.

Graham, Jefferson. "'Common Ground' Does Ask, Then Tells." *USA Today*, January 28, 2000.

Gussow, Mel. "Theater: Fierstein's 'Torch Song.'" *New York Times*, November 1, 1981.

Guzman, Rafer. "Camp 'Kull' Good Trashy Fun with the Stand-in Barbarian." *Buffalo News*, August 29, 1997.

"Harvey Fierstein's Speech." *Arizona Lesbian's List*. (October 15, 1988). www.geocities.com/westhollywood/park/9700/harvey.html

Holden, Stephen. "Always the Lady, Even When He Needed a Shave." *New York Times*, May 5, 2004.

Johnson, Brian D. "Drag Queen Romance; One Man's Search for a Loving Relationship; Torch Song Trilogy." *Maclean's*, February 20, 1989, 53.

Marks, Peter. "Onstage, in a Dress, in His Element." *New York Times*, June 23, 2002.

Singer, Heidi, and Tatiana Deligiannakis. "Pageant's Main Drag; B'way Star Gets Santa Slight." *New York Post*, November 28, 2003.

SEE ALSO

Film Sissies; *In the Life;* Screenwriters; Transvestism in Film; Divine (Harris Glenn Milstead); Warhol, Andy; Waters, John

Film

IN THE SPRING OF 1991, THE PRODUCTION OF CAROLCO'S *Basic Instinct* moved to San Francisco for some necessary location shooting. Directed by Paul Verhoeven, *Basic Instinct* is a nasty drama about a homicidal lesbian and her beautiful, deranged bisexual girlfriend; Michael Douglas plays the hero, a heterosexual investigator.

Even before the crew's arrival, San Francisco's lesbian and gay activist groups were prepared. Earlier complaints about Joe Eszterhas's script—mean and misguided even beyond the standard exaggerations of Hollywood fiction—had received no responses. On the first night, filming was interrupted by a furious crowd of protestors who came armed with ear-splitting whistles. Riot police made a number of arrests.

Despite a court restraining order, local news coverage encouraged protestors' attendance and continued disruption of the shooting. Photocopies of the script were circulated on Castro Street.

The protests against *Basic Instinct* were neither new—New York had seen the same thing in 1980 when William Friedkin began shooting *Cruising* in the gay bars—nor especially successful in effecting changes to the finished film, but they summarize the feeling of American lesbians and gays in the early 1990s. "Hollywood only understands money," declared one speaker at the *Basic Instinct* demonstration. "If they're going to make films that endanger my life, they better budget for my anger."

It is true. If Hollywood merely offered career advice, gay men and women would be better off on unemployment. Mainstream movies have presented gays with a repetitive and sinisterly limited range of job opportunities—as spinster schoolteachers and sly spies; as hairdressers, fashion photographers, gossip columnists, and worried politicians with sweaty brows and secrets to hide; as gossipy best friends, sneaky butlers, poor prostitutes, twisted prison wardens, serial killers, and assorted borderline psychotics.

But this persistent belittling belies Hollywood's real agenda. In films as different as *Adam's Rib* (1949) and *American Gigolo* (1980), *A Florida Enchantment* (1914) and *The Hunger* (1980)—from Laurel and Hardy to lesbian vampires—Hollywood has been fascinated with finding ways of representing gayness since cinema began.

It is a part of popular cultural mythology that homosexuals are meant to be obsessed with Hollywood—all those queens crying for Judy, dykes swooning for Garbo. What is much less remarked upon is precisely the reverse: Hollywood's obsession with homosexuality.

Representations of Gay Men and Lesbians

Confronted by this torrent of lesbian and gay images, subtexts, and sensibilities, the question is not whether Hollywood's homosexuals have matched up to real life, but rather, how has sexuality been represented on the screen? What are the defining characteristics and how do they relate to common ideas about gay men and women?

There are essentially two ideas behind the label *gay cinema*: first, that Hollywood's images of homosexuals are worth investigating and, second, that gay filmmakers themselves have been working independently—and in opposition—to these images.

Thus, there are two strands to gay film history, which only really intertwine in the last three decades, when independent films such as *Longtime Companion* (1990), *Desert Hearts* (1986), and *Parting Glances* (1986) proved that gay and lesbian culture has what Hollywood cutely calls "crossover" potential.

Despite the critical and commercial success of these films, lesbian and gay cinema is not something that has happened only since gay liberation. Politicization has provided the impetus to sift through history and tease out what was previously concealed.

Romance and Sympathy

A 1916 Swedish film, *The Wings*, seems to be one of the first overt gay screen romances; based on Herman Bang's novel, *Mikael*, it races through the melodrama of sculptor Claude Zoret and the elusive youth of the title. Anticipating the dominant theme of mainstream cinema over the next fifty years, their romance ends unhappily, with adopted son Mikael provoking his patron and lover

to a feverish death. In *The Wings*, at least, Zoret dies of a broken heart, a genuinely romantic demise; more often, gay characters have died out of guilt or punishment.

Meanwhile, in Weimar Germany, a second version of homosexual tragedy was being played. Magnus Hirschfeld's Institute for Sexual Science in Berlin initiated the first campaign for decriminalizing homosexuality; *Different from the Others* (1919), starring Conrad Veidt, explicitly pleaded for tolerance. A tale of blackmail and suicide, prefaced by a direct-to-camera monologue by Hirschfeld, *Different from the Others* set the standard for liberal tolerance and for a durable new genre of gay sympathy films.

The Sissy

While Hirschfeld was pleading for tolerance, Hollywood was playing for laughs. Hirschfeld's theories were based on the radical idea of a "third sex," whereas contemporary popular conceptions identified homosexuality as an inversion of ordinary gender: women in men's bodies, men in women's. Hence Hollywood's most enduring stereotype: the sissy.

In his benchmark history, *The Celluloid Closet,* the prodigious researcher and author Vito Russo picked out characters such as the dressmaker in *Irene* (1926), played by George K. Arthur, and Grady Sutton in *Movie*

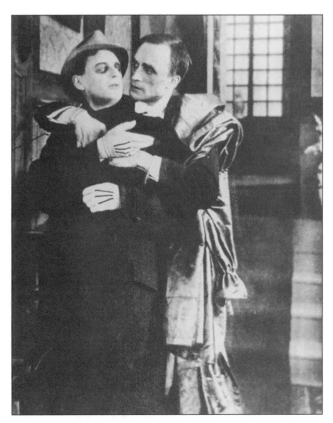

A film still from *Anders als die Andern* (*Different from the Others,* 1919).

Crazy (1932) as early examples of the sissy type. In *Movie Crazy* Sutton shrieks and leaps on a table at the thought of a mouse; it is this sort of incongruous and effeminate behavior that marks early characterizations.

In later films the shading of the sissy becomes more complex; the dialogue often juggles with their sexual ambiguity. Comedians Eric Blore, Edward Everett Horton, and Franklin Pangborn most often occupied these roles.

In *The Gay Divorcee*, Horton plays Fred Astaire's priggish friend Pinky, who enjoys some quick banter with Blore (whose character is tagged as having an "unnatural passion for rocks"); besides the innuendos, the homosexuality of the sissies lies in their easy association and their comic conspiratorial conversation, as compared to the edgy air between the would-be lovers played by Astaire and Ginger Rogers.

Naturally, most gay people would now dispute the causal connection between gender and sexuality, but there is also something to celebrate in the sissy image. There is a flip side to the sissy's intimations of conspiratorial behavior, hyperemotionalism, and frivolous humor: companionship, sensitivity, and backbiting wit. David Wayne as Katharine Hepburn's best friend, Kip, in *Adam's Rib* (1949) is a shining example of these fairly noble qualities.

Women Behaving Like Men

If the sissy was premised on the idea of a man behaving like a woman, it did not work out so well the other way around. In *Turnabout* (1940), a convenient genie enables an overworked husband (John Hubbard) and his jejune wife (Carole Landis) to swap bodies. While Hubbard arrives at work with a clutch bag and enjoys a bit of gossip with the stocking salesman (Franklin Pangborn), Landis takes to full-throated, thigh-slapping behavior, donning men's pants, and mountaineering on the roof of their Manhattan apartment. But the woman-in-man's-clothing gag lacked the longevity or easy humor of the male sissy; as an image it rarely attained a sexual tenor.

According to archivist Andrea Weiss, lesbian interest in early Hollywood figured less on broad comedy and more on drama's major stars such as Garbo, Hepburn, and Dietrich—all of whom had their moments of cross-dressing, in, respectively, *Queen Christina* (1933), *Sylvia Scarlett* (1935), and *Morocco* (1930)—who in their combination of sexual objectification and stage-center action became pinups for women as much as for men.

The Tragic Homosexual

The sissy is something that can be signaled immediately, in the flick of a wrist or a rapid sashay. The other predominant gay image in mainstream movies is a little more elusive. If the sissy belongs to the domain of farce and comedy, the tragic figure haunts the genres of crime, melodrama, and horror. As a stereotype, the tragic homosexual is to be found wherever Hollywood is required to signal shady bars on the wrong side of town, bohemian decadence, or the ill effects of same-sex proximity.

As with the sissy, so much is signaled by certain visual conventions. With Gloria Holden in *Dracula's Daughter* (1936), Judith Anderson in *Rebecca* (1940), and, later, Sal Mineo in *Rebel Without a Cause* (1955) and Robert Walker in *Strangers on a Train* (1951), the tragic homosexual's torture is concentrated in the eyes—sunken, searching out love, or, in the thrillers, young prey.

His or her most common profession is in a role of minor authority (schoolteacher, warden, housekeeper), or some equally small part in the criminal world (blackmailer, getaway-car driver), or perhaps merely playing a devoted mother's boy or best friend. Often the male characters were pictured in a bohemian context—what writer and critic Richard Dyer has identified as the image of "the sad young man."

The Sad Young Man was not merely an invention of Hollywood; like the sissy, which can be traced back to nineteenth-century images of the fop and dandy, it already existed in literary and art history. The Sad Young Man is part Dorian Gray, part Narcissus. In *Now You See It*, his exhaustive study of the American lesbian and gay underground, Dyer finds the image in the films of Kenneth Anger and Gregory Markopoulos.

Anger's *Fireworks* (1947), one of the first widely screened gay underground movies, is the imaginative and seemingly masochistic sex fantasy of its slim solitary dreamer.

Fifteen years later, Markopoulos's New York–set *Twice a Man* (1962) exploits the image seemingly without irony: Paul, the melancholic, suicidal hero, literally weeps his way through the Oedipal drama.

Underground Film

Dyer relates the rise of the male homosexual underground to the popularization of Freudianism (which, however fumblingly, emphasized the idea of unconscious and therefore unwilled attraction), to the war (which brought large numbers of gay men and women together in single-sex environments), and to the boom in paperback publishing (where exposés of homosexual lives were frequently accompanied by the first illustrations of the gay milieu).

The latter two factors also led to the wide-scale distribution and manufacture of gay pornography. From its beginnings with the Athletic Model Guild—a studio devoted to male photography based in Los Angeles—an empire was quickly assembled.

AMG auteur Richard Fontaine started making short, silent posing-pouch snapshot films in the mid-1950s and moved on to sound titles like *In the Days of Greek Gods* (1958) and *Muscles from Outer Space* (1962), which featured narratives as well as nudity.

Fontaine's films were among the first gay advocacy documents in American cinema; he often managed to include references to the lowly status of the homosexual. His first feature-length erotic film, *In Love Again* (1969), is more like propaganda than porn.

Dyer has characterized the gay images—and there are many—of the 1960s underground as "listless and inconsequential." Andy Warhol's films very much capture the essence of this limp mode; his stars are passive hustlers—Joe Dallesandro in *Blow Job* (1969) or drugged, drunken queens (Taylor Mead in any title, but especially in *Tarzan and Jane Regained...Sort Of* and *Lonesome Cowboys*).

In the late 1960s, it was only the works of less well-promoted directors such as George Kuchar, Curt McDowell, and John Waters that allowed the appearance of energetic, lusty gay protagonists.

Lesbian underground filmmakers took a different route. As it has been throughout the history of independent cinema, there is less work by women from this period. Apart from an exceptional moment of semi-seduction in Maya Deren's *At Land* (1945), it was left to 1970s filmmakers such as Constance Beeson and Barbara Hammer to break new ground.

Hammer's films—among them *Superdyke* (1975), *Labryis Rising* (1977), and *Women I Love* (1976)—express a metaphoric, collective lesbian iconography: Instead of the individualistic narratives of the male underground, they try to present new images for all lesbians.

Hammer's work since then persistently continued this devotion to new vocabulary. In the 1980s, she began to look back at the success of the lesbian avant-garde, reprocessing and juxtaposing footage from that decade and the previous one. Hammer's more recent film *Nitrate Kisses* (1993) recuts a classic of the gay male underground: Melville Weber and James Sibley Watson's *Lot in Sodom* (1930).

Sad Young Men (and Women)

For mainstream cinema, as for popular culture in general, the late 1950s and 1960s was a time for the tragedy of the homosexual experience. As the censorship systems in Britain and the United States were found to be more malleable, the image of the Sad Young Man (and Woman) figured in narratives.

Movies were suddenly keener to diagnose the condition of their characters. Studio executives, however, read the boom in pop psychology and hand-me-down Freud a little differently from the intellectuals of the underground. Films such as *Tea and Sympathy* (1956), *The Children's Hour* (1962), *Suddenly, Last Summer* (1959), *The Boys in the Band* (1970), and, from Britain, *Victim* (1961) and *The Killing of Sister George* (1968) set about creating a narrative context for the stereotype of the Sad Young Man.

These films focused on the loneliness of their homosexual figures, but their vision was blurred by a double purpose of sympathy and voyeurism. *Victim* ostensibly credits the anomie of gay men to their illegality and sets out to prove that their susceptibility to blackmail and imprisonment ensures a miserable life. Designed therefore as a campaigning, liberal film, *Victim* also ends on an image of unbearable isolation.

Similarly, in the final frames of *The Children's Hour*, after Shirley MacLaine hangs herself, wrongly labeled lover Audrey Hepburn walks proudly and tearily down a desolate tree-lined avenue; after ejecting and humiliating his dinner party guests, *The Boys in the Band*'s host (Kenneth Nelson) wipes a tear and takes another tranquilizer.

One of the most dour denouements belongs to a British film, *Walk a Crooked Path* (1969), in which a married gay teacher, after having engineered the murder of his wife, is abandoned by the schoolboy he adores. He sits alone in his now still home and the image changes from color to black and white as the film flashes through long shots of each deserted room.

Yet these intensely melancholy fantasies were of course rooted in real-life homophobia, legislation, and social stigma. Just as musicals capture moments of ecstasy and community, *Victim* and *The Children's Hour* exaggerate isolation and injustice to a degree that is recordable, palpable, and undeniable.

Gay Bar Scenes

Another key moment in films of the 1960s and 1970s is the gay bar scene. *The Detective* (1968) pitches Frank Sinatra in pursuit of a homosexual killer and comes up with a crawl tour of New York's gay dives. There is a self-consciousness not just in the representation of "casual" gay social life but also in the camera pans and overhead shots, a sense in which the film is proud to present something so explicitly and yet still be bewildered by what it sees.

The Detective was not the first film to peek inside a gay bar (Vito Russo pinpoints this to *Call Her Savage*, a 1932 Clara Bow drama), but it typified the realist trend of the next decade.

Each gay-themed film made a special claim to authenticity. For example, *Sister George*'s publicity made much of the fact that its bar scenes had been partly filmed at London's famous Gateways Club. Ten years later, William Friedkin took to Manhattan leather bars in search of real-life clubbers for *Cruising*.

The mid-1960s films often used the device of an investigative figure delving into the gay scene in order to resolve a mystery, serving as a commentator to a criminal version of *Lifestyles of the Rich and Famous*. Later, *Investigation of a Murder* (1973), *Partners* (1982), and *Cruising* made their heroes literal detectives.

The bar scene is also constructed to confirm culture's queer conspiracy theory, which goes something like this: *Homosexuals have a secret code and a secret meeting place, just below the surface of ordinary social life.*

Yet, for gay viewers, the bar scene may function as a vision of utopia, a restorative after all the hours of miserable, cinematic isolation. The self-consciously casual scenes of 1970s social life potentially offered the pleasure of recognition for lesbian and gay audiences. Not for the first time, Hollywood's homosexual images could be experienced differently, and in complex ways, by a gay audience.

Making Love

By 1980, however, the curiosity of gay viewers had been both sorely tested and exploited. Twentieth Century Fox released *Making Love* (1982) with much self-generated excitement. Penned by openly gay writer Barry Sandler and promoted as the first honest look at gay relationships, *Making Love* is best remembered for a sex scene of astonishing discretion.

More interesting than the movie itself—a TV-movie tale of broken marriage and bisexuality, with Kate Jackson as the hurt wife on the trail of her husband's nighttime liaisons—was the narrative of the film's marketing. Aside from the standard campaign, which presented *Making Love* as an old-fashioned women's picture and bleached away the gay theme, Fox also ran a separate campaign for the gay community.

This campaign involved preview screenings for gay journalists and other community opinion-makers, as well as a new poster picturing Harry Hamlin undressed and embraced by Jackson's movie husband, with Kate herself banished to the background.

Making Love was a failure with both constituencies, gay and nongay. Against that film's much derided middle-class coziness, the plurality of lesbian and gay lifestyles was apparent in the increasing vigor of the American gay movement.

Documentary Films

In the 1970s, independent documentarians had tried to get at this diversity. *A Position of Faith* (1973), *Gay USA* (1977), and Peter Adair's hands-across-America panorama, *Word Is Out* (1977), all attempted not just to explain the premise of gay liberation but to show it too. When interviewees in *Word Is Out* claimed, "We're just like you," audiences could see that it was true.

Later nonfiction features achieved this mission more succinctly: *The Times of Harvey Milk* (1984) is a persuasive political tearjerker, while *Before Stonewall* (1984), made the same year, is an elegant family album of archival footage; both films, like the documentaries of the 1990s—such as *Tongues Untied* (1990) and *Voices from the Front* (1991)—still rely on the truth of personal testimony to move, or forge identification with, their audiences.

The Blur between Hollywood and Independent Films

In the 1980s and 1990s, gay-themed fiction commanded a high profile. In *Parting Glances* (1986), *Desert Hearts* (1986), and *Lianna* (1986), the blur between Hollywood and the independents produced narratives that addressed both gay and nongay audiences. Many of these were directly the result of filmmakers' experience in the 1970s with international work made and screened exclusively for gay men and women.

For American audiences, annual gay film festivals (in San Francisco, New York, Los Angeles, and other cities) discovered European directors such as Eloy de la Iglesia (*The Deputy*, 1979), Monika Treut (*Seduction: The Cruel Woman*, 1986), and Alexandra von Grote (*November Moon*, 1984) or otherwise reclaimed the lesbian and gay sensibility of avant-gardists like Ulrike Ottinger, Isaac Julien, and Rosa von Praunheim.

Crucially, dedicated researchers such as Richard Dyer, Vito Russo, and Andrea Weiss brought new perspectives to the work of earlier filmmakers.

Eroticism

Eroticism features strongly in today's mainstream gay movies. AIDS has moved gay-themed films once again away from realism, has clarified that films are indeed fictions. Whether it is boredom with heterosexuality or another burst of voyeurism, Hollywood seems captivated by what gay people do in bed; hence, *Lianna, Longtime Companion, Maurice* (1987), and *Torch Song Trilogy* (1988), all made independently but picked up by major distribution companies.

Of course, it would be unfair to claim that eroticism is the sole project of any of these films, but it is true to say that the bed scene has replaced the bar scene.

Gay Themes and Diverse Responses

As Hollywood claws back and reconstitutes the novelty of lesbian and gay culture, and as independent gay filmmakers confess to the pleasure of mainstream genres such as romance, gay themes and influences cluster in increasingly bizarre regroupings.

Among these themes and influences are the adoration of the male body/buddy (Schwarzenegger; Cruise; *My Own Private Idaho*, 1991); the mass marketing of camp (*Too Much Sun*, 1990; *Pee-Wee's Big Adventure*, 1987; *Soapdish*, 1991); ceaseless homosexual subtexts about Oedipal indecision in teen movies such as *Fright Night* (1985) and *Point Break* (1991); the reappearance of the destructive film noir lesbian (*Slamdance*, 1986; *Bellman and True*, 1987; *Basic Instinct*, 1992); the dominance of educational-TV movies (*An Early Frost*, 1986; *Consenting*

Adult, 1985; *Andre's Mother*, 1990); AIDS and associational imagery in horror (*The Fly*, 1986; *Lifeforce*, 1985); homosexual serial killers and their newly graphic crimes (*The Krays*, 1990; *Silence of the Lambs*, 1991).

Oppositional work is also thriving, either as agitprop or avant-garde. Video allows for fairly instant responses to issues: There are now hundreds of tapes around AIDS, and within a few months of Britain's new antigay legislation in 1988, eighteen polemical tapes attacking the outrage had been logged.

At the same time, a new kind of underground cinema is identifiable; filmmakers like Su Friedrich (*Sink or Swim*, 1990), Gregg Araki (*The Living End*, 1991), Tom Kalin (*Swoon*, 1992), and Todd Haynes (*Poison*, 1991) are unarguably at the vanguard of a playful new aesthetic.

Conclusion

The tentative and fractious nature of these recent groupings is proof that heterogeneity is still the norm. For as long as homosexuality occupies the same difficult ideological position that it does—ceaselessly yoked with anxieties about disease, reproduction, and contamination; bound in with legislative and civil rights discourse; shaped by sociological surveys and celebrity scandal—filmmakers will undoubtedly continue to produce provocative and complex images.

—*Mark Finch*

[Originally published as "Gays and Lesbians in Cinema." *Cineaste's Political Companion To American Film*. Gary Crowdus, ed. Chicago: Lake View Press, 1994.]

Bibliography

Bad Object-Choice Collective, eds. *How Do I Look?: Queer Film and Video*. Seattle: Bay Press, 1991.

Dyer, Richard. *Gays and Film*. New York: New York Zoetrope, 1984.

_____. *Now You See It: Studies on Lesbian and Gay Film*. New York: Routledge, 1990.

Russo, Vito. *The Celluloid Closet: Homosexuality in the Movies*. New York: Harper and Row, 1987.

Tyler, Parker. *Screening the Sexes: Homosexuality in the Movies*. New York: Holt, Rinehart and Winston, 1972.

Weiss, Andrea. *Vampires and Violets: Lesbians in the Cinema*. London: Jonathan Cape, 1992.

See also

Bisexuality in Film; Documentary Film; European Film; Film Directors; Film Festivals; Film Noir; Film Sissies; Film Spectatorship; Horror Films; New Queer Cinema; Anger, Kenneth; Araki, Gregg; Crowley, Mart; Dietrich, Marlene; Garbo, Greta; Garland, Judy; Hammer, Barbara; Haynes, Todd; Julien, Isaac; Kuchar, George; Mineo, Sal; Ottinger, Ulrike; Praunheim, Rosa von; Treut, Monika; Warhol, Andy; Waters, John; Weiss, Andrea

Film Actors: Gay Male

FROM THE SILENT ERA FORWARD, GAY FILM ACTORS HAVE made significant contributions to cinematic art and Western culture. While very few gay and lesbian actors have been permitted the luxury of openness, many of them have nevertheless challenged and helped reconfigure notions of masculinity and femininity and, to a lesser extent, of homosexuality.

Because of the peculiar hold of film celebrity on Western popular culture, film actors—particularly film stars—have always been the subject of rumor and gossip, which in turn has affected the way they are perceived by others. Literally scores of actors, ranging from silent stars such as Rudolph Valentino and later screen idols such as Cary Grant and James Dean to contemporary stars such as Tom Cruise, John Travolta, Keanu Reeves, and Tom Selleck, have been rumored to be gay. Sometimes the rumors are true, but often they are not.

Although the most successful gay film actors have achieved success by fulfilling the fantasies of the predominantly heterosexual mainstream audience, some of them have also simultaneously fulfilled the fantasies of gay men.

Any list of gay male film actors is bound to be selective and somewhat arbitrary. It should include accomplished character actors such as Charles Laughton, Clifton Webb, Michael Jeter, Dan Butler, and Simon Callow, as well as handsome hunks such as Rock Hudson and Tab Hunter. The actors mentioned in the following paragraphs are representative and are included because they exemplify in various ways the peculiar difficulties faced by creative artists who were or are homosexual.

For the public, film actors are often expected to be not merely talented performers but also the embodiment of the characters they portray, and for many people an essential characteristic of film stars is their heterosexuality. For most of film history, open homosexuality, or even rumors of homosexuality, could end the careers of actors; hence, it is not surprising that most gay actors have had to expend enormous energy disguising their sexuality.

Today, the question of an actor's homosexuality tends to center on whether the public will accept an openly gay actor in a heterosexual role. Many gay actors refuse to come out because they believe it may limit the kinds of roles they are offered.

The Silent Era and the Coming of Sound

When Rudolph Valentino died on August 23, 1926, he was mourned wildly. Over 100,000 women swarmed his funeral. One month before his death, however, the *Chicago Tribune* called Valentino a "pink powder puff" and announced that if effeminate men like Valentino really existed, it was time for a matriarchy, even if led by "masculine women."

Male audiences were offended by Valentino's extravagant dress, colorful spats, makeup, and willingness to display his body on screen in such films as *The Sheik* (1921) and *Blood and Sand* (1922). Hollywood's first queer film star, Valentino disrupted his era's rigid codes of sex and gender. Valentino's sexuality remains ambiguous, but rumors of his homosexuality were rife in Hollywood gay circles, despite (or because of) his marriages to and divorces from Jean Acker and Natacha Rambova, both lesbian.

Ramón Novarro, who starred in *Mata Hari* (1931) and *Ben Hur* (1926), was an outsider, a Mexican immigrant in a town known for its negative representations of Mexicans. But he brought to the screen a delicate masculine body and boyish eroticism that unsettled male viewers.

Novarro defied Louis B. Mayer, head of Metro-Goldwyn-Mayer Studios, who demanded that the actor marry to deflect rumors of his homosexuality. Defiance of Mayer, as well as internal conflicts over his sexuality, which led to alcoholism, prematurely ended Novarro's career. Many years after he had faded into obscurity, Navarro, at age seventy, was killed by two male hustlers—his death confirming the rumors that had hounded him during his days in the limelight.

By all accounts, William Haines, an MGM star in the 1920s, was the first openly gay actor in Hollywood. Although Haines met his life companion, Jimmy Shields, in 1923, he remained boldly flirtatious on movie sets. Louis B. Mayer again sought to control a star's image by issuing a press release, this time announcing Haines's deep love for actress Pola Negri.

Haines rose to stardom with *Tell It to the Marines* (1927), but, ironically, he plummeted from stardom six years later after he was reportedly arrested with a sailor in a room at the YMCA. Mayer allegedly canceled his contract and prohibited him from ever working in Hollywood, at least as an actor. Haines went on to a successful career as an interior designer.

In 1922, Hollywood established the Motion Picture Producers and Distributors of America, a self-regulating body led by former Congressman Will Hays that functioned as the public relations and lobbying arm of Hollywood. The MPPDA squelched actors, homosexual and heterosexual, who generated bad publicity, and in 1929 it instituted the Production Code, a complex set of moral standards for film content. The banishment of Haines and the establishment of the MPPDA forced actors of ambiguous sexuality, such as Tyrone Power, deeply into the closet.

With masculinity defined in terms of the machismo of Clark Gable and the outdoor ruggedness of John Gilbert, there was little room for film stars who deviated very far from the increasingly rigid American gender and sex roles. The press became bolder, looking with skepticism at any publicity release announcing the imminent marriage of (gay) actors. During the 1930s and 1940s, gay actors were the "Twilight Men."

The Legacy of Stardom in the 1950s

James Dean, Montgomery Clift, and Rock Hudson achieved stardom in the 1950s, each leaving a lasting mark on film history and the public.

When Dean died on September 30, 1955, only one of his films, *East of Eden* (1955), had been released. After his death and the release of *Rebel Without a Cause* (1955) and *Giant* (1956), Dean became an icon of the sensitive and moody young man.

In the decades since Dean's death, rumors of his bisexuality have been repeated in numerous newspapers, magazines, and books. Allegedly, Dean had affairs with prominent men and women in Hollywood and frequented leather and S/M bars. Dean's screen persona, that of a troubled, uncertain, and reckless late adolescent in conflict with 1950s conformist values, fused with the rumors of his personal life and resonated deeply with gay audiences.

"No other star captured the hearts and minds of gay men like Montgomery Clift," proclaims John Stubbard. Clift's persona was sensitive, introspective, fragile, and intense. "Clift was like a wound," Jane Fonda noted, constantly suffering and in psychological turmoil. But with his physically slight body, pretty face, hesitance to take action, and troubled stare, Clift helped reconfigure notions of masculinity in Hollywood.

Gay men of the 1950s may have responded so fully to the suffering of Dean and Clift because they connected it with the degradation they faced everyday in a homophobic society.

Almost every year during the 1950s, *Look*, *Photoplay*, *Modern Screen*, and other movie magazines proclaimed Rock Hudson "most popular star" or "top male star." He was six feet four inches tall, virile, steadfast, with a smooth muscular body and heroic square jaw. The strength of his masculine persona permitted Hudson to feign effeminacy in comedies with Doris Day and Tony Randall and to appear vulnerable and indecisive with women in Douglas Sirk's melodramas.

Fearing imminent outing of his client by *Confidential* magazine, Henry Willson, Hudson's agent, arranged the star's marriage with Phyllis Gates, his executive secretary. It lasted three years.

Obsessed with his image, Hudson supposedly declared he would rather die before fans discovered he was gay. In the 1950s, Hollywood publicists filled magazines with pictures of Hudson in his shorts, frolicking with Elizabeth Taylor and other glamorous female stars. Gay males of the era saw through this facade, however, and, most of them also necessarily closeted, could even identify with it.

In the 1980s, many gay males could also identify with Hudson in another way. Shortly after the news broke in July 1985 that Hudson had AIDS, the writer Armistead Maupin, a friend and briefly a lover of Hudson's, publicly outed him to the *San Francisco Chronicle*. Waking up an apathetic president (and a wider public) may well be the most significant legacy of Hudson's stardom. A *New York Times* headline of September 2, 1989, declared, "Actor's Illness Helped Reagan to Grasp AIDS, Doctor Says."

Troublesome Rumblings from the Closet

Many gay actors invested an enormous amount of energy to remain closeted, but such efforts took their toll physically and psychologically. Raymond Burr, for example, believed he could ensure privacy by creating an imaginary world to hide his homosexuality and his forty-year relationship with Robert Benevides. Burr claimed he was married three times and had a son who died of leukemia at age ten. Only in the late 1990s did his sister admit that Burr was married only once, for a short time, and had no son.

No one can explain with certainty why Burr created such an elaborate facade to keep his life secret, but the actor clearly believed extreme actions needed to be taken. Possibly Burr had found out that, in 1961, at the height of his popularity in television and film, a member of the American Bar Association, an organization Burr frequently addressed by virtue of his famous portrayal of Perry Mason, gave the FBI documents indicating that Burr was "a noted sex deviate."

Anthony Perkins's masculine persona was delicate, timid, and agitated. He suffered psychologically over his homosexuality, and, reportedly, had severe panic attacks in the presence of beautiful actresses when no sexual feelings were generated. Alarmed over possible exposure by *Confidential* magazine, Perkins married Berry Berenson, who had had an adolescent crush on him and was sixteen years his junior.

Some friends believe that Perkins's desperate attempts to develop a heterosexual response were only partly successful. Another casualty of AIDS, Perkins was also a casualty of his internalized homophobia.

If Burr and Perkins are examples of the extremes actors have gone to in an effort to conceal their homosexuality, Tommy Kirk is an object lesson in the dangers of not concealing one's gayness in the early 1960s.

Kirk was a child star in such blockbuster Disney films as *The Absent Minded Professor* (1961) and *The Shaggy Dog* (1959). But in his late teens, despondent over the exploitation of his cute all-American adolescent image, Kirk took a step that most of his gay predecessors in Hollywood never dared. He came out to Disney.

Immediately fired, Kirk briefly received national press coverage but soon passed into obscurity. He joined church organizations working with gay and lesbian youth. He remained furious, and, at times, vocal, about Disney's propaganda mill and discriminatory practices. Unfortunately, Kirk's heroic act has all but disappeared from gay history.

The British Take the Closet in Stride

In 1988, Ian McKellen outed himself as he spoke on BBC Radio against pending antigay government regulations. Still closeted at that time were many other highly respected actors, some of whom, such as Nigel Hawthorne, would later be outed.

Three years later, when McKellen was knighted, gay British filmmaker Derek Jarman attacked him for accepting the honor and for his congenial ties with a homophobic government. Openly gay British actors Stephen Fry, Alex McCowen, and Simon Callow came to McKellen's defense. It would be impossible to conceive of a scenario comparable to this one occurring in Hollywood at that time.

Interestingly, Sir John Gielgud, Dirk Bogarde, and Nigel Hawthorne remained silent during the McKellen controversy, yet they were among the best-known gay actors in England.

Gielgud, one of the greatest stage actors of the century and the winner of an Academy Award for Best Supporting Actor in *Arthur* (1981), had been outed years ago by his arrest in a public restroom. But he had led a circumspect life for many years, his homosexuality widely known and accepted but not discussed. His silence at the time of the McKellen controversy must have been both considered and painful.

Living in rural France, Bogarde remained aloof and distant, offending British actors who wanted his distinguished reputation behind their lobbying efforts. After becoming England's Rock Hudson in the 1950s, starring in comedies and romances, Bogarde had taken a daring step by appearing in the 1961 film *Victim*, in which he played a lawyer who was blackmailed for his homosexuality. Two years later, in *The Servant* (1963), Bogarde portrayed a predatory homosexual who destroys a home's quiet domesticity.

Despite his daring in accepting these parts at a time when they may have damaged his career, Bogarde was notoriously reticent about his private life. He never discussed his homosexuality or his relationship with his manager, Tony Forwood, claiming that who he was could be seen in his movies and discovered in his autobiographies.

Similarly, Hawthorne, who was to receive an Oscar nomination for Best Actor in *The Madness of King George* (1994), professed not to understand why one should be an activist. Even after he was outed by the gay press in 1994 and headlined by the British tabloids ("The Madness of Queen Nigel"; "Yes Minister, I'm Gay"), he merely brushed off the insults as trashy. Hawthorne seems to have felt that carrying on with life in an unassuming manner was a better path for him to take.

Contemporary Debate: To Come Out or Not to Come Out

The British actor Rupert Everett came out publicly in 1989. Rather than ruining his career, however, the revelation seems only to have made him more interesting to audiences. After his success in *My Best Friend's Wedding* (1997), in which he played a gay character, critics predicted that he would become the first openly gay romantic leading man in Hollywood. Everett received such ecstatic audience responses at test screenings of the film that the director shot additional scenes that beefed up his role.

Everett's success rekindled discussion about whether audiences would accept an openly gay actor in heterosexual roles. Ian McKellen's response was blunt: "Bullshit, I think that anyone who believes [that audiences would not accept gay actors] is just battling homophobia within themselves." McKellen has pointed out that one of the first roles offered to him after the public revelation of his homosexuality was that of a notorious womanizer, former British cabinet minister John Profumo.

Similarly, the coming out of Hong Kong actor Leslie Cheung, the acclaimed star of Chen Kaige's *Farewell My Concubine* (1993), did not damage his career. Admittedly, however, Cheung specialized in playing sexually ambiguous roles.

Still, the perception remains that being identified as homosexual can severely limit an actor's career. A lawsuit filed by Tom Cruise, in which he charges a tabloid with falsely alleging that he is a homosexual, contends that such allegations could result in audiences' inability to identify with him as an action hero.

An openly gay casting director seemed to confirm that possibility when he stated recently that he refuses to date gay actors because an actor seen in public with him risked confinement to gay or sexually ambiguous roles.

Indeed, even the initial assumption that Rupert Everett's openness about his homosexuality would not harm his career has recently been challenged. Everett has complained that studio executives have denied him roles because they believe that an audience will not accept an openly gay man in a romantic leading role.

Moreover, director Irwin Winkler, who recently made *De-Lovely* (2004), about Cole Porter's life as a gay composer, acknowledged that the fear of being outed as a gay actor still permeates Hollywood. Winkler confirmed that most gay actors are not openly gay, stating that

some in particular would be quite upset to hear their names discussed in a gay context.

In his 2002 autobiography *Why the Long Face? The Adventures of a Truly Independent Actor*, Craig Chester chronicles the battles lost by being an openly gay actor, and concludes that "being in the closet is good for business." Citing the example of Sean Hayes, who plays an outrageously stereotypical gay character on *Will and Grace*, he notes that if Hayes "can't come out because of the ramifications...then who can?"

Actor Robert Gant stayed in the closet for over a decade while securing roles in such television shows as *Caroline in the City*. After coming out, he landed an important role on *Queer As Folk*. Even so, he believes that openly gay actors will be limited in their choices until one achieves the stature of a romantic lead.

—*Richard C. Bartone*

BIBLIOGRAPHY

Anger, Kenneth. *Hollywood Babylon II*. New York: E. P. Dutton, 1977.

Dyer, Richard. *Stars*. London: BFI Publishing, 1999.

Ehrenstein, David. *Open Secret: Gay Hollywood 1928–2000*. New York: Perennial, 2000.

Hadleigh, Boze. *Conversations with My Elders*. New York: St. Martin's Press, 1986.

"Ian McKellen School of Drama." *The Knitting Circle*. Lesbian & Gay Staff Association, South Bank University, London. http://myweb.lsbu.ac.uk/~stafflag/drama.html

Mann, William J. *Behind the Screen: How Gays and Lesbians Shaped Hollywood, 1910–1969*. New York: Penguin Books, 2001.

Stubbard, John. "Only Monty." *Out/Takes* 3 (1984): 23.

SEE ALSO

Film; Film Actors: Lesbian; Bogarde, Sir Dirk; Burr, Raymond; Butler, Dan; Callow, Simon; Chamberlain, Richard; Chapman, Graham; Cheung, Leslie; Clift, Montgomery; Cumming, Alan; Dean, James; Everett, Rupert; Fry, Stephen; Gielgud, Sir John; Grant, Cary; Haines, William "Billy"; Hawthorne, Sir Nigel; Hudson, Rock; Hunter, Tab; Laughton, Charles; McKellen, Sir Ian; Novarro, Ramón; Sargent, Dick; Valentino, Rudolph; Webb, Clifton; Williams, Kenneth; Winfield, Paul

Film Actors: Lesbian

FROM THE DAYS OF SILENT FILMS TO THE PRESENT, lesbian actresses have played a significant role in Hollywood—both in the movies themselves and outside them—but their contributions have rarely been recognized or spoken of openly.

While female bisexuality and homosexuality are gradually becoming more acceptable in the film world—and sexual identity more of a pressing issue—many queer actresses still fear that openness will damage their careers. The "lavender marriage," a term coined to describe nuptials between gay male and lesbian stars for reasons of career insurance and social approval, is by no means only a relic of the past.

Early Films and the Advent of the Hays Code

The private lives of early film stars Alla Nazimova, Greta Garbo, Marlene Dietrich, and Tallulah Bankhead have long been fodder for public speculation and gossip. Many actresses of the 1930s, 1940s, and 1950s were part of what were then termed in gay argot "sewing circles," a phrase allegedly coined by Nazimova to describe discreet gatherings of lesbians in Hollywood. Unable to be open about their sexuality, these women—with varying degrees of secrecy—nevertheless formed romantic and sexual relationships with each other.

The bisexuality of Nazimova, a Russian stage actress who moved to New York City early in the twentieth century to pursue a career in acting, was fairly well known in the film community, despite her long-term involvement with (gay) actor Charles Bryant. In 1918, she moved to Hollywood, where she bought a large Spanish-style house that would later become the Garden of Allah, a hotel and apartment house where a number of Hollywood luminaries would live.

In the 1920s, Nazimova became one of the most popular movie stars in America. Her film career began with the silent film *War Brides* (1916), continued through such movies as *Camille* (1921), and culminated in *The Bridge of San Luis Rey* (1944). For a while she was Metro-Goldwyn-Mayer's highest-paid actress. She later formed her own motion picture company, which produced a famous (but financially disastrous) all-gay film version of Oscar Wilde's *Salomé* (1922), the failure of which effectively eroded her status as a Hollywood power broker.

Nazimova's lesbian relationships with the writer and lover of female celebrities Mercedes de Acosta, stage actress Eva Le Gallienne, butch film director Dorothy Arzner, and Oscar Wilde's lesbian niece, Dolly, earned her a reputation as something of a ladykiller.

But her film career finally dried up, not only because of the spectacular failure of *Salomé*, but also because of the formation of the Motion Picture Producers and Distributors of America in 1922, which was to institute the infamous Motion Picture Production Code in 1929, and the rise of the studio system.

The Code—also known as the Hays Code after the man who drafted it, former chairman of the Republican National Committee and Postmaster General Will H. Hays—was a major boon to advocates of censorship. It decreed that there would be no "immorality" or "impropriety" on screen—only chaste kisses and heterosexual characters.

Worse, the Code was applied to actors' private lives; and drug use, adultery, sexual promiscuity, and especially homosexuality were grounds for blacklisting. The vulnerability of gay and lesbian actors to blacklisting was exacerbated by the consolidation of the movie industry into a few powerful studios.

The name Alla Nazimova, with its lesbian connotations, became known as "unsafe" in Hollywood. In an increasingly repressive climate, many lesbian actresses retreated ever more deeply into the closet, dating or even marrying men in order to appear heterosexual.

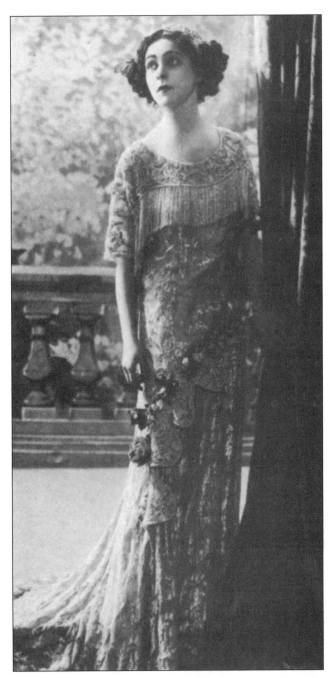

Bisexual actress Alla Nazimova in *Marionettes* (1911).

Yet several actresses in the decades to follow—such as the openly bisexual seductress Marlene Dietrich and the irrepressible Tallulah Bankhead—appeared unconcerned about the gossip surrounding their sexuality. They seemed even to encourage it.

Golden Age Actresses

The underground network of lesbians and bisexual women in the film industry during Hollywood's golden age illustrates how many upper-class lesbians adapted to the restrictions imposed on them. Unlike working-class lesbians, whose socializing largely took place in bars and who had less glamorous careers to lose, Hollywood lesbians tended to socialize at private parties, where they could safeguard their "secret" lives. Absentee or gay husbands made it easy for these women to meet regularly.

Nazimova hosted many a soiree at her home. Salka Viertel, a lesbian screenwriter, also threw notable parties. She is rumored to have been the only person with whom Greta Garbo discussed Marlene Dietrich.

(If legendary screen sirens Garbo and Dietrich had been involved romantically with each other, they were tight-lipped about it to the very end. In fact, throughout their careers, the two women publicly denied having ever met. But, according to Diana McLellan, the two appeared together in the 1925 silent film *The Joyless Street* and enjoyed a brief affair.)

Garbo went on to lead a life entirely different from that of Dietrich: She never married and became famously reclusive after her retirement from film at the tender age of thirty-six. In contrast, Dietrich, who had had a husband and child in her early twenties, maintained her notoriously seductive ways with both men and women throughout her long career.

Despite the differences in their approaches to sexuality, Garbo and Dietrich apparently had, whether knowingly or not, lovers in common. For example, de Acosta and Le Gallienne, aside from their relationships with each other and with Nazimova, both became involved with Garbo at different times; de Acosta also had an affair with Dietrich.

Tallulah Bankhead, primarily a stage actress but also the star of films such as *Tarnished Lady* (1931) and *Lifeboat* (1943), was intimate with one of the few openly lesbian actresses of the time, comedian Patsy Kelly. Bankhead reportedly had affairs with both Dietrich and Garbo and also claimed to have slept with Barbara Stanwyck.

Louise Brooks—the silent-film actress famous for her bobbed hairdo as well as her role as Lulu in *Pandora's Box* (1929)—became outspoken in her later years. In her memoirs and conversations, she reminisced about affairs with women, including a tryst with Garbo.

Aloof from the "sewing circles" were other actresses rumored to be lesbian or bisexual, including Janet Gaynor, star of *A Star is Born* (1937), and Mary Martin, best known for her role as Peter Pan. Reportedly, these "best friends" both had lavender marriages, to a costume designer and an interior decorator, respectively.

Character and supporting actresses also went to great lengths to hide their sexuality, though they usually lived without the constant public scrutiny superstars experienced. Agnes Moorehead, for example, never mentioned her lesbianism, which was widely assumed.

Moorehead appeared in more than sixty films, including *Citizen Kane* (1941), and received several Academy Award nominations for her supporting performances. She is perhaps now best known for her role as Endora, mother of witch Samantha in the 1960s television series *Bewitched*. Despite her reticence, however, she was widely assumed to be lesbian. Gay comedian Paul Lynde proclaimed her "classy as hell, but one of the all-time Hollywood dykes."

Barbara Stanwyck, best known for her steamy roles in such films as *Stella Dallas* (1937) and *Double Indemnity* (1944), also had a booming television career in the 1960s and 1970s. Stanwyck married twice, the first time to vaudevillian Frank Fay and the second time to actor Robert Taylor. Although she rebuffed any questions about her sexuality or her marriages, many observers of the Hollywood scene believed that neither Stanwyck nor either of her husbands was heterosexual.

Throughout their careers, Dame Judith Anderson, Elsa Lanchester, and Sandy Dennis were the subject of persistent rumors that they were lesbian, but they never confirmed the rumors.

The closetedness of lesbians and gay men during the golden age of Hollywood is, of course, quite understandable. Not only were homosexual acts a prosecutable offense in all parts of the United States, but, especially after World War II and the advent of the Cold War, homosexuals became one of the favorite targets of witch-hunts.

Moreover, during this period, scandal magazines became ever bolder. The climate for homosexuals in the United States of the 1950s and early 1960s was oppressive in the extreme. Hence, the fear of exposure for lesbian and gay male actors was by no means paranoid.

Coming Out: Lesbian Actresses to the Present

Although the gay rights movement has helped to improve visibility in industries such as publishing and music, and gay men and women no longer live under quite the same climate of oppression that they did in the 1950s and 1960s, Hollywood has not been liberated from severe heterosexism. There are still only a handful of out lesbians and bisexual women in film, and many of those have only recently come out.

For example, the brilliant stage and film actress Lily Tomlin, whose persistent advocacy for feminism and gay rights led many to suspect her lesbianism for decades, remained hushed about her sexual orientation until early 2001. Even then, the statement she made concerning her thirty-year relationship with writer Jane Wagner was not entirely unambiguous. Moreover, she made it clear that while she does not "disavow [her] private life," she does not "want to become someone's poster girl either."

There is no doubt that television actress and comedian Ellen DeGeneres's public coming-out in 1997 was a landmark in the advancement of lesbians in the entertainment industry. The well-publicized relationship DeGeneres maintained with film actress Anne Heche—who subsequently married a man—made them for a while the only high-profile out lesbian couple in Hollywood.

Before DeGeneres's big announcement, however, Amanda Bearse made one of her own. In 1993, Bearse, a movie and television actress who appeared in films such as *Fright Night* (1985) and *Protocol* (1984) but is primarily known for her portrayal of Marcie D'Arcy on the television show *Married with Children* for over a decade, became the first prime-time television lesbian to come out. She reported that her announcement, prompted by a threat of outing, had no negative repercussions on her career.

Bearse remained comfortably a part of the cast of *Married with Children* until its 1997 finale. In recent years, she has more frequently worked as a director than as an actress.

Female bisexuality generally meets with greater acceptance than lesbianism—especially for those bisexual celebrities who do not appear in public with female companions. For instance, former child star Drew Barrymore and current "It" Girl Angelina Jolie are open about their bisexuality; however, both have married men. In contrast, Ione Skye, known for her romantic lead role in the film *Say Anything* (1989), divorced her husband in 1999 and soon after went public about her relationship with lesbian model Jenny Shimizu.

Comedian/actress/singer Sandra Bernhard has also been forthcoming about her bisexuality—and about her involvement with superstar singer Madonna—for years. Popular comedian and independent film actress Margaret Cho proclaimed herself bisexual in the late 1990s, just as she launched her one-woman show "I'm the One That I Want."

Independent cinema generally puts less pressure on actresses to remain closeted. Out lesbian Guinevere Turner codirected the all-lesbian film *Go Fish* (1994) and also starred in it. Turner went on to appear in more mainstream films such as *Chasing Amy* (1997), *Kiss Me Guido* (1997), and *American Psycho* (2000), which she also cowrote.

Equally out Cheryl Dunye directed and starred in *The Watermelon Woman* (1997), and has gone on to direct *Stranger Inside*, an HBO movie that premiered in June 2001. Leisha Hailey, half of the out lesbian pop duo the Murmurs, appeared in a romantic role opposite Allison Folland—rumored to be a lesbian herself—in the film *All Over Me* (1996).

Many lesbian and bisexual actresses remain secretive for fear of damaging their film careers. While some women simply want to maintain their privacy, or, like Tomlin, worry that they will become a poster girl for Hollywood lesbianism, the notion that acknowledging a same-sex preference will destroy an actress's chances for future (heterosexual) romantic or leading roles is no doubt also a reason. If an actress is publicly identified as a lesbian, then perhaps she will not be convincing (or even cast) in a heterosexual romantic role.

It is worth noting, however, that Anne Heche was cast in a romantic lead opposite Harrison Ford in *Six Days Seven Nights* (1998) after acknowledging her relationship with Ellen DeGeneres. The film was relatively successful, and Heche received critical acclaim for her performance.

The most recent high-profile coming-out was that of actress/comedian/talk show host Rosie O'Donnell. Tabloids had frequently published stories about O'Donnell's sexual orientation and her relationship with Nickelodeon executive Kelli Carpenter. But O'Donnell, who even declared "I love you, Kelli," during her acceptance speech at the Daytime Emmys in 2001, refused to confirm the rumors, saying that her sexuality had no significance for her fans or her career.

However, as part of her advocacy for children and to give a human face to gay parents, who are often discriminated against by adoption agencies and state governments, O'Donnell declared in March 2002, on ABC's *Primetime Thursday*, that she is in fact a lesbian mom. The reaction from her fans was overwhelmingly supportive.

The Usual Suspects

Over the years, rumors of lesbianism or bisexuality have persisted about certain Hollywood actresses—such as Catherine Deneuve, Kristy McNichol, Helen Hunt, actress and musician Queen Latifah, and actress and singer Whitney Houston. The lesbianism of newer actress Clea DuVall, star of the lesbian film *But I'm a Cheerleader* (2000), has also been rumored, but DuVall has made no public statement to date.

The multiple-Academy-Award-winning Jodie Foster occupies a special place in the hearts of many lesbians. She often plays relatively butch on screen but refuses to discuss her private life at all. She has also remained notoriously tight-lipped about who fathered her two children. But, intriguingly, actor Russell Crowe has mentioned that Foster influenced his band's song "Other Ways of

Speaking," which is about "meeting somebody that you think [you] could easily fall in love with...but they...in fact play for a different team." In response, Foster's publicist declared only that "'playing for a different team' could mean a lot of things."

Why Does It Matter?

The eagerness on the part of gay men and lesbians to know the truth about the sexual orientation of public figures such as actors and actresses has little to do with prurience, but much to do with a desire for honesty and a need for self-validation.

The need for validation makes coming out for actresses an important issue to the queer public. Mainstream films reach audiences across a wider spectrum of class and sexual identities than other forms of media, such as gay-themed magazines or books. For gay men and lesbians, particularly those living in oppressive locales, queer movies and actresses themselves can provide much-needed representation.

Because such public figures are often looked up to as role models, the visibility of queer Hollywood actresses— many of them household names—is a crucial step toward more widespread gay acceptance. Conversely, the failure to come out on the part of figures in the public eye sends a message that homosexuality or bisexuality is something shameful that needs to be hidden.   —Teresa Theophano

BIBLIOGRAPHY

"Did Russell Crowe Out Jodie Foster?" Advocate, September 13, 2000: www.advocate.com/html/news/091300/091300ento2.asp

Greenberg, Steve. "Amanda Bearse: Married...with a child." Advocate, September 21, 1993, 39.

Hadleigh, Boze. Hollywood Lesbians. Ft. Lee, N.J.: Barricade Books, 1994.

Hunter, Carson. "Rosie by Any Other Name." Girlfriends, June 2001, 18.

"Lily Tomlin Sort of Comes Out." Advocate, January 12, 2001: www.advocate.com/html/news/011201/011201ento2.asp

McLellan, Diana. The Girls: Sappho Goes to Hollywood. New York: St. Martin's Press, 2000.

Weiss, Andrea. Violets and Vampires: Lesbians in Film. New York: Penguin USA, 1993.

SEE ALSO

Film Actors: Gay Male; American Television: Talk Shows; American Television: Situation Comedies; Arzner, Dorothy; Bankhead, Tallulah; Bernhard, Sandra; Cho, Margaret; DeGeneres, Ellen; Dietrich, Marlene; Garbo, Greta; Moorehead, Agnes; O'Donnell, Rosie; Tomlin, Lily

Film Directors

GAY, LESBIAN, AND BISEXUAL FILM DIRECTORS HAVE been a vital creative presence in cinema since the medium's inception over one hundred years ago. Until the last two decades, however, mainstream directors kept their work (and not infrequently their lives) discreetly closeted, while the films of underground and experimental creators, though often confrontational in theme and technique, had limited circulation and financial support.

More recently, new queer filmmakers have capitalized on increased (though by no means unproblematic) public acceptance to win critical recognition and commercial viability for their projects.

The Hollywood Golden Era

In the so-called golden era of Hollywood, a number of famous directors were privately known for their alternative sexual preferences. These included George Cukor, Edmund Goulding, Mitchell Leisen, F. W. Murnau, Mauritz Stiller, James Whale, and Dorothy Arzner, who functioned with varying degrees of success in the industry.

Cukor (1899–1983) is primarily famous as a prolific and assured director of women's films. His sexuality was a well-known secret in Hollywood, and while it did no substantial harm to his career, his "fairy" reputation is generally believed to have cost him the directorship of Gone with the Wind (1939), following objections from macho star Clark Gable.

Although Cukor's work never overtly addresses gay issues, later critics and viewers have come to appreciate its many queer subtexts: Katharine Hepburn's cross-dressing in Sylvia Scarlett (1935); the gloriously camp bitchiness in the dress and dialogue of the all-women cast of The Women (1939); the effete figure of Kip in the classic Adam's Rib (1949).

Less discreet and, as a consequence, less fortunate than Cukor, James Whale (1893–1957) moved from the English theater to Broadway and then to Hollywood. Although he directed a range of genres, including the first version of the musical Showboat (1936), Whale's reputation as a director rests on his quartet of horror classics: Frankenstein (1931), Bride of Frankenstein (1935), The Dark House (1932), and The Invisible Man (1933). These films, with their grotesque ambience and alienated protagonists, have been interpreted as offering metaphoric expression of queer suffering.

Whale's career collapsed at least in part because of his refusal to tone down his openly gay behavior, and the last two decades of his life were spent on the Hollywood margins. The circumstances of his death by drowning in his swimming pool remained unresolved until only recently, when his suicide note was made public. His last months provided the basis for Bill Condon's 1998 film *Gods and Monsters*, based on the novel *Father of Frankenstein* by Christopher Bram and starring Sir Ian McKellen.

It has sometimes been said that the lesbianism of Dorothy Arzner (1897–1979) afforded her a certain license as "one of the boys" in a fiercely male-dominated profession, but the road for one of only two successful female directors in Hollywood's golden era was not easy.

Censorship codes and convention no doubt prevented Arzner from undertaking overtly lesbian themes. Nevertheless, critics have noted such touches as the sensuous handling of women's friendships in *The Wild Party* (1929) and the focus on such strong, albeit constrained, women as Hepburn's Amelia Earhart-like aviator in *Christopher Strong* (1933) and Joan Crawford's shoulder-padded businesswoman in *The Bride Wore Red* (1937). Forced to retire due to ill health in the 1940s, Arzner made occasional television commercials in the 1950s and later taught film at UCLA in the 1960s.

Avant-Garde, European, and Underground Film

Developments in experimental film from the 1940s onward, as well as the influence of European cinema, led to the formation of what is commonly known as underground cinema—the term coming from the screening context of small, alternative, sometimes illicit venues—that burgeoned in the 1960s.

In this subcultural space, (primarily male) homosexual directors forged a quirky mixture of aesthetic experimentation, kitsch, and homoerotic iconography into what was to become, ultimately, a highly influential set of cinematic techniques.

The doyen of this tradition is undoubtedly Kenneth Anger (b. 1927), a child prodigy who grew up in Los Angeles and started shooting 16 mm shorts at the age of fourteen. While attending the University of Southern California film school, Anger began to create what became an influential series of eclectic films, including *Fireworks* (1947), *Eaux d'artifice* (1953), and *Kustom Kar Kommandos* (1965).

Anger's most famous film is undoubtedly *Scorpio Rising* (1964). Here, Anger anticipates forms subsequently perfected in the music video genre to effect a queer subversion of images of teen romance; for example, he juxtaposes homoerotically charged footage of male bikers with a soundtrack of 1960s pop and rhythm-and-blues songs.

Anger's name is sometimes associated with his University of Southern California film school associate Gregory J. Markopoulos (1928–1992). Like the multitalented Anger, Markopoulos also wrote, edited, produced, and occasionally acted in many of his own works. His aesthetic, however, is markedly more cerebral and lyrical than Anger's, reflecting the influence of Greek myth and classical motifs—as in *Psyche* (1948) and *Lysis* (1948)—and of French literature and avant-garde culture.

Indeed, Markopoulos, like Anger, spent time in Europe in the 1950s and was influenced by writer Jean Genet (1910–1986), as evidenced by the Genet-like title of *Flowers of Asphalt* (1949). Other Markopoulos films of note include *The Dead Ones* (1948) and *Twice a Man* (1963).

The influence of European film has been highly significant in the formulation of a queer cinema aesthetic. Genet's perverse aesthetic of the erotics of the Paris underworld is evident in his own twenty-six-minute silent directorial effort, *Un chant d'amour* (1950). Known primarily as a playwright, Genet was mentored by flamboyant French director Jean Cocteau (1889–1963), who was also responsible for some of the foundational works of gay cinema—*Jean Cocteau, fait du cinema* (1925), *Le Sang d'un poète* (1930), *La Belle et la bête* (1946), and *Orphée* (1950).

The French tradition was a strong influence on the Italian director Luchino Visconti (1906–1976), an aristocrat whose early embrace of Marxism led first to the gritty realism in films such as *Ossessione* (1943) and later to such lavishly staged critiques of the Italian class system as *The Leopard* (1963). In 1971, Visconti made a sensuous adaptation of Thomas Mann's classic homoerotic novella, *Death in Venice*.

Pier Paolo Pasolini (1922–1975) initially established himself as a writer before directing confrontingly queer adaptations of classics such as *Oedipus Rex* (1967) and *Medea* (1970). His final film, the controversial *Salò* or *The 120 Days of Sodom* (1975), was banned in many countries. His murder, shortly after the completion of *Salò*, has never been satisfactorily resolved.

German director Rainer Werner Fassbinder (1946–1982) paired cutting-edge techniques and themes to address postwar German concerns in areas of class, race, and sexuality. His *The Bitter Tears of Petra Von Kant* (1972), staring frequent collaborator Hanna Schygulla, is a powerful study of lesbianism, while *In a Year of Thirteen Moons* (1978) focuses on a doomed transsexual protagonist. Fassbinder's final film, before his suicide by drug overdose, is *Querelle* (1982), an adaptation of the Genet novel that blends film-noir grit with dreamy eroticism to explore the power/desire nexus of the Genet model of masculinity.

In the United States, the burgeoning of underground venues in the 1960s and 1970s provided forums for four multitalented contributors: Jack Smith, Andy Warhol, Paul Morrisey, and John Waters.

A filmmaker, artist, photographer, writer, and occasional actor, Jack Smith (1932–1989) is a significant filmmaker primarily because of his camp hybrid *Flaming Creatures* (1963). This controversial work, subject to a number of legal actions to prevent its screening, was described by critic J. Hoberman as: "a cross between Josef Von Sternberg at his most studiously artistic...and a delirious home movie of a transvestite bacchanal."

In contrast to Smith, the film output of Andy Warhol (1928–1987) was prolific. Already successful in the art world for his pastiches of mass-culture commodities, Warhol (who began his career in advertising) transferred his eclectic pop-art aesthetic to film.

Innately voyeuristic, fascinated with the Hollywood star system and with the technical minutiae of the medium's reproductive capabilities, Warhol explored, sometimes in excruciating detail, the trash and banality of "everyday" life, as experienced by the "superstars" (drag artists like Candy Darling, or socialites like Brigit Berlin) who populated his alternative work space, the Factory.

Warhol's relentless focus on transgressive lives and desires forged an important archive of images for queer culture, from *Blow Job* (1963), a thirty-five-minute single shot focusing on the expressions of a recipient of a blow job, to *My Hustler* (1965), a seventy-minute film about a male hustler, shot on Fire Island, and from *Andy Warhol's Lonesome Cowboys* (1968), a gay take on the Western, complete with ballet dancing cowboys, to the absurd confessional theatrics and squalid lesbian demimonde of *Chelsea Girls* (1968).

Many of the more famous films generally associated with Warhol from the late 1960s onward were in fact primarily the work of his protégé Paul Morrissey (b. 1939). His influence as an assistant is apparent in the more developed narrative structure of the lengthy *Chelsea Girls* (1968). Morrissey went on to direct such underground classics as *Flesh* (1968), *Trash* (1970), *Heat* (1972), and *Blood of Dracula* (1974).

The contemporary heir to the Warhol/Morrissey tradition is John Waters (b. 1946), the Baltimore-based director sometimes referred to as "the Pope of Trash" and "the Sultan of Sleaze." Beginning with innovative shorts after dropping out of film school in the mid-1960s, Waters became a cult figure as a result of a major triumph, the trailer-trash epic *Pink Flamingos* (1972), an exploration of the very queer underside of lower-class suburbia starring such Waters stalwarts as Mink Stole and outrageous drag performer Divine.

Waters, who frequently writes, edits, and acts in his own films, continued his assault on family values in such works as *Desperate Living* (1977) and the hilarious take on 1960s teen conformity, *Hairspray* (1988), which featured Divine as the young Rikki Lake's mother. Recent films include *Serial Mom* (1994), *Cecil B. Demented* (2000), and *A Dirty Shame* (2004).

Feminism and the Rise of Lesbian Experimental Film

Spurred by the rise of the women's liberation movement, with its critique of the structure of patriarchy, lesbian filmmakers came to the fore in the 1970s. They found their central challenge in conceptualizing modes of visual representation that could capture the eroticism of lesbian sexuality without objectifying the female body as spectacle or replicating patriarchal conventions.

Foremost among lesbian feminist filmmakers is the extraordinarily prolific Barbara Hammer (b. 1939). She employed an aesthetic of abstraction in a series of short films to shatter taboos associated with the representation of female bodies. Among the films in this series are *Dyketactics* (1974), *Menses* (1974), and *Multiple Orgasm* (1976).

Hammer has also explored themes of women's spirituality, whether located in primitive rites (*Stone Circles*, 1983), in myth (*Sappho*, 1978), or in nature (*Pearl Diver*, 1984). In her first feature-length film, the semidocumentary *Nitrate Kiss* (1985), Hammer addressed themes of eroticism and aging. Her work in the 1990s included a series of acclaimed documentaries, most notably her study of hidden lesbian histories, *The Female Closet* (1998).

Hammer's early propensities toward abstraction and essentialist symbolism were not always shared by her feminist contemporaries. Jan Oxenberg's influential satirical short *Home Movie* (1972) juxtaposes original home movie footage of the filmmaker's own adolescence (most notably, her activities as a school cheerleader) with an interrogative voice-over and additional footage of contemporary lesbian feminist cultural events to question normative heterosexual socialization.

In subsequent shorts, *I'm Not One of Them* (1974) and *A Comedy in Six Unnatural Acts* (1975), Oxenberg skillfully deploys comedy to explore, challenge, and in some instances rather controversially celebrate lesbian stereotypes. More recently, Oxenberg has moved into a successful television career, working on shows such as *Chicago Hope*.

Lesbian filmmakers building on the work of Hammer and Oxenberg have been united in their aim, in Andrea Weiss's phrase, "to control and define lesbian representation in terms other than those offered by the dominant media."

In the domain of documentary, Weiss (b. 1956) and Greta Schiller (b. 1947) have contributed, via their company Jezebel Productions, numerous innovative documentaries that uncover hidden aspects of gay and lesbian history, including *Before Stonewall* (1984), *Paris Was a Woman* (1995), and *Escape to Life* (2000).

Su Friedrich (b. 1954) and Janet Baus codirected the documentary film *The Lesbian Avengers Eat Fire Too* (1993), which provides entertaining insights on the performative strategies of this radical arm of 1990s lesbian political culture.

Friedrich, as a solo director of short films, has since the late 1970s extended Hammer's techniques of fragmentation, juxtaposition, and abstraction to evoke facets of lesbian identity and desire. Her most acclaimed film, *Damned If You Don't* (1987), uses four contrasting fictional mini-narratives about nuns to explore the conflict between lesbian desire, the lesbian gaze, and religious ideology.

Sheila McLaughlin's 1987 interracial romance *She Must Be Seeing Things* also attempts to subvert conventions of spectatorship in depicting lesbian desire.

Lizzie Borden (b. 1958), in such experimental filmic narratives as *Born in Flames* (1983) and *Working Girls* (1986), addresses social issues such as lesbian identity, racial difference, and the plight of sex workers.

Experimental lesbian filmmakers in America were strongly influenced by international trends, a process exemplified in the work of American-born Yvonne Rainer (b. 1936), who assimilated European trends while initially working there as a choreographer. Rainer's filmic output has moved from general concerns of female sexuality and subjectivity to addressing lesbian themes in later films such as *Privilege* (1990).

Key European figures include Belgian-born Chantal Akerman (b. 1950), whose technically sophisticated and introspective films critically assimilate the aesthetics of French New Wave directors such as Jean-Luc Godard. Akerman's films include such explorations of the complexities of subjectivity and desire as *Je, Tu, Il, Elle* (1974), in which Akerman herself acted a key role, and which had a huge impact upon its release in America, and *Les Rendez-vous d'Anna* (1979).

In an altogether different mold, the surreally parodic historical fantasies of German director Ulrike Ottinger (b. 1942)—*Madame X: An Absolute Ruler* (1977) and *Johanna D'Arc of Mongolia* (1989)—have developed a cult following while forging a distinctive brand of lesbian camp.

Monika Treut (b. 1954), another controversial German director, has celebrated transgressive queer sexuality in films such as *Seduction: The Cruel Woman* (1985), a contemporary tale of sadomasochism. Her documentary *Female Misbehavior* (1992) includes among its subjects academic Camille Paglia and performance artist Annie Sprinkle.

In her first film, *A Question of Silence* (1982), Dutch-born Marleen Gorris (b. 1949) provoked debate with an unsparing critique of patriarchal oppression via a study of women driven to crime. Her other films include the much praised *Antonia's Line* (1995) and a version of Virginia Woolf's *Mrs. Dalloway* (1997), which skillfully employs flashback techniques to bring the novel's lesbian subtext to the fore.

Crossing Over

A major contribution to the integration of gay themes into mainstream cinema has been made by John Schlesinger (1926–2003), the openly gay British director whose films include *Darling* (1965), *Midnight Cowboy* (1969), which won the Best Picture Oscar, and *Sunday Bloody Sunday* (1971), a daring exploration of bisexuality.

Schlesinger's British contemporary, bisexual Tony Richardson (1928–1991), peppered an eclectic and distinguished career, which included a Best Director Oscar for *Tom Jones* (1963), with studies of sexual mavericks, as in his adaptations of Edward Albee's *A Delicate Balance* (1973) and John Irving's *Hotel New Hampshire* (1984).

More overtly avant-garde and less commercially viable than his fellow Britons, Derek Jarman (1942–1994) specialized in visually lavish, outrageous, yet fiercely intelligent productions of classics that brought subtextual queer elements to the fore in a way that emphasized their contemporary relevance: *Jubilee* (1977), *The Tempest* (1979), and *Wittgenstein* (1993).

Edward II (1991), based on Christopher Marlowe's play, exemplifies the Jarman touch via the skillful and provocative linkage of the persecution of Edward and his lover Piers Gaveston to the homophobic platforms of Margaret Thatcher's conservative government.

Another British filmmaker, Terence Davies (b. 1945), came to the fore in the late 1980s with the first of his autobiographical films set in working-class Liverpool, *Distant Voices, Still Lives* (1988). This highly acclaimed film was followed by *The Long Day Closes* (1992). These "memory" films explore the dynamics of family relations in working-class Britain.

Davies went on to make nonautobiographical works, such as *The Neon Bible* (1995), based on the novel by John Kennedy Toole, and *The House of Mirth* (2001), based on the novel by Edith Wharton.

James Bridges (1935–1993) first made his name as a television writer for *The Alfred Hitchcock Hour* during the early 1960s. He made his film directorial debut with *The Babymaker* (1970), which tackled the then controversial subject of surrogate motherhood. Bridges's first big success was *The Paper Chase* (1973), featuring Timothy Bottoms as a first-year law student and John Houseman as his rigorous professor. Bridges had another success with *The China Syndrome* (1979), featuring Jack Lemmon, Jane Fonda, and Michael Douglas.

The film of Bridges that may be the most homoerotic (despite its determinedly heterosexual plot) is *Urban Cowboy* (1980), featuring John Travolta and Debra Winger. Bridges's final film was the disappointing *Bright Lights, Big City* (1988).

While Bridges never made an issue of his homosexuality, he lived openly with his longtime partner, actor Jack Larson. He died of cancer in 1993.

Colin Higgins (1941–1988) may be best remembered for writing the Hal Ashby-directed cult film *Harold and Maude* (1971), a black comedy that violates all kinds of

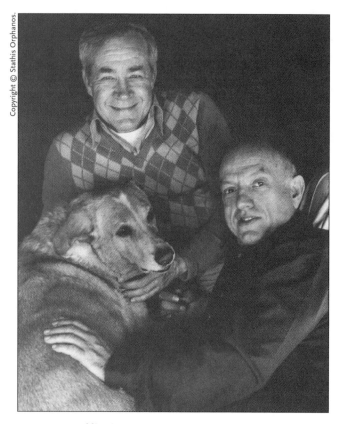

A portrait of film director James Bridges (right) with actor Jack Larson and their dog Max by Stathis Orphanos.

sexual boundaries. He wrote the screenplays for a number of other films, including Arthur Hiller's *Silver Streak* (1976). His directorial debut was *Foul Play,* featuring Goldie Hawn and Chevy Chase, which was a surprise hit. He went on to cowrite and direct two Dolly Parton vehicles, *9 to 5* (1980) and *The Best Little Whorehouse in Texas* (1982). He died from AIDS-related complications in 1988, at forty-seven.

German director Wolfgang Peterson (b. 1941) first gained international attention for *Die Konsequenz* (1977), a discreet and subtle study of homosexuality that he wrote as well as directed. But his great crossover film was *Das Boot* (1981), a nail-biting wartime drama told from the perspective of a German submariner. Peterson has gone on to make a number of mainstream Hollywood films, including *In the Line of Fire* (1993), *Air Force One* (1997), and *The Perfect Storm* (2000).

Randall Kleiser (b. 1946) worked in television during the 1970s. His first feature film was the hit musical *Grease* (1978). This success was followed by such teen (heterosexual) romance films as *Blue Lagoon* (1980) and *Summer Lovers* (1982) and popular comedies such as *Big Top Pee-Wee* (1988) and *Honey, I Blew Up the Kid* (1992).

In *It's My Party* (1996), however, Kleiser abandoned heterosexual comedy to make one of the most powerful AIDS films. Centered on Nick Stark (Eric Roberts), a man who is about to lose his long battle with the AIDS virus and decides to host a two-day farewell party for his family and friends, after which he will commit suicide, the film is emotionally searing but finally consoling. Featuring excellent performances by Roberts, Gregory Harrison (as Stark's former lover), Lee Grant, and Marlee Matlin, among a host of others, the film is based on the death of Kleiser's own lover.

In the late 1990s and the early years of the twenty-first century, writer and director Bill Condon came to prominence with several successful projects based on gay or queer-inflected subject matter. In addition to directing a number of television movies and writing the screenplay for Rob Marshall's *Chicago* (2002), Condon scored hits with *Gods and Monsters* (1998), based on the life of James Whale, memorably portrayed by Ian McKellen, and *Kinsey* (2004), based on the life of sex researcher Alfred Kinsey, brilliantly portrayed by Liam Neeson. Condon wrote the screenplays for both films.

Independent Films

Over the last two decades, a crop of young, openly gay and lesbian directors have achieved success through critically acclaimed independent films, some of which have obtained a degree of mainstream marketability.

The early works of American director Gus Van Sant (b. 1952) include such offbeat films as *Mala Noche* (1985), *Drugstore Cowboy* (1989), and *Even Cowgirls Get the Blues* (1993), based on Tom Robbins's novel. But his masterpiece is *My Own Private Idaho* (1994). Here he expertly blends the genre of the road film with Shakespeare's *Henry IV* to present a compelling study of young gay hustlers, played by Keanu Reeves and the late River Phoenix.

Since *Idaho,* Van Sant has moved more fully into the mainstream, with mixed results. *To Die For* (1995) and the Oscar-winning Ben Affleck/Matt Damon buddy film *Good Will Hunting* (1997) were critically successful. The 1998 remake of Hitchcock's *Psycho*, paying slavish attention to the original, was generally deemed disappointing.

Gregg Araki (b. 1959), another graduate of the University of Southern California School of Cinema and Television, has won critical acclaim for a frequently bleak filmic landscape that explores the post-AIDS experiences of alienated young queers. His work includes a pseudodocumentary, *Totally F***ked Up* (1993), and the road movies *The Living End* (1992), *The Doom Generation* (1995), and *Nowhere* (1997).

Todd Haynes (b. 1961) began his career with the innovative documentary *Superstar: The Karen Carpenter Story* (1987). Featuring Barbie dolls in the central roles, it was subsequently banned via legal technicalities raised by its subject's brother, Richard Carpenter. In the 1990s, Haynes moved on to such hard-edged studies of popular culture as *Velvet Goldmine* (1998), a fictionalized exploration of the polymorphous sexualities of 1970s glam rock.

In his Oscar-nominated *Far From Heaven* (2002), Haynes achieved mainstream success. Paying homage to the style of 1950s auteur Douglas Sirk, he skillfully draws out and makes explicit the homosexual subtexts latent in Sirk's melodramas.

In 1986, director Donna Deitch (b. 1945) adapted Jane Rule's classic lesbian novel *Desert of the Heart* as *Desert Hearts*. A full-length feature, it was perceived by many lesbian critics as too implicated in the aesthetics and values of traditional heterosexual romances; however, it won and maintained a strong following by lesbian viewers.

Deitch, meanwhile, has moved into television work, directing numerous high-profile dramas such as *NYPD Blue, Murder One, ER,* and *Crossing Jordan.* In the television movie *Common Ground* (2000), she returned to gay and lesbian themes.

The success of Rose Troche (b. 1964) was established with the experimental *Go Fish* (1994). Made on a shoestring budget in black and white, it flirted with avantgarde editing techniques and queer sensibilities, examining, for example, a lesbian who sleeps with a man and butch/femme role-playing. Troche's next effort, filmed in Britain, *Bedrooms and Hallways* (1998), was an enjoyable romantic comedy with the focus this time on gay male relationships.

In 2001, Troche scored a critical success with her film, based on A. M. Homes's provocative collection of short stories, *The Safety of Objects.* In the last few years, she has worked mainly in television, most notably as writer and director for the lesbian-focused drama *The L Word.*

Canadian film director Patricia Rozema (b. 1958) began her career with the gentle, offbeat *I Heard the Mermaids Singing* (1987). This film was followed by a depiction of lesbian awakening in *When Night Is Falling* (1995). Rozema's latest work—an intelligent, elegant film of Jane Austen's *Mansfield Park* (1999)—brought the classic novel's queer subtext to the surface, eliciting a mixture of critical alarm and praise.

Lisa Cholodenko (b. 1964) is a newly emerging writer/director. Her 1998 film *High Art* was a big winner at the Sundance Film Festival. It offers witty nods to Warhol and Fassbinder. Her second film, *Laurel Canyon* (2002), starring Frances McDormand as a record producer, focuses on conflicting values in Los Angeles.

Director Kimberly Peirce (b. 1967) has received critical plaudits for her film *Boy's Don't Cry* (1999), based on the case of murdered transgendered lesbian Brandon Teena. After Hilary Swank won the Academy Award for Best actress for her stunning performance as Teena Brandon, the film achieved considerable mainstream success.

Spanish director Pedro Almodóvar (b. 1951) deploys a surreal, iconoclastic blend of comedy and drama to map subcultures of sexual dissidence in post-Franco Madrid. Beginning with the comic short *Film Político* in 1974, Almodóvar has made numerous films, including *Women on the Verge of a Nervous Breakdown* (1988), *Tie Me Up, Tie Me Down* (1990), *The Flower of My Secret* (1995), and *Bad Education* (2004). *All About My Mother* (1999), a tragicomic study of a "straight" woman's love for a transsexual, won the Academy Award for Best Foreign Film.

Almodóvar's distinctively queer filmic universe has obtained widespread critical acclaim and a broad-based following. His success may offer a happy augury for the growing recognition of high-quality gay, lesbian, bisexual, transgender, and queer cinema. —*Deborah Hunn*

BIBLIOGRAPHY

Dyer, Richard. *Now You See It: Studies on Lesbian and Gay Film.* New York: Routledge, 1990.

Gever, Martha, John Greyson, and Pratibha Parmar, eds. *Queer Looks: Perspectives on Lesbian and Gay Films and Video.* New York: Routledge, 1993.

Hadleigh, Boze. *The Lavender Screen: Gay and Lesbian Films, Their Stars, Makers, Characters and Critics.* New York: Citadel Press, 1993.

Hanson, Ellis. *Outtakes: Essays on Queer Theory and Film.* Durham, N.C.: Duke University Press, 1999.

Hoberman, J. "The Big Heat: The Making and Unmaking of Flaming Creatures." *Flaming Creature: Jack Smith, His Amazing Life and Times.* Edward Liffingwell, Carole Kismaric, and Marvin Heiferman, eds. London: Serpent's Tail, 1997. 152–167.

Murray, Raymond. *Images in the Dark: An Encyclopaedia of Gay and Lesbian Film and Video.* Philadelphia: TLA Publications, 1994.

Rich, B. Ruby. *Chick Flicks: Theories and Memories of the Feminist Film Movement.* Durham, N.C.: Duke University Press, 1998.

Russo, Vito. *The Celluloid Closet.* New York: Harper & Row, 1981.

Smith, Paul Julian. *Desire Unlimited: The Cinema of Pedro Almodóvar.* London: Verso, 1994.

Suarez, Juan A. *Bike Boys, Drag Queens and Superstars: Avant-Garde, Mass Culture, and Gay Identities in the 1960s Underground Cinema.* Bloomington, Ind.: Indiana University Press, 1996.

Weiss, Andrea. *Violets and Vampires: Lesbians in Film.* London: Penguin, 1993.

SEE ALSO

Film; Documentary Film; European Film; Film Noir; New Queer Cinema; Akerman, Chantal; Almodóvar, Pedro; Anger, Kenneth; Araki, Gregg; Arzner, Dorothy; Cocteau, Jean; Condon, William "Bill"; Cukor, George; Davies, Terence; Divine (Harris Glenn Milstead); Fassbinder, Rainer Werner; Goulding, Edmund; Hammer, Barbara; Haynes, Todd; McKellen, Sir Ian; Murnau, Friedrich Wilhelm; Ottinger, Ulrike; Pasolini, Pier Paolo; Richardson, Tony; Rozema, Patricia; Schlesinger, John; Stiller, Mauritz; Treut, Monika; Troche, Rose; Van Sant, Gus; Visconti, Luchino; Warhol, Andy; Waters, John; Whale, James

Film Festivals

PARALLELING THE GROWTH OF THE MODERN GAY RIGHTS movement since the 1970s, the diverse collection of glbtq film festivals, now recognized as the queer film festival circuit, came into its own in the early 1990s, just as the New Queer Cinema achieved mainstream recognition. It has now burgeoned into a major international phenomenon.

The New Queer Cinema

The 1990s opened with the 1991 art-house release of such unapologetically queer films as Todd Haynes's *Poison*, Jennie Livingston's *Paris Is Burning*, Gus Van Sant's *My Own Private Idaho*, and Norman René's *Longtime Companion*, which paved the way for the 1992 phenomenon known as the New Queer Cinema.

This term was coined by cultural critic B. Ruby Rich in her seminal *Village Voice* overview of the 1992 Sundance Film Festival. The triad of gay features she identified as characterizing the term—Christopher Munch's *The Hours and Times*, Tom Kalin's *Swoon*, and Gregg Araki's *The Living End*—were the hot tickets on the gay festival circuit for 1992, with both *Swoon* and *The Living End* achieving limited theatrical release from Fine Line Features and Strand Releasing, respectively.

While 1986 had seen a miniboom that was dubbed the "Gay New Wave" by *Film Comment* magazine, few of these films (Donna Deitch's *Desert Hearts*, Bill Sherwood's *Parting Glances*, Arthur Bressan's *Buddies*, Jaime Humberto Hermosillo's *Doña Herlinda and Her Son*) were exhibited at the major gay film festivals of the time.

However, the New Queer Cinema was basically a gay male phenomenon. The real lesbian crossover did not happen until 1994. The Sundance Film Festival was once again the origin of mainstream legitimacy when the Samuel Goldwyn Company acquired worldwide rights for a scrappy lesbian feature out of Chicago, Rose Troche and Guinevere Turner's *Go Fish*.

Although the film was only a moderate success at the box office (with a national gross of just under $2.5 million), it was a major turning point in lesbian cinema. Goldwyn's marketing plan for the film capitalized on the big three summer festivals (New York, San Francisco, and Los Angeles), timing the film's release in each city to make the most of its high profile in the gay film festivals.

On opening night at the 1994 San Francisco International Gay & Lesbian Film Festival, a choked-up Rose Troche explained to 1,500 delighted lesbians (okay, there were lots of gay men there too), "I made this film for you guys." The film opened the next day in San Francisco for a very successful run and remains one of the top ten lesbian releases in terms of box office grosses.

This marketing strategy continues today: Many distributors clamor for opening- and closing-night slots at the major gay film festivals as a means of creating excitement and garnering exposure for their films in an increasingly saturated marketplace.

This is a drastic change from earlier prevailing attitudes, when distributors went to great lengths to avoid having their films pegged as "gay" or "lesbian" and thus avoided gay film festivals. "It's not a gay film, it's universal" was a common refrain of the time.

From Akron to Zurich

There are currently more than 150 glbtq film festivals listed in PlanetOut's PopcornQ Directory of International Lesbian & Gay Film Festivals. These festivals span the globe from Akron, Ohio, to Zurich, Switzerland.

Most festivals are annual events. (More than thirty take place in October, also known as GLBT History Month.) Some take place over the course of a weekend, some last a week to ten days, and some carry on over the course of many weeks, as is the case with touring festivals.

While screenings of new and recent films predominate, the festivals also create additional programming such as archival and repertory film showings, panel discussions, speakers, or clip and comment shows offering overviews of anything from gay film history—the origin of Vito Russo's *The Celluloid Closet* (1981)—to a tongue-in-cheek look at the career of porn star Ryan Idol (Richard Dyer's clever foray at the 1994 San Francisco International Lesbian & Gay Film Festival).

The oldest and largest of the glbtq festivals is the San Francisco International Lesbian & Gay Film Festival, which was established in 1977. The festival's twenty-fifth anniversary in June 2001 was celebrated with an expanded program and a huge international queer film and video conference called *Persistent Vision*.

A random sampling of the festivals conveys a sense of their range and diversity: Tokyo's International Lesbian & Gay Film and Video Festival, Memphis's Twinkie Museum GLBT Film Festival, Cape Town's Out-in-Africa Film Festival, Calgary's Fairy Tales, Kalamazoo's Queer Arts Film Festival, Stockholm's Queer and Feminist Video & Film Festival, Bozeman, Montana's, Lesbian, Gay, Transgender, Questioning, Queer Film Festival, and Berkeley's East Bay Gay Asian Men's Film Festival.

Types of Festivals

There is a considerable diversity of types of festivals within the queer film festival circuit. Over the years, different types of specialty festivals have evolved, the most notable being the strong collection of experimental gay festivals spearheaded by MIX.

MIX: The New York Lesbian & Gay Experimental Film and Video Festival was founded by Jim Hubbard and Sarah Schulman in 1987. The festival is now firmly established as one of the leading gay festivals in the world and has been a pioneer in the fields of digital production, online film exhibition, and interactive multimedia.

The festival originated as an alternative to what was then called the New York Gay Film Festival. (The word *lesbian* found its way into festival titles in the early 1980s, with *bi* and *trans* gaining some ground in the late 1990s.) MIX has also evolved into a groundbreaking international franchise, spawning sister festivals such as MIX Brazil and MIX Mexico, as well as sponsoring a college touring program of MIX highlights.

The mid-1990s also saw the launch of the first Black GLBT Film Festival, in London, as well as an increasing effort on the part of the major queer festivals to address their constituencies of color in programming, staffing, and audience outreach efforts. Again showing its leadership in the field, MIX: The New York Experimental Lesbian & Gay Film Festival was the first of the queer festivals to have codirectors of color, bringing on Shari Frilot and Karim Ainouz in 1993.

Numerous lesbian-specific festivals have thrived over the years, the oldest being Cineffable, the Paris Lesbian Film Festival, established in 1988. The last five years or so has seen a burgeoning trans festival movement, as well; especially notable is London's International Transgender Film & Video Festival and San Francisco's Tranny Fest, both of which held their fourth festival in 2001. Olympia, Washington, hosts Gender-Queer: Northwest Transgender and Intersex Film Festival.

San Francisco is also home to an annual Bi Film Festival, while Sydney, Australia, hosts an annual Queer Documentary Film Festival and Bologna presents an HIV/AIDS film festival.

Many of the larger glbtq film festivals began taking the show on the road in the 1990s. The London Lesbian & Gay Film Festival began touring highlights programs to regional British cinemas as early as 1991. Berlin's Verzaubert festival tours to various German cities, and Sao Paolo–based MIX Brazil tours across Brazil.

The most recent technological innovation for the festival circuit is the advent of the online queer film festival. Pioneered by MIX New York and PlanetOut's PopcornQ in 1998, the Online Queer Digifest lays claim to being the first such festival. Several of the larger gay film festivals have begun showing clips or shorts on their websites as an adjunct to their events. The PlanetOut Short Movie Awards is certainly the largest online festival, with roughly fifty short films and videos being exhibited at the 2000 event.

The Ecosystem

As the glbtq community has evolved and become more tolerated (even embraced) by mainstream society, so the festivals have thrived and flourished. Nonetheless, festival organizers are under immense pressure to justify their existence, as they are forced to compete with the wider availability of gay cinema in general—in theaters, on television, on home video and DVD, and now on the Internet.

A frequent question posed in gay film festival panel discussions is "Are gay film festivals still necessary given the significant number of gay-themed films now seeing wider theatrical distribution?" The answer, of course, is simple: There is nothing like seeing a film at a gay film festival. It is an irreplaceable and unforgettable experience.

The glbtq film festival circuit evolved as part of a queer film ecosystem that continues to grow and evolve today. The film and video makers create the movies, the festival organizers show the movies, the distributors circulate the movies, and the publicists draw attention to them, so that the gay movie lover will plunk down a few dollars to see the movies and the whole process can happen again.

Of course, it is not literally that simple. The truth is, given the economy of the whole enterprise, pretty much every person who makes up this chain is underpaid—an $8.50 ticket price does not go very far divided among that many people.

As a group, we are a diverse and complex people yearning for the experience of community—being together, sharing our different realities, exchanging ideas, cruising each other. Our glbtq film festivals, wherein our lives and aspirations are on display and command the center of attention, are one of the few places where we get to experience community.

—*Jenni Olson*

BIBLIOGRAPHY

PlanetOut's PopcornQ International Directory of Lesbian & Gay Film and Video Festivals: www.planetout.com/popcornq/fests

SEE ALSO

Film; New Queer Cinema; Film Spectatorship; Araki, Gregg; Haynes, Todd; Troche, Rose; Van Sant, Gus

Film Noir

SCHOLARS DISAGREE ON PRECISELY WHEN FILM NOIR originated or what movie deserves recognition as the first film noir. Some have suggested Fritz Lang's *M* (1931), with its expressionist intensity, reigning darkness, and "perverse" subject matter. More frequently cited is John Huston's *The Maltese Falcon* (1941), which presents a gallery of double-crossing molls, fey gangsters, and other grotesques familiar to readers of pulps and *policiers* but less so to moviegoers.

Serendipitously, perhaps, these two films are linked by queer or queer-coded characters, and more specifically by an actor, Peter Lorre, often identified with perverse and otherworldly characters whom attentive viewers have come to recognize as gay. In *M*, Lorre plays the tormented child molester; in *The Maltese Falcon*, he is a mincing criminal.

This connection between two seminal works classified as film noir is more than a rhetorical convenience; queer and queerish characters were a crucial component of the noir landscape, part of the genre's challenge to the complacent America of Currier and Ives and Norman Rockwell.

Film noir's literal darkness provided a hiding place for an assortment of misfits whose presence was disquieting, if not downright disturbing, but also seductive: femmes fatales (or women not domestically minded), weak males, wronged innocents. But it was especially welcoming, if often in subtext, to "perverts."

The latter, already viewed by society as "shadow creatures" hiding from its disapproving eyes, were a perfect fit for a style of film in which vice can trump virtue, all kinds of social norms are routinely ruptured, and the universe is out of control.

The Maltese Falcon and Gilda

The Maltese Falcon is a veritable feast of perversity, though typically the film clouds some of the gay elements. Dashiell Hammett's book was clear about the homosexuality of Joel Cairo (Peter Lorre) and that of the youthful killer Wilmer Cook (Elisha Cook Jr.), derisively called a "gunsel" by straight detective Sam Spade (Humphrey Bogart). *Gunsel* is Yiddish-derived slang for a young gay thug. Wilmer's "patron" is the portly aesthete Casper Gutman, played with arch authority by Sidney Greenstreet.

The film is typical of other noirs from the period that present gay characters as criminally minded dandies who are ultimately tamed by a more manly male. This taming does not occur without some tension around the issue of queerness.

In one of the rare scenes where Spade loses control, he screams at Gutman to stop Cook from following him. His agitated "I'll kill him!" points to emotions beyond the story proper, the fear of a homosexual pursuer that unhinges even an unflappable character like Spade.

The 1940s would seem to be the last place to look for queer male couples, but the elegant gangster Ballin Mundson (George Macready) and his protégé Johnny Farrell (Glenn Ford) in Charles Walters's *Gilda* (1946) can hardly be read otherwise. Johnny is literally a pickup by Ballin, who rescues him from a sailor he has duped.

The script is rife with homoromantic dialogue, as when Johnny says to Ballin, "I was born last night when you met me in that alley" or when Ballin remarks, "Quite a surprise to hear a woman singing in my house, eh, Johnny?"

Even the actors were in on the joke, which indicates that the closet door was often slightly ajar even before the modern era of gay liberation. According to John Kobal (quoted by Richard Dyer), Glenn Ford said flatly: "Of course, we knew their relationship was homosexual."

Noir Lesbians

Lesbians, and certainly lesbian couples, were less evident in noir, just as they were paid less attention to in the culture by those in the medical, social science, and religious fields who were puzzling over the question of homosexuality. When they did appear, they often took the form of the lesbian predator.

In Nicholas Ray's *In a Lonely Place* (1950), a butch masseuse roughly, almost sadistically, handles her female customer and plays to cultural expectations of destructive homosexuality by insidiously undermining the film's major, already troubled, heterosexual relationship.

Another such case is in Michael Curtiz's *Young Man with a Horn*, made the same year. The audience squirms when neurotic bisexual Amy North (Lauren Bacall) tires of her macho musician boyfriend Rick Martin (Kirk Douglas) and brutally abandons him for a willowy young woman.

Some films even had two lesbian predators. John Cromwell's women-in-prison drama *Caged* (1950) divides the queerness between sadistic matron Harper and an aging, lascivious moll who calls the other women "cute tricks." Despite the film's halfhearted attempts to heterosexualize them (via vague mentions of men in their lives), there is little doubt of their lesbianism.

Gay Lovers

By the mid-1950s, and in spite of that decade's reputation for repression, queer motifs were coming into focus. In Joseph H. Lewis's *The Big Combo* (1955), gangsters Fante (Lee Van Cleef) and Mingo (Earl Holliman) are clearly indicated as gay lovers, working (as gangsters) and relaxing together, even sleeping together in the same bedroom.

When the inevitable comeuppance occurs via an exploding box of cigars that kills them both, Mingo's anguished last cry is "Don't leave me, Fante!"

Lewis was also responsible for the noir classic *Gun Crazy* (1949), which featured gay actor John Dall as a vulnerable sharpshooter done in by a femme fatale.

Noir's Queer Victims and Villains

Queer victims and villains served several purposes in these films. They indicated a world in which the basic building block of society, the heterosexual couple, was in question. They made visible, if only in half-light, characters who were treated as invisible in society.

A good example of the erasure of the homosexual in films is offered by the transformation of Richard Brooks's novel *The Brick Foxhole* (1945), about a victimized gay man, into Edward Dmytryk's *Crossfire* (1947), a film about a victimized Jew.

Queer characters also helped give film noir a knowingness, a hip cachet, by challenging the status quo with controversial characters, creating the frisson of a "walk on the wild side" for straight audiences and a sense, however qualified, of empowerment for queer and perhaps other marginalized viewers.

Noir's sometimes indiscriminate doubling of queers with sadists and lunatics (as with *Caged*'s psycho matron Harper, for example) may seem deplorable to modern viewers, but this was a reflection of cultural anxieties around homosexuality and can be consigned to the period. Despite their often baroque treatment, gay characters also helped noir achieve a sense of realism that was crucial in connecting the genre with viewers.

Neonoir

These comments have drawn on classic film noir, often identified as having ended by the late 1950s with Orson Welles's *Touch of Evil* (1958), which featured Mercedes McCambridge as a scary leather-clad biker dyke. By the 1980s and 1990s, the genre had shrunk to its modern variant, the minor form known as neonoir.

In 1996, Andy and Larry Wachowski's neonoir *Bound* decisively reversed the trope of queer as sinister-comic decoration or disquieting-titillating subtext. The film's lesbian lovers were also its stars, indeed its heroines. The fact that it was both a critical success and a mainstream hit showed the culture's readiness for images of gay people out of the shadows, even in a shadow-drenched genre like film noir.

—*Gary Morris*

BIBLIOGRAPHY

Christopher, Nicholas. *Somewhere in the Night: Film Noir and the American City.* New York: Henry Holt, 1997.

Corber, Robert J. *Homosexuality in Cold War America: Resistance and the Crisis of Masculinity.* Durham, N.C.: Duke University Press, 1997.

Dyer, Richard. "Homosexuality and Film Noir." *The Matter of Images: Essays on Representation.* London: Routledge, 1997. 52–72.

Hirsch, Foster. *The Dark Side of the Screen: Film Noir.* San Diego: A. S. Barnes, 1981.

_____. *Detours and Lost Highways: A Map of Neo-Noir.* New York: Limelight Editions, 1999.

Silver, Alain, and Elizabeth Ward, eds. *Film Noir: An Encyclopedic Reference to the American Style.* Woodstock, N.Y.: Outlook Press, 1979.

SEE ALSO

Film

Film Sissies

"I LIKED THE SISSY," HARVEY FIERSTEIN SAID IN AN interview for the documentary *The Celluloid Closet*. This simple sentiment, though rendered apologetically, is hardly surprising coming from an actor who has played his share of such characters over the years.

What is surprising is that mainstream audiences, and sometimes queer viewers who have more at stake in such imagery, have mostly agreed with him, judging from the sheer staying power of the sissy archetype, which can be found everywhere from the earliest silent films (*The Celluloid Closet* includes a sighting from 1895) to recent action movies (*Rush Hour 2*, 2001).

What is it about the sissy that has assured his appeal through world wars and major societal shifts?

As a distorted mirror of masculinity, the sissy fascinates as both a challenge to rigid masculine norms and a reinforcement of them. His mere presence in close proximity to the heterosexual male (or female)—often as a valet, decorator, faithful friend, or, later, in the confusion that erupted around the image, as a romantic rival—subtly reminds the audience that there are other, perhaps more satisfying, ways of being than conventional heterosexuality.

The often riotous humor of character actors such as Eric Blore, Edward Everett Horton, Franklin Pangborn, et al.—beloved fixtures in their films, always eagerly awaited—hints at a carefree world of foolish fun that represents a kind of ideal.

This is especially evident in the Fred Astaire–Ginger Rogers films, which always feature at least one, and sometimes several, sissies who, as much as the "satin and platinum" decor, indicate a desirable world of sophistication and pleasure far from the boring status quo.

The 1930s: The Heyday of the Sissy

The 1930s were the sissy's heyday, and the portrayals are more diverse than might be thought at first glance. Most of director Gregory La Cava's films from that era feature the enchanting Franklin Pangborn, whose roles offer a tidy précis of the possibilities of the 1930s sissy.

In *Bed of Roses* (1933), he is a pure figure of fun, whimsically associated with women's underwear as the fussy, commanding head of the ladies' department in a clothing store. In *Fifth Avenue Girl* (1939), he is unexpectedly pleased with his outsider status, confessing to his surprised wealthy boss: "We servants have all of the luxuries of the rich and none of their problems."

My Man Godfrey (1936) shows the sissy as morally upright arbiter, as Pangborn presides over an absurd scavenger hunt by cheating wealthy "nitwits." *Godfrey* breaks one of the cardinal rules of sissydom by having Pangborn lovingly touch the hero (William Powell), provocatively stroking the latter's face ("Do you mind?" he says seductively) to see if his beard is real.

Despite their outsider status, sissies were not above public service to the culture's needs, sometimes taking on the burden of bringing together a warring heterosexual couple, which not coincidentally was usually part of the process of denying their own sexuality. (Expressions of homosexuality were forbidden by the 1934 Hays Code, though sissies were not.)

In the 1933 *Female*, Ferdinand Gottschalk plays a mincing, homunculus-like secretary to a powerful female executive. While he mostly fawns over "Miss D," he ends up advising both her and her intransigent male love interest on how they can come together. Anxieties around the sissy character are also apparent in his role, as *Female* inexplicably has him courting one of the other secretaries, a woman, though it is treated as more campy than serious.

Other kinds of 1930s sissies were strictly exotic window dressing, brought in as novelties to liven up the "real" characters' lives or a stage show. Two examples are the lewd, prancing queens in the gay bar scene in Clara Bow's *Call Her Savage* (1932) and the Rocky Twins, professional drag entertainers in real life, frolicking onstage in the Marion Davies vehicle *Blondie of the Follies* (1932).

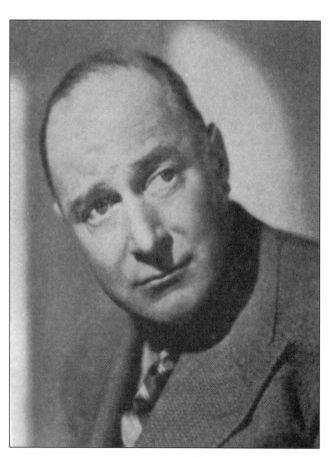

Eric Blore, an actor famous for playing sissy roles.

The 1940s: The Sissy as Threat

By the 1940s, the sissy took off his gloves and shrugged off some of his comic and self-sacrificing impulses. In that era of war and noir, he could turn against the kind of man he once served obsequiously.

Clifton Webb's Waldo Lydecker in *Laura* (1944) shows this scary new sissy, one whose threat to heterosexual norms becomes palpable. Lydecker is treated sympathetically in subtext even as the text shows him as a deranged killer; this is partly because the film endorses the values he imparts to Laura through their apparently sexless relationship—sophistication, deep friendship, an appreciation of beauty—even as it shows that relationship as hopeless.

The nominal hero, the stolid policeman Mark (Dana Andrews), is portrayed as thuggish, dismissive, cold; and for once (but not the last time) the sissy moves from background decoration to the starring role. Webb, unlike the simpering, sometimes frail, or just plain weird sissies of the prior decade, is an attractive, charismatic creature. The title is misleading; *Laura* is really Webb's film, and thus the sissy's.

1950s Sissies

For some observers, the sissy's golden age ended in the 1940s, but the character remained a minor but persistent force.

Vincente Minnelli's *Tea and Sympathy* (1956) was a major postwar text on sissydom, wringing its hands in the manner of the liberal problem picture over the troubling effeminacy of the character dubbed "Sissy Boy" by cruel schoolmates. In the play he was homosexual, in the movie he is "sensitive"—and rescued from sissydom by a sympathetic woman.

Also during this decade, Jerry Lewis perfected what Parker Tyler called the "sissy-boy clown," but Lewis's schtick, derived from vaudeville, was more manic than queer.

1960s Sissies

In two of his 1960s movies, *Lover Come Back* (1961) and *A Very Special Favor* (1965), Rock Hudson pretends to be a sissy in order to win over a woman, a dizzying collision of reality and fiction in the case of a gay actor such as Hudson.

More adventurous sissies arrived with the late-1960s counterculture. William Friedkin's *The Boys in the Band* (1969, based on a play by Mart Crowley), for example, featured a slew of sissies brimming with superb dish and self-hate, dancing, smoking dope, making out, discussing Maria Montez.

For some sissy-watchers this was the ultimate treat, a rare film made up *entirely* of sissies, with only a single disturbed heterosexual to spoil the fun. (And he's soon relegated to the background, where sissies once dwelt.)

More politically minded queers dismissed *Boys* as an unappetizing tableau of self-loathing homosexuals that pandered to heterosexist morality. (Critic Vito Russo called it "a homosexual period piece just as *Green Pastures* was a Negro period piece.")

The 1970s and Beyond

In the gay-inflected prison drama *Fortune and Men's Eyes* (1971), audiences were treated to a previously unthinkable image: the sissy unclothed. The film's Queenie (professional drag entertainer Michael Greer) is in some respects the apotheosis of the threatening effeminate queer, reordering the prison as a kind of personal fiefdom for his own pleasure and, in a startling sequence, entertaining the prisoners, guards, and their families by doing a lewd drag number that ends with him exposing himself and verbally lacerating the audience. Queenie shows the intransigent sissy's resilience, surviving a brutal beating to reclaim his place.

Queenie's legacy of the out-of-control sissy did not last, however, and, aside from the curious conflation of queer and killer that made a popular subgenre in films such as *Silence of the Lambs*, and an occasional perverse-powerful sissy such as Louis XIII in Ken Russell's *The Devils* (1971), mainstream post-1970s films mostly featured more subdued sissies.

From Harvey Fierstein cowering under a desk in *Independence Day* (1996) to the drag queens of *To Wong Foo, Thanks for Everything, Julie Newmar* (1995) who sacrifice their sexuality and transform the lives of small-town heterosexuals, from neurotic Nathan Lane in *The Birdcage* (1996) to Jeremy Piven as a Versace salesman flirting wildly with Jackie Chan and Chris Tucker in *Rush Hour 2*, the modern sissy has returned to more familiar and culturally reassuring territory: a minor but provocative diversion in the comic-decorative mode that he played so memorably in the 1930s.   —*Gary Morris*

BIBLIOGRAPHY

Davis, Ray. "The Sissy Gaze in American Cinema." *Bright Lights Film Journal* 23 (December 1998):
www.brightlightsfilm.com/23/sissy.html

Howes, Keith. *Broadcasting It: An Encyclopedia of Homosexuality on Film, Radio, and TV in the UK 1923–1993*. London: Cassell, 1993.

Murray, Raymond. *Images in the Dark: An Encyclopedia of Gay and Lesbian Film and Video*. New York: Plume, 1996.

Russo, Vito. *The Celluloid Closet: Homosexuality in the Movies*. New York: Harper & Row, 1987.

Tyler, Parker. *Screening the Sexes: Homosexuality in the Movies*. New York: Holt, Rinehart and Winston, 1972.

SEE ALSO

Film; Film Noir; Fierstein, Harvey; Hudson, Rock; Lane, Nathan; Minnelli, Vincente; Webb, Clifton

Film Spectatorship

FILM SPECTATORSHIP IS AN INTEGRAL PART OF QUEER culture, affording a process of self-invention and making possible the coded articulation of queer desires and identities.

The British historian A. J. P. Taylor dubbed film spectatorship "the essential social habit of the age," and there can be little doubt that, for much of the past century, cinema and its various audiovisual offspring have been dominant entertainment forms for audiences around the globe. Glbtq people have been a significant, if not always readily identifiable, segment of those audiences and have made spectatorship an integral part of queer culture.

The image of the movie-obsessed queer has become a veritable staple of homosexual representation, evident in any number of popular cultural texts from *Kiss of the Spider Woman* (1984) to *Billy's Hollywood Screen Kiss* (1998). While it is an image often skewed to the point of grotesque stereotype, it highlights the significance that spectatorship has come to assume for many glbtq people.

Historical Overview

With its unique combination of voyeuristic fantasies on the screen and bodies thrown into close proximity in a darkened auditorium, film spectatorship is a profoundly erotic experience, which is no doubt one of the reasons it has long drawn the anxious gaze of censors and other moral guardians. Historically, glbtq people have been quick to respond to the erotic capacities of spectatorship, deploying it for distinctively queer ends. As early as the 1910s, for example, gay men in the large urban metropolises of Europe and North America routinely used storefront theaters, nickelodeons, and other such places of film viewing for making sexual contacts and socializing with what one disapproving magistrate of the time termed "congenial spirits."

Movies themselves also emerged quite early as important sites of queer engagement, furnishing opportunities for identity building and subcultural exchange. Unlike many other social groups whose sense of identity is openly recognized from birth and cultivated through public systems of kinship, education, and government, queers have largely grown up isolated from each other and have had to invent their own modes of cultural identification. For much of the twentieth century and beyond, the fantasy world of cinema has been a privileged and particularly fertile forum for this process of queer self-invention.

Not only have movies offered glbtq people an avenue of escape and a chance to imagine utopian possibilities "over the rainbow," they also furnished them with a proto–common culture through which to communicate and bond. According to Andrea Weiss, American lesbians of the 1930s would routinely use popular films and stars of the time as a "shared language" with which to "define and empower themselves."

Gay men developed similarly intense investments in and uses of film. Indeed, throughout the midcentury, gay male subcultures developed a finely nuanced taste culture based on Hollywood film. Certain genres such as the musical and the melodrama, and stars such as Judy Garland, Bette Davis, and Joan Crawford, emerged as firm favorites of gay men and were consequently charged with particular queer affect.

In an era when gay men and lesbians were rendered all but invisible, film spectatorship became a symbolic sphere for the coded articulation of queer desires and identities.

In line with broader sociohistorical changes, cinema arguably lost its position of unrivalled primacy in queer subcultures during the latter part of the twentieth century, ceding to newer media forms such as television and popular music and to a host of self-authored subcultural practices from the popular gay press to dance parties. However, film spectatorship continues to function as a significant component of contemporary queer cultural life.

The older traditions of gay and lesbian cinematic taste are kept alive through screenings of "gay cult classics" at repertory theaters or through gay video stores, while new modes of queer spectatorship have developed around recent film forms like documentary, New Queer Cinema, and pornography, or exhibition forums such as film festivals. In addition, new digital media such as computers and the Internet have enabled the emergence of various modes of spectatorship from Net surfing to cyberporn, which, though seemingly far removed from classic models of cinematic viewing, still serve vital functions of self-definition and empowerment for many queer spectators.

The Queer Gaze

While it may have been a cultural lifeline for many glbtq people over the years, cinema has not exactly been a trove of positive queer imagery. For much of its history, mainstream film categorically refused the explicit representation of queer lives and loves, and, even today, queer presences onscreen remain largely exceptional, relegated to the margins of popular cinema and frequently subjected to homophobic stereotyping. As a result, queer viewers have had to develop various modes of oppositional spectatorship through which to combat the heterosexist dynamics of mainstream film and open it up to queer investment and use.

This process of appropriating or "queering" film assumes various forms and uses multiple tactics. At a general level, glbtq spectators are acutely adept at appropriating film to their own frames of reference and imbuing it with specifically queer affect. A pertinent example here would be a film such as *The Wizard of Oz* (1939).

With its status as a mainstay of wholesome "family" cinema, *The Wizard of Oz* seems an unlikely candidate for queer popularization, but generations of glbtq spectators have responded to this film in ways that have rendered it patently queer. Out of the seemingly childish tale of a young girl's trip through a fantasyland, queer spectators have interpreted a mytho-epic journey from heteronormative mundanity into queer difference and have reconstructed the film as an empowering urtext of queer survivalism and community.

Some critics suggest that glbtq spectators learn almost as habit to read film symptomatically, to scour texts for casual signs of queerness—a "colorful" supporting character; an ambiguous line of dialogue; a furtive glance between same-sex characters—that may seem insignificant to the film's immediate narrative function but that enable the production of coded queer subplots.

Others claim that queer spectators prize film not so much for its stories, which are invariably heteronormative, but for its moments of spectacular transcendence and bewitching glamour—Dietrich in top hat and tails stooping to kiss a woman in the audience; Norma Desmond's staircase descent into madness; Mrs. Danvers's frenzied torching of Manderley—and that they value these moments as symbolic gestures of social and sexual defiance.

Other critics again highlight extratextual elements such as star gossip and their use by queer spectators to subvert the heterosexual coding of a given star and his or her roles, thereby rendering the star available for specifically queer identification. In this context, one could consider the films of a star such as Rock Hudson replete with all manner of queer double meanings when read in light of knowledge of his homosexuality. Today that knowledge circulates more or less freely, but during the height of Hudson's stardom in the 1950s it was available to queer spectators only through discourses of subcultural gossip.

The common element across these diverse strategies of queer spectatorship is the desire to remake mainstream film in a way that better accommodates and supports queer interests and desires. Glbtq people have always shown great resourcefulness in making their own cultural meanings and spaces, often out of the very material of dominant culture that would seek to exclude them. Queer spectatorship is a potent example of this resistant creativity at work.

—*Brett Farmer*

BIBLIOGRAPHY

Creekmur, Corey K., and Alexander Doty, eds. *Out in Culture: Gay, Lesbian and Queer Essays on Popular Culture.* Durham, N.C.: Duke University Press, 1995.

Doty, Alexander. *Making Things Perfectly Queer: Interpreting Mass Culture.* Minneapolis: University of Minnesota Press, 1993.

Farmer, Brett. *Spectacular Passions: Cinema, Fantasy, Gay Male Spectatorships.* Durham, N.C.: Duke University Press, 2000.

Hanson, Ellis, ed. *Out Takes: Essays on Queer Theory and Film.* Durham, N.C.: Duke University Press, 1999.

Weiss, Andrea. *Vampires and Violets: Lesbians in the Cinema.* London: Jonathan Cape, 1992.

White, Patricia. *UnInvited: Classical Hollywood Cinema and Lesbian Representability.* Bloomington, Ind.: Indiana University Press, 1999.

Wilton, Tamsin, ed. *Immortal Invisible: Lesbians and the Moving Image.* London and New York: Routledge, 1995.

SEE ALSO

Film; Film Festivals; New Queer Cinema; Documentary Film; Dietrich, Marlene; Garland, Judy; Hudson, Rock

Flowers, Wayland (1939–1988)

THE COMPLEX RELATIONSHIP BETWEEN THE PUPPETEER and his puppet, an inanimate object that he has invested with a life and a personality of its own, can take many bizarre twists. Such is the case of Wayland Flowers and his puppet Madame, who, arguably, was far more famous than her creator.

Indeed, a decade and a half after Flowers's death, there is little biographical information available about him and he would seem a mostly forgotten minor celebrity of the 1970s, while a search of the Internet reveals that Madame still retains a cult following.

Wayland Flowers was born in Dawson, Georgia, on November 26, 1939. He began to practice puppetry at an early age, drawn, perhaps, by a puppet's license to say and do in public a wide variety of things forbidden to its human operator.

In the 1960s, Flowers moved to New York, where he was an assistant puppeteer for a number of children's television shows. But while he entertained children during the day, he also developed Madame, an "adults-only" puppet, a grotesquely ugly and flamboyantly ribald old crone festooned in outrageous evening gowns, tiaras, and rhinestones.

Flowers performed with Madame in nightclubs and gay bars, where her frank and often acerbic observations about sex, men, and life in general, similar to those expressed by drag queens in their acts, gained the "dirty old lady" and—by extension—Flowers a following that led to frequent television guest appearances on variety and talk shows.

By the late 1960s, Flowers and Madame had become regulars on the comedy program *Laugh-In,* one of the most popular television programs at the time and known for its cutting-edge topical humor that frequently challenged network censorship. In this context, Flowers was able to present a campy gay point of view mediated through his puppet.

Naughty old ladies have long been a staple of bawdy comedy, able to indulge sarcastically in double entendre and sexual innuendo and yet be found amusing rather than offensive, if for no other reason than that the audience perceives older women, no matter how stereotypical, as being past any serious sexual interest.

This comedic incongruity, then, could be taken to even greater lengths by means of an old lady who was not only extraordinarily ugly (though pretending to be a great beauty) but who was also, in reality, wood and wire rather than flesh and blood.

In this way, Flowers was able to express on prime-time television the attitudes and desires of many gay men in the early days of gay liberation—views that would otherwise have been regarded as pointedly offensive to mainstream audiences—without censure.

Throughout the 1970s, Wayland Flowers and Madame appeared frequently on television, as the hosts of *Solid Gold,* a weekly popular-music show, and on the game show *Hollywood Squares,* where, after nearly a decade of guest appearances, they succeeded Paul Lynde, a gay comic as bitchy and queeny as Madame, in the all-important center square.

By the early 1980s, the puppet/human relationship had taken a strange turn in Flowers's career. Madame became the star of her own sitcom, *Madame's Place,* in which she played the lead role, interacting with the other actors as if she were human.

Flowers, ironically, remained completely out of sight, his function as Madame's voice the only outward evidence of his presence. Indeed, she seemed to take on a life of her own, eclipsing Flowers until he became invisible—both literally and figuratively—behind her.

As a result of his invisibility, very little attention was drawn to his personal life, and thus it was a surprise to many when Flowers died in Hollywood on October 11, 1988, a victim of the AIDS epidemic. Madame was buried with him.

—*Patricia Juliana Smith*

BIBLIOGRAPHY

Simmons, Gary. *Madame: My Misbegotten Memoirs, as Told to Wayland Flowers.* New York: Dodd, Mead, 1983.

www.jumptheshark.com/m/madamesplace.htm

SEE ALSO

American Television: Situation Comedies; Lynde, Paul

Flynn, Errol (1909–1959)

A

T THE HEIGHT OF HIS CAREER, ERROL FLYNN WAS THE heartthrob of movie fans throughout the world. Handsome, athletic, graceful, and charismatic, Flynn seemed to personify Robin Hood and the other heroic figures that he portrayed onscreen. A highly publicized trial for statutory rape in 1942 tarnished his public image and revealed darker qualities than had been expressed in his previous films. In his final years, Flynn played psychologically complex characters, expressing aspects of his personality not evident in the swashbuckling roles for which he is most famous.

Flynn exuded sexual energy. He tellingly declared in a famous interview of 1950 that he wanted his gravestone to be inscribed: "If It Moved, Flynn Fucked It." This assertion might be regarded as corroboration of persistent and widely disseminated rumors that he was eager to have sex with both men and women. In the aptly titled, posthumously published, but unreliable *My Wicked, Wicked Ways* (1959), Flynn included abundant details about his countless sexual conquests of women. While he emphasized that he enjoyed partying with his male buddies, he never indicated that their interactions had sexual overtones.

However, in his autobiography, Flynn effectively acknowledged—without confirming—the rumors about his sexual exploits with men when he noted that many of his female costars thought he was a "faggot" (his term) because his politeness was interpreted as emotional distance. This explanation for the rumors is utterly unconvincing, since Flynn was notorious for behavior on the sets of his pictures that could hardly be considered either polite or emotionally distant.

Biographers of Flynn, as well as other observers of Hollywood, have claimed that Flynn had sexual (if not romantic) flings with Tyrone Power and numerous other, less well known actors during his Hollywood years. The best cases for Flynn's alleged bisexuality were made by controversial biographers Charles Higham and David Bret. Although Higham's sensational charges that Flynn was a Nazi spy have been thoroughly discredited, his account of Flynn's sex life, while infuriating to many of the actor's fans, has not been. Bret, who emphatically rejected allegations that Flynn was a spy, substantiated Higham's account of the actor's supposed bisexuality by providing fuller information about his sexual escapades with other men. Moreover, Flynn's first wife, Lili Damita, insisted as late as 1994 that Flynn enjoyed sexual encounters with men, and her assertions have been corroborated by some of Flynn's associates in Hollywood, including Marlene Dietrich.

However, other close friends and family members—including actor David Niven, Flynn's roommate during his early Hollywood years; his second wife, Nora Eddington; and his third wife and widow, Patrice Wymore—have emphatically denied that Flynn was bisexual or gay. More disturbingly, many of Flynn's fans have rejected out of hand the possibility of the actor's bisexuality because they think such allegations besmirch their hero's reputation or because they somewhat naively believe that Flynn's well-documented heterosexual activities preclude any interest in homosexual dalliances.

Notwithstanding such protests, it may be telling that in recounting a visit to a brothel in Marrakech, Flynn claimed that he was initially horrified to discover that the establishment was actually a male brothel; but, he says, he quickly came to the realization that everyone had a right to whatever pleasures suit them, and he encouraged his readers to remember the splendors of ancient Greece, which had accepted homosexuality. The anecdote, of course, indicates nothing definite about Flynn's own sexual interests, but the plea for tolerance, coupled with the familiar citation of the glories of Greece, is significant because it challenges the climate of sexual repression that was pervasive in the 1950s.

There is no doubt that Flynn was a compulsive womanizer. The likelihood is that he also had occasional sexual relations with men. While no concrete evidence has been discovered that unequivocally documents Flynn's affairs with men, this is hardly surprising. At a time when homosexual acts were illegal in the United States and Great Britain, and the mere suspicion of homosexuality could destroy careers, such documentation would almost certainly not be preserved. Given the time in which he lived, Flynn probably did not self-identify as a bisexual. However, his exuberant sexual appetites, and his willingness to transgress all kinds of sexual boundaries, increase the likelihood that the widespread rumors of his sexual affairs with men had a basis in fact.

Background and Early Career

Flynn was born on June 20, 1909, in Hobart, Tasmania, in Australia. His father, Theodore Thomson Flynn, a lecturer at the University of Tasmania, already had gained international recognition for his research in marine biology. His mother, Lily Mary Flynn, was a descendent of Fletcher Christian (leader of the Bounty mutiny), whom Errol would portray in his first movie role. From a very young age, Errol showed exceptional athletic ability, but he devoted much of his energy to sometimes cruel pranks on children and adults alike. As a result, he was—despite his father's eminence—expelled from numerous schools in Australia and England.

Dismissed in August 1926 from a prestigious grammar school in Sydney, he worked in a large import–export firm until September 1927, when he was fired for borrowing money from petty cash. Errol attempted to support himself for a while as a semiprofessional boxer, but, in September 1928, he went to New Guinea in hopes of finding a fortune by prospecting for gold. Although his claim produced little gold, Flynn remained in New Guinea for nearly four years, trying his hand at all sorts of legal and illegal activities, including training as a cadet patrol officer, growing tobacco, and even engaging in the slave trade. While in New Guinea, he contracted malaria, which would plague him for the rest of his life.

On a visit to Sydney in 1929, he and some friends bought a fifty-year-old yacht, *Sirocco*. Despite their lack of experience, they decided to sail it 3,000 miles back to New Guinea; their adventures formed the basis of Flynn's novel, *Beam Ends* (1937).

In 1930, Dr. Hermann F. Erben, a medical researcher in tropical diseases and an adventurer, hired Flynn to sail up the Sepik River in order to make a documentary film about those parts of the interior of New Guinea that were still largely unexplored by Europeans. As the captain of the *Sirocco*, Flynn appeared occasionally in the film. In 1932, impressed by Flynn's dashing appearance, motion picture director Charles Chauvel offered him the role of Fletcher Christian in the first Australian sound feature film, *In the Wake of the Bounty* (1933), about the history of Pitcairn Island.

Intrigued by this experience, Flynn resolved to develop a career as a professional actor in Britain. In 1933, accompanied by Erben, he spent several months traveling to Europe through the Philippines, Asia, and North Africa. Unable to find employment in film studios in London, he accepted a position at the Northampton Repertory Company, where he worked from December 1933 to June 1934. Playing a variety of roles, he gained increased skill as an actor.

By fall 1934, Flynn was working as an extra at Warner Brothers' Teddington Studios in London. Impressed with his good looks and charm, Irving Asher, the head Warner executive in Britain, gave him a starring role in *Murder at Monte Carlo* (1935). At Asher's persuasion, Jack Warner viewed a copy of the film and promptly offered Flynn a six-month contract at the American studio. On board ship to New York, Flynn met Lila Damita (1905–1994), a French-born movie star, then under an extended contract to Warner Brothers. They initiated an intense but stormy relationship and married on June 19, 1935.

Initially, Flynn had difficulty getting assignments at Warner Brothers. His first American appearance was as a corpse in the Perry Mason film *The Case of the Curious Bride* (1935). In *Don't Bet on Blondes* (1935), he appeared for about five minutes as a society playboy.

Success in Hollywood, 1935–1942

Flynn got his big break in May 1935, when he was offered the lead role in *Captain Blood*. The film, con-

ceived from the start as a major production, was based on a 1922 Rafael Sabatini novel that had been made into a very successful silent film in 1924.

After negotiations broke down with preferred leading actors Robert Donat, Leslie Howard, and Clark Gable, Warner Brothers conducted an extensive talent search among contract players. From their first look at a screen test made of Flynn (who was being considered for a small role), both studio boss Jack Warner and director Hal Wallis agreed that he perfectly exemplified the masculine but debonair adventurer. Originally intended for Bette Davis, the female lead ultimately was given to an equally unknown actor, Olivia de Haviland, who would costar with Flynn in seven other movies.

Opening in December 1935, *Captain Blood* established Flynn as a major star. Drawing upon his own experiences as an adventurer, he was able to breathe life into the screen image of the swashbuckler. Doing virtually all of his own stunts, he displayed his strength, skill, and grace in fencing and other athletic activities.

As Peter Blood, Flynn plays a seventeenth-century English doctor wrongly convicted of treason. Sent to Jamaica, he is sold into slavery on a plantation owned by the Olivia de Haviland character's uncle. Leading a successful rebellion, Blood becomes the captain of a pirate ship manned by other former slaves. After a series of adventures, Blood provides valuable services to the British crown; he is rewarded with the governorship of Jamaica, where he takes up residence with his new bride (Olivia de Haviland, of course).

This story of an unjustly accused hero who redeems himself through selfless actions is one that would be repeated in numerous other Flynn movies, set in diverse historical and contemporary contexts, including medieval England, nineteenth-century India, the Western frontier, contemporary American small towns, and various battlefields in World War II.

According to Bret and some other biographers, Flynn had an affair with supporting actor Ross Alexander (1908–1937) during the filming of *Captain Blood*. Speculation about their possible relationship seems to be supported by the tenderness and intensity of their onscreen performances. Adding to the script, Flynn constantly referred to Alexander as "dear" and "darling." Intentionally or not, some of the scenes by Flynn and Alexander have a homoerotic aura: for example, Flynn's massage of Alexander's leg, interrupted by the question "What's going on between you two?" as Lionel Atwill enters the set.

A number of Flynn's other screen performances also have homoerotic dimensions, including, for instance, his flirtatious conversations with a decidedly uncomfortable Fred MacMurray in *Dive Bomber* (1941). However, it should be kept in mind that, while these possible queer readings suggest the complexity and richness of Flynn's acting, they do not provide firm evidence about his own sexual orientation or experiences.

Between 1936 and 1942, Flynn was at the pinnacle of his career. He starred in nineteen major films for Warner Brothers during this period. Costing over $2 million, the Technicolor film *Adventures of Robin Hood* (1938) was the most expensive film made up to that point. The role became one of Flynn's signature roles.

Intending to star Flynn and Warner leading lady Bette Davis in *Gone with the Wind*, David O. Selznick signed a very lucrative contract with Warner Brothers for their services. When the deal fell through because Davis refused to act with Flynn (whom she considered untalented), Jack Warner forced her to work with him in two movies: the soapy melodrama *The Sisters* (1938) and the lavish historical romance *The Private Lives of Elizabeth and Essex* (1939).

Although Flynn detested the genre, he was compelled to star in several Westerns during his time at Warner Brothers, beginning with the hugely successful *Dodge City* (1939). In *They Died with Their Boots On* (1942), Flynn expanded the limits of his usual adventurer roles by conveying the complexities and contradictions of General Custer.

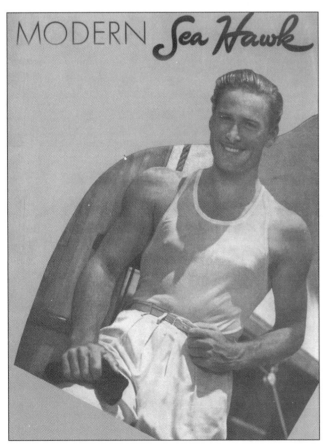

Errol Flynn in a promotional piece for his film *The Sea Hawk* (1940).

Feeling increasingly constrained by his swashbuckler vehicles, Flynn pleaded with the studio to allow him to undertake other types of films. In *The Perfect Specimen* (1937, costarring Joan Blondell) and *Four's a Crowd* (1938, costarring Olivia de Haviland and Rosalind Russell), he demonstrated exceptional comic timing, as well as the sophisticated wit admired by his friends. Many film historians maintain that had Flynn been allowed to perform in more movies of this type, he would have challenged Cary Grant's status as the dominant male star of screwball comedies.

In 1937, already tired of studio efforts to control all aspects of his life and eager for an actual (as opposed to filmed) adventure, Flynn traveled with his old friend Dr. Erben to Spain, then in the midst of a devastating civil war. Although most of his friends insist that Flynn was apolitical, he professed strong support for the Republican cause. It is virtually certain that Flynn was unaware that Erben, though Jewish, was a card-carrying Nazi working as a spy. Erben photographed German dissidents in Spain and gathered other information for the German government.

Flynn placed himself in many dangerous situations, as he and Erben sought to photograph battles in and around Barcelona and Madrid during March and April 1937. At one point, Spanish newspapers published stories of his death and the Spanish government sent condolences to his wife. Because of his association with Erben, the FBI doubted Flynn's loyalty and placed him under constant surveillance during World War II.

Despite the fiasco of the trip to Spain, Warner Brothers Studios succeeded in creating a very positive public image for Flynn throughout the period from 1936 to 1942. A continuous stream of publicity emphasized correlations between his personality and his screen roles. Flynn's youthful adventures were fully exploited for this purpose. In addition, every effort was made to create the impression that he was actually as rigorously virtuous and as conventionally upright as he appeared to be onscreen.

For younger viewers, this conception was reinforced by several series of elementary and high school textbooks of such classic works as *The Charge of the Light Brigade*, which extensively referenced Flynn's screen performances. Until 1942, studio publicists managed to conceal from public view Flynn's seemingly insatiable sexual appetites and the heavy drinking that increasingly affected both his general health and his performances.

Flynn's Final Years at Warner Brothers, 1942–1952

In the early 1940s, several events coalesced to shatter Flynn's carefully crafted public image. At the beginning of World War II, the actor applied for United States citizenship, but he was unable to enlist in the military because of chronic health problems, including recurring bouts of malaria and a diagnosis of tuberculosis. However, eager to preserve Flynn's status as a heroic adventurer, Warner Brothers rigorously concealed from the press all information about his medical condition. Therefore, Flynn's perceived "failure" to participate in the fighting puzzled and disturbed his fans. Flynn was deeply upset by numerous editorials in newspapers of the Hearst Corporation that questioned his patriotism.

In September 1941, Lili Damita left Flynn and took their son, Sean, with her; in November, she initiated divorce proceedings, accusing him of intolerable cruelty. Because Flynn and Damita had quarreled violently for years, most of their acquaintances thought the divorce a good resolution to a bad situation. However, the general public was shocked by the breakup of what had been publicized as a perfect marriage. The settlement, finalized in May 1942, entitled Damita to substantial monthly payments for the rest of her life. In later years, this settlement would contribute to Flynn's economic woes.

On October 18, 1942, the Los Angeles District Attorney's office filed formal charges against Flynn of statutory rape of two women, Betty Hansen (eighteen at the time of the accusation, but seventeen in September 1941 when Flynn was alleged to have had intercourse with her) and Peggy Satterlee (only sixteen at the time of the accusation). All aspects of the trial were reported by international media.

Defending Flynn, Hollywood lawyer Jerry Geisler discredited the character and credibility of both women. For instance, he established that the District Attorney's office had offered them immunity from prosecution for oral sex and abortion (both criminal offenses at the time) in exchange for bringing charges against Flynn.

Although Flynn was acquitted on February 6, 1943, the implication of his guilt remained, and most people did not view him with the same degree of respect that they had previously. Not surprisingly, many women moviegoers were disturbed by the trial, but fan mail suggests that at least some of them were also intrigued by the revelations about his sexual escapades. Further, publicity surrounding the trial gained Flynn grudging admiration among many GIs for his sexual prowess and ability to escape responsibility for his actions. Thus, enlisted men coined the phrase "In like Flynn" to describe examples of sexual boldness and success.

During the course of the trial, Flynn discreetly began an affair with Nora Eddington (1924–2001), who was working at a tobacco stand in the courthouse. When she became pregnant in August 1943, Flynn married her in order to provide their child with a "legitimate" name. Eager to pursue the lifestyle of a bachelor, Flynn publicly denied rumors about the marriage, until the birth of his daughter Deirdre on January 10, 1944, was reported by the Hollywood press. The couple subsequently had another daughter, Rory.

Eddington eventually moved into Flynn's home, and his children remember him as an excellent father. However, with his restless spirit, Flynn could not be contained within the limits of a conventional household. Thus, he continued to pursue sexual liaisons with countless women (and, likely, some men) and indulged in heavy drinking with his male buddies. According to family and friends, his desire for adventure caused him to experiment with drugs; his resulting addiction to morphine created many problems for him in his later years. Increasingly frustrated by Flynn's behavior, Eddington divorced him on July 7, 1949.

Initially, Warner Brothers was wary that the trial for statutory rape would destroy Flynn's box-office appeal. However, *Gentleman Jim* (1942), rushed into release before the trial began, proved to be highly successful. Still, the features that Flynn made during his final decade at Warner's generally did not attract the same degree of enthusiastic fan response that his earlier films had. Furthermore, most of his pictures were given lower budgets than previously, and he was even assigned to several cheaply produced B movies.

An exception to this trend was *The Adventures of Don Juan* (1949), which was intended to give Flynn one last chance at a big-budget epic. As he had in *Captain Blood* and other swashbuckling films, he displayed considerable prowess in swordfights and stunt work, though he looked considerably older than he had in the earlier epics. Most significant, Flynn infused self-conscious humor into the role of Don Juan—creating the archetypal camp (and, undoubtedly, self-mocking) image of the insatiable lover. Although his performance in *Don Juan* remains a favorite among many gay viewers, not least because of Flynn's self-conscious satire of romantic clichés, American audiences in general were disappointed by the film. It did exceptionally well in Europe, however.

In the course of filming *Don Juan,* Flynn's binge drinking and morphine addiction had begun to spin out of control. His prolonged absences from the studio delayed production and greatly inflated costs. After this point, Warner Brothers regarded him as a liability, though they retained him under contract until 1952.

Despite a significant number of inconsequential films, Flynn also gave some outstanding screen performances during the period from 1942 to 1952. For instance, in *Uncertain Glory* (1944), he subtly portrayed a criminal who sacrificed his life to redeem hostages held by the Nazis. Avoiding conventional sentiment, he revealed the petty and cunning aspects of the character, as well as his idealism.

Flynn conveyed the tedium and horror of battle in *Operation Burma* (1945), now regarded as one of the few combat films produced during World War II that still seems credible. But outrage by the British media over the film's presentation of the Burmese operation as an American endeavor caused Warner's to withdraw the film from distribution in the Commonwealth countries and hurt its theatrical run even in the United States. In *That Forsyte Woman* (1949), Flynn, on loan to MGM, played against character as the scheming and possessive Soames Forsyte.

With its stilted script and B-level production, *Rocky Mountain* is typical of the films to which Flynn was assigned during the final years of his contract. However, the project gave him the opportunity to meet singer and actress Patrice Wymore (b. 1926), whom he married in France on October 23, 1950, and with whom he had a daughter, Arnella Roma.

Last Years

In 1952, by mutual agreement, Flynn and Warner Brothers abrogated Flynn's contract. Resolving to demonstrate his ability to create major features on his own terms, he began a lavish European production of *William Tell* in spring 1953. If completed, this would have been the first independent feature to be made in Cinemascope. Unfortunately, his Italian partners withdrew from the production and left Flynn to deal with the legal complications resulting from the deal's collapse. Contributing to Flynn's dismay were the retaliatory legal actions taken by his longtime friend the actor Bruce Cabot, who seized his cars, clothes, and other personal possessions.

Later in 1953, Flynn's financial woes intensified when he discovered that Al Blum, his recently deceased financial manager, had been stealing from him and had left him with a debt of over $1 million to the IRS. Refusing to declare bankruptcy, Flynn sold many of his remaining assets to pay off some of his debts.

In 1955, Damita made claims for additional alimony and won Flynn's house in partial payment; thereafter, his yacht, the *Zaca*, became his primary residence. During the mid-1950s, Flynn made guest appearances on television variety shows; in most cases, he was required to enact caricatures of his earlier heroic roles.

Wymore's appearances in films and television helped the couple to survive financially, and she also offered Flynn great emotional support. However, he separated from her in 1958 and pursued a scandalous affair with a teenager, Beverly Aadland (b. 1942), whom he had met the previous year.

During the mid-1950s, Flynn made a few routine pictures for British studios, including *Let's Make Up* (1955), a sentimental romance costarring the popular English musical star Anna Neagle, and *The Warriors* (1955), his final historical epic.

However, in the final years of his life Flynn experienced a resurgence of his film career, and he gave out-

standing performances that revealed dimensions not expressed in most of his previous roles. His portrayal of a world-weary alcoholic in *The Sun Also Rises* (1957) was widely hailed as a major comeback, and he followed this success with critically acclaimed performances as John Barrymore in *Too Much, Too Soon* (1958) and as a British deserter who devotes himself to preservation of African elephants in *The Roots of Heaven* (1958).

Still eager for adventure, Flynn went to Cuba in 1959 in order to witness the revolution occurring there. For American and Canadian newspapers he wrote enthusiastic reports about Fidel Castro, which he later retracted. He also made a short feature, *Cuban Rebel Girls* (1959), intended both to glorify Castro and to showcase Aadland. The favorable publicity surrounding his Cuban escapade evoked the period of his greatest successes.

Flynn died of a heart attack on October 14, 1959, in Vancouver, where he had gone to sell his boat in an effort to repay some of his debts.

Conclusion

In a tribute to Flynn, Jack Warner vividly characterized his screen performances: "He was all the heroes in one magnificent, sexy, animal package. He showered the audience with sparks when he laughed, when he fought, or when he loved." The dynamism, sexual energy, and charisma evident in his early films still excite viewers of diverse backgrounds and perspectives. In his final films, he revealed a profound awareness of the tragedies and complexities of life.

Flynn deserves a place in glbtq history for several reasons. In *The Adventures of Don Juan*, he devised a thoroughly camp interpretation of the insatiable lover that resonated particularly with gay viewers at a time of great repression, and in other films he added a homoerotic dimension that may have gone over the heads of most of his audience but which thrilled gay fans.

Moreover, in real life, Flynn was a sexual adventurer. He probably had sexual relations with men as well as women. Most important, he exemplifies the fluidity of sexual desire and the somewhat indiscriminate nature of sexual compulsion. The persistent rumors of his dalliances with men, coupled with his own self-description ("If It Moved, Flynn Fucked It"), suggest that his compulsive womanizing may have been related to sexual needs that transcend current categories of sexual orientation (homosexual, heterosexual, and bisexual) and might more appropriately be described as polyamory.

—*Richard G. Mann*

BIBLIOGRAPHY

The Adventures of Errol Flynn. DVD. Directed and written by David Heeley; produced by Joan Kramer and David Heeley. New York: Top Hat Productions and Turner Entertainment, 2005.

Bret, David. *Errol Flynn: Satan's Angel*. New York: Robson Books, 2004.

Flynn, Errol. *My Wicked, Wicked Ways*. Rpt., New York: Buccaneer Books, 1976.

Godfrey, Lionel. *The Life and Times of Errol Flynn*. New York: St. Martin's, 1977.

Higham, Charles. *Errol Flynn: The Untold Story*. New York: Doubleday, 1980.

McNulty, Thomas. *Errol Flynn: The Life and Career*. New York: McFarland & Company, 2004.

Niven, David. *Bring on the Empty Horses*. New York: Putnam, 1975.

Thomas, Tony. *Errol Flynn: The Spy Who Never Was*. New York: Citadel Press, 1990.

———, Rudy Behlmer, and Clifford McCarty. *The Films of Errol Flynn*. New York: Citadel Press, 1969.

Valenti, Peter. *Errol Flynn: A Bio-Bibliography*. Westport, Conn.: Greenwood, 1984.

SEE ALSO

Film; Dietrich, Marlene; Grant, Cary

Fry, Stephen   (b. 1957)

TALL, HEAVY, GAY, AND WITTY, BRITISH ACTOR STEPHEN Fry was told for many years that he reminded people of Oscar Wilde. It is apt, then, that he was cast in the lead role in the film *Wilde* (1997), in which he seemed to embody perfectly the great playwright and victim of intolerance.

Yet there is much more to the versatile Fry than this one role; he is also an accomplished comic, novelist, memoirist, and philanthropist.

Stephen John Fry was born on August 24, 1957, in Hampstead, London, to an affluent family. His father, Alan, is a physicist and inventor; his mother, Marianne, was born in Austria, and her Jewish family immigrated to England to escape Nazi persecution. A bright, inquisitive child, he was educated in private boarding schools.

Fry began to rebel in his teens, after first suspecting that he was gay. By the time he was fifteen, he had been expelled from three schools, and, at sixteen, he attempted suicide. At seventeen, he was arrested for credit card fraud and sentenced to three months in prison, an experience that proved a turning point for the troubled young man. Consequently, he applied himself to his studies, so much so that he won a scholarship to Queens College, Cambridge University.

At Cambridge, he became active in various university drama clubs and performances, and his friends included fellow students Kenneth Branagh, Emma Thompson, and Hugh Laurie, all of whom would be his future professional collaborators. In 1982, he graduated from Cambridge with High Honours and a degree in English literature.

His career blossomed almost immediately thereafter, beginning with the television comedy *Al Fresco*, which also featured Thompson and Laurie. His revised libretto for the 1930s Noel Gay musical *Me and My Girl* was adopted for the hit Broadway revival, making him a millionaire and winning him a Tony Award (1987).

Throughout the 1980s, Fry maintained an almost constant presence in the British media, appearing in stage plays, on radio, and, most extensively, on television, where he was featured in the popular series *Blackadder*, a spoof on British history, and as Jeeves the butler in *Jeeves and Wooster*, a series based on the P. G. Wodehouse novels.

During the late 1980s, Fry began a film career as well, appearing in supporting roles in such films as *A Fish Called Wanda* (1988) and *A Handful of Dust* (1988). His first major film part was that of the eponymous Peter in *Peter's Friends* (1992), which also starred Branagh and Thompson in a tale of a reunion of Cambridge school friends ten years after they had left school.

During this period, Fry embarked on yet another career, that of novelist. His novels, which display his wit and his ability to balance literary astuteness with utter vulgarity, so far include *The Liar* (1991), *The Hippopotamus* (1994), and *Making History* (1996).

Despite his successes, not all was well for Fry by the mid-1990s. Well-publicized personal insecurities had long kept him out of relationships, and a 1995 nervous breakdown brought much unsought media attention. His struggles, however, drew support from members of the public who are likewise afflicted with depression, and thus he was subsequently credited with drawing positive social attention to this greatly misunderstood illness.

The sympathy and empathy that his breakdown elicited were qualities with which Fry endowed his compassionate and very human portrayal of Oscar Wilde. The part, though often witty, allowed the actor to go beyond the comic portrayals with which he was most identified. Fry's layered depiction captured the complexity and contradictions of Wilde himself.

Fry's amusing yet emotionally honest autobiography, *Moab Is My Washpot* (1997), was published at the time *Wilde* was released, and gives the public an intimate portrait of the highly complex actor. Settled in a relationship at last, he lives with his partner in London and in his country home in Norfolk.

Most recently, he has starred in *The Discovery of Heaven* (2001) and was featured in *Gosford Park* (2001). He made an auspicious directorial debut with *Bright Young Things* (2003), based on his own adaptation of Evelyn Waugh's novel *Vile Bodies*.   —*Patricia Juliana Smith*

BIBLIOGRAPHY

Fry, Stephen. *Moab Is My Washpot.* London: Hutchinson, 1997.

Gray, Simon. *Fat Chance: The 'Stephen Fry Quits' Drama.* London and Boston: Faber and Faber, 1995.

SEE ALSO

British Television; Film Actors: Gay Male; Callow, Simon; McKellen, Sir Ian

g

Garbo, Greta
(1905–1990)

ONCE BILLED BY METRO-GOLDWYN-MAYER AS THE "Swedish sphinx," Greta Garbo is perhaps best known for her mystery. Raised in a culture that did not pursue or value celebrity, Garbo was frightened and horrified by the almost predatory interest that the American public took in movie stars.

Although she was a skilled and complex actress who created many memorable screen personae, she retired, not only from films but from any kind of public life, when she was only thirty-six.

Afterward, she lived in New York City in virtual seclusion for almost fifty years, refusing interviews or photographs and emerging from her apartment only when protected from public view by big hats and sunglasses.

Still, in spite of, or perhaps because of, the way she withheld herself, the public was mesmerized by her in a unique way. One need exclaim only the name Garbo! to evoke a gentle, passionate dignity as deep and complex as the Swedish sphinx herself.

Garbo began life in poverty as Greta Lovisa Gustafsson, the daughter of a janitor in Stockholm, Sweden. When her father died in 1919 of tuberculosis, Greta, just fourteen, had to quit school and go to work.

Her good looks helped her get jobs in a couple of advertising films before she was discovered in 1922 by unabashedly homosexual Swedish filmmaker Mauritz Stiller. He cast her as the female lead in *Gosta Berling's Saga* (1924) and got her a role in a German film, *The Joyless Street* (1925).

Stiller took control of the actress's career, changing her last name to Garbo. When he went to the United States to work for Louis Mayer at Metro-Goldwyn-Mayer, Stiller took his protégée along.

Mauritz Stiller did not succeed in Hollywood, but Greta Garbo was destined to become a star. She made fourteen silent films, among them *The Torment* (1926) and *Flesh and the Devil* (1927), in which she tended to play the beautiful femme fatale, luring men into passion.

Garbo made the rocky transition from silent films to talkies flawlessly. Her husky, accented voice fitted intriguingly with her ethereal beauty, enabling her to create more complex characters than she ever had in silents.

In *Anna Christie* (1930), *Anna Karenina* (1935), *Camille* (1936), and other films, she played a tragic heroine, passionate but doomed. In the delightful 1939 comedy *Ninotchka*, she mocks this gloomy sensuality with charming self-deprecation, causing MGM to tout the film with the single headline "Garbo Laughs!"

In 1941, prompted perhaps by the failure of *Two-Faced Woman*, her comedy follow-up to *Ninotchka*, Garbo took a break from filmmaking. Although she reportedly considered several projects for a comeback, the title roles in *Hamlet* and *The Portrait of Dorian Gray* among them, her break turned into permanent retirement.

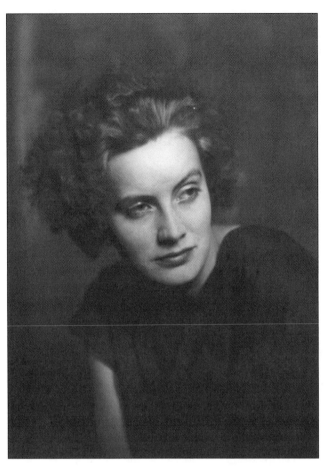

A portrait of Greta Garbo by Arnold Genthe (1925).

Garbo's smoldering aloofness, combined with her penchant for cross-dressing, ignited the passions of men and women alike. Although she never married or settled down, she had famous relationships with actor John Gilbert (whom she stood up at the altar in 1926), photographer Cecil Beaton, and businessman George Schlee, among many.

Garbo almost certainly had lesbian affairs as well, including well-known liaisons with actress Louise Brooks and writer Mercedes de Acosta, and perhaps also an affair with Marlene Dietrich.

For seven decades, lesbian audiences have drooled over the dashing figure of Garbo in drag as she appeared in *Queen Christina* (1933), dressed in pirate's garb, loose pants and shirt, with soft suede boots to the knee. In this film, through her butch mannerisms and cross-dressing, Garbo conveys a lesbian subtext that undermines the heterosexual plot. —*Tina Gianoulis*

BIBLIOGRAPHY

Daum, Raymond. *Walking with Garbo.* New York: HarperTrade, 1992,

Horton, Robert. "The Mysterious Lady." *Film Comment* 26.4 (July–August 1990): 30–33.

Karren, Howard. "The Star Who Fell to Earth." *Premiere* 4 (Winter 1991): 54–59.

Swenson, Karen. *Greta Garbo: A Life Apart.* New York: Simon & Schuster. 1997.

Vickers, Hugo. *Loving Garbo: The Story of Greta Garbo, Cecil Beaton, and Mercedes de Acosta.* New York: Random House, 1994.

SEE ALSO

Film; Film Actors: Lesbian; Transvestism in Film; Bankhead, Tallulah; Dietrich, Marlene; Goulding, Edmund; Murnau, Friedrich Wilhelm; Stiller, Mauritz

Garland, Judy　　　　　　(1922–1969)

To call Judy Garland an icon of the gay community is a massive understatement. Garland's fragile but indomitable persona and emotion-packed singing voice are undeniably linked to modern American gay culture and identity. This is especially true for gay men, but lesbians also are drawn to identify with Garland's plucky toughness and vulnerability.

Garland's signature song, "Over the Rainbow," is the closest thing we have to a gay national anthem, and many have claimed that it was grief over Garland's death from an overdose of drugs in June 1969 that sparked smoldering gay anger into the Stonewall riots and fueled the gay liberation movement. Whether true or not, this story has such poetry that one feels it ought to be true.

After all, in the intensely closeted pre-Stonewall days, gays often identified themselves to each other as "friends of Dorothy," referring to Garland's 1939 role in *The Wizard of Oz.*

Garland was virtually born a performer. Her parents owned a theater in Grand Rapids, Minnesota, where little Frances Gumm was born on June 10, 1922. She began singing and dancing on stage at the age of four. She toured in vaudeville, performing with her sisters, before being discovered in 1935 and signed to a contract with the Metro-Goldwyn-Mayer film studio.

She changed her name to Judy Garland and starred with Mickey Rooney in the *Andy Hardy* film series before being cast in her career-defining role in *The Wizard of Oz.*

Early in her career, studio doctors began giving Garland prescription drugs. The "speed" she took to lose weight made her too nervous to sleep, so she was given tranquilizers and sleeping pills, beginning a destructive cycle that would continue throughout her life and finally kill her.

Garland was painfully insecure; and, unfortunately, she began her career at a time when performers worked under contract to powerful studios and had little control over their careers. Her attempts to take charge of her career caused the studios to reject her as a troublemaker, but Garland's powerful talent and sheer heart propelled her through comeback after comeback.

After Garland's childhood career ended, she wowed audiences in her first adult role in *Meet Me in St. Louis* in 1944. In 1954, after more difficult years, she starred powerfully in *A Star is Born* with James Mason.

When the film roles were not offered, she went back on the concert stage, performing long runs at New York's Palace Theater. Despite an Academy Award nomination for a stunning performance in *Judgment at Nuremberg* (1961) and a brief but memorable television show on CBS (1963–1964), Garland found herself nearly penniless. Near the end of her life, she performed anywhere she could, even in piano bars when she could find no other work.

Garland was adored by gay fans throughout her career, but her connection to the world of homosexuality did not stop with her fans. Her beloved father, Frank Gumm, had been a closeted gay man, and Roger Edens, her strongest supporter in the early days at MGM, was also gay.

Even two of Garland's husbands, Vincente Minnelli and Mark Herron, were gay, which made possible an intergenerational *ménage* when Herron had an affair with Peter Allen, who was married to Garland's daughter Liza Minnelli.

Garland is surely one of the most memorable and indefatigable performers in the history of American popular entertainment. She made over thirty feature films, received a special Academy Award, and was nominated for two others. She also garnered several Emmy nominations and a special Tony Award.

Garland made numerous recordings, including the Grammy Award–winning *Judy at Carnegie Hall*, which has never been out of print. Her concert appearances became legendary, both for their triumphs and their spectacular failures.

Perhaps the most touching, and telling, image of Judy Garland, embedded in the memories of gay men and lesbians of a certain age, is the way she ended many of her concerts. Dressed in drag as a hobo, her smudged face showing the pathos of the eternal outsider, she approaches the audience and sits on the edge of the stage. Looking far into the distance, she sings "Somewhere Over the Rainbow" with intense, lonely sweetness, longing for that impossible land where dreams come true. —*Tina Gianoulis*

Bibliography

Clarke, Gerald. *Get Happy: The Life of Judy Garland*. New York: Random House, 2000.

DiOrio, Al, Jr. *Little Girl Lost: The Life & Hard Times of Judy Garland*. Greenwich, Conn.: Kearny Publishing, 1975.

Gross, Michael Joseph. "The Queen Is Dead." *Atlantic Monthly*, August 2000, 62.

Guly, Christopher. "The Judy Connection." *Advocate*, June 28, 1994, 48.

Vare, Eehlie A. *Rainbow: A Star Studded Tribute to Judy Garland*. New York: Boulevard Books, 1998.

See also

Film; Edens, Roger; Minnelli, Vincente

Gielgud, Sir John (1904–2000)

Sir John Gielgud has long been acknowledged as one of the greatest British actors of the twentieth century. A highly versatile performer, he played leading and character roles on both stage and screen, in every genre from classical tragedy to low comedy. While he was in many ways reticent about his sexuality, his experiences illustrate the significant changes in public attitude toward homosexuality over the decades.

Arthur John Gielgud was born in London on April 14, 1904, to a family with theatrical backgrounds on both sides. His father was the son of a Lithuanian actress, and, through his mother, he was the great-nephew of Dame Ellen Terry, the most renowned British actress of the nineteenth century.

Gielgud began acting in his teens, joining the Old Vic theater company in 1921, and making his film debut in the silent picture *Who Is That Man?* (1923). Soon thereafter, Gielgud became Noël Coward's understudy, eventually taking over the lead roles in Coward's play *The Vortex* (1924) and Margaret Kennedy's *The Constant Nymph* (1924).

Other successes followed quickly, as Gielgud began to play major Shakespearean roles at the Old Vic, beginning with Romeo, and, before he was thirty, the more mature lead roles in *Richard II*, *The Tempest*, *Macbeth*, *Hamlet*, and *King Lear*.

During this time, he began his first major romantic relationship. Actor John Perry lived with him until their separation in the early 1940s.

By the 1930s, Gielgud was a box-office idol—a rather unlikely one, given his bulbous nose and unprepossessing figure; indeed, his detractors thought his Romeo "feminine." His great gifts were his catlike mobility and, most notably, his expressive voice, which fellow actor Alec Guinness described as being "like a silver trumpet muffled in silk."

Gielgud also became a respected stage director, launching his own distinguished company in 1937 at the Queen's Theatre. He directed and often performed in productions of Shakespeare and such classics as *School for Scandal*, *Three Sisters*, and *The Importance of Being Earnest*.

In 1953, Gielgud was named in Queen Elizabeth's Coronation Honors List as the recipient of a rather belated knighthood. That this honor came about at all was the result of two of his knighted colleagues, Laurence Olivier and Ralph Richardson, pleading with Prime Minister Winston Churchill to remedy the grievous oversight.

As Gielgud's homosexuality was generally known if not publicly acknowledged in a time when sexual acts between men were still a criminal offense in Britain (and remained so until 1967), the government had been reluctant to bestow its approval on him.

Given the controversy over his knighthood, it was cruelly ironic that, within months of receiving the honor, Gielgud was involved in an embarrassing incident that might have been fatally damaging to his career.

During the early 1950s, British legal authorities conducted a veritable persecution of gay men that resulted in criminal charges against a number of prominent figures. Gielgud was arrested outside a public lavatory in Chelsea for "importuning for an immoral purpose," and the press conducted a vitriolic campaign against him.

Gielgud nonetheless received a standing ovation upon his next stage appearance, and his arrest is thought to have been instrumental in starting the process of decriminalization. (The incident did not, moreover, prevent the Queen from granting him two further distinctions, the Companion of Honour in 1977 and the Order of Merit in 1996.)

But, having been so deeply humiliated, Sir John never spoke publicly about the matter or his sexuality again, and he was banned from entering the United States for the next four years.

After World War II, Gielgud's career shifted, as he began to appear with greater frequency in the character roles for which he is now best remembered. With the advent of the Angry Young Men of the 1950s, Gielgud's acting style was greatly out of fashion on the British stage, and, accordingly, he appeared more frequently in motion pictures.

He acted in more than 130 films in his long career, the greater portion of which were made between the 1960s and the 1980s; and in 1982 he received the Academy Award for Best Supporting Actor for his portrayal of the sardonic butler in *Arthur*.

Finding it increasingly difficult to commit lengthy dialogue to memory, Gielgud retired from the stage in 1988, but continued to perform in films nearly until the end of his life. At the age of eighty-six, he had his first nude scene in *Prospero's Books* (1991), and he subsequently appeared in *Shine* (1996), *The Portrait of a Lady* (1996), and *Elizabeth* (1998).

In 1999, he was deeply bereaved by the death of his partner, Martin Hensler, with whom he had lived for nearly forty years. Within months, on May 21, 2000, Gielgud himself passed away quietly at his home in Aylesbury, Buckinghamshire, at age ninety-six.

—*Patricia Juliana Smith*

Bibliography

Brandreth, Gyles. *John Gielgud: A Celebration*. Boston: Little, Brown, 1984.

Croall, Jonathan. *Gielgud: A Theatrical Life*. London: Methuen, 2000.

Francis, Clive. *Sir John: The Many Faces of Gielgud*. London: Robson, 1995.

Gielgud, John. *An Actor and His Time*. London: Sidgwick & Jackson, 1979.

_____. *Backward Glances*. London: Hodder & Stoughton, 1989.

_____. *Distinguished Company*. London: Heinemann, 1972.

Harwood, Ronald, ed. *The Ages of Gielgud: An Actor at Eighty*. New York: Limelight Editions, 1984.

Morley, Sheridan. *John Gielgud: A Biography*. London: Hodder & Stoughton, 1995.

Tanitch, Robert. *Gielgud*. London: Harrap, 1988.

See also

Film Actors: Gay Male; British Television

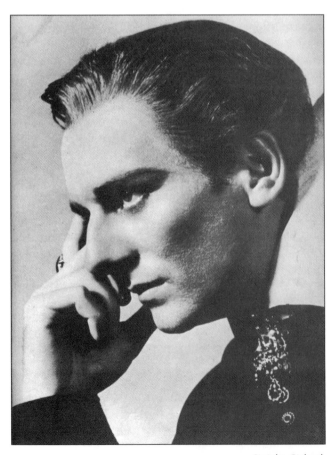

Sir John Gielgud.

Goulding, Edmund (1891–1959)

EDMUND GOULDING WAS ONE OF THE MOST TALENTED and eccentric characters of golden age Hollywood. He was a singer, actor, composer, screenwriter, and novelist, but he primarily excelled as a director. His romantic nature and sexual attraction to men endeared him to actresses, and for a time he was considered a great "woman's director," the equal of George Cukor.

Goulding was born in London on March 20, 1891, during the twilight of the Victorian age. The son of a butcher, Goulding began acting in amateur theatricals and by 1909 began appearing on the West End in productions such as *Gentlemen, The King* (1909), *Alice in Wonderland* (1909), and a notorious presentation of Oscar Wilde's *The Picture of Dorian Gray* (1913), adapted for the stage by G. Constant Lounsbery.

Goulding served in World War I, then emigrated to the United States to become a singer. He was a fine idea man, and could crank out a silent screen scenario very quickly. His writing talents were in demand by producers at Paramount and Famous Players–Lasky, and so his singing aspirations were shelved. He wrote for several early film stars, and he met his greatest success as coauthor of Henry King's *Tol'able David*, a 1921 silent masterpiece.

Goulding directed Joan Crawford in her first substantial role, in *Sally, Irene and Mary* (1925), and Greta Garbo and John Gilbert in the smash hit *Love* (1927), before writing the script for *Broadway Melody* (1929), the first film musical.

Goulding directed Gloria Swanson in her first talkie, *The Trespasser* (1929), and Nancy Carroll in *The Devil's Holiday* (1929). However, his greatest triumph came as director of Metro-Goldwyn-Mayer's *Grand Hotel,* winner of the 1932 Academy Award as Best Picture and granddaddy of the all-star ensemble story format.

Subsequent assignments at MGM include *Blondie of the Follies* (1932), with Marion Davies and Robert Montgomery, and *Riptide* (1934), with Norma Shearer, the latter from a Goulding script.

Goulding moved to Warner Brothers in 1937, where he directed some of his best movies: *Dawn Patrol* (1938), *White Banners* (1938), and four outstanding melodramas with Bette Davis: *That Certain Woman* (1937), *Dark Victory* (1939), *The Old Maid* (1939), and *The Great Lie* (1941).

The Constant Nymph (1943), with Joan Fontaine, *Claudia* (1943), with Dorothy McGuire, and *Of Human Bondage* (1946), with Eleanor Parker were further testimonies to Goulding's adept direction of actresses.

After World War II, Goulding was hired at Twentieth Century Fox and made two excellent movies of starkly contrasting themes: *The Razor's Edge* (1946), based on a novel by Somerset Maugham, and the noir thriller

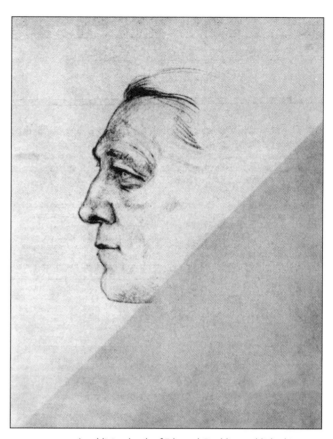

A publicity sketch of Edmund Goulding published in 1939.

Nightmare Alley (1947), both featuring Tyrone Power at his best.

Goulding's output after that was uneven. He made the comedies *Everybody Does It* (1949); *Mr. 880* (1950), with Burt Lancaster; and *We're Not Married* (1952), with Marilyn Monroe and Ginger Rogers. His last movie was *Mardi Gras* (1958), a dismissible musical starring Pat Boone.

By then, the man who directed the great stars of early moviedom was old, tired, and alcoholic. He died of a heart attack in 1959.

Goulding's style as a director is distinguished by brisk pacing and an ability to elicit honest emotion from his players. He mastered a number of genres—comedy, romance, musicals, noir, and the war picture—and he adapted well to the personnel and conditions of each studio for which he worked.

There is a paradox to Goulding. His sensitivity to women's emotions brought him enduring success, as witnessed by his swooning melodramas, but his private life reflects a lack of sensitivity. Goulding was bisexual, with a decided taste for promiscuity and voyeurism. His sex parties and casting couch were notorious.

But he cannot be dismissed simply as a sex addict or sexual exploiter. For every excoriation of his morals, there are accounts of his loyalty to friends, generosity to family, gentlemanly manner on the set, and preternatural ability to bring out the best in his actors.

He never had a long-lasting romance. A marriage to dancer Marjorie Moss ended quickly with her premature death of tuberculosis. He maintained brief love affairs with younger men and women throughout his life, but either did not want or proved unable to sustain a long-term relationship.

The real romance in Edmund Goulding's life is found in his movies.   —*Matthew Kennedy*

BIBLIOGRAPHY

Brooks, Louise. "Why I Will Never Write My Memoirs." *Focus on Film* 15 (March 1978): 29–34.

Katz, Ephraim. *The Film Encyclopedia.* New York: Harper Perennial, 1994.

Meyer, William R. *Warner Brothers Directors.* New Rochelle: Arlington House, 1978.

Swanson, Gloria. *Swanson on Swanson.* New York: Random House, 1980.

Walker, Michael. "Edmund Goulding." *Film Dope* 20 (April 1980): 32–34.

SEE ALSO

Film Directors; Cukor, George; Garbo, Greta

Grant, Cary   *(1904–1986)*

CARY GRANT EMBODIED THE ELEGANCE, CHARM, AND sophistication of Hollywood in its golden years. His good looks, charisma, and ambiguous sexuality enchanted women and men alike. As the starstruck comedian Steve Lawrence once said, "When Cary Grant walked into a room, not only did the women primp, the men straightened their ties."

Born Archibald Alexander Leach on January 18, 1904, near Bristol, England, Grant began his career in vaudeville. In 1932, he signed with Paramount and moved to Hollywood, where he developed the debonair persona that made him famous.

After appearing in half a dozen films, his big break came when the sultry Mae West handpicked him to star with her in *She Done Him Wrong* (1933). Based on West's Broadway hit *Diamond Lil*, the film made Grant a bankable star.

Appearing in seventy-two films from 1932 to 1966, Cary Grant combined urbanity with a down-to-earth charm. Starring with the most ravishing female stars of the time, such as Katharine Hepburn, Sophia Loren, Deborah Kerr, Ingrid Bergman, and Audrey Hepburn, Grant exuded romance, refinement, and, perhaps most

surprisingly, humor. As C. K. Dexter Haven in George Cukor's *The Philadelphia Story* (1941), with Katharine Hepburn, he added the crucial sophistication necessary to screwball comedy.

Most directors Grant worked with, including the celebrated Howard Hawks, Frank Capra, and Peter Bogdanovich, were content simply to use Grant as the elegant leading man audiences adored. But Alfred Hitchcock was attracted to the actor's darker side. Grant gave some of his best performances in *Suspicion* (1941), *Notorious* (1946), *To Catch a Thief* (1955), and *North by Northwest* (1959), playing brooding, enigmatic, and troubled characters.

Rumors of Grant's homosexuality swirled early in his career and followed him throughout his life. Grant and his close friends consistently denied rumors of his homosexuality or bisexuality. Although he had many failed relationships with women (he married five times) and numerous gay friends, including actor William Haines and Australian artist Jack Kelly (later a set designer professionally known as Orry Kelly), with whom he lived briefly in Greenwich Village, there is no conclusive evidence that Grant was bisexual.

The rumors of Grant's bisexuality were sparked principally by his close friendship with Randolph Scott, his live-in companion and costar in *My Favorite Wife*

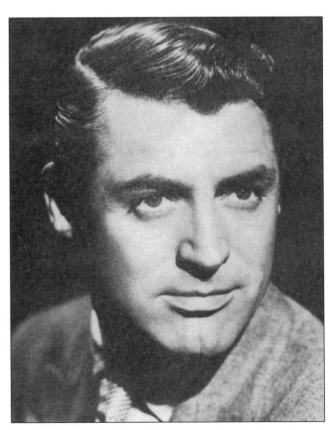

A portrait of Cary Grant published in 1946.

(1940). The two shared a Santa Monica beach home from 1935 to 1942.

Paramount started an intense publicity campaign, including photos of them in domestic scenes, promoting Grant and Scott as the epitome of Hollywood's new young man. More camp than intimate, these staged photos offer no real insight into the private nature of their relationship. They stopped living together when Grant married his second wife, Barbara Hutton, but the two remained close friends throughout their lives.

Although most of his career was spent playing a static archetype, Grant was unafraid to take risks, professionally or privately. He is credited with using the word *gay* for the first time in a homosexual context on screen. In *Bringing Up Baby* (1938), Grant plays a shy paleontologist against Katharine Hepburn's spoiled New York heiress. During one scene, Grant appears in a frilly pink dressing gown and to incredulous observers delivers his famous line "because I just went gay all of a sudden."

Grant sported women's clothing again in the lesser-known film *I Was a Male War Bride* (1949). He also became the first Hollywood star to admit to using LSD as part of psychotherapy in the late 1950s.

Knowing his audience did not want to see him age, Grant retired from films in the 1960s, secure as one of Hollywood's brightest stars. He died on November 29, 1986.

—Julia Pastore

BIBLIOGRAPHY

Higham, Charles, and Ray Moseley. *Cary Grant: The Lonely Heart.* New York: Harcourt Brace, 1989.

McCann, Graham. *Cary Grant: A Class Apart.* New York: Columbia University Press, 1996.

Wansell, Geoffrey. *Cary Grant: Dark Angel.* New York: Arcade Publishing, 1996.

SEE ALSO

Film; Film Actors: Gay Male; Transvestism in Film; Cukor, George; Haines, William "Billy"

Greyson, John   (b. 1960)

INTERNATIONALLY RECOGNIZED AS AN AVANT-GARDE filmmaker and video artist, John Greyson was born in Nelson, British Columbia, but spent most of his childhood and teenage years in London, Ontario. He lived in New York for a brief time during the 1970s, but in 1980 moved to Toronto, where he wrote for *The Body Politic* and local art and cultural magazines.

Greyson began as a video and performance artist before taking up cinema as a full-time vocation. Although

he was a resident at the Norman Jewison Canadian Film Centre in 1990, he is largely self-taught as a filmmaker.

Greyson has never flinched from confronting contentious topics. The vast majority of his work, the earliest of which dates from 1978, boldly presents socially relevant themes, especially issues related to homosexuality, gay rights, and AIDS activism.

His films document the trials and tribulations of Toronto's gay community, while also dealing with such topics as race (*A Moffie Called Simon,* 1986), censorship and copyright (*Uncut,* 1997), police harassment and surveillance (*Breathing Through Opposing Nostrils,* 1982; *Urinal,* 1988), and the AIDS crisis (*The AIDS Epidemic,* 1987; *Angry Initiatives, Defiant Strategies,* 1988; *The World Is Sick (Sic),* 1989; *The Pink Pimpernel,* 1989; and *Zero Patience,* 1993).

Recently, Greyson has begun to deepen his already wide repertoire of themes to include focused studies of love and relationships (*Lilies,* 1996; *Law of Enclosures,* 1999). Stylistically, his work runs the gamut from the whimsical (*Zero Patience*) to the poetic (*Lilies*). His films often interweave multiple story lines and are exceedingly involved compositionally.

Greyson's work may best be understood in terms of the drama theory advanced by Bertolt Brecht (1898–1956), who believed that the goal of drama was not to evoke an emotional response or identification with the figures who appear on stage but to cause an audience to think critically. Brecht thought that the use of historical characters in contemporary drama would prevent an audience from overly identifying with characters and induce them to contemplate the underlying message of a work.

Thus, Greyson features historical figures in many of his films and videos. For example, *Urinal,* the story of police control of public-washroom sex in Ontario, features such historical and fictional figures as Dorian Gray, Frances Loring and Florence Wyle, Langston Hughes, Frida Kahlo, and others.

In *Zero Patience,* Greyson confronts the topic of AIDS through an unlikely genre, the musical comedy. In this feature-length work, the filmmaker responds to the sudden glut of death by navigating a plethora of emotional and intellectual concerns and pronouncements regarding individual and media representations of AIDS, while also attempting to maintain a critical distance from other films that sentimentalize the disease.

Critics have not always responded positively to Greyson's films. However, *Lilies,* based on a play by the openly gay Quebec playwright Michel Marc Bouchard (b. 1957), is the exception.

A historical dramatization of a schoolboy love story, it is set primarily in a Quebec prison in the 1950s and tells the story of Bishop Bilodeau, who, having gone to hear a dying convict's confession, is held captive by conspiring guards and prisoners and forced to reveal his own sins. As the bishop watches through the confessional's keyhole, scenes from his past are brought to life, including his love for a fellow classmate and the tragedy that followed.

The film received four Genie Awards from the Academy of Canadian Cinema and Television, including one for Best Picture.

Greyson's most recent feature, *Proteus* (2003), is based on the transcript of a 1735 sodomy trial. It explores an interracial relationship in the South African prison on Robben Island.

In addition to his film work, Greyson has also directed for television, including an episode of the American version of *Queer As Folk*.   —*Eugenio Filice*

BIBLIOGRAPHY

Gever, Martha, John Greyson, and Pratibha Parmar. *Queer Looks: Perspectives on Lesbian and Gay Film and Video.* Toronto: Between the Lines, 1993.

Greyson, John. *Urinal and Other Stories.* Toronto: Art Metropole + The Power Plant, 1993.

Klusacek, Allan, and Ken Morrison, eds. *A Leap in the Dark: AIDS, Art and Contemporary Cultures.* Montreal: Artexte Information Centre and Véhicule Press, 1993.

Miller, James, ed. *Fluid Exchanges: Artists and Critics in the AIDS Crisis.* Toronto: University of Toronto Press, 1992.

SEE ALSO

New Queer Cinema; Screenwriters; Praunheim, Rosa von

Grinbergs, Andris   (b. 1946)

DIFFICULT AS IT IS TO OVERSTATE THE HAZARDS OF making art that positively, compellingly expresses homosexual desire within a Western homophobic society, the risks that Soviet artists faced if they dared to express affirmative homosexual content were horrific, including incarceration in a psychiatric prison or a staged "suicide" at the hands of KGB agents.

Despite the potentially lethal consequences of living as a bisexual and working as a nonconformist artist under totalitarianism, Latvian performance artist Andris Grinbergs pioneered Happenings, body art, and underground filmmaking in Soviet-occupied Latvia from the late 1960s onward.

Born on March 3, 1946, Grinbergs was training as a clothing designer at Riga's Applied Arts School when the so-called youthquake brought international hippie fashion to cities on the western periphery of the Soviet Union. Before long, he was outfitting his fellow flower children in bell-bottomed jeans and lacy, unisex blouses—that is, if they chose to wear anything.

When these aspiring artists, writers, and musicians participated in the numerous Happenings organized by Grinbergs, he designed their highly imaginative costuming, much of which was designed to come off.

From the beginning—including the 1972 Happening *The Wedding of Jesus Christ*, during which Grinbergs married his lifelong (female) partner Inta Jaunzeme—these performances celebrated same-sex passion.

In 1972, a time when even representations of heterosexual eroticism were curbed by Soviet censors, Grinbergs directed the short film *Self-Portrait*, which forthrightly depicted his bisexuality. The artist tenderly kisses a man in a public toilet, enfolds a near-naked youth in his fur coat, and cuddles in bed with another man, both of them nude, while a party proceeds around them.

Elsewhere in this carnivalesque setting, a trio of naked women dance together, one of them deflating a man's balloon phallus with a burning cigarette when he amorously approaches her; and a homoerotic vignette recalls the martyrdom of St. Sebastian.

The central third of the film features Grinbergs and Jaunzeme copulating, seen from the shoulders up in the reticent manner of Andy Warhol's film *Blow Job*. The montage of campy artifice and nude performance-art documentation resumes in the final third of *Self-Portrait*, concluding with a playful shot of Grinbergs in bed with his wife and his male cinematographer.

Two weeks after the film's completion, its sole print escaped discovery when KGB agents raided Grinbergs's flat during a private, unsanctioned photography exhibit. For twenty-three years, *Self-Portrait* remained concealed in fragmentary form in Riga.

After its 1996 restoration and premiere at Anthology Film Archives in New York, filmmaker and independent film authority Jonas Mekas proclaimed *Self-Portrait* "one of the five most sexually transgressive films ever made." Mekas's judgment is all the more impressive in light of his own arrest record for screening landmarks of queer cinema in the mid-1960s. *Self-Portrait* must be placed in the company of films by Warhol, Kenneth Anger, Jean Genet, and Jack Smith.

Throughout the 1970s and 1980s, Grinbergs defied official Soviet proscriptions with performances inspired by phenomena as disparate as medieval sacral mysteries, the Baader-Meinhof Gang, and Bo Widerberg's film *Elvira Madigan*. After Communism's demise, Grinbergs marked his forty-fifth birthday and Latvia's passage to democracy by staging an event at which cake was served from the nude torso of the prime minister's son.

Grinbergs remains active today, his art's homoerotic content steadily expanding not only in the performance genre, but also in collages that combine gay porn magazines, classic disco album sleeves from Casablanca Records, and photographs of his male lovers.   —*Mark Allen Svede*

BIBLIOGRAPHY

Bilzens, Indulis, ed. *RIGA. Lettische Avantgarde.* West Berlin: Elefanten Press, 1988.

Svede, Mark Allen. "All You Need is Lovebeads: Latvia's Hippies Undress for Success." *Style and Socialism: Modernity and Material Culture in Post-War Eastern Europe.* David Crowley and Susan Reid, eds. London: Berg, 2000. 189–208.

_____. "'Blue' Filmmaker, 'Blue' Milieu." "Gay and Lesbian Art." Chris Reed, ed. New York and London: Thames & Hudson, forthcoming.

_____. "Twiggy & Trotsky: Or, What the Soviet Dandy Will Be Wearing This Five-Year Plan." *Dandies: Fashion and Finesse in Art and Culture.* Susan Fillin-Yeh, ed. New York: New York University Press, 2001. 243–269.

SEE ALSO

Film; Anger, Kenneth; Warhol, Andy

h

Haines, William "Billy"   (1900–1973)

MORE THAN THIRTY YEARS AFTER THE STONEWALL riots, it is difficult to conceive of creating an openly gay identity in a world with few precedents or examples, but such was the world in which actor and decorator William Haines was born.

As a motion picture actor, William "Billy" Haines is largely forgotten today, but in 1930 he was the number one box-office draw and was among the top five motion picture actors from 1928 to 1933. After the end of his acting career, he became one of the country's most successful interior decorators.

Haines was born in Staunton, Virginia, on January 1, 1900. The eldest of four children, he was a product of a respected upper-middle-class family. At the age of fourteen, he ran away from home, accompanied by a boy Haines in later life referred to as "his first boyfriend." After a brief return to Virginia, Haines became a resident of Greenwich Village, where he pursued a life unfettered by provincial constraints.

In New York, he became friends with Boston-born Mitchell ("Mit") Foster and Australian artist Jack Kelly (professionally known as Orry Kelly), who was then the boyfriend of English circus performer Archie Leach, later known as Cary Grant. These early friendships became significant lifelong relationships.

Foster moved to California and in 1928 became Haines's business partner in an antique store there, which evolved into Haines's decorating business. Orry Kelly also went to Hollywood, where he become an Oscar-winning costume designer for such films as *An American in Paris* (1951), *Les Girls* (1957), and *Some Like It Hot* (1959).

Haines's journey to Hollywood films began in New York, where he won a national talent search, the "new faces" of 1922, sponsored by Samuel Goldwyn Studios. After a successful screen test, he was signed as a contract player; and in 1922 he departed for California with the female winner, Eleanor Boardman.

Boardman and Haines arrived in Los Angeles amid studio-orchestrated fanfare that presaged Boardman's immediate placement in a starring vehicle. Haines's welcome was less auspicious, as he was given uncredited and nonspeaking bit parts from 1922 to 1924. His first real opportunity was four and a half minutes of credited screen time, ironically in an Eleanor Boardman vehicle, *Souls for Sale* (1923).

Haines's first success and leading role came in 1924 with *Midnight Express*. The melodrama offered a glimpse of the character who would be his trademark: the irresponsible or easygoing smart aleck who is redeemed by crisis or tragedy.

Haines's status as a leading man was not confirmed until *Brown of Harvard* and *Mike* in 1926. These films, and *Tell It to the Marines* the following year, propelled him to the top of his profession.

Haines was one of the few silent film actors to make the transition to sound with little trauma. He possessed an easy Southern-edged baritone that matched his affable movie persona. His sound debut, *Alias Jimmy Valentine* (1929), was a financial as well as artistic triumph for MGM.

Subsequently, Haines's films became formulaic, but they remained popular. By 1930, he was receiving more mail than any other male star at MGM.

Despite his successful transition to talking pictures, however, his career was cut short. According to Hollywood legend, Metro-Goldwyn-Mayer studio chief Louis B. Mayer allegedly forced Haines to choose between his film career and his homosexual lifestyle. It may be, however, that Haines himself decided to retire gracefully from films when he began to lose his youthful good looks. He had always wanted to pursue his other love, interior design.

Beginning in 1926, Haines lived openly as a couple with Jimmy Shields (a former movie stand-in). The public relations "solution" for most acknowledged gay actors and actresses in the studios was the conspiratorial sham marriage affecting an outwardly "respectable" and heterosexual facade. Haines, however, refused to give up Jimmy Shields for the sake of his film career, and the relationship endured until Haines's death in 1973.

Haines's transition to full-time interior designer coincided with the loss of his MGM contract in 1934. Using his antique business as a base, Haines became a prominent interior decorator whose clients included the elite of Hollywood's golden age: Carole Lombard, Joan Crawford, Claudette Colbert, William Powell, George Cukor, and Jack Warner.

Haines exorcised the pseudo-Spanish motif that had dominated the grand movie-industry residences since the 1920s. He single-handedly created the "California Style": one in which pristine antiques and his signature hand-painted Chinese wallpapers and ceramics coexisted in astute eclecticism with the West Coast lifestyle, incorporating modern Art Deco materials and movie-star splendor.

In addition to decorating the homes of Hollywood royalty, Haines decorated the homes of other high-profile wealthy clients. For example, he decorated several residences of retail magnates Alfred Bloomingdale and Tom May and their wives.   —*Benjamin Trimmier*

Bibliography

Mann, William J. *Wisecracker: The Life and Times of William Haines, Hollywood's First Openly Gay Star.* New York: Viking Penguin, 1998.

Wentink, A. M. "Haines, (Charles) William ('Billy')." *Who's Who in Gay and Lesbian History from Antiquity to World War II.* Robert Aldrich and Garry Wotherspoon, eds. London and New York: Routledge, 2001. 197–198.

See also

Film Actors: Gay Male; Bankhead, Tallulah; Cukor, George; Grant, Cary; Webb, Clifton

Hammer, Barbara   (b. *1939*)

BARBARA HAMMER HAS CREATED OVER EIGHTY EXPERImental shorts, videos, and features to date. She is the most prolific lesbian feminist filmmaker in the history of cinema.

Hammer was born in Hollywood on May 15, 1939. She did not formally study film; she was educated in psychology, art, and English literature at UCLA and San Francisco State University.

Hammer combined some of her early activist and aesthetic interests as a teacher at Marin County (California) Juvenile Hall, but in 1967—at the age of twenty-eight—she shot her first film, *Schizy*, about her own coming-out process. This template proved to be a durable one; most of Hammer's work is both personal and political. She uses cinema to inspire viewers to "leave the theater with fresh perceptions and emboldened to take active and political stances for social change in a global environment."

The formerly heterosexual Hammer, who divorced her husband a year after *Schizy*, has worked exclusively in experimental, nonlinear forms as a means of overcoming the patriarchal bias in conventional filmmaking and its attendant processes of marketing and distribution.

Hammer's radical separatist stance triggered a controversy early in her career. For the debut of her sexually explicit 1974 short *Dyketactics*, generally cited as the first film celebrating lesbian love to be made by a lesbian, she insisted that the film be seen only by female audiences.

Hammer's desire to reach larger audiences soon led her away from radical separatism into a more inclusive, often lyrical approach. She has cited pioneering feminist auteur Maya Deren as an influence in this transformation, particularly Deren's dreamlike *Meshes of the Afternoon* (1943).

Hammer's "goddess" films, such as *Women's Rites* (1974) and *Sappho* (1978), are typical of this stage of her work. These films intermingle erotic imagery with a sense of fantasy to create a lesbian cinema that avoids the objectifying male gaze. Also during the 1970s, the director continued her explorations of female sexuality in works such as *Multiple Orgasm* (1977).

Hammer can be said to have constructed, in what she has called her "alternative autobiographies," an alternative lesbian gaze. She is most often her own subject, from this early period, with works like *I Was/I Am* (1973), where she appears in both motorcycle drag and a gown, to the later, more ambitious films such as *Tender Fictions* (1995), whose goal is to reassert the presence of the lesbian in cinema.

Tender Fictions typifies Hammer's sometimes dazzling formalism, and like much of her work it demands, and rewards, a close reading. The film is built from a vast array of raw materials: scratchy home movies; snapshots; voice-overs from academic texts; interviews; skewed television

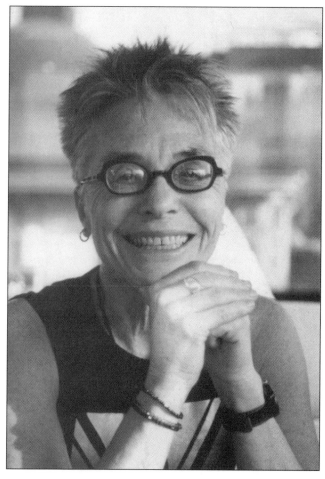

Barbara Hammer.

programs; interviews with family and friends and a string of ex-girlfriends.

The film is fearless in probing its author–subject. In a sequence on the influence of the mother–daughter relationship on lesbians, she recalls rejecting her dying mother's plea that she climb in bed with her: "That's incest—I can't!"

Hammer's most famous work is probably *Nitrate Kisses* (1992), like *Tender Fictions* a striking attempt to restore a lost queer history, this time by intermingling images of lesbian and gay male lovemaking with aural and visual collages of concentration camps, the Hollywood Hays Code that banned "perversion," and snippets from what is often regarded as the first queer film made in the United States, *Lot in Sodom* (1933) by James Watson and Melville Weber.

Part of the importance of *Nitrate Kisses* is in its double breakthrough in showing not only lesbians, but mature lesbians, making love.

Recent works such as *History Lessons* (2000) effectively mine some of the same areas. They wittily weave clips from Hollywood melodramas, high school sex-education pictures, and excerpts from newsreels and nudist films into a sweeping canvas of the history of queer sexuality and identity.

Hammer is both a filmmaker and a theorist (see, for example, her important essay "The Politics of Abstraction" in *Queer Looks: Perspectives on Lesbian and Gay Film and Video*), but while her films have political and theoretical underpinnings, they are also among the most thoughtful and unabashed celebrations of queer life.   —*Gary Morris*

BIBLIOGRAPHY

Hammer, Barbara. "The Politics of Abstraction." *Queer Looks: Perspectives on Lesbian and Gay Film and Video*. Pratibha Parmara, Martha Gever, and John Greyson, eds. New York: Routledge, 1993. 70–75.

Harvey, Dennis, "History Lessons." *Variety*, July 10, 2000.

Kaplan, E. Ann. *Women and Film: Both Sides of the Camera.* New York: Methuen, 1983.

Morris, Gary. "Tender Fictions: Barbara Hammer's Truth Club." *Bright Lights Film Journal* 17: www.brightlightsfilm.com/17/08c_tender.html

Zita, Jacqueline. "Counter Currencies of a Lesbian Iconography: The Films of Barbara Hammer." *Jump Cut* 24 (1981).

SEE ALSO

Film; Film Directors; Documentary Film

Hawthorne, Sir Nigel   *(1929–2001)*

BEFORE HIS 1994 PERFORMANCE IN THE TITLE ROLE IN Nicholas Hytner's film *The Madness of King George*, Nigel Hawthorne's reputation was that of a highly professional and versatile character actor. His long career comprised mostly supporting roles for stage, film, and British television.

In March 1995, in the wake of tremendous critical acclaim for his most noted role thus far, the *Advocate* described Hawthorne as "the first openly gay actor to be nominated for a Best Actor [Academy] Award." This article resulted in his unlikely and apparently reluctant self-outing.

Nigel Barnard Hawthorne was born on April 5, 1929, in Coventry, England, and emigrated with his family to South Africa at the age of two. He was educated at a strict Catholic school for boys, where the faculty's favored mode of discipline was corporal punishment. It was here, according to his recollections, that he first realized he was gay.

In 1951, after a short stint at the University of Cape Town, Hawthorne made his acting debut in a South African theater. He moved to England the following year and made his London debut in the musical comedy *You Can't Take It With You*. Success and significant roles eluded him, so he returned to South Africa, only to return to England once again in 1962.

Throughout the 1960s and 1970s, Hawthorne appeared in numerous British stage productions, demonstrating his versatility in Shakespearean roles as well as in contemporary drama and light comedy. His motion picture career began inauspiciously with an uncredited role in Richard Attenborough's *Young Winston* (1972), and he occasionally played character roles in film and on British television over the next two decades.

Although success did not come to Nigel Hawthorne during the first quarter century of his career, the second quarter century proved very different. In 1977, he received his first major recognition as the recipient of the Clarence Derwent Award and the Society of West End Theatres Award for Best Supporting Actor in Peter Nichols's *Privates on Parade*.

Subsequently, he began what would be his most enduring role, that of the scheming Sir Humphrey Appleby in the popular British television comedy series *Yes, Minister* (later *Yes, Prime Minister*), which ran from 1980 to 1992. When these series were aired on PBS, Hawthorne's bravura performance as Sir Humphrey made him a familiar face to American audiences.

In 1989, Hawthorne starred as C. S. Lewis in the London production of *Shadowlands*; he then earned the 1991 Tony Award for his performances in the play's two-year run on Broadway. (Anthony Hopkins, for reasons of name recognition, was chosen as the lead for the film version.)

Hawthorne's sensitive portrayal of a man awakening to love in middle age garnered him the lead (as George III) in Nicholas Hytner's 1992 London staging of Alan Bennett's *The Madness of King George*, for which he won the Olivier Award. He was subsequently cast in the same director's 1994 film version, and received the British Academy Award for Best Actor as well as a nomination for the American Academy Award.

Beginning in the late 1970s, Hawthorne lived openly with his partner, writer Trevor Bentham. While never exactly closeted about his sexuality, Hawthorne had chosen to protect his private life from the intrusion of the press.

Shortly before the 1995 Academy Awards ceremony, however, he granted an interview to the *Advocate* in which he discussed his life and relationship. Although the ensuing article was sympathetic, Hawthorne has stated that the magazine did not honor his request that his privacy be respected, and he was apparently traumatized by the sensational press coverage that resulted from the article.

Following that traumatic outing, Hawthorne spoke more openly and freely about his personal life and made a notable film appearance as an unambiguously gay character in Hytner's *The Object of My Affection* (1998). Moreover, his outing did not diminish or alter the success for which he strove over nearly five decades. Indeed, in 1999, he was knighted by Queen Elizabeth II.

Hawthorne also contributed an acclaimed performance as the authoritarian father in David Mamet's 1999 film adaptation of Terence Rattigan's *The Winslow Boy*, a study of a family under the stress of public scrutiny.

After battling pancreatic cancer for two years, Hawthorne died of a heart attack on December 26, 2001.

—*Patricia Juliana Smith*

BIBLIOGRAPHY

Barber, Lynn. "The King and I." *Observer Magazine*, September 5, 1999, 14.

Clarkin, Michelle. "Acting Out." *Advocate*, April 4, 1995, 45.

Koenig, Rhoda. "Mad About the Boy." *Independent Weekend Review*, October 16, 1999, 5.

SEE ALSO

Film Actors: Gay Male; British Television

Haynes, Todd   (b. 1961)

SINCE HIS 1991 FILM *POISON* WON THE GRAND JURY Prize at the Sundance Film Festival, innovative filmmaker Todd Haynes has emerged as the leading figure of the New Queer Cinema.

Haynes's body of work to date includes four feature-length films, *Poison*, *Safe* (1995), *Velvet Goldmine* (1998), and *Far From Heaven* (2002); and three shorts, *Superstar: The Karen Carpenter Story* (1987), *Assassins: A Film Concerning Rimbaud* (1985), and *Dottie Gets Spanked* (1993).

Only *Poison*, *Velvet Goldmine*, and *Far From Heaven* deal directly with homosexuality. But all of Haynes's films subvert conventional narrative structure, a structure he associates with the dominant heterosexual culture and its artifacts. The experimental, nonlinear, and complex narrative designs of his films qualify them all as queer, according to Haynes.

Haynes was born on January 2, 1961, in Los Angeles. He remembers making his first film at age ten. As a child, Haynes was moved and inspired by Robert Stephenson's *Mary Poppins* (1964), and, as a teenager, by Nicholas Roeg's *Performance* (1970), which stars Mick Jagger as a mysterious and androgynous rock star who provides sanctuary to a criminal. These diverse influences may help account for his films' melodramatic flair and excessive stylization.

Haynes attended Brown University, where he developed a love for the American avant-garde cinema and from which he graduated with a degree in art and semiotics. After graduation, he became a founding member of Apparatus Productions in New York City, an organization that promotes independent filmmaking.

He also became a member of ACT UP in the mid-1980s, and credits AIDS activism with "instigating" the early films of the New Queer Cinema.

Superstar, depicting Karen Carpenter's death from anorexia nervosa, begins an investigation of identity that permeates Haynes's films. The singer's self-consciousness of body image and eventual death are partly attributed to a manipulative mother. But the film takes a broader perspective, examining social norms that commodify women's bodies and exposing the danger of equating body image with identity.

By animating Karen's melodrama with puppets that closely resemble Barbie and Ken dolls, Haynes provides a campy edge to tragedy. His unauthorized use of idyllic songs by the Carpenters led A&M Records and Richard Carpenter to file suit against him and the film's distributors, which resulted in the film's abrupt withdrawal from distribution.

Haynes credits the writings of Jean Genet for inspiring the three tales of *Poison*, "Hero," "Horror," and "Homo." The last tale directly employs Genet's writings to illustrate the consequences of disguising one's homosexuality in a prison environment rife with erotic tension.

All three tales, directly or indirectly, explore the consequences of repressing self-identity and the fear and discontent of gays in society.

After discovering that Haynes received National Endowment for the Arts funds for *Poison*, Reverend Donald Wildmon of the American Family Association wrote Congress warning of its "explicit porno scenes of homosexuals engaged in anal sex." With the New Queer Cinema then in its infancy, the response of NEA chair John Frohnmayer, who noted that *Poison* "illustrates the destructive effect of violence and is neither prurient nor obscene," helped give credibility to serious films on queer issues.

Void of explicit "homosexual" content, *Safe* chronicles the process of an unnamed disease that wastes the body of an upper-middle-class woman. The gay community could not fail to notice the parallels between the woman's disease and AIDS and its cultural significance. Haynes criticizes the debilitating effect of finding identity through disease, as well as organizations that make deceptive claims for cures.

Velvet Goldmine, awarded the Special Jury Prize for Artistic Contribution at Cannes, depicts the tumultuous rise and fall of glam rockers through a fantastical fusion of performance and sexual identity. Haynes recognized that an underground gay subculture used glam to celebrate the defiance of social regulations through an excessive display of sexuality and to blur the boundaries of masculine and feminine, gay and straight.

In *Velvet Goldmine*, Haynes evokes the writings of Oscar Wilde and the cult of the personality to place flamboyant and theatrical images of androgyny in historical context. Camp, which exists to some degree in all Haynes's films, is most evident in *Velvet Goldmine*, a film that has foundation, Haynes notes, "in a long tradition of gay reading(s) of the world."

Far From Heaven (2002) pays tribute to one of the most commercially successful directors of 1950s Hollywood, Douglas Sirk. But *Far From Heaven* depicts in a stark and unsettling manner repressed homosexual desire and rampant racism, issues that Sirk could only hint at in the 1950s. Dennis Quaid excels in the role of a husband tormented by his homosexuality. The film garnered four Academy Award nominations, and Haynes suddenly felt disconcerted by Hollywood's acceptance of an experimental and misunderstood queer filmmaker.

Currently, Haynes is ecstatic that Bob Dylan has agreed to cooperate with him on his next film, to be titled *I'm Not There: Suppositions on a Film Concerning Dylan*. According to Haynes, the film is structured as a "multiple refracted biopic" that reconstructs and reinvents Dylan in different time periods by seven actors, including a woman.

Each of Haynes's films is unique, each employing a distinctly experimental structure. Yet they are united by a common concern with the problem of identity and by their relentless opposition to the dominant discourses and images of heterosexual Hollywood.

—Richard C. Bartone

BIBLIOGRAPHY

DiStefano, Blase. "Briefs, Barbies, & Beyond: An Interview with Todd Haynes." *OutSmart*, August 15, 1995, 34.

Gross, Larry. "Antibodies." *Filmmaker* 3.4 (Summer 1995): 39–42, 52–54.

Mitchell, John Cameron. "Flaming Creatures." *Filmmaker* 7.1 (Fall 1998): 56–58, 99–101.

Saunders, Michael William. *Imps of the Perverse*. Westport, Conn.: Praeger, 1998.

Stephens, Chuck. "Gentlemen Prefer Haynes." *Film Comment* 31.4 (1995): 76–81.

SEE ALSO

Film; New Queer Cinema; Film Directors; Screenwriters; Film Festivals; Vachon, Christine

Hong Kong Film

WHEN IT COMES TO QUEER SUBJECTS, HONG KONG cinema has enjoyed, and perhaps has suffered from, a special historical and political position. On the one hand, Hong Kong is the inheritor of the traditional Chinese aesthetics of theatrical transvestism and transgenderism. On the other hand, a Westernized, colonial

Hong Kong had adopted both the homophobia of European culture and the only slightly lesser homophobia of neo-Confucianism.

As these various cultural and historical strands continued to intertwine in light of the decriminalization of homosexuality in 1991 and Hong Kong's reversion to China in 1997, filmmaking in Hong Kong eventually came to terms with, exploited, and often blurred the lines between Chinese traditions of gender ambiguity and Westernized, out politics.

The Opera-Film

First, the tradition of the opera-film, a dominant genre of Hong Kong cinema in the 1950s and 1960s, had established a cinematic tradition of cross-dressing arguably more transgressive than any of the out queer films that came decades later.

Opera actresses such as Yam Kim-fai and Ivy Ling-boh starred in hundreds of stagey film versions of traditional operas such as *The Purple Hairpin* and *Lady General Hua-Mulan,* where they performed cross-dressed in heroic male roles.

Unlike the parody of a drag show, in Chinese opera the audience is supposed fantastically to suspend its disbelief and accept whatever gender is being performed, suggesting that the performativity espoused by Western queer theory is not such a novel idea.

Years later, director Shu Kei's out lesbian film *Hu-du-Men* (1996) would provide a rich account of a Cantonese opera actress coping with her lesbian daughter, joining traditional and modern notions of Chinese queerness in the same family.

The New Wave Period

The peak of Hong Kong's cinematic artistry is usually considered to be its New Wave period—from about 1977 to the early 1990s—when Western-schooled directors infused Hong Kong cinema with cosmopolitan technology and an eye for naturalism. Two basic trends notable during this era were the social realism exemplified by directors such as Ann Hui and Allen Fong and the wild, kaleidoscopic fantasies purveyed by Tsui Hark and Ching Siu-tung.

Neither of these trends, however, managed to engage queer subjects seriously, and when homosexuality did rear its head, it was framed within terms as homophobic as those of Hollywood during the same period, even in an "important" film such as Tsui Hark's political allegory *Don't Play with Fire* (1980).

Apart from the homoerotic male bonding of the John Woo–style gangster film, the only legitimate appeals to queerness in the 1980s were references to homosexual patronage in films set in the world of Chinese opera, such as Sammo Hung's *The Prodigal Son* (1981), Tsui

Hark's *Peking Opera Blues* (1986), and Jacob Cheung's *Lai Shi: China's Last Eunuch* (1988).

The one notable exception here is the work of Clarence Fok (aka Clarence Ford), whose *On Trial* (1980) stars a young Leslie Cheung in a blatantly homoerotic story of unrequited schoolboy longing, and whose seedy *Before Dawn* (1984) portrays the lethal relationship between an awkward young man and a gay killer.

In later, more liberated years, Fok would emerge as a cult director with the erotic lesbian thriller *Naked Killer* (1992), as well as *Cheap Killers* (1998), a rare genre film that positively portrays openly gay action heroes.

The 1990s Period Costume Film

In the early 1990s, producer-director Tsui Hark's obsession for commedia dell'arte–style comedies of disguise would make cross-gender disguise and intrigue a standard part of the reinvented period costume film. Unlike the "permanent" cross-dressing of the traditional opera-film, however, this new costume film would involve only *diegetic* cross-dressing, where we are fully aware that a character cross-dresses solely to fulfill some purpose of the plot.

Usually, this involves a girl in disguise for reasons of self-interest (as in Shakespeare). This is the case in films such as *Dragon Inn* (1992), *Magic Crane* (1993), *The Lovers* (1994), and the *Swordsman* trilogy (1990–1993), which adds a supernaturally transgendered antihero(ine) to the mix.

Yet Tsui's treatment of his latently queer material is often coy, and many of the period martial arts films influenced by Tsui are more open about their transgressive possibilities. For example, frankly lesbian complications ensue between a disguised Josephine Siao and the woman who falls in love with her/him in Yuen Kwai's *Fong Sai Yuk* (1993), and campy homosexual kisses between top male stars highlight costume farces such as Wong Jing's *Flying Dagger* (1992) and Jeff Lau's *Eagle Shooting Heroes* (1993).

The period costume trend—every film of which invariably mandated that some character appeared cross-dressed—climaxed around 1993, the year that also saw Chen Kaige's controversial, gay-themed mainland opera tale *Farewell My Concubine* (1993).

Following on the popularity of these films, a new liberal trend emerged, resulting in countless contemporary, urban, middle-class films with glbtq themes or openly glbtq characters. These include Lawrence Cheng's *He and She* (1993), Peter Chan's *Tom, Dick, and Hairy* (1993), Derek Chiu's *Oh My Three Guys!* (1994), Leonard Heung's *Love Recipe* (1994), Peter Chan's *He's a Woman, She's A Man Pts. 1–2* (1994, 1996), Joe Hau's *Boys* (1996), Lee Lik-chi's *Killing Me Tenderly* (1996), and many others.

The Emergence of Queer Films

Yet, as the 1997 deadline for the handover to China ticked away, and as Hong Kong film directors worried about what censorship the future might hold, a more focused, less apologetic batch of queer films emerged, films poised to challenge the mainland's official denials of Chinese homosexuality.

These films include Cheung Chi-sing's slyly political bisexual seriocomedy *Love and Sex among the Ruins* (1996), Shu Kei's coming-out narrative *A Queer Story* (1997), Wong Kar-wai's highly publicized *Happy Together* (1997), Jacob Cheung's lesbian romance *Intimates* (1997), and Yim Ho's disarming transsexual drama *Kitchen* (1997).

Also during this period, Stanley Kwan, Hong Kong's foremost gay director, decided to come out cinematically with his fascinating semiautobiographical documentary *Yang and Yin: Gender in Chinese Cinema* (1996). Previously, Kwan's gayness as a director had been limited to a hint of transvestism in *Rouge* (1987) and Maggie Cheung's subdued portrayal of a lesbian in *Full Moon in New York* (1990), a rarity for its time.

Category 3 Films

Paralleling these trends was the creation of a new censorship category in 1989 to allow for more sexually explicit films. Predictably, queer images in Hong Kong's category 3 films tend toward lesbian erotica aimed at the fantasies of a heterosexual male audience, as in the *Sex and Zen* series (1991–1996), the *Erotic Ghost Story* series (1990–1992), the *Raped by an Angel* series (1993–2000), or Ho Shu Pau's lesbian thriller *The Love That is Wrong* (1993).

On the other hand, lesbianism in these films is often vibrant, unashamed, and (somewhat) liberated, and we should not overlook the probability that lesbian audiences have covertly, subversively enjoyed such films.

Furthermore, a few of these films offer some politically incorrect surprises, from a mafia syndicate populated by real-life transsexuals in Lau Siu Gwan's *Hero Dream* (1993) to a homophobic male hero becoming the sex object of a diabolical bisexual rapist in Wong Ying Git's *The Sweet Smell of Death* (1995).

Moreover, marginal, low-budget category 3 thrillers such as Joe Hau's *Passion Unbounded* (1995), Lo Gin's *Spider Woman* (1995), and Joe Hau's *Crazy* (1999) offer both gay and lesbian characterizations that are more nuanced than the stereotypes often found in bourgeois, assimilationist fare.

The "One Country, Two Systems" Policy

While filmmakers' fears of what would follow 1997 were justified, the production of queer films continued according to the "one country, two systems" policy, whereby the mainland government would not interfere with Hong Kong's social fabric until 2047.

Recent queer films have been as diverse as Stanley Kwan's existential *Hold You Tight* (1998), Yip Wai-man's lesbian gangster epic *Portland St. Blues* (1998), Yonfan's Japanese *manga*-inspired *Bishonen* (1998), Julian Lee's category 3 art film *The Accident* (1999), and Stanley Kwan's controversial *Lan Yu* (2001), a sexually explicit romance set against the backdrop of Tiananmen Square.

While Hong Kong's film industry is not as strong as it was before the handover, and while production of films overall has lessened considerably, the openness of queer themes in Hong Kong cinema is apparently here to stay.

—*Andrew Grossman*

BIBLIOGRAPHY

Grossman, Andrew, ed. *Queer Asian Cinema: Shadows in the Shade*. Binghamton, N.Y.: Harrington Park Press, 2000.

Kwan, Stanley, dir. *Yang and Yin: Gender in Chinese Cinema*. Documentary film. Hong Kong: Media Asia 1996.

Sandell, Jillian. "Reinventing Masculinity: The Spectacle of Male Intimacy in the Films of John Woo." *Film Quarterly* 49.4 (Summer 1996): 23–42.

Tan See Kam. "Delirious Native Chaos and Perfidy: A Post-colonial Reading of John Woo's The Killer." *Antithesis* 6.2 (1993): 53–66

www.hkmdb.com

www.planetout.com/popcornq

SEE ALSO

Asian Film; Japanese Film; Cheung, Leslie

Horror Films

THE COUPLING OF HOMOSEXUAL AND MONSTER HAS been an enduring, if not always consciously acknowledged, cultural motif. Cinema has been an especially welcoming venue in this regard, populated as it is by a disproportionate number of queer artists working as directors, writers, and set decorators, and ideally positioned as a space in which gender anxieties can be explored and vented on a mass scale.

Coding the Queer as Monster

The monsters of cinema, indeed of popular culture in general, are troubled, and troubling, outsiders, their sexuality thwarted or altered, sometimes seductive and suave, other times repulsive and terrifying, but always threatening to the social and sexual order.

They can easily be read as doubles for societal views of homosexuals as predatory, amoral, perverse, possessed of secret supernatural powers, capable of—and very interested in—destroying "normal life" and toppling such vulnerable institutions as the nuclear family, the church, capitalism, the heterosexual paradigm, or a combination thereof.

Coding the queer as monster allows viewers the catharsis of experiencing the terror of a threat to "normal life," while insulating them against that threat by presenting it as a fantasy character or *demimondain* usually destroyed by film's end.

Queer Couples

One of the major strategies in the perceived queer monster's arsenal is replacing straight couples with gay or gay-coded ones. This was evident even in the silent era, in films such as Robert Wiene's *The Cabinet of Dr. Caligari* (1919), which presents one of the earliest of cinema's many "unwholesome" male couples—a sensitive, vulnerable younger man under the control of an older, more sophisticated "mentor" who lures his protégé into a terrifying dream world far from normalcy, that is, far from the heterosexual norm.

Gay director James Whale's *Bride of Frankenstein* (1935) is one of the most direct expressions of this trope, with aged, corrupt, effeminate Dr. Praetorius (married but gay Ernest Thesiger) luring the nervous, neurotic Dr. Frankenstein (rumored bisexual Colin Clive) into a heady world of "gods and monsters."

But *Bride* also presents intriguing variations on the theme that would persist. It shows two major male couples in blasphemous alliance: Praetorius and Frankenstein, whose collaboration results in the unholy progeny of the "Bride" (who makes a memorable appearance in the film's witty assault on marriage); and a partnership of outsider-equals in the Frankenstein monster and the blind hermit, who briefly set up what is in effect a loving homosexual household before it is literally destroyed by the meddling of two straight townsmen.

Whale's *Old Dark House* (1932) has a similarly threatening male couple in the two main outsiders, the inchoate butler Morgan (Boris Karloff) and the insane Saul (Brember Wills), whose death unleashes Morgan's deepest anguish and violence.

A subset of the queer male relationship is the basis of Tod Browning's *Dracula* (1932), that is, master and slave in a sadomasochistic relationship. Renfield's perpetually apologizing, groveling posture is contrasted throughout the film with Dracula's rigid uprightness as he commands, degrades, and ultimately enslaves Renfield, forcing him into all manner of depravities.

Queer Monsters as Predators

Society's idea of the homosexual as a kind of virus that wastes its victims and spreads its monstrosity unchecked requires that there be multiple—in fact, endless—victims. (David Skal has explored the link between societal views of vampirism and AIDS.) Thus, the predatory

Dracula must conquer London neck by neck, exercising his penetrative, pleasure-and-survival needs on men, women, and children; and, as Judith Halberstam has pointed out, in a way that is emphatically antiprocreation and antifamily.

The queer monster/corrupted-straight-victim relationship reappeared in further variations in later decades, where the corrupter is more of an authority figure than a monster, but is still coded as queer.

During the 1950s, the low-budget studio American International Pictures specialized in a subgenre of horror in which a successful, middle-aged professional, often a scientist or trusted teacher, transforms a maladjusted youth under his (or her) care into a monster, playing off the then current notion that older homosexuals were driven to "recruit" the young and vulnerable into their lifestyle.

I Was a Teenage Werewolf (1957) and *How to Make a Monster* (1958) present both a perverse male couple (a scientist and assistant in the former, a makeup artist and assistant in the latter) and a robust but troubled youth who is forced to act out the couple's gruesome antisocial agenda.

Just as Dracula was compelled to find fresh victims, the scientist in *How to Make a Monster* demands a string of "boys" on whom to work his lethal magic. A lesbian variant on this conceit from the same period can be found in Herbert L. Strock's *Blood of Dracula* (1957), in which an unmarried female science teacher hypnotizes a female student into becoming a violent monster who does her bidding.

Lesbian Monsters

Until the 1970s, lesbian monsters were less visible in cinema than their male counterparts. The most important early image of the dyke vampire is in Lambert Hillyer's *Dracula's Daughter* (1935), which presents Countess Zaleska's (Gloria Holden) vampiric encounter with a beautiful, innocent young woman as an unmistakable homosexual seduction.

The female vampire who preys on other women has long been a staple of literature high and low, and is probably the most common image of the queer female monster in cinema.

In the 1960s and 1970s, this character resurfaced in stylized but surprisingly sensual portrayals in films such as Roger Vadim's *Blood and Roses* (1961) and Harry Kumel's *Daughters of Darkness* (1971), in which the lesbian vampire is presented as irresistibly beautiful and stylish—and unapologetic—rather than homely and tormented as in *Dracula's Daughter*.

More model-beautiful vampires (some of the actresses had been *Playboy* bunnies) appear in Hammer Studio's "Carmilla" trilogy (based on J. Sheridan Le Fanu's famous

1872 novel). Roy Ward Baker's *The Vampire Lovers* (1970), Jimmy Sangster's *Lust for a Vampire* (1971), and John Hough's *Twins of Evil* (1972) titillated both heterosexual male and lesbian audiences with images of sharp female teeth sinking into heaving breasts.

1980s and 1990s Horror

Cultural anxieties around the queer monster continued in films throughout the 1980s and 1990s, and persist today. The sleek, sexy female vampires of the 1960s continued to set the standard in films such as Tony Scott's *The Hunger* (1982), but queer horror could be found more often in subtext than text, despite a general loosening of cinematic standards.

Wes Craven's *Nightmare on Elm Street 2* (1982) features both an out homosexual in the form of a sadistic gym coach (who is brutally dispatched in a Grand Guignol shower scene) and a coded/closeted queer boy, Jesse (Mark Patton), whose outsiderness attracts the attention of the monster Freddy Krueger (Robert Englund).

Harry Benshoff reads the scene of the coach's death—which occurs through Freddy's inhabiting, that is, penetrating, Jesse—as a version of homosexual panic that results in Jesse's becoming a murderer. Freddy's function is both to unleash Jesse's potential homosexuality and to possess Jesse himself, an extension of the 1950s theme of the sophisticated older homosexual taking charge of a vulnerable, wavering younger man.

Queer auteur Joel Schumacher's *Lost Boys* (1987) transformed the teen drama popular in that decade into an ensemble of queer-coded vampire boys who often seem more interested in each other—after all, they have to seduce new "recruits" into their ranks—than in their nominal heterosexual relationships.

Neil Jordan's *Interview with the Vampire* (1994) exposed many of the tensions around the queer monster, both tantalizing viewers with a series of obviously queer relationships and dancing nervously around the details, as when it almost, but not quite, has Louis (Brad Pitt) and Armand (Antonio Banderas) kiss.

Porn, Exploitation, and Independent Horror Films

Queer horror has often found a warmer haven in porn, exploitation, and independent films than in mainstream cinema. Hard-core porn titles such as James Moss's *Dragula, Queen of the Vampires* (1973) and Roger Earl's *Gayracula* (1983) show that the vampire remains the gay monster of choice, even in disreputable genres.

A gay werewolf cult is the subject of Will Gould's sympathetic independent film *The Wolves of Kromer* (1998). Most recently, David DeCoteau, a former director of gay and straight porn, has expropriated formerly straight cultural spaces in a series of luridly homoerotic teen-horror programmers.

The Brotherhood (2000), *The Brotherhood 2: Young Warlocks* (2001), and *Voodoo Academy* (2000) are as much unabashed paeans to the postadolescent underwear-clad male physique as they are horror films. (One critic disparagingly likened them to feature-length Calvin Klein commercials.)

Voodoo Academy is particularly outrageous in this regard, with a gay priest working for a female demon, both of whom caress their charges before transforming them into voodoo dolls. In the director's cut, the camera lovingly lingers on the handsome students as they writhe possessed in their beds in self-stimulating poses that recall the teasing postures found in porn films.

The fact that these films went directly to video without a regular theatrical release suggests the culture's reluctance to acknowledge such blatant displays of homoerotic horror in "approved" mainstream venues. The fact that they have been successful on video, acquiring a minor cult reputation, points to the culture's continued, if uneasy, accommodation of queer horror.   —*Gary Morris*

BIBLIOGRAPHY

Benshoff, Harry M. *Monsters in the Closet: Homosexuality and the Horror Film.* Manchester, UK: Manchester University Press, 1997.

Doty, Alexander. *Flaming Classics: Queering the Horror Canon.* New York: Routledge, 2000.

Halberstam, Judith. "On Lesbians, Vampires, and Coppola's Dracula." *Bright Lights Film Journal* 11 (1993): 7–9.

Morris, Gary, "Queer Horror: Decoding Universal's Monsters." *Bright Lights Film Journal* 23: www.brightlightsfilm.com/23/universalhorror.html

Murray, Raymond. *Images in the Dark.* New York: Plume, 1996.

Skal, David. *The Monster Show: A Cultural History of Horror.* New York: Faber & Faber, 2001.

Skal, David. *V Is for Vampire: The A-Z Guide to Everything Undead.* New York: Plume, 1996.

Weiss, Andrea. *Vampires and Violets: Lesbians in Film.* New York: Penguin, 1990.

SEE ALSO

Film; Vampire Films; Whale, James

Hudson, Rock   (1925–1985)

HOLLYWOOD'S STAR SYSTEM WAS STILL IN FORCE AT THE start of the 1950s; tall, dark, and very handsome Rock Hudson was totally a product of it. His limited talent was mainly nurtured within the strict confines of a studio (Universal) contract and a series of B pictures.

After playing bad boy redeemed in *Magnificent Obsession* (1954), Hudson's popularity soared, consolidated by a number of successful melodramas, such as *All That Heaven Allows* (1955) and *Written on the Wind* (1956), which were directed by Hudson's mentor, Douglas Sirk.

Hudson was born Roy Harold Scherer Jr. in Winnetka, Illinois, on November 17, 1925. When his mother divorced his father, an auto mechanic, and married a man named Wallace Fitzgerald, the future actor became known as Roy Fitzgerald.

After high school and military service, he moved to Hollywood to pursue a movie career. Agent Henry Willson named him "Rock Hudson."

The Sirk films and an Oscar nomination for *Giant* (1956) notwithstanding, Hudson was not taken seriously as an actor until, ironically, he turned his hand to light comedy in *Pillow Talk* (1959), costarring with Doris Day. Other comedies with Day soon followed, including *Lover Come Back* (1962) and *Send Me No Flowers* (1964).

Throughout the 1960s, he alternated frothy sex comedies with action dramas. His one challenging role—that of a man who changes identities, in *Seconds* (1966)—caused little excitement and the film failed at the box office. A few years later, he was starring as a police commissioner in the long-running television series, *McMillan and Wife* (1971–1977).

The glossy hothouse melodrama that Hudson helped popularize in the 1950s had, by the early 1980s, become a world television phenomenon. Hudson joined the cast of one of these super-rich sagas, *Dynasty*, in late 1984. His drawn features aroused comment, and by mid-1985 photographs of the spectral, virtually unrecognizable star were flashed across the world. Rumors that he was suffering from AIDS were confirmed when he sought treatment in Paris.

Hudson's death, a few months later, focused world attention on the AIDS virus and its sufferers, enabling Hudson's friend Elizabeth Taylor and others to gain the ear of government and moneyed people who had hitherto been deaf and mute to the subject.

Hudson's sex life received detailed attention posthumously when a lover, Marc Christian, whom he had not informed of his diagnosis, successfully sued his estate.

Onscreen, Rock Hudson was the epitome of the movie star: upright, virile, unassuming. His screen partnership with Doris Day further boosted his popularity as a wolfish playboy with a mischievous little-boy charm. It could be claimed that Rock Hudson was one of the greatest actors who ever lived: a gay man who became an unassailable international symbol of heterosexuality.

Rock Hudson was probably the last of the manufactured stars, his screen presence bolstered by beefcake photographs, fan clubs, and an eternal bachelorhood briefly interrupted by an arranged marriage to Willson's secretary Phyllis Gates in 1955. (They were divorced in 1958.)

However, in the more open 1970s, Hudson did become more visible in gay bars and bathhouses on the West Coast, and was even included postcoitally—anonymously but with his blessing—in Armistead Maupin's newspaper serial *Tales of the City*.

Hudson's charismatic mixture of seeming guilelessness and single-minded ambition, wearing a public mask until it was savagely ripped off him, places him firmly among the great American glamour icons: James Dean, Marilyn Monroe, Elizabeth Taylor, and President John F. Kennedy.

—*Keith G. Howes*

Bibliography

Davidson, Sara, and Rock Hudson. *Rock Hudson: His Story.* New York: Bantam, 1986.

Royce, Brenda Scott. *Rock Hudson: A Bio-Bibliography.* Westport, Conn.: Greenwood Press, 1995.

See also

Film; Film Actors: Gay Male; Film Sissies; Documentary Film; Dean, James; Liberace; Nader, George

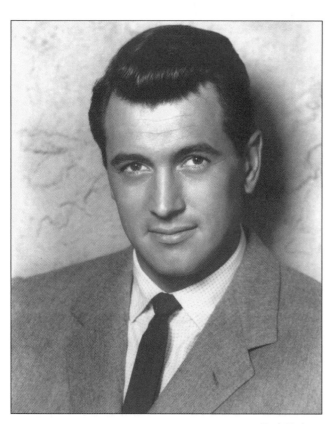

Rock Hudson.

Hunter, Tab   (b. 1931)

Y OUNG TAB HUNTER'S BLOND GOOD LOOKS MADE HIM
a movie idol in the 1950s. His romantic heterosexual
roles on screen concealed his true identity as a gay man.

The actor was born Arthur Kelm in New York City
on July 11, 1931. A few years later, his mother, Gertrude
Gelien Kelm, divorced her abusive husband, Charles
Kelm, and moved to California with her two young sons.
She resumed her maiden name and changed the chil-
dren's surname as well.

Hunter left school at fifteen to join the Coast Guard,
lying about his age in order to be accepted, but was dis-
charged when the deception was discovered. He returned
home and went to work at a riding academy.

Horsemanship had long been Hunter's passion. As a
young teen, he had frequented a riding school, where he
met an actor named Dick Clayton. After Hunter's dismissal from the Coast Guard, Clayton encouraged him
to try his hand at acting and introduced him to agent
Henry Willson, who represented Rock Hudson, among
others.

Willson decided that the aspiring actor needed a new
name, declaring, "We've got to tab you something."
When Clayton volunteered that the young man was a
horseman who rode hunters and jumpers, Arthur Gelien
(né Kelm) became Tab Hunter.

Hunter's film debut, in Joseph Losey's *The Lawless*
(1950), was less than auspicious: His only line was cut.
His first major role came in Stuart Heisler's *Island of
Desire* (1952) opposite Linda Darnell. Often half-naked
in this film, Hunter attracted the attention of gay men
across the country, who were to become some of his
most loyal fans. He rose to stardom in 1955 when he
appeared in Raoul Walsh's *Battle Cry*, playing a marine
in a love triangle.

In September 1955, with the release of *Battle Cry*
imminent, *Confidential*, a Hollywood magazine known
for exposing closeted gay celebrities, ran an article about
the arrest by the Los Angeles vice squad of Hunter and
about two dozen others who were attending a "pajama
party" in suburban Walnut Park in 1950.

Since the police found nothing more than dancing by
same-sex couples in progress, the partygoers were at first
charged as "idle, lewd or dissolute persons," and even
that was reduced to "disorderly conduct." Hunter was
assessed a fifty-dollar fine.

In a 1974 interview, Hunter downplayed the incident, claiming that he had only gone to the party—which
was not, he insisted, a pajama party—at the casual suggestion of a friend and that he was surprised to find gay
men and lesbians in attendance. He added that he was in
the kitchen innocently preparing a peanut-butter sand-
wich when the raid by the vice squad occurred.

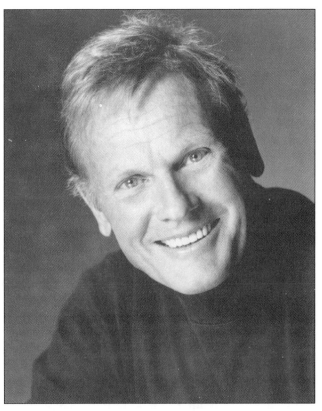

A portrait of Tab Hunter by Greg Gorman.

Since *Confidential* had a limited circulation and the
national press did not pick up the story, Hunter survived
the 1955 outing and his career did not suffer. In addition,
he used the common ruse of "dates" with actresses—duly
photographed and reported by popular fan magazines—
to mask his true personal life.

While America was reading that Hunter was enamored with Debbie Reynolds, Dorothy Malone, or Natalie
Wood, Hunter was actually pursuing an affair with actor
Anthony Perkins, a tortured homosexual who eventually
(though apparently not successfully) attempted to become
heterosexual. Hunter and Perkins were involved with
each other for several years.

Although the public remained in the dark, members
of the entertainment industry were aware of Hunter's
sexual orientation. His sexual orientation was also widely
suspected by members of the glbtq community, who were
among his most ardent fans.

Hunter solidified his image as a golden boy and teen
idol by recording the pop tune "Young Love" (by Carole
Joyner and Ric Carty), which topped the charts for over
a month in 1957. Gifted with a pleasant voice, but not
great musical talent, Hunter subsequently recorded other
singles and albums, their successes due more to his
celebrity as an actor than to his musicianship.

His movie career prospered for a while. He enjoyed
notable success in the 1958 films *Damn Yankees* (directed

by George Abbott and Stanley Donen) and *Lafayette Escadrille* (directed by William J. Wellman) and in Sidney Lumet's *That Kind of Woman* in 1959.

As he matured and was no longer suited to "boy next door" roles, he worked increasingly in television. His own *Tab Hunter Show* (1960–1961) was short-lived, but he continued to appear on the small screen in both dramas and comedies and occasionally on game shows. Even as his spectacular looks faded, Hunter remained popular by virtue of his ability to project a sweet nature.

Hunter had a brief turn on Broadway in 1963 playing opposite Tallulah Bankhead in a production of Tennessee Williams's *The Milk Train Doesn't Stop Here Anymore*. A legendary disaster, the show closed after five performances.

In the 1970s, as his career as a movie star declined, Hunter toured in dinner-theater productions.

He continued acting in films, some produced in Europe and most not particularly memorable. In 1981, however, he appeared with transvestite actor Divine in John Waters's *Polyester*, which has become a cult classic. Four years later, Hunter again teamed with Divine in *Lust in the Dust*, a spoof of cowboy pictures, directed by Paul Bartel and coproduced by Hunter and Allan Glaser.

In association with Republic Pictures International and Bonnie Sugar, Hunter and Glaser made the 1992 film *Dark Horse*, described as a "touching family drama." The story was by Hunter, Glaser was the principal producer, and David Hemmings directed.

Hunter's love of horses drew him to another project, a series on the HorseTV cable network called *Hollywood on Horses*. The show debuted in June 2002 with Hunter as host and executive producer.

Hunter and Glaser, along with Neil Koenigsberg, have been in negotiations with director Peter Bogdanovich to make a film to be called *Blues in the Night*, based on a story by Evelyn Keyes.

In fall 2005, Hunter published a memoir, *Tab Hunter Confidential*, in which he discusses his life as an actor and a gay man.

Hunter has acknowledged that he and Glaser have lived together as life partners "for many years."

—Linda Rapp

BIBLIOGRAPHY

Archerd, Army. "Just for Variety." *Variety*, August 7, 2003, 2.

Ehrenstein, David. *Open Secret: Gay Hollywood 1928–1998*. New York: William Morrow and Company, 1998.

Hunter, Tab. *Tab Hunter Confidential: The Making of a Movie Star*. With Eddie Muller. Chapel Hill, NC: Algonquin Books, 2005.

Weinraub, Bernard. "A Star's Real Life Upstages His Films; Tab Hunter Looks Back on Sadness and Success and Ahead to a Book." *New York Times*, September 9, 2003.

www.tabhunter.com

SEE ALSO

Film Actors: Gay Male; Bankhead, Tallulah; Bartel, Paul; Divine (Harris Glenn Milstead); Hudson, Rock; Waters, John

i

Iglesia, Eloy de la   (b. 1944)

ELOY DE LA IGLESIA WAS AMONG THE FIRST SPANISH directors to make films with homosexual themes. Although he enjoyed commercial success, critics dismissed his work as sensational, melodramatic, and violent. More recently, however, film scholars have begun to reevaluate his work, in particular his depictions of socially and politically marginalized groups.

De la Iglesia was born in Larautz in the Basque region of Spain on January 1, 1944. As a young man, he hoped to enter the Escuela Oficial de Cinematografía, but, not being old enough, began working in the Teatro Popular Infantil (youth theater) instead. He remained interested in directing, however, and in 1966 made his first film, *Fantasía...3*. The eighty-five-minute film is a collection of three stories for children.

De la Iglesia's major body of work consists of twenty films made between 1968 and 1986. His movies are very much a product of and reaction to his place and time.

During the Franco regime, Spanish cinema was dominated by films with religious or historical themes and low-budget comedies. The state, heavily influenced by the Catholic Church, exercised strict censorship over what Spanish audiences were allowed to see. Political views inimical to the government were not permitted. Representation of sexual relationships outside of marriage were relatively rare, and the few that were allowed invariably involved heterosexual couples.

The political climate was repressive to homosexuals, especially men. *La Ley de Peligrosidad y Rehabilitación* ("The Social Danger and Rehabilitation Law") made homosexual acts illegal, allowed police to arrest men suspected to be homosexual, and imposed penalties of up to three years in prison.

In the latter years of the Franco regime, which ended in 1975, as the dictator's power ebbed, filmmakers began taking more risks and found slightly greater latitude than before. Nevertheless, when de la Iglesia made his first feature film, *Algo amargo en la boca*, in 1968, he encountered problems with the censors even though the film dealt with heterosexual attraction.

De la Iglesia's first international success came in 1972 with *La semana del asesino* (*The Week of the Murderer*), which included an element of homosexual attraction. Like many of his films, particularly the earlier ones, it contained an amount of violence that many viewers found disturbing.

With the death of Franco in 1975 came new freedom for Spanish filmmakers. During the period known as the transition, approximately 1975 to 1978, many moved away from the former norms of Spanish cinema. Whereas the family had previously been the central unit in the filmic narrative, focus now shifted to the couple, including homosexual couples.

Two of de la Iglesia's best-known films, *Los placeres ocultos* (*Hidden Pleasures*, 1976) and *El diputado* (*Confessions of a Congressman*, 1978), date from this time.

The first, initially banned by the censors, is the story of a closeted banker attracted to a poor youth who is heterosexual. The banker attempts to create a new model of the family by spending time with the young man and his fiancée. He takes on a traditional paternal function by giving the youth a job in the bank and improving his education, but his true wish is for the two of them to be a couple.

Because of personal, social, and economic tensions that arise, it appears that he may fail in both roles. The end of the film, however, has the banker smiling as he answers a doorbell rung by an unseen person, leading viewers to believe that he has at least the possibility of achieving happiness as part of a homosexual couple.

In *El diputado* de la Iglesia also creates an atypical family—a gay Socialist congressman, his wife, and the young man (again, poor) with whom he is in love. The congressman plays the roles of both fatherly mentor

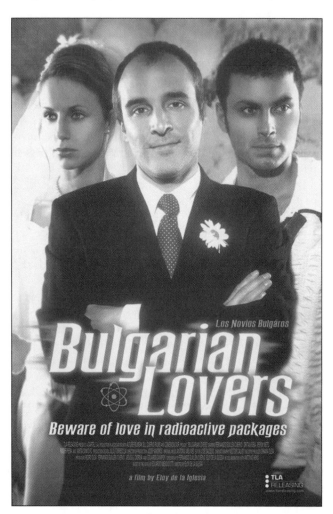

A promotional poster for Eloy de la Iglesia's film *Bulgarian Lovers* (2003).

and lover to the youth. In this film the love affair ends tragically.

De la Iglesia's films deal with those who have been marginalized by society for various reasons—sexual orientation, politics, economics, ethnicity, and participation in the drug culture. In one of his later films—and his greatest commercial success—*El pico* (*The Shoot*, 1983), de la Iglesia treats three such marginalized groups, homosexuals, heroin users, and the Basque minority in Spain.

De la Iglesia's films were long either ignored by serious critics or condemned as "sensationalistic and commercial" and frequently violent—for example, *Una gota de sangre para morir amando* (*A Drop of Blood to Die Loving*, 1973) and *Navajeros* (*Knife Fighters*, 1980). In recent years, however, commentators have begun to reexamine his work and its relationship to the social and historical context in which it was produced.

While making *El pico*, de la Iglesia began using heroin, to which he became addicted. After an almost decade-long absence from the public, he reemerged at the 1996 San Sebastián film festival, which featured a tribute to his work.

In 2001, he made his first film for television, an adaptation of Albert Camus's *Caligula*, which was broadcast on Spain's TVE-1 network. He also began collaborating with Fernando Guillén Cuervo on a screenplay based on *Los novios búlgaros*, a novel by Eduardo Mendicutti.

Released in 2003, *Bulgarian Lovers* is characteristic of de la Iglesia's work in that it deals with a story of homosexual love set in the context of a marginalized group, in this case eastern European immigrants in Spain. In the film, a middle-aged attorney falls in love with a macho Bulgarian hustler who draws him into a world of shady business dealings.

—*Linda Rapp*

BIBLIOGRAPHY

Cervino, Mercedes. "Eloy de la Iglesia: Dirigir es como andar en bici, no se olvida." *Efe News Services* (U.S.) (June 10, 2001): https://web.lexis-nexis.com/universe/docuA1&_md5=7ced3078 eld7a8d0dab7160ff7b2a;

"Eloy de la Iglesia." *El Mundo* (Madrid), March 25, 2001: www.el-mundo.es/magazine/m78/textos/eloy1.html

G., R. "Diez años de reflexión." *El País* (Madrid), May 5, 1996.

Larraz, Emmanuel. *Le cinéma espagnol des origines à nos jours.* Paris: Les Éditions du Cerf, 1986.

Smith, Paul Julian. *Laws of Desire: Questions of Homosexuality in Spanish Writing and Film 1960–1990.* Oxford, UK: Clarendon Press, 1992.

Tropiano, Stephen. "Out of the Cinematic Closet: Homosexuality in the Films of Eloy de la Iglesia." *Refiguring Spain: Cinema/Media/ Representation.* Marsha Kinder, ed. Durham, N.C., and London: Duke University Press, 1997. 157–177.

SEE ALSO

Film; European Film; Film Directors

In the Life

AMERICA'S ONLY NATIONALLY BROADCAST GAY AND LESbian newsmagazine, *In the Life* began in 1992 as a variety show, but has since evolved into an acclaimed public-affairs program, hosted by such luminaries as Kate Clinton, Harvey Fierstein, Cherry Jones, and B. D. Wong.

Although *In the Life* is presented by Thirteen/WNET, the New York Public Broadcasting System flagship station, and is distributed by the American Program Service, a major source of programming for public television stations, the show receives no federal funding from PBS or the Corporation for Public Broadcasting.

Produced by In the Life Media Inc., a nonprofit educational organization, the program is supported largely by membership dues from nearly 5,000 individuals and by foundations such as the Gill Foundation and the van Ameringen Foundation.

When it debuted in 1992, *In the Life* aired on only six television stations. Now broadcast on over 125 public television stations in thirty states, it plays in the country's top twenty television-viewing markets. This penetration is remarkable considering the fact that when it was launched it roused immediate controversy. Even before the first episode was aired, Senator Robert Dole denounced the program from the floor of the United States Senate.

Now each episode of the program is seen by more than one million viewers, which makes *In the Life* the world's most widely distributed gay and lesbian media project. However, dozens of PBS stations still refuse to air the program, and many of those that do schedule it during late-night and early-morning hours and fail to promote it.

In most markets, the program airs monthly, in a one-hour format, featuring five or six stories. There are usually six new episodes per year.

In the Life is dedicated to presenting a uniquely gay and lesbian perspective on issues and news relevant to gay men and lesbians and to documenting the gay and lesbian civil rights movement. It also aims to educate both heterosexual and homosexual audiences about the diversity and variety of the gay and lesbian community.

In the Life features stories on a wide range of topics, from AIDS to same-sex marriage and from "Don't Ask, Don't Tell" to gay and lesbian parents. It has been particularly praised for its coverage of events such as the 1993 March on Washington and the 1994 Gay Games and for its attention to youth and global issues. The acclaimed April–May 1998 episode entitled *In the Life Goes Global* reported on the progress of gay rights internationally.

Although many of the episodes feature cameo appearances by gay and lesbian (or gay-friendly) celebrities,

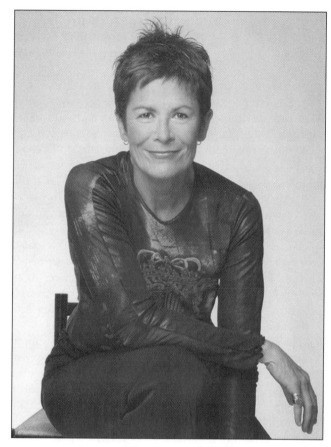

A portrait of frequent host Kate Clinton by David Rodgers.

and due attention is given to the accomplishments of artists, writers, and entertainers, *In the Life* is dedicated to the real-life issues and concerns of grassroots people. Hence, the emphasis is less on glitz and glamour than on the struggles of ordinary individuals who have performed extraordinary achievements.

A recent show, for example, featured stories about a gay couple who had been honored as Indiana's Foster Parents of the Year and a group of lesbians who were helping the people of Nicaragua recover from a hurricane. Other stories have examined gay and straight high school groups, the Names Project AIDS Memorial Quilt, and lesbian and gay journalists.

In the Life has grown to become a valuable resource for the gay and lesbian communities of the United States. For many viewers, it has also become a significant presence on PBS, however reluctant the broadcasting corporation may be to acknowledge the fact.   —*Claude J. Summers*

BIBLIOGRAPHY

www.inthelifzetv.org

SEE ALSO

American Television: News; Fierstein, Harvey; Jones, Cherry; Wong, B. D.

Ivory, James, and Ismail Merchant
James Ivory (b. 1928)
and Ismail Merchant (1936–2005)

PERHAPS THE MOST ENDURING AND INFLUENTIAL GAY partnership in film history, James Ivory and Ismail Merchant are known for their visually sumptuous period pieces based on familiar literary works. So closely intertwined was this team that many assume that "Merchant Ivory" is the name of one individual. But while associated in many minds with British literary and cultural traditions, their professional and personal relationship actually brought together diverse elements of American and Indian culture.

James Francis Ivory, who is the director in Merchant Ivory Productions, was born in Berkeley, California, on June 7, 1928. After graduating from the University of Oregon, he received an advanced degree from the University of Southern California School of Cinema and Television in 1957.

His first film was an acclaimed documentary about Venice, and his second, *The Sword and the Flute*, examined Indian art. In 1960, at a New York screening of the latter film, he met his future partner and collaborator.

Ismail Noormohamed Abdul Rehman, later Merchant, was born on December 25, 1936, in Bombay, India. He came to the United States as a student and earned an M.B.A. degree at New York University, a background that prepared him for his role as the producer and business mind of the partnership.

While working for an advertising agency, he produced a film based on Indian myth, *Creation of Woman* (1961), which earned an Academy Award for Best Short Subject. In that year, he and Ivory formed Merchant Ivory Productions.

The Householder (1963), their first feature film, was set in India and based on a novel by Ruth Prawer Jhabvala, who has since written the screenplays for most of their productions. Their early films, as well as some of their more recent ones, focused on the culture clash between East and West in India. These include *Shakespeare Wallah* (1965), *The Guru* (1969), *Bombay Talkie* (1970), *Heat and Dust* (1982), and *Cotton Mary* (1999). By the mid-1970s, however, they began to branch out so as to attract larger audiences.

After critical and commercial mishaps with *Savages* (1972) and *The Wild Party* (1975), Merchant and Ivory found what would become their characteristic mode with *The Europeans* (1979), a cinematic adaptation of Henry James's novel. Subsequently, their most notable films have been settings of canonical literary works, usually by gay or lesbian authors and with significant gay or lesbian plots or subplots.

In *The Bostonians* (1984), Vanessa Redgrave sympathetically portrays James's protagonist Olive Chancellor, a woman caught in a rivalry with a man for the love of another woman, while *Maurice* (1987) created a new audience for E. M. Forster's long-suppressed novel of love between men.

Other works based on queer literary sources include their adaptations of Forster's *A Room with a View* (1986) and *Howards End* (1992), Carson McCullers's *The Ballad of the Sad Café* (1991), and James's *The Golden Bowl* (2001).

By bringing controversial issues of sexuality and race into films accessible to a mainstream audience, Merchant and Ivory, often in subtle ways, made advances in cinematic representations of social difference. Although often produced on modest budgets, their films are visually stunning and they frequently showcase leading actors.

The two men shared residences on the three continents that shaped their work, including a home in Claverack, New York.

After forty-five years of collaboration in life and in art, the Merchant Ivory partnership ended on May 25, 2005, when Ismail Merchant died in London of complications from stomach surgery.

—*Patricia Juliana Smith*

BIBLIOGRAPHY

Long, Robert Emmet. *The Films of Merchant Ivory.* New York: H. N. Abrams, 1997.

Pym, John. *Merchant Ivory's English Landscapes: Rooms, Views, and Anglo-Saxon Attitudes.* New York: H. N. Abrams, 1995.

_____. *The Wandering Company: Twenty-One Years of Merchant Ivory Films.* London: British Film Institute, 1983.

SEE ALSO

Film; Callow, Simon

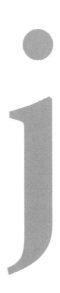

Japanese Film

WHILE ALTERNATIVE SEXUALITIES HAVE LONG PLAYED a role in Japan's literary history, from bisexuality in Lady Murasaki's eleventh-century *Tale of Genji* to Saikaku's seventeenth-century *Great Mirror of Male Love*, homosexuality in Japanese cinema, except for rare feudal-era gay films such as Oshima Nagisa's *Gohatto* (1999), has been mostly informed by twentieth-century modernity.

Also, the odd experimental film such as Ichikawa Kon's *An Actor's Revenge* (1963) notwithstanding, post-MacArthur Japanese cinema never really created film genres derived from native traditions of theatrical transvestism in the way that Hong Kong films did.

Rather, queer themes in Japanese cinema have drawn upon a cross section of leftist political filmmaking, pornography, and popular trends in *manga* (comics) and *anime* (animated films), a complex of factors that continues to make problematic all attempts to read contemporary queer Japanese films in terms of Western, post-Stonewall politics.

Indeed, only in the 1990s did Westernized gay liberation movements gain momentum in Japan, in part because Buddhist Japan has only recently adopted the Western notion of gayness and never had to deal directly with the homophobia underlying Christian sexual attitudes.

The 1960s New Wave Films

Although the *samurai* (warrior) and *yakuza* (gangster) genres have always been open to homoerotic interpretation, the first authentic queer films in Japan were products of the 1960s New Wave, a leftist movement concurrent with New Wave cinemas in the West. Films such as Imamura Shohei's *The Profound Desire of the Gods* (1968), Hani Susumu's *Nanami: First Love* (1967), and Terayama Shuji's *Emperor of Tomato Ketchup* (1970) dealt with incest, child sexuality, and other taboos.

In this radical atmosphere, a few queer films, such as Masumura Yasuzo's lesbian-themed marital satire *Passion* (1964, based on an early story by Tanizaki Jun'ichiro) and Matsumoto Toshio's transvestite black comedy *Funeral Procession of Roses* (1969), caused quite a stir.

But like many portrayals of deviant sexuality in the Japanese New Wave, homosexuality in these films arguably amounted only to another means of shocking the bourgeoisie, rather than an attempt to establish a transgressive queer cinema.

One exception, perhaps, is Fukasaku Kinji's brilliant *Black Lizard* (1968), a baroque transvestite burlesque whose main concerns are the gender ambiguities of romantic attraction, unalloyed by sexual exploitation or politics.

Pink Films

Around 1963, Nikkatsu studios fostered a new film genre, the "pink film" (*pinku eiga*). At first an artsy kind of soft-core sadomasochistic pornography, by the late 1960s the pink film had accrued radical political themes.

The best-known practitioner of pink films was Wakamatsu Koji, who, like Oshima Nagisa and other Japanese New Wavers, was heavily influenced by the radical student movements of late-1960s Japan, and whose depictions of anarchic sexuality became metaphors for the era's revolutionary politics.

Pink films—and there are thousands of them—are low budget, quickly produced, usually about one hour in length, and frequently feature lesbian images aimed, unsurprisingly, at heterosexual male audiences.

There are, however, some pink films of legitimate homosexual interest: Nakamura Genji's *Beautiful Mystery* (1983), a satire of Mishima Yukio's "Shield Society"; Shimada Koshi's gay romance *More Love* (1984); Sato Hisayasu's surreal, Pasolini-obsessed *Muscle* (1988); and Oki Hiroyuki's *Melody for Buddy Matsumae* (1992) and *I Like You, I Like You Very Much* (1994).

It should be noted, however, that some of these directors are not necessarily gay themselves—Nakamura Genji was a prolific director of heterosexual erotica and Sato Hisayasu is best known for his sadoerotic horror films (such as *Naked Blood*, 1995).

Indeed, with the exception of directors such as Oki Hiroyuki or Hashiguchi Ryosuke, most Japanese directors of gay films are not gay identified. We should remember that even seventeenth-century writer Saikaku wrote both hetero- and homosexual stories to please different audiences.

Manga and Anime

It is impossible to discuss queer Japanese cinema without emphasizing the importance of *manga* and *anime*. Since the late 1980s, animated erotica such as *LA Blue Girl* (1992), *Demon Beast Invasion* (1993), *Twin Angels* (1995), and hundreds of others have flooded video shops in both Japan and the West. Falling under the subgenre of *hentai* ("pervert"), these cartoons usually feature young lesbians with mystical powers and a penchant for blushing onanism.

While such lesbian-themed erotica for heterosexual male audiences is common wherever there is pornography, Japan is unique in that it also produces a prolific amount of young male homoerotic stories (*shonen ai*, literally, "boys' love"), usually written by women for the voyeuristic consumption of young, heterosexual women.

Shonen ai themes in *anime* can include anything from the coy homoeroticism and transvestism in *Here is Greenwood* (1991) to "taboo" gay romances such as *Wind and Trees Song* (1987, based on Takemiya Keiko's *manga*), Kigurashi Teruo's *Homosexual White Paper: Man's Decision* (1992), and Michihari Katsumi's *Love's Wedge* (1992), or the more aggressive gay erotica of Kodaka Kazuma's *Kizuna* (1995).

Japan has been most comfortable with queerness in *manga* and *anime*, perhaps because male and female characters are drawn similarly anyway, often with only hairstyles distinguishing genders. Furthermore, because Japanese censorship laws prohibit the "threat" of frontal nudity, the genital region is rendered as a blank slate, and what the artists draw is effectively a "neutered" or third gender.

This gender ambiguity has allowed for queer or gender-ambiguous characters to become a regular part of animated series popular with adolescents: an incidentally gay cop in the *Bubblegum Crisis* series (1987–1988), an ambisexual assassin in the *Cyber City Oedo* series (1990–1991), the transsexual farce of Takahashi Rumiko's *Ranma 1/2*, and even same-sex desire in the children's cartoon *Sailor Moon*.

Live-action versions of *manga* and *anime* are also common, such as Kaneko Shusuke's *Summer Vacation 1999* (1988, based on the 1974 manga *Heart of Toma*), in which the first-love yearnings of four teenage boys alone on summer break are enacted by four cross-dressed female actresses; and Hosoyama Tomoaki's outrageous satires *Weatherwoman* (1995) and *Weatherwoman Returns* (1996), which play like absurdist lesbian porn versions of Paddy Chayefsky's *Network*.

The "Gay Boom"

In the early 1990s, Japan experienced a so-called gay boom, with homosexuality becoming a standard topic on television talk shows and in tabloid magazines, just as it was in the West, and Japan witnessing its first Gay Pride marches.

Gay novels such as Hiruma Hisao's sensationalistic *Yes, Yes, Yes*, Nishino Koji's coming-out narrative *When I Met You in Shinjuku Ni-chome*, and Fushimi Noriaki's *Private Gay Life* were popular with both curious straight women and gay men, and the television serial *Dosokai* (1993) marked a kind of watershed in gay visibility.

During this period, a number of generically gay (male) films were released: Kojima Yasushi's *Rough Sketch of a Spiral* (1990), a landmark documentary about the lives of urban gay men; Matsuoka Joji's fake marriage drama *Twinkle* (1992); Nakajima Takehiro's *Okoge* (1992); Hiroki Ryuichi's *800 2 Lap Runners* (1994); and Hashiguchi Ryosuke's *Slight Fever of a Twenty Year Old* (1990) and *Like Grains of Sand* (1995), the latter promoted as the first commercial feature-length Japanese film about teenage male homosexuality.

While these films often do consider Western notions of gay rights, many are also framed in the *shonen ai* terms of the female spectator; for example, *Okoge*, the only one of these films to have been widely distributed in North America to date, is told from the point of view of a young woman fascinated by her gay male friends. Some gay rights activists in Japan, in fact, have criticized this trend for objectifying and trivializing the lives of gay men.

Furthermore, as the male homoeroticisms of the gay boom catered to the curious gaze of heterosexual audiences, lesbianism received short shrift, and one must look back to Yazaki Hitoshi's wistful romance *Afternoon Breezes* (1980) or ahead to Shindo Kaze's *Love Juice* (2000) and Shu Lea Cheang's experimental sci-fi porn *I.K.U.* (2000) for sincere representations of lesbian desire.

The Future of Japanese Queer Cinema

It remains to be seen what course Japanese queer cinema will take after the gay boom, whose films—with the exception of the upbeat *Okoge*—often seem more interested in creating a minimalist aesthetic of melancholy rather than expressing overt political points of view.

Furthermore, even allegedly outré Japanese cult films, rather than challenging bourgeois sensibilities in the style of the 1960s New Wave, tend to appease heterosexual bourgeois audiences by presenting homosexuality as a curious, "taboo" spectacle.

For example, the gay kiss between two criminals in Ishii Takashi's *Gonin* (1995) is not really as shocking as it is meant to be, and Miike Takashi's *Fudoh* (1996) presents a nihilistic, *manga*-inspired world where queer characters exist mainly to add another sensationalistic color to the film's spectrum of wild sex and violence.

The Uniqueness of Japanese Queer Cinema

Queer themes in Japanese films, then, cannot be framed solely in terms of Western gay liberation politics, which is still a new phenomenon in Japan. Yet it is precisely because of these differences that queer Japanese cinema is unique, offering visions of sexual transgression divorced from Western political correctness and assimilationist civil rights ideals.

While the idea of the female consumer of gay male images may seem grounded in a cultural misogyny—the female spectator perhaps imagines herself to be a man loving another man because loving as a woman is insufficient—it also fundamentally challenges the usual construction of same-sex desire.

Perhaps most significant, Japan's is the only world cinema that mass-produces sexually transgressive films, in the form of gender-bending *anime*, for children and adolescents. So while we should first appreciate such cultural differences on their own terms, we should also realize that Japanese cinema can offer queer alternatives more imaginative, more playful, and possibly more transgressive than those that conventional Western identity politics frequently allows.

—*Andrew Grossman*

BIBLIOGRAPHY

Desser, David. *Eros Plus Massacre: An Introduction to the Japanese New Wave.* Bloomington, Ind.: Indiana University Press, 1988.

Grossman, Andrew, ed. *Queer Asian Cinema: Shadows in the Shade.* Binghamton, N.Y.: Harrington Park Press, 2000.

Miller, Stephen, ed. *Partings at Dawn: An Anthology of Japanese Gay Literature.* San Francisco: Gay Sunshine Press, 1996.

McCarthy, Helen. *The Anime Movie Guide.* Woodstock, N.Y.: Overlook Press, 1996.

_____, and Jonathan Clements. *The Erotic Anime Movie Guide.* Woodstock, N.Y.: Overlook Press 1999.

Weisser, Thomas, and Yuko Mihara Weisser. *Japanese Cinema Encyclopedia: The Sex Films.* Miami: Vital Books, 1998.

SEE ALSO

Asian Film; Hong Kong Film

Jeter, Michael   *(1952–2003)*

VERSATILE CHARACTER ACTOR MICHAEL JETER PLAYED a wide variety of roles on stage, in movies, and on television. He was also a dedicated fundraiser in the cause of AIDS research.

Michael Jeter came from a family of health-care professionals, and it was expected that he, like his father, would go into medicine. Thus, when he left Lawrenceburg, Tennessee, the small city where he was born on August 26, 1952, it was to enroll as a premed student at Memphis State University.

Leaving Lawrenceburg was a relief for Jeter. He had always known that he was gay, but growing up in "a very conservative Southern Baptist family" in a generally conservative community caused him to have "a particularly traumatic time accepting" the fact. "I knew instinctually that I had to get out of there if I was ever going to understand what [my] difference was and get comfortable with it," he recalled.

As a student at Memphis State, Jeter discovered theater and soon developed a lively interest in pursuing an acting career. He abandoned his medical studies and transferred to the arts program.

After graduation in 1974, Jeter headed for New York, where he worked as a secretary at a law firm to support himself while he sought out acting jobs.

A small role in Milos Forman's *Hair* (1979) gave Jeter his first movie credit. He worked for Forman again in *Ragtime* (1981).

Jeter also found some work in off-Broadway theater productions, beginning with a role as a bellboy in Moss Hart and George S. Kaufman's *Once in a Lifetime* (1978).

After appearing in several other stage shows, Jeter joined the cast of Caryl Churchill's *Cloud 9* (1981–1983), directed by Tommy Tune.

It was in another production directed by Tune, Vicki Baum's *Grand Hotel* (1989), that Jeter had his greatest success on the stage, winning an Outer Critics Circle Award for Outstanding Actor in a Musical, a Drama Desk Award for Featured Actor in a Musical, the Clarence Derwent Prize for most promising actor on the metropolitan scene, and a Tony Award for Best Performance by a Featured Actor in a Musical.

At the 1990 Tony Awards ceremony at the Lunt-Fontanne Theater, Jeter stopped the show with his Charleston number from *Grand Hotel*, a piece that was not even in the original play. Jeter praised Tune, the choreographer as well as director, for creating a number suited to him even though he was not trained in dance. "I think that's one of Mr. Tune's little bits of specific brilliance," said Jeter. "That he can look at the way your body moves, and he can find the medium, in dance, within which to move it."

The dance was also ideally suited to Jeter's character, Otto Kringelein, a dying bookkeeper who, having led a sad and boring life, goes to Berlin "for a first and last fling." Jeter portrayed Kringelein, Mervyn Rothstein wrote, "breaking loose, with arms and legs gyrating in unexpected moments of sheer, uninhibited joy."

In his acceptance speech at the Tony Awards ceremony, Jeter said, "If you've got a problem with alcohol and drugs and think you can't stop, I stand here as living proof" (to the contrary). Afterward, he declined to speak in detail about his problems, saying only that they had begun when he was trying to gain acceptance by his peers at around age fourteen, and that he had been in recovery for some nine years.

Jeter became familiar to millions of television viewers when he appeared on the CBS situation comedy *Evening Shade*, starring Burt Reynolds. In the show, which ran from 1990 to 1994, Jeter played Herman Stiles, a wimpy and high-strung high school math teacher tapped to be the assistant football coach. Jeter won an Emmy for his role in 1992 and was nominated again in each of the next two years.

Jeter explained the appeal of the Stiles character by saying, "He is not perfect in any sense of the word. Everyone is Herman on some level." He went on to note that he had become comfortable with being less than perfect himself, saying, "I know that I am not what one normally thinks of as, let's say, fit for fantasy. I am not a romantic lead, and that's fine.... There was a time in my life when I hated myself for being so sort of squirrelly looking and odd."

Jeter gained fans in a younger generation of the television audience in 1998, when he joined the cast of the PBS children's series *Sesame Street*, appearing as the well-intentioned but bumbling Mr. Noodle in the "Elmo's World" segment.

Jeter appeared on television frequently in the 1990s, earning two more Emmy nominations for roles as a guest star on *Chicago Hope* and *Picket Fences* (both CBS). The role of an eccentric frog-breeder in the episode of *Picket Fences* was written especially for him.

He also performed in the PBS miniseries *Tales of the City* (1993), based on the stories of Armistead Maupin and directed by Alastair Reed, as well as in a number of made-for-television movies.

Jeter's long list of film credits is a testament to his versatility as a character actor. A cartoonish bad guy in the Disney movie *Air Bud* (1997, directed by Charles Martin Smith), Whoopi Goldberg's comic sidekick priest in the slapstick *Sister Act 2: Back in the Habit* (1993, directed by Emile Ardolino and Bill Duke), and a kindly mental patient in *Patch Adams* (1998, directed by Tom Shadyac), Jeter also gave a poignant performance as a homeless cabaret singer with AIDS in Terry Gilliam's *The Fisher King* (1991).

The movie role Jeter is perhaps best known for is kind-hearted Cajun death-row inmate Edward Delacroix in Frank Darabont's *The Green Mile* (1999). Critics raved about his performance, and Darabont concurred, commenting, "It's a hell of an indication of how good someone is when you see some big, hairy grip wiping his eyes after you cut."

Jeter had just completed filming his scenes for Robert Zemeckis's *The Polar Express* (2004) when he died in Hollywood on March 30, 2003.

Jeter was diagnosed as HIV-positive in the mid-1990s. He spoke publicly of his condition at an HIV/AIDS symposium at the Academy of Television Arts and Sciences in April 1997 and discussed it again a few months later on the syndicated television program *Entertainment Tonight*.

Jeter was an active supporter of AIDS charities, particularly AIDS Project Los Angeles, and appeared frequently at fund-raisers and benefits.

Jeter also had a "mission...to win over homophobic minds." His own parents were slow to accept his sexual orientation. They had never met a partner of their son until 1999, when Jeter introduced them to Sean Blue, his lover of four years. He called the occasion "really quite momentous in my life."

Jeter noted that photos of him at movie premieres were rarely published because he and Blue routinely held hands as they walked down the red carpet. He found, however, that most fans were accepting when they met the pair. Jeter observed, "The most effective way to do anything about the perceived differences between us is to say, 'This is the person I love, and we're happy to meet you.' And people are happy to meet us back." —*Linda Rapp*

BIBLIOGRAPHY

"Actor Michael Jeter Comes Out—as HIV-positive." *Advocate*, September 2, 1997, 22.

"Actor Michael Jeter, 50, Dies." *Advocate*, April 2, 2003. www.advocate.com/new_news.asp?id=8216&sd=04/02/03

Epstein, Jeffrey. "He Walks the Mile." *Advocate*, February 1, 2000, 46.

"Michael Jeter, 50, Dies; Won Acting Prizes." *New York Times*, April 3, 2003.

Oliver, Myrna. "Michael Jeter, 50; 'Mr. Noodle' on Sesame Street." *Los Angeles Times*, April 1, 2003.

Rothstein, Mervyn. "Tony Winner's Journey from Rock Bottom to Top." *New York Times*, June 5, 1990.

SEE ALSO

Film Actors: Gay Male

Jones, Cherry   (b. 1956)

CHERRY JONES BECAME THE FIRST OUT LESBIAN TO WIN a Tony Award when she was chosen as Best Actress in 1995. Classically trained and notably versatile, she has performed in a wide range of stage and film roles, gaining admiration for her professionalism.

Onstage, as Nicholas Martin, the director of the Huntington Theatre Company, comments, Jones "has a direct connection from the playwright's voice to the audience." Because she values being able to relate to the spectators, Jones particularly relishes working onstage, but she has also appeared in a number of films, including a television movie about a lesbian couple and the legal battle to retain custody of their daughter.

Jones began acting at an early age, "playing everything from Tarzan to cowboys-and-Indians to *Romeo and Juliet*" in the woods in Paris, Tennessee, the town where she was born on November 21, 1956. Her parents encouraged her interest by sending her to classes with Ruby Crider, a local drama teacher.

Seeing Colleen Dewhurst in Eugene O'Neill's *A Moon for the Misbegotten* caused Jones, then sixteen, to aspire to be a professional actress herself. Her grandmother, Thelma Cherry, supported her in this ambition, and Crider helped her get into the acting program at Carnegie Mellon University.

After she graduated, Jones moved briefly to New York before joining the American Repertory Theater (ART) in Cambridge, Massachusetts, in 1980. Jones calls her ten years at the ART a particularly valuable apprenticeship, by the end of which she "could finally hang out [her] shingle as a mature, seasoned actor."

As a member of the ART company, Jones appeared in works by Shakespeare, Chekhov, Molière, Brecht, Shaw, García Lorca, and others. At the same time, she was gaining experience and attention through performances off-Broadway and in regional theater.

After making her Broadway debut as the Angel in Tony Kushner's *Angels in America*, Jones had her first major Broadway role in Timberlake Wertenbaker's *Our Country's Good* in 1991, for which she earned a Tony nomination. She was also nominated in 2000 for her performance in *A Moon for the Misbegotten*.

In 1995—after fifteen years onstage—Jones became an "overnight sensation" with a powerful lead performance in a revival of Ruth and Augustus Goetz's *The Heiress*, and she also became the first openly lesbian actress to win a Tony Award. In her acceptance speech, she thanked architect Mary O'Connor, her partner since 1986.

Jones realized as a girl back in Paris, Tennessee, that she was a lesbian. Although she regards her hometown with affection, calling it "a wonderful little town…a wonderful mix of tolerant and intolerant people," she acknowledges feeling like an outsider at times, such as when, at age twelve, she felt alienated from her church because "they could never embrace me because of my homosexuality."

Her family, however, has been supportive. Jones says that her parents have taken pride in her professional accomplishments and that "they worshipped Mary [O'Connor] on sight."

Jones came out publicly at the very beginning of her career.

Some of her acting projects have had gay or lesbian themes. In 1992, she won an Obie Award for her performance in the off-Broadway production of lesbian playwright Paula Vogel's *The Baltimore Waltz*, about a seriously ill woman whose brother—dying of AIDS, unbeknownst to her—takes her on a fantasy trip to Europe to fulfill their long-held dream.

Jones also costarred with Brooke Shields in the television movie *What Makes a Family* (2001, directed by Maggie Greenwald), a dramatization of the story of a lesbian couple and the obstacles faced by one of the women when she must fight homophobic laws in order to adopt their daughter after her partner, the birth mother, dies.

Jones has hosted several episodes of *In the Life*, the glbtq newsmagazine that airs on many PBS stations.

She has appeared in a number of films as well. She had small parts in *A League of Their Own* (directed by Penny Marshall) and *Housesitter* (directed by Frank Oz) in 1992. Her performance in Alan Wade's *The Tears of Julian Po* (1997) was described by one reviewer as "the only memorable element of the film."

Her other film credits include *The Horse Whisperer* (1998, directed by Robert Redford), *The Cradle Will Rock* (1999, directed by Tim Robbins), *Erin Brockovich* (2000, directed by Steven Soderbergh), *The Perfect Storm* (2000, directed by Wolfgang Peterson), *The Divine Secrets of the Ya-Ya Sisterhood* (2002, directed by Callie Khouri), *Signs* (2002, directed by M. Night Shyamalan), *The Village* (2004, directed by M. Night Shyamalan), and *Ocean's Twelve* (2004, directed by Steven Soderbergh).

Although Jones acknowledges that film work is more lucrative, she prefers playing before live audiences instead of cameras. She won a Jason Robards Award "for artists devoted to live theater" in 2001, the inaugural year of the prize.

Jones won kudos in late 2002 for her seductive performance on Broadway as Mary McCarthy (opposite Swoosie Kurtz's Lillian Hellman) in Nora Ephron's "play with music," *Imaginary Friends,* an exploration of the famous literary feud between the two writers.

In 2004, Jones starred in the Manhattan Theatre Club's production of John Patrick Shanley's *Doubt,* which moved to Broadway in 2005 and won the Pulitzer Prize for Drama. Hailed by critics as mesmerizing and powerful, Jones's intense performance as a nun suspicious that a priest might be abusing students was rewarded with her second Tony Award.

Jones's road to stardom has not been without bumps. In the early 1990s, she suffered a bout of clinical depression and drank heavily, but she has overcome these problems.

Colleagues are impressed by her presence both onstage and off. Director Robert Falls, with whom she worked in Tennessee Williams's *Night of the Iguana,* speaks of her "absolute command of the stage." Playwright Tina Howe, in whose *Pride's Crossing* Jones starred in New York, adds that "she's always adding feeling and color and light into any room she walks.... [Jones] is a very healthy woman and sort of shines, as if she has all these klieg lights inside her."

Quick to learn lines, eager to accept challenges, and generous in her appreciation of those with whom she works, Jones is considered a consummate professional. Andre Bishop, the artistic director of the Lincoln Center Theater, states, "Everyone adores Cherry because, number one, she's a first-rate person. Number two, she's a first-rate actress. And, number three, she's hardworking to a fault."

Jones has also been described as "genuinely and deeply modest." Indeed, she eschews the glamour that can come with stardom in favor of a simpler lifestyle. She and O'Connor live in a small studio apartment and travel around New York City on bicycles.

After Jones received her first Tony Award, the couple celebrated her win—and coincidentally O'Connor's fortieth birthday—by driving to the home of some friends and drinking coffee in their farmyard as the sun came up.

Jones called the experience of being the first out lesbian to win a Tony "humbling," and spoke of the importance of the award to others, saying that "it means the world to all of those people in all of those places who can't be out."

—*Linda Rapp*

BIBLIOGRAPHY

Dezell, Maureen. "Cherry's Jubilee: With a Return to ART, Jones Puts the Topping on Broadway, Hollywood Acclaim." *Boston Globe,* May 10, 2002.

Hoffman, Jan. "A Luminous Path Navigated by Stage Lights." *New York Times,* January 7, 1998.

"Jones, Cherry." *Current Biography Yearbook 1998.* Elizabeth A. Schick, ed. New York and Dublin: The H. W. Wilson Company, 1998. 324–327.

Pacheco, Patrick. "She's in L.A., Not Hollywood; Cherry Jones Comes to Town with 'The Heiress,' But She's Not Looking for Great Fame and Fortune. You Can Catch Her Onstage at the Ahmanson (Or Perhaps Trying to Sneak out the Back Door)." *Los Angeles Times,* September 8, 1996.

"Role Models: Two Theatrical Treasures, Playwright Paula Vogel and Actor Cherry Jones, Talk about Women in the Arts, Lesbians Having Babies, and Ageism in America." *Advocate,* February 2, 1999, 42.

Scanlon, Dick. "Cherry Jones: Basking in Broadway Raves and a Girl-friend's Love, History's First Out Lesbian Tony Winner Remembers Her Fabulous 1995." *Advocate,* January 23, 1996, 76.

Stockwell, Anne. "One Family's Value: Exclusive; Advocate Cover Girl Brooke Shields and Gay Acting Goddess Cherry Jones Touch Hearts and Minds as Lesbian Moms in What Makes a Family." *Advocate,* January 30, 2001, 28.

SEE ALSO

In the Life

Julien, Isaac   *(b. 1960)*

FILMMAKER, ARTIST, AND CULTURAL CRITIC ISAAC JULIEN is the most prominent member of a new wave of black artists and filmmakers involved in examining black and gay representation.

Born in London in 1960 to parents from St. Lucia, Julien studied painting at St. Martin's School of Art in London.

Julien's first film, *Who Killed Colin Roach?* (1983), made at St. Martin's, shows many of the distinguishing features of the works that would follow, particularly a concern with the politics of representation. The film investigates the suspicious death of a black youth on the council estate where Julien lived. It draws upon the British tradition of documentary filmmaking, but abandons any pretense to objectivity in order to make a strong political statement.

Films that followed include *Territories* (1984) and *Passion of Remembrance* (codirected with Maureen Blackwood, 1986), which explore the history and representation of blacks in Britain. Both of these films were made with the groundbreaking black film and video collective Sankofa, which Julien cofounded.

Julien's first film to explore gay themes, *This Is Not an AIDS Advertisement* (1987), attempted to counter the antisex rhetoric of the 1980s and to promote more diverse representations of gay men on the screen.

Julien's next film is perhaps his best known, *Looking for Langston* (1989), produced for British television. This work, a lush and evocative meditation on the life of the African American poet Langston Hughes, is at the same time a sensuous portrayal of the black male body and black homosexuality.

Young Soul Rebels (1991), Julien's first feature film, is aimed at a younger and more mainstream audience than his previous works. Although not a commercial success, it won the Critics Prize at Cannes.

Set during the patriotic fervor of the Queen's Silver Jubilee in 1978, the film uses the explosion of punk and soul in the British music scene to deal with a series of controversial issues, including racism, interracial sex, and homophobia in the black community. It intertwines the narrative of the murder of a black man in a cruising park with the story of two black youths, one gay and one straight, who run a pirate radio station.

The disagreement between the two about how best to increase the station's profile can be seen as a debate about the most productive relation of minority groups to the nation. Criticizing those who insist on the purity of minority identity categories and minority politics, the film uses the space of the dance floor to argue for an intermixing of identities and for a coalitional approach to oppositional politics.

In 1993, Julien established, with three friends—singer Jimmy Somerville, filmmaker Steve McLean, and writer/producer Mark Nash—a production company they named Normal Films. The company is dedicated to producing queer documentaries and films. Among their productions are Julien's *The Attendant* (1993) and *A Darker Side of Black* (1994).

The Attendant portrays the interracial, sadomasochistic fantasies of a black museum guard, while *The Darker Side of Black* is a documentary about homophobia in the music of dance-hall star Shabba Ranks and others.

Frantz Fanon: Black Skin White Mask (1996) is once again a blend of documentary and fiction, looking at the life and works of the seminal theorist of colonial resistance.

Julien was also the senior producer of the four-part documentary series *The Question of Equality*, a history of the gay and lesbian movement in America.

In 2000, Julien collaborated with Venezuelan choreographer Javier de Frutos on *Cinerama*, a gallery installation, with the main feature a video entitled *The Road to Mazatlán*, which gives a stylized view of the cowboy. The title of the video is from a line in Tennessee Williams's *The Night of the Iguana*.

For almost as long as he has been making films, Julien has been a prominent cultural theorist in Britain and has for some years also worked as a visual artist. Since 1995, he has taught film and cultural theory, most recently at Harvard.

Throughout his career, Julien has experimented with fictional and nonfictional forms in order to challenge the dominant representations of both black men and homosexuality, as well as the dividing lines between various identity categories.

—Jim Ellis

BIBLIOGRAPHY

Diawara, Manthia. "The Absent One: The Avant-Garde and the Black Imaginary in Looking for Langston." *Representing Black Men.* Macellus Blount and George P. Cunningham, eds. New York: Routledge, 1996. 205–224.

———. "Black British Cinema: Spectatorship and Identity Formation in Territories." *Black British Cultural Studies: A Reader.* Houston A. Baker Jr., Manthia Diawara, and Ruth H. Lindeborg, eds. Chicago: University of Chicago Press, 1996. 293–305.

Grundmann, Roy. "Black Nationhood and the Rest in the West: An Interview with Isaac Julien." *Cineaste* 21.1–2 (1995): 28–31.

Jackson, Lynne, and Jean Rasenberger. "Young, British and Black." *Cineaste* 16.4 (1988): 24–25.

Julien, Isaac, and Colin MacCabe. *Diary of a Young Soul Rebel.* London: British Film Institute, 1991.

Mercer, Kobena. "Dark and Lovely Too: Black Gay Men in Independent Film." *Queer Looks: Perspectives on Lesbian and Gay Film and Video.* Martha Gever, John Greyson, and Pratibha Parmar, eds. New York: Routledge, 1993. 238–256.

Orgeron, Devin. "Re-Membering History in Isaac Julien's *The Attendant.*" *Film Quarterly* 53.4 (2000), 32–40.

SEE ALSO

Film Directors; Documentary Film; Film; British Television

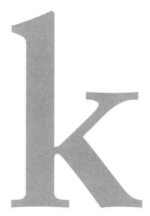

Kuchar, George (b. 1942)

FILM HISTORIAN JACK STEVENSON TELLS THE STORY OF how George Kuchar dealt with a problem that many directors have faced: a recalcitrant actor. On the set of his 1961 *Night of the Bomb*, the film's Puerto Rican female star refused to do the nude scene the script called for. Without hesitating, George substituted his own buttocks for hers. Born in 1942, he was at least about the right age.

This "can-do-in-the-face-of-chaos" attitude informs all the work of one of the founding fathers of underground cinematic camp. He and his twin brother, Mike, were born on August 21, 1942; they have been making innovative, if engagingly threadbare, epics since 1954, when *The Wet Destruction of the Atlantic Empire* saw the light of day. In that instance, the boys' appropriation of all available materials included their mother's nightgown.

According to George, "At the age of twelve I made a transvestite movie on the roof and was brutally beaten by my mother for having disgraced her, and also for soiling her nightgown." Mrs. Kuchar's reaction was the Kuchars' first bad review, but it is a testimony to the endearing quality of her sons and of their work that by the mid-1960s she was making regular cameo appearances in it.

Devotees of comic books, pornography, and commercial Hollywood cinema, George and Mike tried to replicate on film what they saw in their working-class lives—or filter it through their own gay sensibilities—using their 8 mm camera and whatever locations, props, friends, and family members were available.

In a 1998 essay, "Schooling," Kuchar recalls his artistic beginnings in language as lurid as his work: "After school my twin brother and I would escape to the cinema, fleeing from our classmates; urban urchins who belched up egg creams and clouds of nicotine. In the safety of the theater we'd sit through hour upon hour of Indian squaws being eaten alive by fire ants, debauched pagans coughing up blood as the temples of God crashed down on their intestines, and naked monstrosities made from rubber lumbering out of radiation-poisoned waters to claw the flesh off women who had just lost their virginity."

Wet Destruction was followed by many other works in the comic chaos mode, torrid two-dollar melodramas based on Kuchar favorites such as Douglas Sirk's *Written on the Wind* (1956). Some of the titles are as notorious as the films themselves: *Corruption of the Damned* (1967), *Pussy on a Hot Tin Roof* (1961), *Hold Me While I'm Naked* (1966). Many featured shoestring special effects that included floods, earthquakes, and tornadoes, rendered with stock footage, backyard assemblages, and matte paintings by the talented duo.

The Kuchars were innovative exhibitors as well, setting up informal cinema clubs to show their work, which scandalized some of the attendees with its sexual frankness, anarchistic air, laughable plots, and grade-Z special effects.

Eventually, members of the haute underground—Andy Warhol, Ken Jacobs, Jack Smith—took notice, and the Kuchars' films became both infamous in creating their legend and influential in showing others that neither a large budget nor good taste was a necessary condition of film art. John Waters cites them as a major inspiration.

In the 1960s, the brothers began to work separately. George refined the steamy camp melodrama, using a stock company of friends, and later worked in a diary format, which allowed him to record with droll humor the nuances of his daily life and his self-proclaimed favorite topic, midwestern tornadoes. In the early 1970s, he became a cartoonist in the underground comics scene but continued to make films.

In 1975, George Kuchar collaborated with the late gay filmmaker Curt McDowell on what would become one of underground cinema's best-known titles, *Thundercrack!*, a lewd send-up of the "old dark house" genre from 1930s Hollywood, which Kuchar cowrote and acted in.

Since 1971, Kuchar has taught filmmaking to scores of students at the San Francisco Art Institute, often collaborating with them on their projects and corralling them into working on his.

A scan of Kuchar's titles from the past several decades shows that his sensibility has remained pure, as evidenced by such titles as *The Devil's Cleavage* (1975), *Ascension of the Demonoids* (1985), *Summer of No Return* (1988), and the unusual self-portrait *I, An Actress* (1977).

Kuchar's latest major work, funded by the Rockefeller Foundation, carries his obsession with earthly, fleshly things into the literal stratosphere. *Secrets of the Shadow World* (2000) is a 140-minute digital video epic ostensibly tracking his attempts to make a "big UFO movie," but it is really an excuse to display the filmmaker's scintillating sensibility and eccentric gallery of friends.

In a bizarre tableau that reaches the giddy heights of camp, Kuchar shows the famed alien of Roswell, New Mexico, as a sex fiend, stretched out on top of a woman (Kuchar's friend Linda Martinez) who thrills to the touch of its plastic paw and moody, ovoid bedroom eyes.

—*Gary Morris*

BIBLIOGRAPHY

Kuchar, George, and Mike Kuchar. *Reflections from a Cinematic Cesspool*. Berkeley, Calif.: Zanja Press/Dangerous Concepts, 1997.

Murray, Raymond. *Images in the Dark: An Encyclopedia of Gay and Lesbian Film and Video*. New York: Plume, 1996.

Stevenson, Jack. "The Day the Bronx Invaded Earth: The Life and Cinema of the Brothers Kuchar." *Bright Lights Film Journal* 26 (November 1999): www.brightlightsfilm.com/26/kuchar1.html

Taubin, Amy. "Video Vanguard." Village Voice, July 25, 2000, 124.

SEE ALSO

Film; Film Directors; Warhol, Andy; Waters, John; Wood, Ed

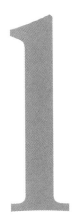

LaBruce, Bruce

(b. 1964)

BRUCE LABRUCE HAS BECOME ONE OF THE MOST CON-troversial and influential members of the queercore, or homocore, movement of extreme or guerrilla-type homosexual artistic expression. A writer, editor, actor, and photographer, LaBruce is most widely known as a director whose films consistently challenge and invert the way queer culture is depicted and celebrated.

Born Justin Stewart in Southampton, Ontario, in 1964, LaBruce experienced an "idyllic" and "isolated" childhood. His career in queercore began in his early twenties, when he became editor and producer of the homo punk fanzine *J.D.* (1985–1991).

In the late 1980s and early 1990s, he surfaced as the producer/director/writer/star of several Super 8 mm films, including *Boy/Girl, I Know What It's Like to Be Dead, Bruce and Pepper Wayne Gacy's Home Movies*, and *Slam!*

In 1991, LaBruce released his first feature-length film, *No Skin Off My Ass*. This film explores the relationship between an effete hairdresser (played by LaBruce) and a mute skinhead. The film quickly became a favorite of the independent film circuit and a cult hit.

LaBruce's next film was *Super 8?* (1994), an admonitory biopic about the rise to cult stardom of a rapidly aging porn actor/director and the underground filmmaker who exploits him. *Super 8?* played at film festivals worldwide, and was followed by *Hustler White* (1996), which LaBruce codirected with Rick Castro.

Hustler White tells the story of a Santa Monica Boulevard street hustler (Tony Ward) who is being pursued by a love-struck writer (LaBruce). The film intersperses parodic treatments of Billy Wilder's *Sunset Boulevard* (1950) and Robert Aldrich's *Whatever Happened to Baby Jane?* (1962) with graphic depictions of hard-core, underground sex. The most notorious scene in the film depicts a man being anally penetrated by the stump of an amputee's leg.

In 1999, LaBruce made the small but significant transition from queercore independent film to pornographic movies, directing *Skin Flick*, released by Cazzo Films. Recently, LaBruce has worked as a photographer and columnist for magazines such as *Honcho, Inches*, and *Index Magazine*.

In an interview, LaBruce explained why he entitled his 1997 memoir *The Reluctant Pornographer*. He remarked, "I think you'd be crazy not to be reluctant with regard to working in pornography. It is a very strange and harsh world which attracts a lot of interesting but sometimes insane and freaked out people. I choose to work in pornography because it is one of the few remaining places where homosexuals can express themselves freely and radically without fear of censure."

As a founder of the queercore movement, LaBruce has been instrumental in reaffirming and celebrating the outsider status of homosexuals. His films depict worlds inhabited by marginalized people such as street hustlers, porn stars, skinheads, drag queens, sadists, masochists, and others who exhibit an atypical sexuality. LaBruce believes these figures are in danger of disappearing in this new conformist century.

Regarding the movement he helped found, LaBruce said in an interview with *Oasis* magazine, "I think gay culture is more bourgeois than ever because now that it has been identified as a demographic which can be economically exploited by corporations, it is to the advantage of those who can capitalize on its commodification to make it as innocuous and non-threatening as possible in order to market it. Queercore was and probably remains a form of rebellion against this process."

An iconoclast and provocateur, LaBruce, through his work, remains committed to pushing the boundaries of cinema, society, moral comfort, and, yes, even taste, in his desire to demystify and explore worlds many might deem taboo.

—*Michael G. Cornelius*

BIBLIOGRAPHY

Gonick, Noam, ed. *Ride, Queer, Ride!* New York: Plug-In Editions, 1997.

Hannaham, James. "A Fellating Fellini." *Village Voice,* March 14, 1995, 56.

LaBruce, Bruce. *The Reluctant Pornographer.* New York: Gutter Press, 1997.

Thibault, Simon. "Bruce LaBruce: Reluctant Pornographer or Cinematic Idiot Savant?" *Oasis,* April 2000: www.oasismag.com/Issues/0004/cover2.html

SEE ALSO

Film; Pornographic Film and Video: Gay Male

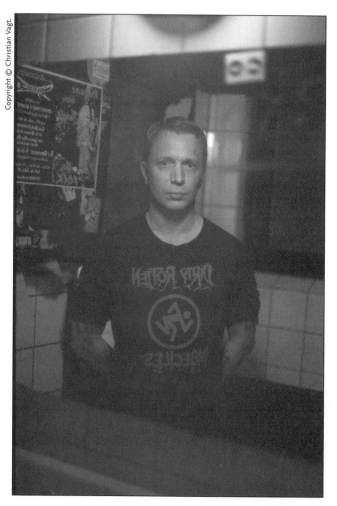

A portrait of Bruce LaBruce by Christian Vagt.

Lane, Nathan   (b. 1956)

A HIGHLY ACCLAIMED ACTOR, NATHAN LANE HAS appeared on stage, screen, and television. He has starred in Broadway productions of *Guys and Dolls, A Funny Thing Happened on the Way to the Forum, Love! Valour! Compassion!,* and *The Producers.* He has received numerous acting honors, including two Tony Awards. Openly gay himself, he has portrayed gay characters in several plays and also on screen in *Frankie and Johnny* and *The Birdcage.*

One of the most accomplished comic actors of his generation, Lane has an appealing presence that has earned him the admiration of legions of fans and critics. Although his métier is that of comedy, he is remarkably versatile. As Alex Witchel has observed, "Lane is an outsize talent who can belt it to the balcony and back, cajoling and beguiling with song, laughs, a few lumps in the throat. With his classic clown's face, part bulldog, part choirboy, he can be good and evil, smart and stupid, funny and sad, sometimes all in one number."

The youngest of three sons of Daniel Lane, a truck driver, and Nora Lane, a secretary, he was born Joseph Lane on February 3, 1956, in Jersey City, New Jersey. Around the time of his birth, his father's eyesight began to fail. Unemployed, the father fell victim to alcoholism and eleven years later "drank himself to death," according to his son.

When Lane was in his early teens, his mother began to suffer from manic depression severe enough to require occasional hospitalization. Lane's older brother Daniel became a surrogate father to him and encouraged his love of reading and theater.

Lane began acting while attending St. Peter's Preparatory School in Jersey City. He won a drama scholarship to St. Joseph's College in Philadelphia, but even with the award, the family could not afford the expense of college, and so he began working as an actor.

As Lane established himself in the profession by performing in dinner theater and children's productions, he supplemented his income with various jobs, including telemarketing, conducting surveys for the Harris poll, and delivering singing telegrams.

At the age of twenty-two, Lane registered with Actors' Equity. Since there was already a performer listed as Joe Lane, he changed his first name from Joseph to Nathan after the character Nathan Detroit in *Guys and Dolls*, whom he had played in dinner theater the previous year.

With Patrick Stark, Lane formed a comedy team called Stark and Lane. The duo, based in Los Angeles, worked at clubs, opened concerts, and made occasional television appearances. After a couple of years, Lane quit the act, which was not particularly profitable because of the travel expenses involved. In addition, Lane wanted to return to New York.

Before leaving California, Lane auditioned for and won a part in *One of the Boys*, a situation comedy starring Mickey Rooney. The series, which was filmed in New York, ran for only thirteen episodes in 1982, but it brought Lane to the attention of the public.

In the same year, Lane made his Broadway debut, playing Roland Maule in Noël Coward's *Present Laughter*, directed by George C. Scott. His performance met with critical approval, and he went on to appear in a number of plays, including Goldsmith's *She Stoops to Conquer* (1984, directed by Daniel Gerroll), Shakespeare's *Measure for Measure* (1985, directed by Joseph Papp), Simon Gray's *The Common Pursuit* (1986–1987, directed by Simon Gray and Michael McGuire), and August Darnell and Eric Overmyer's *A Pig's Valise* (1989, directed by Graciela Daniele), as well as two unsuccessful musicals, Elmer Bernstein and Don Black's *Merlin* (1982–1983, directed by Frank Dunlop) and William Perry's *Wind in the Willows* (1985–1986, staged by Tony Stevens).

In 1987, Lane made his film debut playing a ghost in Hector Babenco's *Ironweed*, based on the novel by William Kennedy.

In 1989, Lane played his first gay role, as Mendy in Terrence McNally's *The Lisbon Traviata*, directed by John Tillinger. His performance earned him the Drama Desk Award for best actor in a play.

Lane's association with McNally has been long and successful. In 1990, he acted in McNally's *Bad Habits* (directed by Paul Benedict), and in 1991, he appeared in the playwright's *Lips Together, Teeth Apart* (directed by Tillinger). In the latter he played a homophobic character.

In the early 1990s, Lane had roles in half a dozen films, including *Frankie and Johnny* (1991, directed by Garry Marshall), which was based on a play by McNally. In it he played the gay friend of Frankie, the female lead.

In 1992, Lane returned to Broadway in a revival of Frank Loesser's *Guys and Dolls*, directed by Jerry Zaks.

His performance as Nathan Detroit earned him rave reviews and another Drama Desk Award, this one for best actor in a musical, as well as a Tony nomination. The next year, he was well-received as the star of Neil Simon's *Laughter on the 23d Floor*, also directed by Zaks.

In 1994, Lane supplied the voice of Timon the meerkat in Rob Minkoff's *The Lion King*. Lane teamed with Ernie Sabella, who voiced Pumbaa the warthog, on the movie's extremely popular song "Hakuna Matata." Lane has since been the voice of other animated characters, including a cat in the film *Stuart Little* (1999, directed by Minkoff) and a dog in the Disney cartoon show *Teacher's Pet*, for which he won a Daytime Emmy Award.

In 1994, Lane worked in another play by McNally, *Love! Valour! Compassion!* (directed by Joe Mantello). He earned a Drama Desk Award as best featured actor in a play for his complex and moving portrayal of a gay man with AIDS.

Lane next appeared in a 1996 revival of Stephen Sondheim's *A Funny Thing Happened on the Way to the Forum*, directed by Zaks. Starring as Pseudolus, a Roman slave, Lane garnered enthusiastic reviews and a Tony Award for best performance by a leading actor in a musical.

In 1996, Lane played drag queen Albert opposite Robin Williams's Armand in Mike Nichols's film *The Birdcage*, a remake of Edouard Molinaro's 1978 film based on Jean Poiret's play, *La Cage aux Folles*. The film, with a script by Elaine May and Mike Nichols, was set in Miami's South Beach. Although controversial in a number of quarters, especially for its stereotypical portrait of a gay couple, the film was a commercial success, and Lane's performance was described as "wide-ranging [and] inventive."

Lane starred in a CBS situation comedy entitled *Encore! Encore!* in 1998–1999. He played a retired opera singer who returns to his home in the Napa Valley to assume management of his family's winery. Lane's original concept for his character was that of a "diva chef in a five-star restaurant" who had come out and was raising his son.

As it turned out, however, his character was entirely heterosexualized and he played an (unlikely) womanizer. Despite his own good acting (and the presence of veteran actress Joan Plowright, who played his mother), the show failed to attract an audience and was soon canceled.

Lane's recent work has included a 2000 production of Moss Hart and George S. Kaufman's *The Man Who Came to Dinner* (directed by Zaks) and, most successfully, a starring role in Mel Brooks's *The Producers* (2001, directed by Susan Stroman), described as "the biggest hit on Broadway in more than a decade." Lane won a Tony Award for best actor in a musical for his hilarious performance as Max Bialystock.

In 2002, Lane appeared as Mr. Crummles in Douglas McGrath's film version of Dickens's *Nicholas Nickleby*.

The actor, who has a "talent holding deal" with CBS, also was chosen to star in a comedy series in which he will play a gay congressman. The show has not yet been scheduled.

In 2004, Lane opened to mixed reviews in a musical adaptation of Aristophanes' *The Frogs*, with a book by Bert Shrevelove and music and lyrics by Stephen Sondheim. The show was originally produced in 1974 at the Yale School of Drama; for the 2004 production Lane freely adapted Shrevelove's book and starred as Dionysos, the god of theater.

Lane has never made a secret of his homosexuality. He came out to his family when he was twenty-one and about to move in with a lover. He did not comment publicly on his sexual orientation until 1999, however.

Lane has been criticized by some activists in the gay community for waiting so long to come out publicly. In an interview in the *Advocate* he explained that he "[found] it difficult to discuss [his] personal life with total strangers" but was moved to speak out after the murder of gay college student Matthew Shepard. "At this point it's selfish not to do whatever you can," said Lane. "If I...say I'm a gay person, it might make it easier for somebody else. So it seems stupid not to."

In other interviews Lane has alluded to an "on-again-off-again relationship with an actor who lives in Los Angeles," but has otherwise maintained privacy about his personal relationships.   — *Linda Rapp*

BIBLIOGRAPHY

"Lane, Nathan." *Current Biography Yearbook 1996*. Judith Graham, ed. New York: The H. W. Wilson Company, 1996. 286–289.

"Lane, Nathan." *Contemporary Theatre, Film and Television*. Michael J. Tyrkus, ed. Detroit: Gale Group, 2000. 201–203.

Vilanch, Bruce. "Citizen Lane." *Advocate*, February 2, 1999, 30.

Witchel, Alex. "'This Is It–As Happy as I Get, Baby.' Nathan Lane." *New York Times*, September 2, 2001.

SEE ALSO

Film Actors: Gay Male; Film Sissies

Laughton, Charles   (1899–1962)

CHARLES LAUGHTON WAS A DISTINGUISHED ANGLO-American stage and screen actor and director, as well as a noted orator and storyteller. He was also a tormented soul who, for much of his life, suffered from self-loathing and internalized homophobia. While his unhappiness may have contributed to his mastery as an actor, it in many ways poisoned his life.

Deeply ashamed of his desires, Laughton died at the age of sixty-two without ever having publicly discussed or declared his homosexuality—a state of affairs that was pretty much the norm for individuals of his generation. He disclosed it to his wife, Elsa Lanchester, in 1930, after a year of marriage, and she publicly discussed it for the first time in her 1983 book *Elsa Lanchester, Herself*.

Working in Britain as well as the United States, Laughton appeared in thirty-eight plays and fifty-two films, and gave hundreds of readings in one-man shows. For all his successes, however, he seemed to have most fully defined himself in terms of his failures.

The Night of the Hunter (1955), the only film Laughton directed, failed commercially and perplexed critics. Today it is considered a brilliant work of art, years ahead of its time; but its failure added to Laughton's sense of inadequacy. This sense of inadequacy was further fueled by his spectacular disaster on stage in 1959 in the role of Shakespeare's King Lear, the part he had set as his goal since becoming an actor.

Horrified at his homosexuality, Laughton lived with self-loathing, torturous shame, and constant fear of public exposure. Accepting and intensifying society's prejudices against homosexuals, Laughton turned against himself.

In *Charles Laughton: A Difficult Actor*, openly gay actor, director, and writer Simon Callow theorizes that Laughton channeled his pain and suffering into his stage and screen characterizations, using his "inner tensions in service of his art."

Born on July 1, 1899, in Yorkshire, England, Laughton was the son of Eliza Conlon and Robert Laughton, who owned the Victoria Inn in Scarborough. Charles attended the Jesuit Stonyhurst College, Lancastershire, where he excelled in mathematics. A brief involvement with theater ignited his passion for acting. He received his certificate in 1915, and went into the family business and then into the British Army.

Returning from World War I in 1919, Laughton worked for over five years in a family hotel until finally receiving his father's permission to enroll in the Royal Academy of Dramatic Arts in 1925. In 1926, he debuted in London's West End in Gogol's *The Government Inspector*.

After scoring a series of successes in London, Laughton appeared on Broadway in 1931 and then made the journey to Hollywood. His first film role was in gay director James Whale's comedy-horror movie, *The Old Dark House* (1932).

By 1936, critics noted that the characters Laughton selected were "downright repellent." Laughton preferred to describe his screen persona as "wicked, blustering, and untidy."

Although journalists did not address Laughton's homosexuality directly, they had no qualms about discussing his corpulence. Laughton responded by boasting

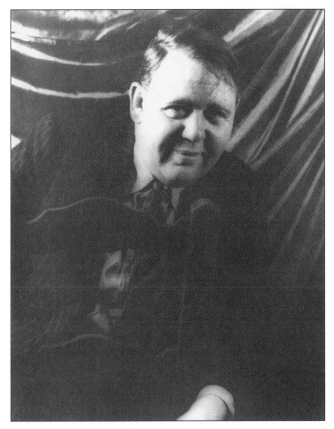

A portrait of Charles Laughton by Carl Van Vechten (1940).

that "having poundage has meant a succession of good roles."

Yet the bravado barely hid his hatred of his own body. When Laughton said he would never be a "romantic blade," he added, "sadism is more my type"; in that addition, perhaps more revealingly than he intended, he indicated the consequences of his homosexuality and obesity on his self-image.

Laughton won an Academy Award for *The Private Life of Henry VIII* (1933). In the title role, he created an "impulsive, tender, generous" portrait of a monarch.

But this role was the exception to the lonely, alienated, depraved villains that were more typical of Laughton's choices. He received acclaim for these characters in such plays as *A Man with Red Hair* (1928), *On the Spot* (1930), and *Payment Deferred* (1931), and in such films as *Devil and the Deep* (1932), *Sign of the Cross* (1932), and *The Barretts of Wimpole Street* (1934).

Laughton was a popular star after his Oscar-winning performance. His international fame and high critical regard were secured by his intense interpretations of Captain Bligh in *Mutiny on the Bounty* (1935) and Quasimodo in *The Hunchback of Notre Dame* (1939).

Laughton played Quasimodo as the horrific "other," thrown out and tortured by society. On a personal level, Laughton heaped additional—even unnecessary—cruelty

upon himself, demanding excessive makeup and an unreasonably heavy hump that made movement difficult and exhausting. In his role as Quasimodo he tapped into his guilt and suffering and exposed his inner conflicts in a brilliant interpretation.

Laughton's passionate performances almost certainly were motivated by an attempt to capture the love and admiration of audiences, qualities he believed were impossible for him to attain in his personal life.

To dissipate his loneliness, he sought the companionship of beautiful young men, many of whom began as his masseur or personal assistant. With a few of these men, he developed long and deeply romantic relationships. He was happy and productive when involved in these affairs, but when certain men parted, work was disrupted and loneliness returned.

Many of the actors and actresses with whom Laughton worked knew of his homosexuality, and it was rarely an issue on set or stage. But Laughton felt that his homosexuality rendered him vulnerable to attack by others. On the set of *Mutiny on the Bounty* (1935), Clark Gable's alleged homophobia and Laughton's apparently detached attitude created so much tension that producer Irving Thalberg had to intervene and restore order.

Although Laughton trembled at a possible public scandal, he always brought lovers on the sets of films to help him relax. Laughton's worst fear materialized while directing Henry Fonda in the play *The Caine Mutiny Court Martial* (1954). Fonda, angry at the play's development and execution, lashed out after Laughton made an unprovocative statement, saying, "What do you know about men, you fat faggot?"

Although Laughton generally played unsympathetic characters, he did so with passion and imagination. His acting was a means of escaping himself and disappearing into another personality. He used those things he despised most in himself to formulate characters so memorable that an audience would love—or at least admire—him for creating them.

In his later years, Laughton appeared less frequently in films, and then most often in smaller roles. Among his later successes were his memorable characterizations of Sir Wilfred Robarts in *Witness for the Prosecution* (1957) and Senator Seabright Cooley in *Advise and Consent* (1962).

In the early 1950s, Laughton embarked on reading or storytelling tours, bringing alive the works of writers he loved to audiences in relatively small venues. Laughton valued these "one-man guided tours," as he preferred to call them, believing Americans had a thirst for literature and knowledge.

Of equal importance to Laughton was the context, alone on a bare stage, that allowed closer contact with people. His personal comments and observations, the bridges between stories, intensified the intimacy of his relationship with his audiences. Audiences responded enthusiastically, offering the recognition, love, and companionship he needed.

Some of Laughton's internalized homophobia was also alleviated in 1960, after he and his wife bought a house in Santa Monica next door to writer Christopher Isherwood and artist Don Bachardy. The two couples became close friends, and Isherwood's and Bachardy's gay militancy and pride helped Laughton achieve a degree of acceptance.

Decades after Laughton's death, gay film critics and queer theorists appreciate especially the subtlety and brilliance of a wide range of Laughton's roles, including his work in *The Old Dark House* (1932) and *The Island of Lost Souls* (1933)—which have been characterized as "homo-horror" films—and in *The Sign of the Cross*, where he plays an effeminate Nero.

In Laughton's career, one failure was the most physically and psychologically debilitating, and one great success kept him alive. All serious actors, Laughton believed, conquered Shakespeare. But *Macbeth* and *King Lear* could not inhabit the poundage of Laughton's body, and he was unable to speak Shakespeare's verse authoritatively and rhythmically. The failure of his performance as Lear in Stratford in 1959 was crushing.

However, his supreme acting success as a happily married man sustained him. As prominent actors, Laughton and Lanchester were scrutinized by the press, reported on regularly in entertainment and mass-market magazines. Although their marriage was far from ideal, it satisfied certain needs of each of them. A measure of Laughton's success in the role of husband for thirty-two years is that in 1962 the press proclaimed him and Elsa the screen's happiest couple.

Laughton died in Hollywood on December 15, 1962.

—*Richard C. Bartone*

Bibliography

Callow, Simon. *Charles Laughton: A Difficult Actor.* London: Methuen, 1987.

Higham, Charles. *Charles Laughton: An Intimate Biography.* New York: Doubleday, 1976.

Lanchester, Elsa. *Elsa Lanchester, Herself.* New York: St. Martin's Press, 1983.

——. *Charles Laughton and I.* New York: Harcourt Brace, 1938.

McVay, Douglas. "Intolerant Giant." *Films and Filming* (March 1993): 20–24.

See also

Film; Film Actors: Gay Male; Horror Films; Callow, Simon; Whale, James

Laurents, Arthur (b. 1918)

P LAYWRIGHT, LIBRETTIST, SCREENWRITER, AND DIRECtor, Arthur Laurents brought an independent sensibility to some of the most important works of stage and screen in the post–World War II era.

He dared to live openly with a male lover in Hollywood in a period when the studios insisted upon the appearance of sexual conformity. And, in prime examples of what theorist Wayne Koestenbaum has termed "male double writing," Laurents collaborated with such major gay talents as Stephen Sondheim, Leonard Bernstein, Jerry Herman, Harvey Fierstein, and Jerome Robbins on musicals that challenged audiences to accept an unorthodoxy that goes against the grain of the American success myth.

In Laurents's *The Time of the Cuckoo* (1952), the courtly Renato Di Rossi, asked by a judgmental American spinster to justify the dishonesty required for his extramarital affairs, replies simply, "I am in approval of living." So, apparently, is Laurents.

Laurents was born on July 14, 1918, in the Flatbush section of Brooklyn to middle-class Jewish parents from whom he inherited socialist leanings.

Following graduation from Cornell University, Laurents served during World War II in an army film production unit in Astoria, Queens, where he wrote scripts designed to educate servicemen going overseas, as well as radio plays intended to foster civilian support for the war.

The success of Laurents's first commercially produced play, *Home of the Brave* (1945)—written in nine days and critically applauded for addressing the issue of anti-Semitism in the armed forces—encouraged him to move to Hollywood, then in its heyday.

In the film industry, Laurents quickly became known for his deftness with psychological themes. He wrote the scripts for *The Snake Pit* (1948), the story of a woman's emotional collapse and recovery, set in a mental asylum, with scenes considered shockingly realistic at the time; and Alfred Hitchcock's *Rope* (1948), a psychological thriller with a powerful homosexual subtext, which starred Laurents's then lover, Farley Granger.

Although Laurents was never blacklisted himself, his opposition to the studio heads' support of the communist witch hunts weakened his status in Hollywood.

He returned to New York, where he enjoyed success as a playwright (*Time of the Cuckoo*, 1952; *A Clearing in the Woods*, 1957; *Jolson Sings Again*, 1999), librettist (*West Side Story*, 1957; *Gypsy*, 1959; *Anyone Can Whistle*, 1964; *Do I Hear a Waltz?*, 1965; *Hallelujah, Baby!*, 1967; *Nick and Nora*, 1992), and director (*I Can Get It for You Wholesale*, 1962; the 1973 London premiere and 1989 Broadway revival of *Gypsy*; *La Cage aux Folles*, 1983).

Although he returned to Hollywood to work on the films *The Way We Were* (1973) and *The Turning Point* (1977), he has lived contentedly with his lover, Tom Hatcher, on a beachfront property in Quogue, Long Island, for almost fifty years, since 1955.

Laurents's experience of discrimination as both a Jew and a gay man—intensified by his experience during the Hollywood blacklist period—infuses his work with a strong social conscience.

In *The Way We Were*, Katie Morosky is marginalized both by her Jewish ethnicity and by her unflagging pursuit of social justice; her tragedy is to fall in love with Hubbell Gardner, a WASP who assimilates social norms so effortlessly that, finally, he has no principles.

Laurents also treated the subject of blacklisting in *Jolson Sings Again*, which dramatizes the sacrifices of life and integrity made to the McCarthyite drive to root out possible subversives.

Laurents's musical *Hallelujah, Baby!*, written for his good friend Lena Horne, looks at sixty years of race relations in America and was advertised as a "civil rights musical."

While Laurents followed the basic plot of Shakespeare's *Romeo and Juliet* in his book for *West Side Story*, he made two significant changes in the story. Rather than chance, it is the racial prejudice of the Jets/Montagues that prevents Anita/the messenger from delivering to Tony/Romeo the assurance that Maria/Juliet is still alive; and Maria/Juliet lives to confront the survivors with the evidence of what their hatred has cost the community.

Laurents suggested the "Officer Krupke" scene in *West Side Story*, which comically analyzes society's inability to deal with the juvenile delinquents who have been created by the mainstream's own misguided values.

Laurents's willingness to challenge social conventions makes him particularly interested in the relative values of madness and sanity. The relativity of normalcy is clear in *Time of the Cuckoo*, where Laurents satirizes American tourists in Venice who are unimaginative, insensitive, and self-centered, yet certain of their own superiority to the supposedly childlike, sexually undisciplined, immoral—yet clearly happier—Italians.

More provocatively, one of the settings for *Anyone Can Whistle* is a sanitarium called The Cookie Jar, described as catering to "the socially pressured"; the brilliant "Cookie Chase" scene underscores the contradictions in the American pursuit of success and happiness, which drives social authorities to attempt to destroy any instance of potentially subversive originality. Rose's breakdown in the climactic scene of *Gypsy* dramatizes the consequence of striving for success at any cost.

Laurents is at his best when depicting a female character's search for liberation from the social strictures that demand conformity. In *Gypsy*, Rose angrily protests

to her father that her own two daughters will "have a marvelous time! I'll be damned if I'm gonna let them sit away their lives like I did. And like you do—with only the calendar to tell you one day is different from the next!"

Laurents's most daring decision was to focus *Gypsy* not on the title character, on whose memoirs the play was based, but on Gypsy Rose Lee's mother, making the play the portrait of a woman so determined to break free of the humdrum that she is unaware of the moral monster she becomes in the process.

In *The Turning Point*, middle-aged friends Deedee Rogers and Emma Jacklin are forced to confront the choices made earlier in life that led one to leave the ballet stage to marry and raise a family in obscurity, and the other to become an internationally famous ballerina with an unsatisfying private life.

In *A Clearing in the Woods*, Virginia learns that "an end to dreams isn't an end to hope." And in *Time of the Cuckoo*, Leona Samish must let go of her unrealistic romantic expectations and accept the moment as life offers it. As Di Rossi advises Leona, "You are a hungry child to whom someone brings—ravioli. 'But I don't want ravioli, I want beefsteak!' You are hungry, Miss Samish! Eat the ravioli!"

Daring to aspire to a life beyond the humdrum, yet courageous enough to resist the corresponding temptation to be blinded by romantic illusion, Laurents's female characters are portraits of human resilience. They spoke strongly to the pre-Stonewall generation of gay men, themselves experimenting with constructing an alternative, more satisfying existence.   —*Raymond-Jean Frontain*

BIBLIOGRAPHY

Laurents, Arthur. *Original Story by Arthur Laurents: A Memoir of Broadway and Hollywood.* New York: Applause Theatre Books, 2000.

Mann, William J. *Behind the Screen: How Gays and Lesbians Shaped Hollywood, 1910–1969.* New York: Viking Penguin, 2001.

Miller, D. A. "Anal Rope." *Inside/Out: Lesbian Theories, Gay Theories.* Diana Fuss, ed. New York: Routledge, 1991. 119–141.

Mordden, Ethan. *Coming up Roses: The Broadway Musical in the 1950s.* New York: Oxford University Press, 1998.

———. *Open a New Window: The Broadway Musical in the 1960s.* New York: Palgrave, 2001.

SEE ALSO

Film Directors; Screenwriters; Fierstein, Harvey

Liberace   *(1919–1987)*

Mr. Showmanship, the Candelabra Kid, Guru of Glitter, Mr. Smiles, The King of Diamonds, and Mr. Box Office, Wladzui "Walter" Valentino Liberace was for many the epitome of camp, excess, and flamboyance, yet he was also a gay man who steadfastly refused to acknowledge publicly his sexual identity.

Born into a musical family on May 16, 1919, in West Allis, Wisconsin, Liberace learned to play the piano by ear at the age of four. As a teenager, he played popular tunes in local Milwaukee movie theaters and nightclubs as Walter Buster Keys. He also continued his classical training, debuting as a soloist with the Chicago Symphony in 1940.

After a brief stint with the Works Progress Administration Symphony Orchestra, Liberace attended the Wisconsin College of Music on scholarship.

An encore request after a 1939 classical recital altered Liberace's career path. His performance of the popular tune "Three Little Fishes" in a semiclassical style proved an immediate audience favorite.

Soon armed with his trademark candelabra on the piano, Liberace found himself booked into dinner clubs and hotels from coast to coast. Audiences immediately responded to his unique musicianship, which blended classical and popular music with glamour and glitter.

In 1950, Walter Valentino Liberace officially changed his name to Liberace. With an act that now included witty banter and some singing, the performer positioned himself to tackle a new market: television.

Begun in 1952 as a summertime replacement for *The Dinah Shore Show,* within two years *The Liberace Show* was the most watched program in the country. The show was on the air until 1956 and garnered Liberace a huge fan base. By 1954 he was earning over $1 million a year, with sixty-seven albums on the market, outselling even pop sensation Eddie Fisher. Although he made several movies, the performer was far more successful on the small screen than on the big one.

Liberace's appearance at the Hollywood Bowl in 1952 was the beginning of another Liberace trademark: elaborate clothes. Fearful he might get lost in the sea of black tuxedos worn by members of the Los Angeles Philharmonic, Liberace wore a custom-made white suit of tails.

Soon Liberace was spending a small fortune on flashy costumes. His elaborate costumes almost killed him in 1963 when he collapsed backstage after inhaling carbon tetrachloride, a cleaning chemical used on his soiled costumes.

Even though Liberace made his Carnegie Hall debut on September 25, 1953, his true home was not the concert hall, but the Las Vegas showroom. He opened the new Riviera Hotel in 1955, becoming the highest-paid entertainer in Las Vegas, with a weekly salary of $50,000.

Liberace's enormous popularity and exposure made him the object of speculation and interest on the part of gossip columnists, who could hardly fail to note his fey mannerisms and effeminacy.

When he arrived in London for a 1956 appearance at Festival Hall, the *Times* of London noted that he was welcomed by over 3,000 girls and young women and "some ardent young men."

When the London tabloid the *Daily Mirror* called him a "deadly, winking, sniggering, snuggling, chromium-plated, scent-impregnated, luminous, quivering, giggling, fruit-flavored, mincing, ice-covered heap of mother love" and "a sugary mountain of jingling claptrap wrapped in such a preposterous clown," Liberace sued for libel, stating that the tabloid insinuated that he practiced homosexuality, then a criminal offense.

In court, the performer repeatedly lied about his sexual life and thereby won the case. Liberace's lies about his sexual life may have been a calculated response to the virulent homophobia of the 1950s. One can hardly blame him for wanting to strike back at his persecutors.

Still, the lies established a pattern of denial and evasion that Liberace practiced for the rest of his life. In his four autobiographical books there is not a word of his homosexuality, which may suggest not merely discretion, but internalized homophobia.

In the 1960s, Liberace, now a fixture in Las Vegas, made his performances increasingly outrageous. In addition to the fantastic costumes, he made spectacular entrances, sometimes driving onstage in a custom car and then exiting by seeming to fly away.

In 1979, he opened The Liberace Museum in Las Vegas. It soon became the third-most-popular attraction in Nevada. It features eighteen of Liberace's thirty-nine pianos, numerous costumes, pieces of jewelry, and many of the performer's one-of-a-kind automobiles, including the "Stars and Stripes," a hand-painted red, white, and blue Rolls-Royce convertible.

All of Liberace's efforts to maintain his closet collapsed when Scott Thorson sued the entertainer for $113 million in palimony in 1982. Dismissing Thorson as a disgruntled employee who was fired for alcohol and drug use, Liberace denied in court that the two had been lovers for five years. Ultimately, the matter was settled out of court for $95,000.

Thorson, whom Liberace sent to a plastic surgeon to have Thorson's face remodeled in the performer's own image, was replaced by eighteen-year-old Cary James, who shared Liberace's life and bed until the performer's death five years later. James and Liberace both tested HIV-positive in 1985; James died in 1997.

In spite of his ill health and having lost fifty pounds, the sixty-seven-year-old Liberace honored his contract to appear at Radio City Music Hall in 1986, his third record-breaking engagement there. Horrified by Rock Hudson's recent outing and death, Liberace steadfastly refused to disclose anything about his sexuality or health. He told close friends, "I don't want to be remembered as an old queen who died of AIDS."

Liberace died at the age of sixty-eight on February 4, 1987. He left the bulk of his estate to the Liberace Foundation for the Performing and Creative Arts.

Despite the railing of critics that he was a failed artist who debased music, Liberace remains popular: As of 1994, thirty-one new editions of his records had been issued since his death only seven years earlier.

Liberace was not only immortalized by a star on the Hollywood Walk of Fame, but by two television biographies: *Liberace* (ABC) and *Liberace: Behind the Music* (CBS), both in 1988.   —*Bud Coleman*

BIBLIOGRAPHY

Faris, Jocelyn. *Liberace: A Bio-Bibliography*. Westport, Conn.: Greenwood Publishing Group, 1995.

Hadleigh, Boze. *Hollywood Gays*. Barricade Books, 1996.

Liberace. *An Autobiography*. New York: G. P. Putnam's Sons, 1973.

———. *Liberace Cooks*. New York: Barricade Books, 1970.

———. *The Things I Love*. New York: Grossett and Dunlap, 1976.

———. *The Wonderful Private World of Liberace*. Tony Palmer, ed. New York: Harper & Row, 1986.

Miller, Harriet H. *I'll Be Seeing You: The Young Liberace*. Las Vegas: Leesson Publishers, 1992.

Mungo, Ray. "Liberace." *Lives of Notable Gay Men and Lesbians*. New York: Chelsea House Publishing, 1995.

Pyron, Darden Asbury. *Liberace: An American Boy*. Chicago: University of Chicago Press, 2000.

Thomas, Bob. *Liberace: The True Story*. New York: St. Martins Press, 1988.

Thorson, Scott, with Alex Thorleifson. *Behind the Candelabra: My Life With Liberace*. New York: Dutton, 1988.

SEE ALSO

Film Actors: Gay Male; Hudson, Rock

Lucas, Craig   (b. 1951)

A LEADING CONTEMPORARY AMERICAN PLAYWRIGHT, Craig Lucas integrates high-spirited, kaleidoscopic storytelling with provocative explorations of the meaning of family and love in all its varieties. With the almost simultaneous successes of the Broadway romantic comedy *Prelude to a Kiss* and the landmark AIDS film *Longtime Companion* in 1990, he gained access to a platform for speaking out; he has continued to use that

forum for discussing the role and responsibilities of gay artists in society.

Born in Atlanta, Georgia, on April 30, 1951, Lucas was abandoned that very day in the backseat of a car parked at a gas station. Before he was ten months old, however, he was adopted into a Pennsylvania family; his adoptive father was an FBI agent, and he was raised in a very conservative home and community.

During the political, sexual, and creative ferment of the late 1960s and 1970s, Lucas was drawn to the political left and came to terms with his attraction to other men. To this day, he contends that only after he came out could he embark on a course of emotional healing that was essential to his growth as a writer. The freedom he has achieved to create work on his own terms appears not only in plays that include gay and lesbian characters and issues (*Blue Window* and *The Dying Gaul*), but also in plays that concern characters with quite different profiles (*Reckless* and *Prelude to a Kiss*).

After he graduated from Boston University in 1973 with a bachelor's degree in theater and creative writing, his teacher and mentor the poet Anne Sexton urged him to pursue his writing ambitions in New York. While he worked at various day jobs, his acting, singing, and dancing talents helped him land small parts in Broadway musicals, including *Shenandoah*, *On the Twentieth Century*, and *Sweeney Todd*.

Early Work

When Lucas was rewriting a play about a family's Thanksgiving dinner that eventually emerged as *Missing Persons* (1991), a friend showed a draft to director Norman René. That play centered on Gemma, a reclusive literary critic and the kind of person who can't keep from telling her son how his poetry fails; the wary family members and sparring friends in *Missing Persons* are typical of the mix of characters Lucas loves for his casts. René, who promised to produce the completed play, became his closest collaborator over the next fifteen years; he directed all of the early plays, as well as the films from Lucas's screenplays for some of those works.

As Lucas was working on *Missing Persons*, he and René also developed *Marry Me a Little*. In this cabaret revue of little-known Stephen Sondheim songs, a man and woman living in apartments next to each other without ever meeting sing of yearning and failure to connect. A favorite with show-tune enthusiasts, the original cast album features Suzanne Henry and Lucas in a rare recording of his way with a song.

Blue Window (1984) and *Reckless* (1988) showcase Lucas's talent for fusing meditations on personal identity with exuberant, often zany, satire. *Blue Window* follows seven people (including a lesbian couple and the probably gay character Griever) before, during, and after a comically tense New York dinner party; its spiky collage-like structure, with songs and side trips into dreams and memories, injects fresh energy and surprising resonance into a comedy of yuppie manners that is both funny and thoughtful.

The hostess, Libby, breaks a cap on a front tooth before her guests arrive; she goes through much of the party trying to be the perfect hostess while hiding the broken tooth from everyone. This scenario of an absurd accident and its awkward aftermath enables a mercurial actor to jump back and forth between anxiety and comedy as Libby's story of her recovery from an earlier, more serious, injury unfolds.

Lucas's determination to present multiple facets of his characters in a highly theatrical way is also evident in his treatment of Griever. On the one hand, he offers a private moment in which Griever delivers an over-the-top imitation of Diana Ross's response to the torrential rain at her infamous 1983 Central Park concert; later, he shows how deeply attuned Griever is to Libby's anxiety and struggle to reconnect with others. In *Reckless*, Lucas once again balances comic routines with heartbreak. This black comedy in the John Waters vein introduces us to Rachel, one of the world's most trusting and long-suffering women. Driven from her home on Christmas Eve and forced to leave her baby son by a husband who has ordered a hit on her, she wanders abroad, like Voltaire's Candide, amid horrors and catastrophes.

The play's antic spirit, with a surrealistic conjunction of TV game shows and threats to its heroine's life, keeps audiences laughing while Lucas assesses the toll that being alone and on the run takes on Rachel. The film version (1995), with Mia Farrow in a performance that downplays the spunky exuberance found in most staged versions, illuminates Lucas's statement that he wrote *Reckless* to explore his feelings about his early abandonment; in the film the deeply affecting performance of Stephen Dorff as Rachel's grown son stands out more clearly because of Farrow's interpretation.

Prelude to a Kiss and Longtime Companion

The pop-culture references, sassy humor, and fluid scene movement of *Blue Window, Three Postcards* (a 1987 collaboration with composer Craig Carnelia about three women's uneasy but enduring friendship), and *Reckless*—not to mention Lucas's ability to rethink *Blue Window* cinematically in his screenplay for its *American Playhouse* telecast—soon attracted the attention of Hollywood producers. This would lead to two of his greatest successes, *Prelude to a Kiss* and *Longtime Companion*.

The play *Prelude to a Kiss* (1990, directed by Norman René) is a romantic comedy about a marriage challenged from its first moments. At her wedding reception, Rita is kissed by a mysterious stranger, an elderly man. As if by magic, the kiss enables the stranger's personality to move into Rita's body and vice versa. The physical Rita, inhabited by the alien spirit, and her new husband, Peter, go off on a honeymoon to Jamaica; needless to say, Peter is perplexed by the odd changes in the woman he married. The play nods to the storytelling tradition of the fairy tale when the forces of true love, goodness, faith, and persistence eventually reverse the mysterious transmigration of souls.

Before that happens, however, the Spirit of Rita, resident in the stranger's body, begs, "So we might as well have a good time while we're here, don't you think?" This plea could serve as a motto for more than one of Lucas's put-upon survivors. Playing Rita, endearingly complex in her original state and comically cantankerous later on, when occupied by the stranger's personality, Mary-Louise Parker received wide acclaim and became a Broadway star; the play itself became Lucas's biggest Broadway success to date.

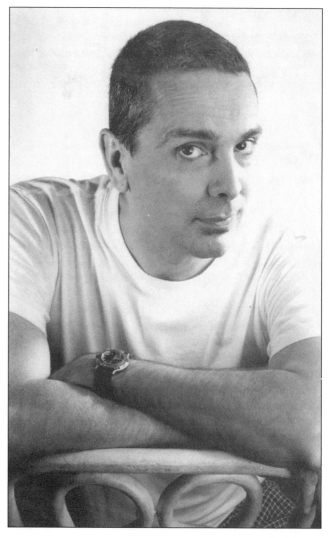

Craig Lucas.

When Hollywood producers began asking for film projects from Lucas, he proposed one about the impact of AIDS on a group of friends in the early 1980s. Revisiting the making of *Longtime Companion* in a 2002 article in the *Advocate*, Lucas spoke of the chilling silence that filled one conference room after another at this suggestion. He also gives full credit to Lindsay Law, producer of PBS's *American Playhouse* at the time, for determining to bring that landmark film to the screen in 1990.

Almost simultaneously with the commercial success of *Prelude to a Kiss*, *Longtime Companion*, with Lucas's original screenplay directed by Norman René, debuted in movie theaters. In contrast to Lucas's effervescent, even fantastical, stage work up to that time, this film, about a circle of friends in New York City in the 1980s, is a naturalistic chronicle of the impact of the AIDS pandemic. Encompassing the period from July 3, 1981, the day the *New York Times* first ran an article on a mysterious syndrome appearing in homosexual men, through July 19, 1989, when only three members of the work's original circle of eight characters survive, the movie portrays the way the world abruptly changed for gay men and their families and friends.

With its attention to everyday details within the circle, *Longtime Companion* reflects Lucas's own experience. (He was a volunteer for Gay Men's Health Crisis in New York and lost many lovers and friends to AIDS.) The film, as a result, carries the emotional power of witness testimony: It depicts all the stages of the pandemic, from early fear and denial through the years of caregiving and loss to the shell shock and exhaustion of those who survive.

Near the end of the film, the three surviving characters—Willy (Campbell Scott), Alan/Fuzzy (Stephen Caffrey), and Lisa (Mary-Louise Parker)—are strolling on the beach at Fire Island; their mood is subdued compared to that of the summer of 1981. Willy, once the wide-eyed innocent, now weary, notes that his one wish after seeing so many of his friends die is "to be there if they ever find a cure." The vision that the three friends share of what such a day would be like is the basis for one of the film's few flights of fantasy, and it is exceptionally moving: Everyone they have lost comes racing down to the beach for a joyous reunion. Then, in an instant, the imagined celebration dissolves. As the film ends, the three friends are back in their reality of grief and loss.

The success of two such different projects, onscreen and onstage, ignited media interest in Lucas, and brought him some curious criticism as well. For example, one queer critic attacked him for being "a closeted gay writer" because *Prelude to a Kiss* did not focus on gay and lesbian characters. Others took Lucas to task for *Longtime Companion*: One prominent movie reviewer

dismissed its characters as devoid of interest, while a gay critic criticized Lucas for not using an all-gay cast.

Defending his creative rights against such criticism, Lucas has given notice that the popularity of some of his work would not "prevent [him] from writing other, perhaps even different, plays as time goes on." He has stated, "The business of artists is to offer what they have seen and to imagine what they cannot truly know.... I believe I can speak sympathetically toward [straight people's] hopes and fears as well as to the issues facing queer people."

Following these media dustups, Lucas moved on to write the screenplay for *Prelude to a Kiss*. The 1992 film, also directed by René, starred Meg Ryan as Rita, in a performance that drew ire from many fans of the play. The experience of making a major Hollywood movie proved to be another eye-opener for Lucas.

Later Work

Whether in reaction to the sniping of reviewers in 1990 or the commercial pressures he felt during production of the film version of *Prelude to a Kiss*, a new, angrier playwright emerged in Lucas's next play. *The Dying Gaul* (1998) follows the journey of Robert, a screenwriter grieving his lover's death of AIDS. The play is savage in its portrait of the film industry and the compromises demanded of artists who wander into it unprepared. If Rachel, the innocent survivor of *Reckless*, seemed only moderately tarnished by her run-ins with an absurdly harsh world, Robert is clearly damaged goods in *The Dying Gaul*, and he admits it.

As Lucas has written, "My lover, my best friend, my closest colleague over decades...and...several dozen friends, ex-lovers and colleagues all died rather horrible deaths in rapid succession, and I did not find myself ascending into a compassionate, giving place, but instead a significantly meaner and less generous one." Not surprisingly, his later dramatic work is informed by searing anger and grief and is set in eerier territory than his early romantic comedies.

Since 1998, Lucas has also been expanding his theatrical reach. As director and writer of musical theater pieces in various stages of development, he has collaborated with a number of composers (Adam Guettel in *The Light in the Piazza* and Jeanine Tesori in *Don Juan de Marco*, among others). He has directed productions of classics by his theatrical idols, including August Strindberg's *Miss Julie* and Joe Orton's *Loot*. On the film front, he has written the award-winning screenplay for Alan Rudolph's *The Secret Lives of Dentists* (2002), adapted from Jane Smiley's novella *The Age of Grief*, and has directed his own screenplay of *The Dying Gaul*. Concurrently with these collaborations, Lucas was also developing a major new work for the stage. *Singing*

Forest (2004) charts one family's history, which spans a forced march from Nazi-infested Vienna in the 1930s to their appearance in celebrity-intoxicated New York City in the year 2000. While exploiting these two geographical and temporal settings for farcical and tragic dramatic effects, Lucas casts a cold eye on psychotherapy (Freud appears as a friend of the family in 1930s Vienna)—dramatizing how it has succeeded in some of its aspirations to enrich lives yet has fallen short in others.

Lucas's comparison of the two eras and places also throws into high relief the changes in the status of gay men. In 1930s Vienna, same-sex relationships could lead lovers to Nazi death camps; in millennial New York, Lucas seems to indicate, homosexuals are now just as likely as their heterosexual brethren to lead comically complicated love lives, but without fatal results.

Yet Lucas, for all his comic flair, clearly intends more than zany antics for the conflicted, struggling survivors of *Singing Forest*. His ability to portray these characters with equal measures of affection, empathy, and irony is what keeps him at the forefront of contemporary American playwrights.

In 2005, *The Light in the Piazza*, featuring music by Adam Guettel and a book by Lucas, opened on Broadway to enthusiastic reviews. Based on Elizabeth Spencer's 1953 novel, the musical has been praised for its psychological complexity, and for the sophistication of Lucas's adaptation of his source.

—*John McFarland*

BIBLIOGRAPHY

DeGaetani, John L. *A Search for a Postmodern Theater: Interviews with Contemporary Playwrights.* New York: Greenwood, 1991.

Hopkins, Billy. "Craig Lucas." *Bomb* 28 (Summer 1989): 56–59.

Lucas, Craig. "Equality in the Theatre," *Bomb* 57 (Fall 1996): 66–70.

———. "Justifying Our Love." *Advocate*, November 12, 2002, 87.

———. *Prelude to a Kiss and Other Plays.* New York: Theatre Communications Group, 1992.

———. *Reckless and Blue Window: Two Plays.* New York: Theatre Communications Group, 1989.

———. *What I Meant Was: New Plays and Selected One-Acts.* New York: Theatre Communications Group, 1999.

Swartz, Patti Capel. "Craig Lucas." *Gay & Lesbian Literature.* Vol 2. Tom Pendergast and Sara Pendergast, eds. Detroit: St. James Press, 1998. 232–34.

SEE ALSO

Screenwriters; Film; Waters, John

Lynde, Paul   *(1926–1982)*

OUT MAGAZINE, WRITING AFTER THE DEATH OF PAUL Lynde, said that the comedian, most famous for occupying the crucial center square on the game show *Hollywood Squares*, made the world "a safer place for sissies."

Yet, in spite of (or perhaps because of) his visibility and immense popularity, Lynde was fiercely closeted during his lifetime, and even known to denigrate gay audiences as a whole. Moreover, despite the campy, bitchy comic image he displayed to the public, Lynde was a tormented individual troubled by chronic alcoholism, weight problems, and loneliness.

Paul Edward Lynde was born on June 13, 1926, in Mount Vernon, Ohio. His father was a butcher and also, for a time, the local sheriff. His mother was known for her cooking, as Lynde would be later in life. Indeed, Lynde's early inclination toward overeating led to obesity by his teens; he weighed over 250 pounds when he enrolled as a freshman at Northwestern University in 1944.

Lynde majored in theater at college, where his classmates included Cloris Leachman and Charlton Heston, and while he aspired to be a "serious" screen actor, his manic persona consistently earned him comic roles. To some extent, this typecasting was one of the frustrations that lasted Lynde's entire life.

In 1949, both Lynde's parents died, apparently from the emotional stress of the recovery of the body of his soldier brother, who had been killed in the Battle of the Bulge in 1944 and who had been classified as missing in action for five years. Rather than affording the closure that such recoveries often provide, in this case the recovery opened new wounds, and the parents died within weeks of each other.

In the wake of this grief, Lynde devoted all his energies to his career; and, after a stint of stand-up comedy in New York clubs, he landed a part in the legendary revue *New Faces of 1952* that earned him great acclaim.

Despite such a seemingly auspicious beginning, Lynde found work hard to come by until 1960, when he won the role of Harry McAfee in the Broadway musical *Bye Bye Birdie*, which he repeated in the film version (1963).

After this turning point, Lynde had recurring roles and appearances on various television programs, including *The Perry Como Show*, *The Munsters* (as Dr. Dudley), and *Bewitched* (as Uncle Arthur). He also had roles in various light-entertainment films, including *Under the Yum Yum Tree* (1963), *Beach Blanket Bingo* (1965), and *The Glass Bottom Boat* (1966).

In 1968, Lynde began his long-running engagement as the center square on *Hollywood Squares*, and soon became a favorite television star for his queeny, campy, and naughty responses to the host's questions, some of them ad-libbed.

Although Lynde acquired fame and wealth during this period, happiness eluded him. He drank heavily, and, in 1965, he was involved in an incident that threatened to destroy his public image.

Jim Davidson, an aspiring young actor, fell or jumped to his death from the eighth-floor window of Lynde's San Francisco hotel room, after a night of drinking and pub-crawling. The matter was kept quiet by the police and the press, as it could have served to out Lynde in a very grotesque manner just as he was developing a large straight following by acting gay but never admitting the fact.

Throughout the 1970s, Lynde was one of television's most popular performers. He made numerous guest appearances as well as a couple of TV movies, and he starred in a short-lived series of his own (*The Paul Lynde Show,* 1972), in addition to his regular role on *Hollywood Squares.* He was dismissed from the latter program in 1979, however, when his drinking made him increasingly belligerent to his fellow performers and to contestants during taping.

After a year, though, the show slipped significantly in ratings, as Lynde had been one of its main draws. He was brought back in 1980, but by then game shows had become passé. *Hollywood Squares* went off the air in 1981.

Lynde's last days were spent in ill health. He was rumored to have cancer or some mysterious disease that was never disclosed to the public. On the night of January 9, 1982, he died in his Beverly Hills home after a sudden cardiac arrest, the result of decades of substance abuse.

—*Patricia Juliana Smith*

BIBLIOGRAPHY

Hadleigh, Boze. *Hollywood Gays.* New York: Barricade Books, 1996.

SEE ALSO

American Television: Situation Comedies; Flowers, Wayland; Moorehead, Agnes; Sargent, Dick

m

Marais, Jean

(1913–1998)

JEAN MARAIS BECAME ONE OF THE MOST CELEBRATED stars of French movies, theater, and television partly because of the early sponsorship of writer and film director Jean Cocteau. In a career that lasted over sixty years, Marais's blond, classical good looks and—with experience—skillful acting were seen in more than seventy movies and numerous plays and television programs.

Onstage, Marais achieved his greatest success in classical roles. Onscreen, he established himself as a romantic leading man in poetic dramas, light comedies, crime melodramas, and, perhaps especially, swashbuckling adventure stories.

Marais was born Jean-Alfred Villain-Marais on December 11, 1913, in Cherbourg to a shoplifting, sometimes violent, sometimes loving mother. Growing up in Cherbourg, the future actor was a poor student but always interested in drama.

He was expelled from high school when, to amuse his friends, he masqueraded as a girl and flirted with a male teacher. After leaving school, Marais worked at various jobs, including newspaper boy, photographer, and sketch artist.

An early interest in painting, which would become a lifelong avocation, led to the twenty-year-old Marais's first opportunity in movies. After purchasing one of his paintings in 1933, director Marcel L'Herbier offered Marais small parts in several of his films.

Marais's career breakthrough came a few years later, with Cocteau's help. The twenty-four-year-old actor first met the forty-eight-year-old poet in 1937, when Marais auditioned for a supporting role in a revival of Cocteau's play *Oedipe-roi* (*Oedipus Rex*, 1927).

Besides giving Marais the part, Cocteau fell instantly in love with the young man. Marais later remembered that, for him, the encounter marked the moment of a "second birth."

Marais and Cocteau became partners in both their personal and their professional lives. At Marais's suggestion, Cocteau wrote a screenplay designed as a vehicle for the ambitious actor, *L'Éternel retour* (*The Eternal Return*, 1943). The film turned out to be both a commercial success and a critical triumph for both its author and its star.

Marais continued to perform in movies and plays while German troops occupied France during World War II. He joined France's Second Armored Division after the liberation of Paris, however, and drove trucks carrying fuel and ammunition to the front during the Allied invasion of Germany. Marais was eventually awarded the Croix de Guerre for his wartime service.

After the war, *La Belle et la bête* (*Beauty and the Beast*, 1946), directed by Cocteau, introduced Marais to American audiences and cemented his international fame. His face and physique became favorite pinup images not

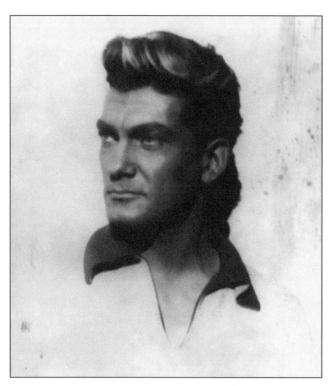

A portrait of Jean Marais by Carl Van Vechten (1949).

only for teenage girls, but also for gay fans aware of his unpublicized relationship with Cocteau.

Marais went on to make four more films with Cocteau: *L'Aigle à deux têtes* (*The Eagle Has Two Heads*, 1947), *Les Parents terribles* (*The Storm Within*, 1948), *Orphée* (*Orpheus*, 1949), and *Le Testament d'Orphée* (*The Testament of Orpheus*, 1960). He also starred in films by such celebrated directors as René Clément, Marc Allégret, Jean Renoir, Luchino Visconti, and Claude Lelouch.

Although the romantic relationship between Marais and Cocteau began to cool by 1949, the two men remained close friends until Cocteau's death in 1963.

When his acting career lost momentum in the 1970s, Marais lived in semiretirement on the French Riviera. He returned to painting and took up sculpture as alternative means of artistic expression, and also wrote several volumes of memoirs.

Marais appeared in his final screen role in 1996, in Bernardo Bertolucci's *Io ballo da sola* (*Stealing Beauty*). The same year, he was awarded the Legion of Honor for his contribution to French cinema.

He died on November 8, 1998, aged 84, survived by his adopted son, Serge Marais.   —*Charles Krinsky*

BIBLIOGRAPHY

Cocteau, Jean. *Jean Marais*. Paris: Calmann-Levy, 1951.

Krinsky, Charles. "Marais, Jean." *Gay Histories and Cultures: An Encyclopedia*. George E. Haggerty, ed. New York: Garland Publishing, 2000. 562–563.

Marais, Jean. *Histoires de ma vie*. Paris: A. Michel, 1975.

Steegmuller, Francis. *Cocteau: A Biography*. Boston: Little, Brown, 1970.

SEE ALSO

Film Actors: Gay Male; European Film; Cocteau, Jean; Visconti, Luchino

McDowall, Roddy   *(1928–1998)*

FOR MANY—PERHAPS MOST—CHILD STARS, LIFE AFTER adolescence means a decline in fame, financial and personal disaster, and, in all too many cases, substance abuse and premature death. Roddy McDowall was one of the great exceptions to the rule.

The British-born actor not only made a graceful transition from juvenile roles to a career as a highly versatile character actor on both stage and screen, but he also enjoyed acclaim for his photographic portraits of his peers.

Roderick Andrew Anthony Jude McDowall was born in London on September 17, 1928, to a Scottish father and an Irish mother. His mother, who had aspired to be an actress herself, enrolled him in elocution lessons at the age of five; and at the age of ten he had his first major film role as the youngest son in *Murder in the Family* (1938). Over the next two years he appeared in a dozen British films, in parts large and small.

McDowall's movie career was interrupted, however, by the German bombardment of London in World War II. Accompanied by his sister and his mother, he was one of many London children evacuated to places abroad.

As a result, he arrived in Hollywood in 1940, and the charming young English lad soon landed a major role as the youngest son in *How Green Was My Valley* (1941). The film made him a star at thirteen, and he appeared as an endearing boy in numerous Hollywood movies throughout the war years, most notably *Lassie, Come Home* (1943), with fellow English child star Elizabeth Taylor, and *My Friend Flicka* (1943).

By his late teens, McDowall had outgrown the parts in which he had been most successful. Accordingly, he went to New York to study acting and to hone his skills in a wide variety of roles on the Broadway stage, where he made his debut in 1953 in a revival of George Bernard Shaw's *Misalliance*.

McDowall was praised for his performance as a gay character in Meyer Levin's *Compulsion* (1957), a fictionalized account of the Leopold and Loeb murder case; and he won a Tony Award for best supporting actor as Tarquin in Jean Anouilh's *The Fighting Cock* (1960).

After a decade's absence, McDowall returned to Hollywood, and over the last four decades of his life he appeared in more than 100 films, encompassing a wide range of genres, from sophisticated adult comedy to children's fare, horror, and science fiction, usually as a character actor.

His best-known appearances were in *The Subterraneans* (1960), *Midnight Lace* (1960), *Cleopatra* (1963), *The Loved One* (1965), *Inside Daisy Clover* (1965), *Lord Love a Duck* (1966), *Planet of the Apes* (1968) and its various sequels, *Bedknobs and Broomsticks* (1971), *The Poseidon Adventure* (1973), *The Legend of Hell House* (1973), *Funny Lady* (1975), *Mae West* (1982), *Fright Night* (1985), *Fright Night II* (1987), *Carmilla* (1989), *Only the Lonely* (1991), *Last Summer in the Hamptons* (1993), and *It's My Party* (1996). His last film role was the voice of Mr. Soil, an ant, in *A Bug's Life* (1997).

Although McDowall never officially came out, the fact that he was gay was one of Hollywood's best known secrets. It is a tribute to his characteristic discretion and the respect with which "Hollywood's best friend" was regarded by his peers that his homosexuality was never really an issue or used against him in his six decades in the entertainment business.

McDowall died of cancer at his home in Studio City, California, on October 3, 1998. At the time of his death, he held several elected posts in the Academy of Motion Picture Arts and Sciences and was a generous benefactor of many film-related charities.   —*Patricia Juliana Smith*

BIBLIOGRAPHY

Aylesworth, Thomas G. *Hollywood Kids: Child Stars of the Silver Screen from 1903 to the Present.* New York: Dutton, 1987.

Castell, David. *The Films of Roddy McDowall.* London: Barnden Castell Williams, 1975.

Moore, Dick. *Twinkle, Twinkle, Little Star (And Don't Have Sex or Take the Car).* New York: Harper & Row, 1984.

Parish, James Robert. *Great Child Stars.* New York: Ace Books, 1976.

SEE ALSO

Film Actors: Gay Male

McKellen, Sir Ian   (b. 1939)

WHILE SIR IAN MCKELLEN IS CERTAINLY NOT THE FIRST gay British subject to be knighted by his monarch, he is nonetheless the first to receive this honor after making a public acknowledgment of his homosexuality. Ironically, McKellen's knighthood became a greater issue of controversy within the British gay cultural community than in the mainstream.

Ian Murray McKellen, arguably the finest Shakespearean actor of his generation, was born on May 25, 1939, in Burnley, Lancashire. His earliest acting experiences came while he was yet in grammar school. He attended St. Catharine's College, University of Cambridge, on scholarship and earned a baccalaureate degree in English in 1961.

While at Cambridge, he performed in numerous student dramatic productions, which earned him an acting apprenticeship at the Belgrade Theatre in Coventry, where he made his professional acting debut in 1961. Over the next three years, he played a wide variety of roles in various regional repertory theaters.

He made his London debut in 1964, as Godfrey in James Saunders's *A Scent of Flowers*, for which role he received the Clarence Derwent Award for best supporting actor.

In 1965, McKellen made the first of many appearances at the National Theatre, London, as Claudio in Franco Zeffirelli's production of Shakespeare's *Much Ado About Nothing*. His film debut came the following year in Waris Hussein's *A Touch of Love*, which featured a screenplay by McKellen's friend from Cambridge, Margaret Drabble; in the film, based on Drabble's novel *The Millstone*, McKellen played a gay character opposite Sandy Dennis.

During the 1960s, McKellen's career branched out into stage direction as well, at first in regional theaters. In 1972, he directed his first London production, a revival of Joe Orton's *The Erpingham Camp*; later that year he cofounded the Actors' Company, a group based on the principle of equality among and management by its members.

McKellen's debut with the Royal Shakespeare Company came in 1974, with his performance in the title role in Christopher Marlowe's *Doctor Faustus*; other roles with the company include Romeo, Leontes (in *A Winter's Tale*), Macbeth, and Sir Toby Belch (*Twelfth Night*).

Over the course of his distinguished career on the British stage, he has received the prestigious Olivier Award five times, and in 1981 received the Tony Award for his portrayal of Mozart's nemesis Salieri in the Broadway production of Peter Shaffer's *Amadeus*.

Until the 1980s, McKellen's career focused primarily on the stage, a medium in which he remains energetically involved. In 1981, he made his first film appearance in a starring role, as D. H. Lawrence in *Priest of Love*.

Other major parts followed in *Plenty* (1985) and *Scandal* (1989). In the latter film, he played the disgraced 1960s British cabinet member John Profumo (a role a number of other British actors turned down) because, as McKellen states, he wanted to prove after coming out publicly that he could convincingly play a character remembered only for being a "raging heterosexual."

While McKellen had quietly lived a gay life for many years, he came out during the course of a 1988 British radio program in response to the host's homophobic comments. He has subsequently been active as a member of Arts Lobby against Section 28 (British legislation, finally repealed in 2003, that forbade "intentional promotion of homosexuality" by local governments), and he cofounded the gay lobbying group Stonewall.

The Queen's 1991 New Years Honours List named McKellen a Knight Commander of the British Empire for services to the arts. Yet, in spite of his highly visible work as a gay activist, his knighthood was the source of considerable controversy and divisiveness within days of its announcement, as director Derek Jarman, then dying of AIDS, publicly and bitterly denounced him.

Jarman equated McKellen's acceptance of the honor with collaboration with the decidedly homophobic Tory government of Prime Minister Margaret Thatcher. This polemic was countered almost immediately by an open letter in the *Guardian*, signed by such noted British gay and lesbian artists as Simon Callow, Nancy Diuguid, Stephen Fry, Bryony Lavery, John Schlesinger, and Antony Sher.

Despite this controversy, McKellen has remained a highly visible champion of gay rights, and he has used his prominence as an actor to draw attention to the social intolerance that homosexuals routinely bear.

In 1994, he premiered his one-man show, *A Knight Out*, which incorporates his reminiscences as an actor and gay man with the words of various gay or bisexual authors. He has also appeared in a number of gay roles and gay-themed films and television productions, including *Six Degrees of Separation* (1993), *And the Band Played On* (1993), *Bent* (1997), and, most notably, *Gods and Monsters* (1998).

In Bill Condon's *Gods and Monsters*, based on Christopher Bram's novel *Father of Frankenstein*, McKellen played James Whale, the British-born gay Hollywood director best known for such 1930s horror films as *Frankenstein* and *The Bride of Frankenstein*. For his performance in this role, McKellen was nominated for the Academy Award for Best Actor.

Among his other films are *Richard III* (1996), *Apt Pupil* (1998), and *X-Men* (2000).

As his acting career entered the twenty-first century, McKellen starred as the wizard Gandalf in the ambitious three-part film adaptation of J. R. R. Tolkien's fantasy epic, *The Lord of the Rings*. His portrayal of the wizard in *Fellowship of the Ring* (2001) received accolades from critics and earned him the Screen Actors Guild Award for Best Supporting Actor and an Academy Award nomination. He also appeared in *Asylum* (2004).

For the past decade, he has lived with his partner, actor Sean Mathias, who directed him in Martin Sherman's *Bent* (1990) and in August Strindberg's *Dance of Death* (2001).

McKellen was Grand Master of the 2002 San Francisco Gay Pride Parade. —*Patricia Juliana Smith*

BIBLIOGRAPHY

Bronski, Michael, Christa Brelin, and Michael J. Tyrkus, eds. *Outstanding Lives: Profiles of Lesbians and Gay Men*. Detroit: Visible Ink, 1997.

Gibson, Joy Leslie. *Ian McKellen*. London: Weidenfeld and Nicolson, 1986.

Russell, Paul Elliott. *The Gay 100: A Ranking of the Most Influential Gay Men and Lesbians, Past and Present*. New York: Birch Lane Press, 1994.

SEE ALSO

Film Actors: Gay Male; British Television; Callow, Simon; Condon, William "Bill"; Fry, Stephen; Schlesinger, John; Whale, James; Wong, B. D.; Zeffirelli, Franco

Mineo, Sal (1939–1976)

ALTHOUGH ACTOR SAL MINEO WAS TWICE NOMINATED for an Academy Award, and enjoyed success as a stage director and recording artist, he is remembered chiefly for his performance in *Rebel Without a Cause* and for the brutal murder that ended his life just as he was on the verge of reinventing himself and his career.

He was born Salvatore Mineo Jr. in the Bronx, New York, on January 10, 1939. His parents, who had emigrated from Sicily, made caskets for a living.

The actor began his career playing sad-eyed juveniles and progressed to leading stage, film, and television roles. Following dismissal from a parochial school at eight as a troublemaker, Mineo attended dancing classes and was cast two years later as a child in the Broadway production of Tennessee Williams's *The Rose Tattoo* (1951).

He made his first film appearance in 1955, and subsequently appeared in many screen productions, typically portraying troubled youths. Yet Mineo's career was dominated by a single role that swiftly achieved mythic status: his Plato in Nicholas Ray's *Rebel Without a Cause* (1955).

In his provocative analysis, Robin Wood argues that *Rebel Without a Cause* is the only film in which Mineo's character is clearly coded as gay. The film deals with a disturbed teenager, Jim (James Dean), who moves into town with an ineffective father (Jim Backus) and a domineering mother (Ann Doran) and becomes friends with two confused adolescents, Judy (Natalie Wood) and Plato (Mineo).

Although *Rebel* intermittently transcends its textbook-sociology basis, it is a striking example of a great opportunity missed: It opens up the possibility of constructing an alternative, nonrepressive and nonauthoritarian sexual/familial structure, then opts for restoring "normality" at the end.

The three teenage characters move toward creating an alternative, mutually caring and protective, family, with Jim as father, Judy as mother, and Plato as child. Yet this archetype is disturbed and complicated by the continual threat (produced as much by the sexual ambiguity of the Dean persona as by the presence of Mineo) of a sexual dimension in the men's relationship.

To repudiate (rather than resolve) those implications, the film has Jim become preoccupied with Judy. Significantly, the vital move for completing this operation is the elimination of Plato, the character who—far more than Jim or Judy—resists assimilation into bourgeois culture.

Typically, as with the film's other teenage characters, Plato's "problem" is explained in terms of an unsatisfactory family background; nevertheless, during the central sequences in the abandoned mansion, his gayness achieves a resonance that escapes the film's glib sociologizing. For his role as Plato, Mineo received an Academy Award nomination as best supporting actor.

Mineo's screen persona had two aspects: vulnerability and aggressiveness. If *Rebel Without a Cause* offered the most complete realization of the former, the latter perhaps received fullest expression in *Cheyenne Autumn* (1964), where Mineo played a transgressive and intractable Native American brave.

In directing Mineo as Dov Landau in *Exodus* (1960), Otto Preminger made possible the ideal fusion of these two aspects. Landau is surely Mineo's finest performance, though, ironically, it is achieved by the explicit repudiation of the character's gay connotations.

The extraordinary intensity of the interrogation scene, in which Landau shamefully and painfully admits, "They used me as you would use a woman," is due primarily to Mineo's combination of vulnerability and aggression.

Other films in which Mineo appeared include *Giant* (1956), *The Gene Krupa Story* (1959), *Who Killed Teddy Bear?* (1965), and *The Greatest Story Ever Told* (1965). He also had a modest success in the 1950s as a rock-and-roll singer.

Mineo received his second Oscar nomination for his supporting performance in *Exodus*. Nevertheless, despite this recognition, his film career declined precipitously thereafter, as he was mostly limited to playing ethnic characters.

Mineo's homosexuality was a fairly open secret even at the height of his Hollywood success. He was rumored to have pursued numerous affairs, including one with Nicholas Ray during the filming of *Rebel Without a Cause*.

With maturity, he sought to explore his homosexuality more fully in both his life and his art. Although he appeared in several television productions and films, in his latter years he increasingly found the theater more supportive of his aspirations.

In 1969, he directed the Broadway and West Coast productions of *Fortune and Men's Eyes*, John Herbert's exploration of power roles in situational homosexuality

at a Canadian prison. Mineo's production was controversial for its nudity and simulated sex.

In 1976, Mineo was cast in a Los Angeles production of James Kirkwood's *P. S. Your Cat Is Dead*. As he returned to his West Hollywood apartment from a rehearsal on February 12, 1976, he was stabbed to death. The murder remains cloaked in mystery. A suspect who initially confessed later recanted, but was nevertheless convicted.

Over the years, some of Mineo's friends and relatives have claimed that the authorities, eager to solve a high-profile murder case, charged the wrong man.

—*Peter J. Holliday*

BIBLIOGRAPHY

Braudy, Susan. *Who Killed Sal Mineo? A Novel.* New York: Wyndham Books, 1982.

Jeffers, Paul H. *Sal Mineo: His Life, Murder, and Mystery.* New York: Carrol & Graf, 2000.

Wood, Robin. "Mineo, Sal." *International Dictionary of Films and Filmmakers. Vol. 3. Actors and Actresses.* 2nd ed. Nicholas Thomas, ed. Chicago and London: St. James Press, 1991. 680–681.

SEE ALSO

Film Actors: Gay Male; Screenwriters; Dean, James

Minnelli, Vincente (1913–1986)

DAPPER VINCENTE MINNELLI WAS ONE OF HOLLYWOOD'S greatest directors, renowned for his skilled use of color and light and his precise attention to detail. He achieved recognition not only for the new life he injected into movie musicals such as *Meet Me in St. Louis* (1944) and *Gigi* (1958), but also for emotionally complex comedies such as *Father of the Bride* (1950) and lushly conceived melodramas such as *Lust for Life* (1956).

Minnelli's campy vision and lavish productions were well suited to the 1940s and 1950s, but his style did not long survive the end of Hollywood's structured studio system. Although he continued to make films into the 1970s (such as *A Matter of Time*, with his daughter Liza Minnelli in 1976), his later films did not gain the popularity or acclaim of his earlier work.

Minnelli was born on February 28, 1903, in Delaware, Ohio, into a family of traveling entertainers. Although his early years were spent on the road learning show business, he settled in Chicago at age sixteen.

He took a job as a window decorator for Marshall Field's department store, where he began to develop his sense of design. He soon took his new knowledge back to the theater, where he worked as an assistant photographer, costume designer, and set decorator. His originality and sharp eye for the details of design soon took him to the Broadway stage, where he was a successful costume and set designer.

Metro-Goldwyn-Mayer producer Arthur Freed discovered Minnelli on Broadway and brought him back to work his magic designing dance numbers for musicals at MGM. He worked on several films, including *Strike up the Band* (1940) and *Babes on Broadway* (1941) with Judy Garland and Mickey Rooney, before he was given the directorship of an all-black musical entitled *Cabin in the Sky* (1943). The stylish and inventive *Cabin in the Sky* was a success, and the window dresser from Chicago was now a Hollywood director.

Minnelli's next film, *Meet Me in St. Louis*, was a tour de force and a milestone in American filmmaking. Not only was it a textured look at turn-of-the-century Americana that spoke poignantly to a country in the midst of World War II, but it was also a showcase for Minnelli's flamboyant camera techniques and powerful use of color.

Meet Me in St. Louis was child star Judy Garland's first adult film. It led to the star's marriage to her director.

Although he married four times, Minnelli was widely known to be gay. In the deeply closeted world of 1950s Hollywood he kept his sexual orientation quite private, though his gay sensibility is visible in many of his films.

In his 1956 film version of Robert Anderson's exploration of masculinity and homophobia, *Tea and Sympathy*, Minnelli worked around the restrictions of the Motion Picture Association of America's production code to recreate the play's ambiguities without ever using the word *homosexual*.

In the little-noticed *Goodbye Charlie* (1964), Minnelli exploits the lighter side of gender confusion with a frothy comedy about a murdered womanizer who returns to earth in the body of a woman.

With the advent of a harsher realism in the movies in the 1960s and 1970s, Minnelli's dream sequences and fanciful use of color came to seem old-fashioned and out of date. He wrote his memoirs in 1974 and retired after the failure of *A Matter of Time* in 1976.

He died in Beverly Hills on July 26, 1986.

In 1999, Liza Minnelli premiered a tribute to her father called *Minnelli on Minnelli*, in which she performed many of the best-known and most beloved songs from his musicals, some of which had been made famous by her mother, Judy Garland, interspersed with loving reminiscences.

—*Tina Gianoulis*

BIBLIOGRAPHY

Gerstner, David. "Queer Modernism: The Cinematic Aesthetics of Vincente Minnelli." www.eiu.edu/~modernity/gerst—html

———. "The Production and Display of the Closet: Making Minnelli's Tea and Sympathy." *Film Quarterly* 50.3 (Spring 1997):13–27.

Harvey, Stephen. *Directed by Vincente Minnelli*. New York: Harper & Row, 1989.

Minnelli, Vincente, with Hector Arce. *I Remember It Well*. Hollywood, Calif.: Samuel French Trade, 1990.

Naremore, James. *The Films of Vincente Minnelli*. New York: Cambridge University Press, 1993.

SEE ALSO

Film; Film Directors; Set and Costume Design; Garland, Judy

Mitchell, John Cameron   (b. 1963)

WHILE HE HAD ALREADY ACHIEVED RECOGNITION AS an actor, the multiple talents of performer, writer, and filmmaker John Cameron Mitchell came to wide public notice in 2001 with the release of his prize-winning film *Hedwig and the Angry Inch*. Based on his successful 1998 musical of the same name, *Hedwig* presents Mitchell in the title role as an "internationally ignored song stylist" who has an "angry inch" of vestigial male anatomy as the result of a botched sex change operation. With songs by Stephen Trask, the musical showcases smart rock tunes written in a range of styles, from pop ballads to punk anthems.

One of Trask's songs, "The Origin of Love," was written after Mitchell asked him to adapt the fable spun by Aristophanes in Plato's *Symposium* to explain what we now call sexual orientation. According to this fable, human beings were originally bundled in pairs of various genders, then split down the middle by an angry god. Since that time, Aristophanes posited, men and women have searched, with varying degrees of success, for their other half. In this charming way, Aristophanes accounts for the existence of gay men, lesbians, and heterosexuals. Mitchell (and Trask) use the fable as a means of commenting on Hedwig's existential dilemma.

Hedwig is a creature divided. As a boy in East Germany, she was named Hansel. After falling in love with an American soldier, Hansel is persuaded to undergo a sex change operation so that he will be able to marry and leave the country. The operation is botched; as Hedwig later sings, "My guardian angel fell asleep on the watch. Now all I've got is a Barbie doll crotch—I've got an angry inch." She tells her story with a liberal sprinkling of humor: "When I woke up from the operation, I was bleeding down there—from a gash between my legs. It's my first day as a woman, [and] already it's that time of the month."

Through music, comedy, and the pathos of her unusual but compelling story, Hedwig challenges prevailing gay norms, which are sometimes codified into rigid orthodoxies, and makes the deeply moral point that even society's outsiders are deserving of love. Stephen Trask's supercharged music and incendiary lyrics for "Freaks" deliver the show's musical manifesto: "We are freaks! We fuck who we please and do what we choose. We're not bad. We're not diseased or confused."

As the drag creation of an openly gay actor and as a transsexual character, Hedwig is the revolutionary embodiment of Mitchell's desire to increase popular acceptance of difference. His utter believability in the role left many observers surprised to learn that Mitchell had never done drag prior to assuming the persona of Hedwig.

After meeting Stephen Trask on a plane in 1997 and inviting him to create songs for the character of Hedwig, Mitchell first appeared in the character at a drag punk club in New York City. Combining Trask's songs with his stand-up monologue, Mitchell used these early appearances as Hedwig to develop the character.

Incorporating Trask's songs, Mitchell eventually had enough material for a full-length show, which was presented off-Broadway in 1998 and became a surprise hit. Hailed as one of the best rock musicals ever produced, it ran for three years at the Jane Street Theater. Various actors, Michael Cerveris and Ally Sheedy among them, have succeeded Mitchell in the stage role in productions all over the country.

When producer Christine Vachon saw the show, she was captivated by it. Her company, Killer Films, produced the movie version. The film won the Best Director award (for Mitchell) and the Audience Favorite award at the Sundance Film Festival in 2001.

Mitchell was born on April 21, 1963, in El Paso, Texas, the son of an army officer and a Scottish-born housewife. An "army brat," he lived in various places around the world; his father, by then a general, was United States military commander in West Berlin from 1984 to 1988. (The character of Hedwig is based, in part, on an East German woman who babysat for the children of military personnel, including Mitchell's brother, and also worked as a part-time prostitute.)

Although he grew up full of self-loathing because of his sexuality, Mitchell came out to his parents at age twenty. They have been largely supportive of him and are proud of his success.

Mitchell studied theater at Northwestern University in the 1980s. Leaving college before graduating, he understudied the role of Huckleberry Finn in the musical *Big River* (1985) and then went to California, winning bit parts in various television shows. Back in New York, he appeared in the original cast of John Guare's *Six Degrees of Separation* in 1990. The following year, he was in the Broadway cast of the musical *The Secret Garden*. In 1992, he earned positive reviews and an Obie

Award for his performance as the young Ned Weeks in Larry Kramer's *The Destiny of Me*. At Lincoln Center in 1994, he was in the original cast of Michael John LaChiusa's stunning musical *Hello Again*, in which he played two gay male characters.

In addition, Mitchell appeared on television sitcoms and did voice-overs and commercials to earn money to finance his pet project, which finally materialized as *Hedwig and the Angry Itch*.

His faith in that project vindicated by the success of both the stage musical and the film, Mitchell hopes in the future to concentrate on filmmaking. He is currently developing a project under the title "Shortbus," about the search for love and sex in New York City, for which he plans to film actual sex scenes.

—Greg Varner

BIBLIOGRAPHY

Berson, Misha. "Man behind Hedwig Captures Her on Film." *Seattle Times,* August 3, 2001.

Covert, Colin. "His Better Half." *Minneapolis Star Tribune,* August 10, 2001.

Dudek, Duane. "In Tune with 'Hedwig': Star Isn't Angry about Gender-bending Role." *Milwaukee Journal Sentinel,* August 14, 2001.

Mitchell, John Cameron, and Stephen Trask. *Hedwig and the Angry Inch.* DVD. New Line Home Entertainment, 2001.

_____. *Hedwig and the Angry Inch.* Original Cast Recording. CD. Atlantic, 1999.

_____. *Hedwig and the Angry Inch.* Original Motion Picture Soundtrack. CD. Hybrid, 2001.

Smith, Dinitia. "Nothing Simulated About It: The Creator of 'Hedwig' Has a New Opus in the Works, and It's Just Full of Sex." *New York Times,* August 19, 2004.

Schaefer, Stephen. "'Hedwig' Creator Inches Forward." *Boston Herald,* August 4, 2001.

Said, S. F. "The Other Half of Hedwig: As John Cameron Mitchell Turns His Cult Musical 'Hedwig and the Angry Inch' into a Must-see Film, He Explains the Origins of His Outrageous, Transsexual Drag Queen." *Daily Telegraph* (London), August 28, 2001.

Varner, Greg. "Freak Show: Given an Inch, Hedwig Goes Miles." *Washington Blade,* August 3, 2001, 31.

Wolf, Matt. "He's Not as Other Men: In Hedwig, John Cameron Mitchell Has Created a Touching, Subversive Character, a Cult Figure with Mainstream Appeal." *Observer* (London), August 12, 2001.

SEE ALSO

New Queer Cinema; Screenwriters; Vachon, Christine

Moorehead, Agnes   *(1900–1974)*

AGNES MOOREHEAD IS PROBABLY BEST KNOWN FOR her role as Endora, the tart-tongued mother-in-law on the situation comedy *Bewitched*. When she took on that part, however, she had already had a long, varied, and distinguished acting career.

Sources often give the year of Moorehead's birth as 1906. Like many actresses of her era, she shaved a few years off her age in order to remain in contention for good parts. Agnes Robertson Moorehead was in fact born on December 6, 1900, in Clinton, Massachusetts, where her father was serving as a Presbyterian minister. His pastoral assignments took the family to Hamilton, Ohio, in 1904, and to St. Louis eight years later.

Moorehead spent four years in the ballet and chorus of the St. Louis Municipal Opera Company. By the time she graduated from high school, she was considering a career on the stage. Her parents did not discourage her ambitions, but her father insisted that she receive a sound education first. She enrolled at Muskingum College, a Presbyterian school in New Concord, Ohio, that had been founded by her uncle. She appeared in student plays there before graduating in 1923. She then continued her studies at the University of Wisconsin, from which she

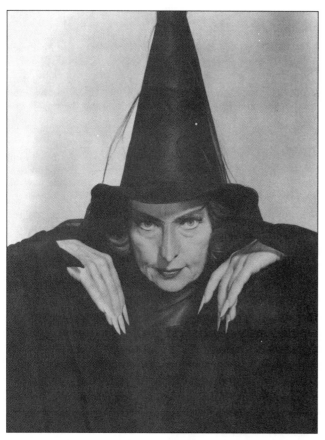

Agnes Moorehead as Endora in *Bewitched*.

graduated with a master's degree in English and public speaking. While studying at Wisconsin, she also worked as a high school English teacher and drama coach.

In 1926, Moorehead went to New York, where she auditioned successfully for the American Academy of Dramatic Arts. While pursuing her course there, she taught acting at a private school and appeared in several plays. She graduated from the Academy with honors in 1929.

The following June, she married John Griffith Lee, who had been a fellow student at the Academy. Finding no success as an actor, Lee took over the management of the large Ohio farm that had been in Moorehead's family since her great-grandparents' day.

Moorehead, meanwhile, was embarking on a theatrical career. She toured with several companies, but when the Depression made opportunities scarce, she turned to radio. Her talents were much in demand. She was featured on many shows, sometimes as many as seven or eight in a day.

Among the most memorable of Moorehead's radio performances came in *Sorry, Wrong Number* (1943) on the *Suspense* program. In a role written especially for her by Lucille Fletcher, Moorehead portrayed a bedridden woman who is going to be murdered. She was severely disappointed when the lead role of the film version of the play went to Barbara Stanwyck.

Moorehead's radio work included several performances with Orson Welles. Beginning in 1937, she spent two years acting on the extremely popular program *The Shadow,* and she also had an uncredited bit part in the Welles classic *War of the Worlds* (1938).

In addition, Moorehead participated with Welles in the Mercury Theatre Group, memorably appearing in a modern-dress production of Shakespeare's *Julius Caesar* in 1937. When the company moved to California in 1939 to work with RKO films, Moorehead traveled west and began her screen career.

Moorehead would appear in more than sixty films over three decades. She was nominated for the Academy Award for best supporting actress four times (1942, 1944, 1948, and 1964).

Morehead's first cinematic role was as Charles Foster Kane's mother in Welles's *Citizen Kane* (1941). Welles also directed her in her second film, *The Magnificent Ambersons* (1942), for which she garnered her first Academy Award nomination and won the New York Film Critics Award.

At the same time Moorehead was appearing in films, she made occasional returns to the stage, including a performance as Lady Macbeth in a 1947 production directed by Welles.

Moorehead's busy professional schedule kept her from spending much time with her husband, but fan magazines alluded to her eagerness to take every opportunity to return to Ohio and work beside him on the family farm. The stories are reminiscent of those that portrayed Alfred Lunt and Lynn Fontanne as delighting in agrarian domesticity.

Moorehead divorced Lee in 1952. She complained that her husband—by then estranged—called her his "meal ticket."

The following year, she married Robert Gist, who was some twenty years her junior. The union was short-lived. The couple separated in 1954 amid charges by Moorehead that Gist had been unfaithful. They eventually divorced, in 1958.

While Moorehead continued to appear in numerous films, she also had a successful turn as a director in a 1955 stage production of George Bernard Shaw's *Don Juan in Hell*. The play opened in San Francisco and then toured Canada and the Pacific Northwest to enthusiastic audience response.

Moorehead also had great success with a one-woman show in which she toured both in the United States and abroad from 1954 until 1970. Her readings included selections from the works for which she was best known, including *Sorry, Wrong Number*, *Don Juan in Hell*, and later *Hush...Hush, Sweet Charlotte* (1964, directed by Robert Aldrich), for which she received a Golden Globe Award and an Academy Award nomination. Among the other sources from which she read were the Bible and the works of Edna St. Vincent Millay, Marcel Proust, James Thurber, and Robert Frost.

Moorehead made numerous television appearances beginning in 1953 and won an Emmy Award for her guest performance on *The Wild, Wild West* in 1967, but many viewers remember her primarily for her role as Endora, the acerbic witch mother-in-law on the situation comedy *Bewitched* (1964–1972). The part brought her five more Emmy nominations. Moorehead's costars on *Bewitched* included gay actors Paul Lynde and Dick Sargent. The role of Endora was a campy romp, with Moorehead arrayed in extravagant costumes and displaying the personality of an imperious diva.

Moorehead starred in a revival of *Don Juan in Hell* in 1973 and continued to work in television, movies, and on the musical stage (in Alan Jay Lerner and Frederick Loewe's *Gigi*) until ill health forced her to retire. She died of lung cancer in Rochester, Minnesota, on April 30, 1974.

There had long been rumors in Hollywood about lesbian relationships involving Moorehead, but she was consistently circumspect in commenting on her personal life. She admitted "a certain amount of aloofness on [her] part at times, because an actor can so easily be hurt by unfair criticism," adding that "an artist should...maintain glamour and a kind of mystery."

No doubt Moorehead's circumspection was also motivated by the knowledge that openness as a lesbian would have had disastrous consequences for her career.

Her *Bewitched* costar Lynde, himself closeted, was less reticent, saying, "The whole world knows that Agnes was a lesbian—I mean classy, but one of the all-time Hollywood dykes." He further stated, "When one of her husbands was caught cheating, so the story goes, Agnes screamed at him that if he could have a mistress, so could she!"

Patricia White calls Moorehead's body of work her "queer career," pointing out that her roles "encompassed a gallery of types connoting female difference." These include a WAC officer, a madam, and the superintendent of a women's prison. Moorehead often played unmarried women—spinster aunts, nuns, governesses, and ladies' companions. In White's analysis, these "character types...connoting 'asexuality' or 'masculinity' have qualities that significantly overlap with those attributed to lesbians" and "connote, if not lesbian identity, at least the *problem* of heterosexual identity."

Such roles made Moorehead a lesbian icon on stage, screen, and television.

—Linda Rapp

BIBLIOGRAPHY

Freeman, William M. "Agnes Moorehead Dies at 67; Acclaimed in a Variety of Roles." *New York Times*, May 1, 1974.

Kear, Lynn. *Agnes Moorehead: A Bio-Bibliography*. Westport, Conn.: Greenwood Press, 1992.

Madsen, Axel. *The Sewing Circle: Hollywood's Greatest Secret: Female Stars Who Loved Other Women*. New York: Carol Publishing Group, 1995.

White, Patricia. *Uninvited: Classical Hollywood Cinema and Lesbian Representability*. Bloomington, Ind.: Indiana University Press, 1999.

SEE ALSO

Film Actors: Lesbian; American Television: Situation Comedies; Lynde, Paul; Sargent, Dick

Morrissey, Paul (b. 1938)

FILMMAKER PAUL MORRISSEY WAS THE AUTEUR WHO created many of the "Andy Warhol films." His works unflinchingly document modern urban subcultures, including the lives of drag queens, hustlers, and addicts.

Born in New York City on February 23, 1938, Morrissey was the son of a Bronx lawyer. He grew up in Yonkers, New York, and was educated at Catholic schools. He studied cinema at Fordham College and began making short experimental films as early as 1961.

A chance visit to a Manhattan screening of Andy Warhol's *Sleep* in 1963 led to a more purposeful trip to

Warhol's Factory, where Morrissey's combination of business savvy and creativity soon gained him considerable control over the day-to-day operations at that legendary space. Those attributes eventually made him the driving force behind the majority of what were known then, and continue to be viewed by many, as "Andy Warhol films."

These include such legendary works as the double-projected *The Chelsea Girls* (1966), early Joe Dallesandro epics such as *Bike Boy* and *The Loves of Ondine* (both 1967), and the first of the commercially released features, *Lonesome Cowboys* (1968).

Morrissey's claim to auteur status is confirmed simply by looking at a list of his duties on these films, which encompassed almost everything except the acting. Even on the high-profile *Trash* (1970), he directed, wrote the story and screenplay, and served as both cinematographer and camera operator.

Morrissey was literally the straight man in the Factory. His unfazed occupation of that fabled space, with its parade of damaged denizens, from disreputable drag queens to dream-boy hustlers, is reflected and extended in his best films, which take an unflinchingly vérité look at a variety of modern subcultures, most tellingly the daily life of junkies and hustlers, as in *Flesh* (1968), *Trash*, and *Mixed Blood* (1984).

Some of his work represents a breakthrough in detailing the lives of the urban walking wounded, as, for example, the clinically recorded process of shooting up heroin in *Trash*. Typical of Morrissey's complex worldview, *Trash* is equal parts comedy and tragedy, reveling in the absurd activities of the drag queen–hustler couple, while bringing a surprising poignancy to their lives.

Other Morrissey films are viciously funny, decidedly politically incorrect takes on subjects the director clearly finds troubling or irritating, as in the 1971 *Women in Revolt*, a camp-drenched send-up of women's liberation played by drag queens.

It is a tribute to Morrissey's skill with actors that these films have an almost documentary reality, as if Morrissey, like his mentor, simply turned the camera on his subjects and left the room, though this was far from what happened.

Morrissey's best films are the queer or queer-inflected works that feature powerful, shrill, unassimilable personalities starving for self-expression and respect. Examples of these memorable portraits include Sylvia Miles's washed-up B-movie slut in *Heat* (1971), Udo Kier's queenly vampire in *Blood for Dracula* (1974), and that Tom of Finland drawing come to life Joe Dallesandro, in all their films together.

A quintessential image in the Morrissey canon is that of a beautiful, passive, nude or nearly nude male (often Dallesandro) surrounded by powerful predatory females or drag queens, who delight in undermining the masculine posing and stupidity of these presumed paragons of heterosexuality. *Flesh, Trash, Heat,* and *Mixed Blood* figure prominently here.

While this trope can be traced to Warhol's use of the debased, self-consumed, passive hunk in his earliest, pre-Morrissey films (for example, *Horse* or *My Hustler*), the fact that it recurs so often in Morrissey's own career suggests the hold it has on his—and the culture's—imagination, a curiosity worth exploring given Morrissey's heterosexuality.

During Morrissey's most productive period, from 1968 to 1973, he brought Warhol's innovations—ordinary people as "superstars," a fixed camera objectively recording a scene, the episodic or nonlinear narrative, cinematic camp, and indifferent nudity—to much larger audiences, middling commercial success, and favorable critical comment.

His films have been a decisive influence on the independent film movement, particularly on the New Queer Cinema of the 1990s, but, unlike other independent icons of the 1960s and 1970s such as John Cassavetes, he remains a marginalized figure. Unheralded except in cult circles, he has been unable to get financing for a film since *Spike of Bensonhurst* (1988).

Part of Morrissey's marginalization is attributable to his political stance—he agrees with the label applied to him by critic Maurice Yacowar, "reactionary conservative"—which seems to contradict the spirit of the independent film movement and calls into question the validity of his own films as shrill but heartfelt celebrations of the outsider.

Part of the problem may also be his abandonment of the queer/camp ethos in most of the work following his two European horror films. The critical and commercial failures of *Madame Wong's* (1981), *Forty Deuce* (1982), *Beethoven's Nephew* (1985), and *Spike of Bensonhurst* may indicate that, separated from his strident "superstars" and perhaps from the blessing or curse of Warhol's imprimatur, he simply lost interest.

—*Gary Morris*

BIBLIOGRAPHY

Bruno, E. "A Warhol Pix Vet, Morrissey Shifts to Horror Films." *Variety* (New York), February 27, 1974.

Ford, Greg. "You Name It, I'll Eat It." Interview with Paul Morrissey. *Cinema* 1 (1973).

Morris, Gary. "Slapstick Realist: The Cinema of Paul Morrissey." *Bright Lights Film Journal* (1996): www.brightlightsfilm.com/17/03_morrissey.html

Stein, Elliott. "Flesh and Fantasy." *Village Voice*, January 2, 1996, 56.

Yacowar, Maurice. *The Films of Paul Morrissey.* New York: Cambridge University Press, 1993.

SEE ALSO

Film Directors; Film; New Queer Cinema; Warhol, Andy

Murnau, Friedrich Wilhelm   *(1888–1931)*

Acclaimed as the greatest director of the German Expressionist period (1919–1933), F. W. Murnau created the first masterpiece of the horror film, his exquisitely stylized *Nosferatu, eine Symphonie des Grauens* (1921).

Shooting on location, Murnau employed the limited special effects available at that time to create an atmosphere of genuine disquiet. The performance of Max Schreck remains unparalleled in its eerie malevolence.

Because of copyright difficulties with the Bram Stoker estate, *Nosferatu* had limited release worldwide. No such problems impeded the release of another masterpiece of silent film, *Der letzte Mann* (1924; American title: *The Last Laugh*), widely acclaimed as possibly the greatest film yet made upon its worldwide release.

What is remarkable about *Der letzte Mann* is that the story is told without titles: This tale of an elderly man's demotion from his position as doorman (epitomized by the elaborate uniform he wears for his job) to a subsidiary position as lavatory attendant (symbolized by the stripping of his uniform) is told with brilliant incisiveness through camera movement, visual composition, and lighting, all employed to provide a subjective perspective to the narrative.

This film established its star, Emil Jannings, as a major international film actor, and led to his coming to America (where he would win the first Academy Award for Best Actor). Jannings's status was further established in Murnau's film of *Tartuffe* (1925), a fluid but somber version of the Molière play.

The success of *Der letzte Mann* enabled Murnau to make *Faust* (1926), the most expensive movie made in Germany to that time, in which Murnau was able to create an entire medieval universe with monumental sets, sweeping locations, and elaborate costumes. The expenses were so overwhelming that the film proved unsuccessful financially, which might have marked the end of Murnau's career if he had not already accepted an offer to go to the United States.

The director's contract with William Fox stipulated that Murnau would be allowed to make a film with no interference; the result was *Sunrise* (1927). Working with many of his colleagues from Germany, including scenarist Carl Mayer, cameraman Karl Struss, and art director Rochus Gliese, Mernau created a "song of two humans" that remains one of the most beautiful films ever made, a magical parable about a peasant couple whose love is threatened but who find renewed commitment.

The enormous sets (the "big city" set was the largest ever built in the United States up to that time) made *Sunrise* a financial disaster upon release; its status as a silent film just when sound was coming in did not help.

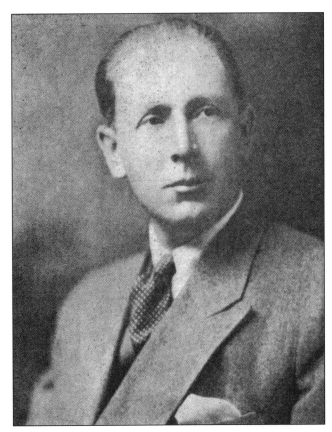

Friedrich Wilhelm Murnau.

Nevertheless, the film was widely acclaimed, and won several Academy Awards during the first year of those awards, including Best Actress for Janet Gaynor, Best Cinematography for Karl Struss and Charles Rosher, and a special award for "Artistic Quality of Production."

The financial failure of *Sunrise* imposed compromises on Murnau's next two productions for Fox. Failures on every level, *Four Devils* (1928) and *City Girl* (1929) caused Murnau to seek to reestablish his career.

In 1930, Murnau set out to form a production company with the documentary filmmaker Robert Flaherty. However, once on location in the South Pacific, Flaherty backed out of the production, leaving the film entirely in Murnau's hands. The resulting work, *Tabu*, proved to be magnificent, a tragic love story in which the location shooting pioneered in *Nosferatu* found its culmination.

Murnau died in a car crash a week before the premiere of *Tabu* in 1931; the movie would go on to win an Academy Award for Best Cinematography for Floyd Crosby, the father of rock musician David Crosby.

An imposingly tall, thin man of aristocratic demeanor, Murnau (born Friedrich Wilhelm Plumpe on December 28, 1888, in Bielefeld, Germany) was the product of the artistic ferment of the Weimar Republic. Before embarking on his career as a filmmaker, he trained as an art historian, which may explain the painterly images of his films and the primacy he accorded to the visual. He also worked under the legendary theater director Max Reinhardt.

In Berlin, Murnau moved in artistic circles, where homosexuality was accepted as a matter of course. In Hollywood, however, Murnau's homosexuality was the cause of much gossip, including the infamous rumor that his death in an automobile accident on March 11, 1931, was precipitated by his fellating his chauffeur while the latter was driving.

All evidence has shown this rumor to be false, yet it persists. Similarly, the recent film *Shadow of the Vampire* (2000), which stars John Malkovich as Murnau, depicts the director as a man so driven that he willingly allows murder. The need to defame gay artists itself demands a psychological study.

While the scandalous rumors surrounding Murnau's death resulted in the appearance of only a handful of mourners at his funeral, one of those was Greta Garbo. She requested that a death mask be made, which she kept on her desk throughout her life.   —*Daryl Chin*

BIBLIOGRAPHY

Collier, Jo Leslie. *From Wagner to Murnau: The Transposition of Romanticism from Stage to Screen.* Ann Arbor, Mich.: UMI Research Press, 1988.

Eisner, Lotte. *The Haunted Screen: Expressionism in the German Cinema.* Berkeley: University of California Press, 1969.

_____. *Murnau.* Berkeley: University of California Press, 1973.

Kracauer, Siegfried. *From Caligari to Hitler: A Psychological History of the German Film.* Princeton, N.J.: Princeton University Press, 1966.

Shepherd, Jim. *Nosferatu.* New York: Alfred A. Knopf, 1998.

SEE ALSO

Film; Film Directors; Horror Films; Vampire Films; Garbo, Greta

n

Nader, George (1921–2002)

ACTOR GEORGE NADER WAS A POPULAR LEADING MAN of the 1950s and 1960s, with over fifty films to his credit. Tall and handsome, he had a beefcake image.

Although he lived openly with his partner, Mark Miller, Nader did not publicly acknowledge his sexual orientation during his acting career; and Universal, the studio for which he worked, went to great pains to hide it, arranging for him to be seen on dates with beautiful female stars. Only in 1986, after the death of their friend Rock Hudson, did Nader and Miller come out.

Nader was born in Los Angeles on October 19, 1921. He became interested in acting while he was in school. He pursued this interest at Occidental College, from which he earned a degree in English in 1943. After graduation, he joined the navy and served as a communications officer in the Pacific Theater.

When the war ended, Nader returned to California and studied acting at the Pasadena Playhouse. There, in 1947, he met Mark Miller, who had one of the lead roles in a production of *Oh, Susannah!* Nader was in the chorus.

The two fell in love and established a household together. Miller had intended to go to New York to study opera but abandoned his plans in order to stay in California and help Nader launch his career. Miller took various jobs, including working as a carhop and a shoe salesman, in order to provide income while Nader established himself as an actor. By 1952, Nader was successful enough that Miller began working as his business manager.

Nader appeared in his first film, *Rustlers on Horseback* (directed by Fred C. Brannon), in 1950. His first starring role came the next year, in Rod Amateau's *Monsoon*.

Another of his early films was the 3-D *Robot Monster* (1953, directed by Phil Tucker). Shot in only four days for a mere $16,000, it took in over a million dollars in its first run but also earned the dubious distinction of being named one of the fifty worst movies in history. It has become a cult classic.

In 1954, Nader won a Golden Globe Award as Most Promising Male Newcomer of the year. He went on to leading or costarring roles in several major pictures, such as *Six Bridges to Cross* (1955) and *Away All Boats* (1956), both directed by Joseph Pevney.

Often, however, Universal used him in second features. Choicer roles frequently went to more heavily promoted stars such as Rock Hudson and Tony Curtis.

Although Nader and Miller were living together, neither publicly acknowledged his homosexuality. The studio, eager to project a heterosexual image for their beefcake star, used various ploys such as arranging dates for Nader with actresses Mitzi Gaynor, Martha Hyer, and Piper Laurie.

One publicist even went so far as to suggest that to avoid being outed by a scandal sheet such as *Confidential*, Nader should marry and then get a divorce a few years later. A female secretary was willing to participate in the scheme. Nader and Miller discussed the possibility, but Nader could not bring himself to take part in such a sham.

In 1958, Nader decided to leave the studio and work freelance. He landed lead roles in three television series, all short-lived. He played the detective hero in *The Further Adventures of Ellery Queen* during the 1958–1959 season. The next year, he portrayed a scientist in *The Man and the Challenge*. In 1961, he played the title role in *Shannon*, a program about an insurance claims investigator.

Not satisfied with professional opportunities in the United States, Nader decided to explore the European market. In 1964, he and Miller moved to Germany, where Nader made a dozen films, including a series of eight in which he played a tough FBI agent. Although the films were popular, they were not of especially good quality. In 1972, Nader and Miller moved back to the United States.

Nader resumed his Hollywood career, but when he suffered a detached retina in an automobile accident, he was no longer able to work under the lights. Miller planned to get a job in real estate to support the couple, but Rock Hudson hired him as his secretary.

Hudson had known Nader and Miller since 1951, when, as a newcomer to Hollywood, he was befriended by the couple; they remained close over the years. Nader and Miller would provide important support to Hudson, particularly in his final battle against AIDS, of which he died in 1985. Hudson left most of his estate to Nader and Miller.

In 1978, Nader wrote his first novel, a homoerotic science-fiction work entitled *Chrome*, which has gone to six printings. The story of forbidden love between a young man and a beautiful male robot, who are eventually exiled to different parts of the universe, can be read as a metaphor for the societal pressures on gay men.

Nader and Miller collaborated on a second novel, "The Perils of Paul," about gays in Hollywood. Rumored to be based on the couple's actual experiences, it is forthcoming.

In retirement, Nader and Miller lived in Palm Springs, California. In September 2001, Nader contracted a bacterial infection. He died on February 4, 2002. —*Linda Rapp*

BIBLIOGRAPHY

Bergan, Ronald. "George Nader: Gay Actor Comfortable in Beefcake Roles." *Guardian* (London), February 8, 2002.

Davidson, Sara. *Rock Hudson: His Story.* New York: William Morrow, 1986.

Mann, William J. *Behind the Screen: How Gays and Lesbians Shaped Hollywood 1910–1969.* New York: Viking, 2001.

Smyth, Mitchell. "Rock Left Actor Millions." *Toronto Star,* May 10, 1992.

Woo, Elaine. "Gerge Nader, 80; Star of '50s Movies." *Los Angeles Times,* February 6, 2002.

SEE ALSO

Film Actors: Gay Male; Hudson, Rock

New Queer Cinema

THE TERM *NEW QUEER CINEMA* WAS COINED BY B. Ruby Rich in several publications (including the British film journal *Sight & Sound*, as well as the New York weekly the *Village Voice*) to describe the appearance of certain films at Sundance Film Festivals in the early 1990s that evinced a politicized stance toward queer culture.

In 1991, Todd Haynes's *Poison* won Sundance's Grand Jury Prize for Best Film; the next year saw the inclusion of Tom Kalin's *Swoon*, Gregg Araki's *The Living End*, and Christopher Munch's *The Hours and Times*.

These young directors, along with the producers Christine Vachon (who produced *Poison* and *Swoon*) and Andrea Sperling (who produced *The Living End* and *The Hours and Times*), were the vanguard of what seemed to be a movement, though it was never really an organized movement as such.

The term *New Queer Cinema* would soon be used indiscriminately to denote independent films with gay and lesbian content. Nevertheless, Rich's assessment centered on what she perceived as a commitment to queer culture in those particular films by Haynes, Kalin, Araki, and Munch.

Independent films made on small budgets and often financed by foundation and arts council grants, the New Queer Cinema can be seen as the culmination of several developments in American cinema and American culture.

Background

There have always been American movies made outside the commercial studio system; by the 1940s, a very active and coherent experimental film culture developed, with many gay artists, such as Kenneth Anger, Gregory Markopoulos, and Curtis Harrington, among those who created an American avant-garde cinema.

Independent, low-budget films made without commercial studio backing gained notice in the 1950s; often, these films dealt with themes deemed too controversial for mainstream cinema.

By the 1960s, the cinematic avant-garde was making what were called "underground films." Many gay artists, including Jack Smith, Warren Sonbert, and Andy Warhol, were among the most prominent creators of underground films. Works such as Kenneth Anger's *Scorpio Rising* (1963) and Andy Warhol's *The Chelsea Girls* (1966) were especially influential in establishing an iconography of homoeroticism that would eventually be replicated in mainstream commercial cinema.

Although homosexual themes had appeared in mainstream commercial films in the 1960s (most notably, *Advise and Consent*, 1962; *The Children's Hour*, 1962; and, most spectacularly, John Schlesinger's Academy

Award–winning *Midnight Cowboy*, 1969), independent gay films made the greatest impact, especially *The Boys in the Band* (1970) and *A Very Natural Thing* (1973).

During the 1970s, arts funding helped to launch several festivals devoted to gay and lesbian films, which in turn helped cultivate an audience for gay and lesbian films. In the 1980s, many of the most adventurous lesbian and gay filmmakers, such as Su Friedrich, Michael Wallin, Peggy Ahwesh, Jack Walsh, and Sheila MacLaughlin, began to experiment with narrative form, a tendency that also characterizes the directors associated with New Queer Cinema.

In addition, the AIDS crisis provoked a large body of activist video productions, exemplified by the work of Gregg Bordowitz, Jean Carlomusto, and Ellen Spiro, among others. The accessibility of video allowed many gay and lesbian artists of color, such as Marlon Riggs, Richard Fung, Michelle Parkerson, Shari Frilot, and Cheryl Dunye, to create work that might not otherwise have found sufficient backing.

All of these artists, and the conditions under which their work was produced, distributed, and exhibited, provided the background and set the precedents for the emergence of New Queer Cinema.

Immediate Precursors

Gus Van Sant's *Mala Noche* (1985) and Bill Sherwood's *Parting Glances* (1986) were the most direct precursors of the New Queer Cinema. Both films had only limited releases, but were nevertheless enormously successful critically. In addition, these two films set important examples for the New Queer Cinema in their modest budgets and mixture of funding sources.

The production history of *Parting Glances* is directly connected with the production histories of *Poison* and *Swoon*; Christine Vachon and the late Brian Greenbaum, who coproduced *Poison*, met while both were working on the production of *Parting Glances*.

Self-Identified Queer Filmmakers

The New Queer Cinema may, ultimately, be described in terms of a number of talented filmmakers who self-identified as queer. A number of these individuals were associated with ACT UP and its artistic ancillary, Gran Fury. Assuming the self-proclaimed gay aesthetic found in European directors such as Pier Paolo Pasolini, Rainer Werner Fassbinder, and Werner Shroeter during the 1970s, these young Americans shared a post-Stonewall openness to questions of gay politics and identity.

Most tellingly, they assumed a queer audience for their productions, so there was no need to "explain" homosexuality and gay men and lesbians to a presumably straight audience. Thus, they were not concerned with presenting a politically correct image of gay men

and lesbians; and they even appropriated and reclaimed negative stereotypes.

They also tended to embrace experimental structures and techniques in telling their stories, sometimes necessitated by the exigencies of low budgets but also for ideological and aesthetic reasons. Some films associated with New Queer Cinema, for example, are in black and white, utilize a large number of interior shots, and feature a limited number of actors. Most important, however, they unapologetically, and sometimes defiantly, present queer subject matter.

The Aggressiveness of New Queer Cinema

It is, in fact, the aggressiveness with which the core films of New Queer Cinema assert homosexual identity and queer culture that distinguishes them from earlier queer films such as *Parting Glances* and *Mala Noche*.

In *Poison*, for example, the prison sequence includes fairly graphic depictions of intense sexual relationships among inmates confined in an all-male environment. In *The Hours and Times*, the homosexuality of Brian Epstein is foregrounded, placed at the very center of the narrative rather than relegated to the margins. In *Swoon*, the Leopold–Loeb murder case of the 1920s is reinterpreted to explore the connections between homosexuality, repression, and criminality.

In *The Living End*, the couple-on-the-run genre is redefined by featuring two young HIV-positive men, whose marginality by virtue of their HIV status and queerness is itself the subject. They act out their marginality as aggression toward social norms of all kinds.

These films not only aggressively assert queer identities, but they also demand an acknowledgement of queer culture.

The Influence of New Queer Cinema

Because the term *New Queer Cinema* is sometimes used indiscriminately to refer to any recent film with gay or lesbian content, it has lost some of its specificity. Still, the broader application of the term is understandable, for the movement it defines has been very influential.

Perhaps most crucially, the critical and commercial success of the core films has helped other independent films with gay and lesbian content find theatrical distribution. In relying on foundation and arts council grants for funding, the New Queer Cinema also established a fund-raising model that has benefited subsequent gay and lesbian films and filmmakers.

Among those who have benefited from the new openness made possible by New Queer Cinema are Rose Troche, whose lesbian love story *Go Fish* (1994) was produced by Tom Kalin and Christine Vachon; Mary Harron, whose *I Shot Andy Warhol* (1996) was produced by Vachon; Kimberly Peirce, whose *Boys Don't*

Cry (1999) was also produced by Vachon; Steve McLean, whose *Postcards from America* (1994), a biographical film about the gay artist and AIDS activist David Wojnarowicz, was produced by Vachon and Tom Kalin; and Nigel Finch, whose *Stonewall* (1995), about the events leading up to the Stonewall riots of 1969, was also produced by Vachon and Kalin.

Certainly the hits of the 2001 Sundance Film Festival, such as the musical *Hedwig and the Angry Inch* (directed by John Cameron Mitchell and winner of the Audience Award for Best Film) and the documentary *Southern Comfort* (directed by Kate Davis and winner of the Grand Jury Award for Best Documentary), may also be seen as part of the efflorescence of queer cinema initiated a decade earlier by the New Queer Cinema.   —*Daryl Chin*

BIBLIOGRAPHY

Gever, Martha, John Greyson, and Pratibha Parmar, eds. *Queer Looks: Perspectives on Lesbian and Gay Film and Video.* New York: Routledge, 1993.

Lippy, Tod, ed. *Projections 11: New York Film-makers on Film-making.* New York: Farrar, Straus & Giroux, 2000.

Pierson, John. *Spike & Mike, Slackers & Dykes: A Guided Tour Across a Decade of American Independent Cinema.* New York: Hyperion, 1996.

Rich, B. Ruby. *Chick Flicks: Theories and Memories of the Feminist Film Movement.* Durham, N.C.: Duke University Press, 1998.

Vachon, Christine, with David Edelstein. *Shooting to Kill: How an Independent Producer Blasts Through the Barriers to Make Movies That Matter.* New York: Avon Books, 1998.

SEE ALSO

Film; Film Festivals; Anger, Kenneth; Araki, Gregg; Fassbinder, Rainer Werner; Haynes, Todd; Mitchell, John Cameron; Pasolini, Pier Paolo; Riggs, Marlon; Schlesinger, John; Troche, Rose; Vachon, Christine; Van Sant, Gus; Warhol, Andy

Novarro, Ramón   *(1899–1968)*

Ramón Novarro became the romantic idol of Hollywood silent films in the 1920s. At the height of his career, his fame almost rivaled that of Rudolph Valentino. Although his persona was usually that of "a boy in love," some moviegoers may have found in him a distinctly androgynous quality similar to Valentino's.

Following Valentino's death in 1926, Novarro became the biggest name in a group of "Latin lovers" that included Antonio Moreno and Ricardo Cortez.

Novarro was born Ramón Samaniego in Durango, Mexico, on February 6, 1899. In 1916, he moved to Los Angeles, where he took jobs as a model and a singing waiter. In 1917, he broke into films as an extra; he further developed his acting skills with a stint in vaudeville.

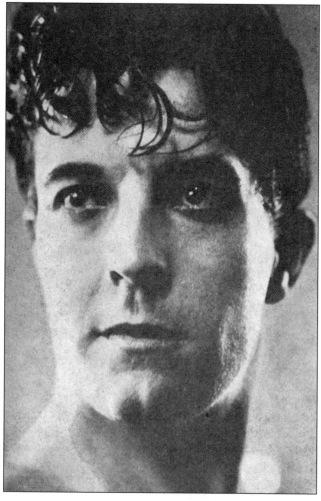

A portrait of Ramón Novarro published in 1929.

Rex Ingram, who had directed Valentino in *The Four Horsemen of the Apocalypse* (1921), discovered Novarro and worked hard to make him a screen idol. In 1922, studio publicity touted Novarro as the new Valentino, but he was always overshadowed by the original.

Ingram directed Novarro in roles as various as that of the villainous Rupert of Hentzau in *The Prisoner of Zenda* (1922) and the tragic lover in *Trifling Women* (1922), and costarred him in three romantic pictures with his wife, Alice Terry.

Novarro reached the pinnacle of his career with the title role in the monumental production of *Ben-Hur* (1926), though he gave a better performance the following year in Ernst Lubitsch's *The Student Prince in Old Heidelberg* (1927). He also directed and starred in the Spanish and French versions of *Call of the Flesh* (*La Sevillana* and *Le Chanteur de Seville*, respectively, 1930).

Novarro was less pretentious than Valentino, and there was a natural style to his acting that distinguished him from other young actors. Contemporary critics praised the ease and charm of his performances.

Although his boyish looks did not adversely affect the critical estimation of his talent during his heyday as a star, retrospectively some film historians find him almost too beautiful to be taken seriously, and he has consequently been perceived as a decidedly effeminate performer. Perhaps that is why he has never quite attained the renown of Valentino or the other reigning romantic lead of the era, John Gilbert.

Novarro continued playing romantic leads into the early 1930s. Age began to take its toll, however, despite Novarro's desperate attempt to look youthful in his early talkies. He later became a parody of his earlier self in such films as *The Sheik Steps Out* (1937). Except for occasional appearances in character parts, his career ended in the 1930s.

Novarro's homosexuality was a fairly open secret in Hollywood. Combined with his androgynous beauty, it not only challenged prevailing norms of masculinity in the 1920s and 1930s, but it has also profoundly affected the critical estimation of his talent.

Some critics have argued that his sexuality influenced his acting style, as they search for feminine qualities in his acting as evidence of his homosexuality. Others have even (somewhat anachronistically) attributed to his homosexuality his apparent propensity for too much makeup (a common effect of the rather primitive lighting on stage makeup in early films) and for seminude posing.

On October 31, 1968, Novarro was found dead in his Hollywood Hills home, having been beaten to death by one of two hustlers he picked up. False rumors still linger that Novarro's killers choked him with a lead dildo replicating the penis of Valentino, supposedly a gift from his former lover.

Joel Harrison assessed the evidence for these rumors in his book *Bloody Wednesday;* and André Soares, in his more recent biography of the star, presents further evidence for their speciousness (including interviews with principals at the subsequent murder trial). The incident also inspired the story of "Willie" in Thomas Tryon's *Crowned Heads* (1976).   —*Peter J. Holliday*

BIBLIOGRAPHY

Ellenberger, Allan R. *Ramon Novarro: A Biography of the Silent Film Idol, 1899–1968.* With a Filmography. Jefferson, N.C.: MacFarland, 1999.

Harrison, Joel L. *Bloody Wednesday.* Canoga Park, Calif.: Major Books, 1978.

Slide, Anthony. "Novarro, Ramón." *International Directory of Films and Filmmakers, vol. 3. Actors and Actresses.* 2nd ed. Nicholas Thomas, ed. Chicago and London: St. James Press, 1991. 741–742.

Soares, André. *Beyond Paradise: The Life of Ramón Novarro.* New York: St. Martin's Press, 2002.

SEE ALSO

Film; Film Actors: Gay Male; Valentino, Rudolph

Novello, Ivor   (1893–1951)

SHOW-BUSINESS RENAISSANCE MAN EXTRAORDINAIRE, Ivor Novello not only composed the scores of musical comedies but also acted in films, while dominating the London stage as a playwright and handsome romantic leading man for three decades.

He was born David Ivor Novello Davies in Cardiff, Wales, on January 15, 1893. His mother was a choir director and celebrated vocal coach. Through her, young Novello developed his deep interest in music and by age fifteen had published his first song.

He attended Magdalen College, Oxford, where he was a chorister. He served in World War I, first as an entertainer in France, then as a pilot in the Royal Naval Air Service. During the war, he composed scores for several musical comedies, but his biggest hit came with the patriotic song "Keep the Home Fires Burning" (1914).

Novello's persona was that of a handsome bachelor made for romantic melodrama and adventure. As such, he dominated the English stage from the 1920s until his death in 1951, rivaled only by another notably versatile actor/writer/composer, Noël Coward.

The lesbian writer and socialite Mercedes de Acosta, in her memoir *Here Lies the Heart* (1960), described Novello's beauty and élan: "A uniquely handsome man, his sensitive face had perfectly balanced features, the dark eyes beautifully cut into it and set off by black and shining hair. He wore his uniform with style and dash and altogether looked enchanting."

Novello made his film acting debut in *The Call of the Blood* (*L'Appel du Sang*, 1919), followed by *Miarka: the Daughter of the Bear* (*Miarka, Fille de L'Ourse*, 1920), both produced in France.

Novello debuted onstage in London in *Deburau* (1921). He then starred onscreen in *Carnival* (1921), *The Bohemian Girl* (1922), *The Man Without Desire* (1923), and D. W. Griffith's *The White Rose* (1923).

A homosexual with no desire to become a family man, Novello thrived professionally in multiple careers. His stint as playwright, and frequent actor of his own words, took off in 1924 when he wrote and performed in *The Rat*. Back onscreen, he acted against type, playing a psychopath in Alfred Hitchcock's *The Lodger* (1926).

Other screen credits include *The Vortex* (1927), from a Noël Coward play; *Downhill* (1927), again for Hitchcock; and *The Constant Nymph* (1928). These were followed by stage runs of *Symphony in Two Flats* (1930), *The Truth Game* (1930), and *I Lived with You* (1932).

The press linked him romantically to *Bohemian Girl* costar Gladys Cooper, but the real love of his life was actor Robert Andrews, with whom he lived from 1917 until his death in 1951.

Novello never hid his homosexuality through marriage or denial, but his women fans adored him anyway, primarily for his striking good looks and remarkable stage presence.

His sophisticated and urbane social circle was peopled with leading homosexuals in the arts, including Noël Coward, Clifton Webb, and Somerset Maugham.

It is likely that the open secret of Novello's homosexuality played a part when a notoriously homophobic judge sentenced him to a month's imprisonment during World War II for evading wartime restrictions on the use of gasoline.

In 1931, Novello went to Hollywood and cowrote several film scripts, including *Mata Hari* (1931) and *Tarzan, the Ape Man* (1932), but he preferred the theater to movies.

In addition to tackling Shakespeare with *Henry V* in 1938, he wrote, composed, and starred in four successful musicals at Drury Lane: *Glamorous Night* (1935), *Careless Rapture* (1936), *Crest of the Wave* (1937), and *The Dancing Years* (1939).

In the late 1930s, British theater critic W. A. Darlington remarked that "without Mr. Novello, Drury Lane is a white elephant; with him it is a gold mine. He writes plays, composes music and acts the principal male parts. Anybody who can do this successfully is a craftsman of the highest order."

Novello's work is rarely revived, as his unashamedly romantic style is far out of fashion. Perhaps it is time for rediscovery. He was amazingly prolific, publishing 250 songs, fourteen plays and eight musicals, in addition to maintaining an active career as an actor.

Ivor Novello died in London on March 6, 1951, from a coronary thrombosis, just four hours after appearing in a performance of *The King's Rhapsody*, a play he wrote. He was fifty-eight.

—*Matthew Kennedy*

BIBLIOGRAPHY

Harding, James. *Ivor Novello*. London: W. H. Allen, 1987.

Macqueen-Pope, Walter James. *Ivor, The Story of an Achievement: A Biography of Ivor Novello*. London: Allen, 1951.

Noble, Peter. *Ivor Novello: Man of the Theatre*. London: Falcon Press, 1951.

Rose, Richard. *Perchance to Dream: The World of Ivor Novello*. London: Leslie Frewin, 1974.

Wilson, Sandy. *Ivor Novello*. London: Michael Joseph, 1975.

SEE ALSO

Film; Film Actors: Gay Male; Webb, Clifton

O'Donnell, Rosie

(b. 1962)

COMEDIAN, ACTRESS, TELEVISION TALK SHOW HOST, and now openly gay mom, Rosie O'Donnell has achieved monumental success in her relatively brief career. Long rumored to be lesbian, she came out publicly in March 2002 in a much-publicized interview with Diane Sawyer on *Primetime Thursday*.

The host of *The Rosie O'Donnell Show* from 1996 to 2002, O'Donnell built a loyal following among viewers of daytime television, including many mainstream Americans. Debuting with the largest ratings of any talk show in a decade, *The Rosie O'Donnell Show* was a phenomenal success and made its host a genuine star. O'Donnell and her show were the recipients of numerous Emmy Awards.

To her chagrin, early in her talk show career, *Newsweek* responded to her homespun humor by dubbing her "The Queen of Nice." Actually, however, her "niceness"—which is often communicated through Broadway show tunes—is an important key to her likability and to her success in rescuing television talk shows from the shock and schlock in which many of her predecessors and competitors were mired. O'Donnell returned civility and fun to a genre that had become dominated by "trash TV."

For all her sentimentality and civility, however, O'Donnell has emerged as one of the most vocal, outspokenly liberal celebrities of the past decade. Devoted to figures such as Hilary Clinton and Barbra Streisand, she has brought before her audiences political discussions on topics as various as gun control, welfare reform, and Rudolph Giuliani. The cause she most passionately espouses is child advocacy.

Interest in the lives of foster children in Florida prompted her decision to come out. Learning of the plight of Steve Lofton and Roger Croteau, a gay couple unable to adopt a foster child in that state, despite having raised him from infancy when no one else would foster him, O'Donnell decided it was time the public added her face to their mental images of gay parents. As she told Diane Sawyer in March 2002, "I don't think America knows what a gay parent looks like: I am a gay parent."

Cynics wondered if O'Donnell's timing was influenced by the scheduled end of her show in May 2002, and if her high-profile coming-out was part of the promotional effort for her new book, *Find Me* (2002). But she maintained that she needed a specific political reason to disclose her sexual orientation publicly.

The staggering number of foster children in the United States motivated her to protest the state law barring gay and lesbian parents from adopting them. "I don't think," she said to Sawyer, "that restricting the pool of adoptive parents is beneficial."

O'Donnell's interest in children's welfare and her desire to provide a loving home for her own three adopted children stem from her own difficult childhood. The third of five children, she was born on March 21, 1962, to Edward and Roseann O'Donnell. She grew up in Commack, New York, on Long Island.

At the age of ten, O'Donnell lost her mother to cancer, though she did not learn the cause of her mother's death until she was sixteen. She has described the period after her mother's death as extremely difficult and her father as having emotionally abandoned his five children. Out of her sense of loss evolved a fierce desire to create her own loving family, regardless of her sexual orientation.

O'Donnell also credits her difficult childhood in part for her interest in the entertainment industry. In high school, she masked her unhappiness with humor. She was not only homecoming queen, prom queen, and senior class president, but also class clown. She attended college briefly after high school (Dickinson College and Boston University), but soon left to begin working comedy clubs.

In the mid-1980s, after winning the Comedy Champion title five times on *Star Search*, she hosted and produced *Stand-up Spotlight* on VH1. The secret to her success as a comedian was her ability to relate to other people and to project an empathetic, nonthreatening persona—the same qualities that made her a successful talk show host.

In the early 1990s, she landed her first film roles in *A League of Their Own* (1992) and *Sleepless in Seattle* (1993), in which she became known for playing the no-nonsense best friend to the female star. Her other films include *Another Stakeout* (1993), *The Flintstones* (1994), *Exit to Eden* (1994), and *Harriet the Spy* (1996).

She has also appeared on Broadway in a revival of *Grease* (1995), among other productions. Her support for Broadway manifests itself not only in her vast store of Broadway tunes, but also in having hosted the Tony Awards. Among her television acting appearances have been guest spots on *Stand by Your Man* and *Will and Grace*.

In 1995, she adopted her first child, son Parker Jaren, and soon afterward, to spend more time with him, she decided to stop working in films and host her own television show. In 1997, she adopted a daughter, Chelsea Belle, and in 1999, another son, Blake Christopher.

O'Donnell has been with her life partner, Kelli Carpenter, since 1998. On November 29, 2002, Carpenter gave birth to the couple's fourth child, Vivienne Rose O'Donnell. O'Donnell and Carpenter were married in San Francisco on February 26, 2004, though their marriage, like other same-sex marriages performed in San Francisco at that time, were invalidated by the California Supreme Court.

In addition to raising her children and hosting her television show, O'Donnell has established her own charity organization, For All Kids Foundation, and launched her own magazine, *Rosie*.

In a flurry of charges and countercharges, O'Donnell ended her association with the magazine in mid-2002.

The departure led to a suit and countersuit between O'Donnell and publisher Gunner + Jahr. The bitter legal dispute ended in November 2003 with a judge's ruling that neither party deserved damages.

In 2003, O'Donnell produced *Taboo*, a musical about the life of fashion designer and performance artist Leigh Bowery, with music by Boy George. The show opened to tepid reviews, but ran for some 100 performances on Broadway.

Among O'Donnell's other recent projects is her participation, with Carpenter and travel industry veteran Gregg Kaminsky, in R Family Vacations, a company that arranges family vacations for the glbtq community.

—*Geoffrey W. Bateman*

BIBLIOGRAPHY

Goodman, Gloria. *The Life and Humor of Rosie O'Donnell: A Biography.* New York: William Morrow, 1998.

Hunter, Carson. "Rosie by Any Other Name." *Girlfriends*, June 2001, 18.

Nordlinger, Jay. "Rosie O'Donnell, Political Activist." *National Review*, June 19, 2000, 33.

O'Donnell, Rosie. *Find Me.* New York: Warner Books, 2002.

Raphael, Rebecca. "Rosie's Story: O'Donnell Talks About Being a Gay Mom." *LGBT Entertainment News* (March 14, 2003): http://lezpride.tripod.com/entertainmentnews.html#2

Tauber, Michelle. "Oh By the Way—." *People*, March 18, 2002, 80.

SEE ALSO

American Television: Talk Shows; Film Actors: Lesbian; American Television: News

Ottinger, Ulrike   (b. 1942)

AVANT-GARDE GERMAN FILMMAKER ULRIKE OTTINGER creates both fictional fantasy worlds that shatter traditional gender constructions and documentaries that examine marginalized peoples.

Born Ulrike Weinberg on June 6, 1942, in Konstanz, Germany, Ottinger studied painting and photography at the Academy of Arts in Munich from 1959 through 1961. She moved to Paris, where she worked as a painter and photographer, before returning to Germany in 1969 to start Visuell, a film organization that she ran until 1972.

With the money earned from painting in Paris, she made her first film, *Laokoon und Söhne* (*Laocoön and Sons*, 1972–1973), starring Tabea Blumenschein, an underground film actress, set and costume designer, and Ottinger's lover at the time.

Ottinger again collaborated with Blumenschein on *Madame X—eine absolute Herrscherin* (*Madame X: An Absolute Ruler*, 1977), now a cult classic and regularly referred to as the "lesbian feminist pirate movie." In this work, six women abandon the oppressive, dull, and materialistic life to seek freedom, danger, and love on the ship *Orlando* led by Madame X. Lesbian lust permeates the journey, and erotic alliances lead to jealousy and death.

Although she refers to herself as an ethnographer, Ottinger makes films that take two distinct paths: documentaries and tales of the fantastic.

The tales are set in futuristic, colorful worlds, populated by extravagantly dressed characters wearing vibrant and surreal costumes, adorned with jewelry. The stunning and otherworldly mise-en-scènes of her films have been characterized as lesbian punk and traced to surrealism and the Baroque grotesque. Fiercely independent, Ottinger writes, photographs, designs, and produces her films, which helps account for their distinctive style.

The sexual attractions and tensions between women in her work are always present but never overt, allowing lesbian audiences the viewing pleasure of recognizing the sometimes subtle codes of lesbian desire.

The fantastic landscapes in *Freak Orlando* (1981), *Dorian Gray im Spiegel der Boulevardpresse* (*The Image of Dorian Gray in the Yellow Press*, 1984), and *Bildnis einer Trinkerin* (*Portrait of an Alcoholic*, 1979) are populated with outcasts and informed by a distinct camp aesthetic. Characters are self-consciously arranged. They posture and strike poses in a visual composition that creates an artificial theatrical space.

Freak Orlando, a loose adaptation of Virginia Woolf's novel, contains midgets, giants, transvestites, and obese and limbless men and women, as well as Orlando, who is an androgyne, both male and female.

Many feminists took offense at what they saw as the exploitation of the human body in this film. But the posturing of freaks in striking settings lets viewers look in awe at images both beautiful and repulsive. Ottinger, concerned with the oppressed position of the "other," noted that it is "deeply disturbing seeing someone of our own species" who is so radically different, but she includes these images to break our resistance to viewing and accepting different bodies.

Feminists have also been critical of "beauty fetishism" in her films, and especially the image of Madame X as a leather-clad dominatrix with a whip. Ottinger dismisses these criticisms, noting that the characters are exaggerated and ironic stylizations.

Ottinger's films shatter traditional gender roles and identity with androgynous and gender-ambiguous characters. Using role reversals, women in *Madame X* and *Johanna d'Arc of Mongolia* (*Joan of Arc of Mongolia*, 1988) are adventurers of sea and land. In *Johanna,* a matriarchal Mongolian tribe captures passengers from a Trans-Siberian Railway train and initiates them into a new female culture. Because of its geographic scope and

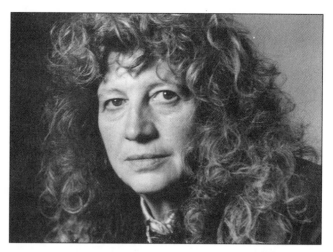

Ulrike Ottinger.

clash of cultures, the film has been characterized by critics as a "lesbian *Lawrence of Arabia.*"

In *Dorian Gray im Spiegel der Boulevardpresse,* the title character, played by ex–fashion model Veruschka von Lehndorff, is coerced into a life of decadence by a female media mogul, Frau Dr. Mabuse.

Countdown (1991) records life in Berlin in the final ten days before monetary unification. The film concentrates on the minorities and nomads of Berlin, including Romanians, Turks, Poles, and homosexuals, and explores their exclusion by the government from a voice in unification issues. The constant examination of outsider status in Ottinger's films has been recognized by glbtq audiences.

For the last twelve years, Ottinger has concentrated on documentaries that examine foreign cultures and marginalized people. *Taiga* (1992), an eight-hour film, focuses on northern Mongolia's nomadic tribes, while *China—die Künste, der Alltag* (*China—The Arts—The Everyday*, 1985), presents almost five hours of daily existence in remote areas of China. These films depict both universal and traditional aspects of life; as a result, the status of these people as outsiders, or "others," is shattered.

The outcasts in *Exile Shanghai* (1996) are Sephardic, Russian, German, and Austrian Jews, who tell of their journeys to Shanghai during the Nazi era and their eventual settlement in the United States. When one of the Jews briefly mentions a relative with AIDS, Ottinger suggests a connection of outsiders from generation to generation.

In *Southeast Passage: A Journey to the New Blank Spots on the European Map* (2002), three two-hour films integrated within larger museum installation projects, Ottinger travels from Wroclaw, Poland, to Varna, Bulgaria, and through Odessa and Istanbul, capturing both the mundane activities of villages and extravagant rituals and festivals.

Ottinger's fictional films, such as *The Specimen* (2002), which is set in the pre- and postrevolutionary Soviet Union, and *Zwolf Stuhle* (*Twelve Chairs*, 2004), which is set in the Ukraine in the 1920s, also employ nonfictional elements. Thus, they share with the documentaries a mingling of the imaginative and the ethnographic.

Ottinger has also presented numerous photographic exhibits featuring images from her films and her travels. Her latest large-scale photographic exhibit, "Faces, Found Objects and Rough Riders" (2004), focuses on the heritage of Mexican American cowboys in San Antonio, Texas.

Ottinger embraces people and activities "unnoticed or denied by the international gaze," and at "the mercy of the law of forgetting." All of her works, the artist notes, are aligned with "the practice of queering," of depicting "the world from a different perspective than mainstream perceptions."

—*Richard C. Bartone*

BIBLIOGRAPHY

Carter, Erica. "An interview with Ulrike Ottinger." *Screen Education* 41 (1982): 34–42.

Friedan, S., R. W. McCormick, V. R. Petersen, and L. M. Vogelsang, eds. *Gender and German Cinema: Feminist Interventions Volume I.* Providence, R.I.: Berg Publishers, 1993.

Grisham, Therese. "An interview with Ulrike Ottinger." *Wide Angle* 14.2 (1992): 28–36.

Grundmann, R., and J. Shulevitz. "Minorities and Majority: An Interview with Ulrike Ottinger." *Cineaste* 18.3 (1991): 40–41, 116.

Kaplan, Janet A. "Johanna d'Arc of Mongolia: An Interview with Ulrike Ottinger." *Art Journal* 61.3 (Fall 2002): 7–22.

Longfellow, Brenda. "Lesbian Fantasy and the Other Woman in Ottinger's Johanna d'Arc of Mongolia." *Screen* 34.2 (1993): 124–136.

SEE ALSO

Film; European Film; Film Directors; Documentary Film

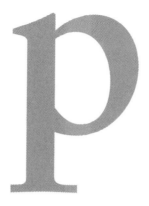

Paradjanov, Sergei (1924–1990)

"SURREALISM," "INCITEMENT TO SUICIDE," "TRAFFIC IN art objects," and "leaning toward homosexuality" all sound like respectable weapons in the modern art arsenal. In the case of director Sergei Paradjanov, however, they were grounds for fifteen years of forced inactivity and, by the director's own reckoning, eight years of imprisonment in some of Russia's many pre-*glasnost* hard-labor camps.

What was it about this jovial, bearlike man that invoked the unending wrath of censors? It may have been his abandonment of wife and children to live the unapologetic gay life he had apparently always desired.

Even more damning, perhaps, were his films, a dozen features unabashedly celebrating Armenian (that is, non-Russian) folk culture, a Dionysian (some would say delirious) approach to his material, an indifference to social realism, and an air of rapturous and whimsical indulgence in color and sound—hardly the stuff to further the revolution.

Paradjanov, an ethnic Armenian, was born on March 18, 1924, in Tiflis, the capital of the Georgian Republic. His first ambition was to be a singer, and to that end he attended the Tiflis Conservatoire from 1942 to 1945.

However, an interest in cinema preempted these studies. He entered Moscow's State Institute in Cinematography, counting Lev Kuleshov and Alexander Dovzhenko among his teachers, and graduated in 1951.

During the next ten years, Paradjanov made a series of Ukrainian-language films based in the social realist tradition but containing subtle signs of a powerful visual imagination trying to break through. By 1964, Paradjanov brazenly abandoned state-dictated style entirely in favor of a purely celebratory folkloric approach. *Shadows of Forgotten Ancestors,* shot in the Carpathian mountains, features wild camera movements (including hand-held) and overripe color.

This widely acclaimed film both put him on the international cinema map and brought him to the attention of Russian authorities, who could approve or reject his projects.

Paradjanov's increasingly high profile as "anti-Russian," homosexual, and activist culminated in his first arrest, in 1968. In 1974, he was sentenced under Russia's antigay law, Article 121, to five years at hard labor.

In prison, Paradjanov created hundreds of artworks, some of them collages made from bits of wire, nails, flowers, and dried grass. "I can create beauty out of rubbish," he said. (Some of the works would have reinforced authorities' fears about him: Paradjanov made friends with other inmates and apparently sketched both their faces and their genitals.)

Released a year early due to international protests, Paradjanov saw most of his proposed projects rejected, but he managed to make three features before his death in 1990.

Sympathetic response to this visionary's work requires an open mind and a willingness to be transported by his captivating imagery and lush scores, which evoke both the richness of Georgian-Armenian folk music and the high-art sounds of the great Russian composers.

None of his films feature overtly gay themes, but they are infused with Paradjanov's queer sensibility, which manifests itself in lyrical tableaux of a vibrant minority culture whose mere existence stands in opposition to a repressive status quo.

The Color of Pomegranates (1972) is considered Paradjanov's masterpiece, but it is also one of his most challenging works. Nominally a biography of Armenian poet and troubadour Sayat Nova, the film opens with a series of striking *tableaux vivants*, most notably one in which the youthful Nova lies down in what looks like a concrete gully with seemingly endless books arranged around him, their pages fluttering fantastically in the breeze.

Books are crucial in Paradjanov, not only because they contain and hold much of the world's artistic history, but also because much of his imagery is inspired by the ancient illuminated manuscripts to which he always managed to obtain access. (The Armenian church apparently liked him more than the Russian government did.)

Nova's history is rendered as a kind of interiorized bildungsroman, or coming-of-age story, tracing the boy's progress from early bookworm to apprentice rug maker to devotee of the female body. "I am the man whose life and soul are tortured," reads a subtitle repeated throughout the film, but Paradjanov's colorful vision of a rich culture in which every dress is a tapestry and every man a handsome devil is far more upbeat than the phrase suggests.

Paradjanov's much-remarked hubris is evident from the start of *Pomegranates* when he aligns himself with the Christian God by invoking the creation of the world. *The Legend of Suram Fortress* (1984) is less grandiose though no less mesmerizing.

This charming picaresque tells of a plebe who gets his freedom and sets off to buy that of his wife, a fortune-teller. The film pivots on the concept that the Georgian way of life, symbolized by the besieged fortress of the title, can be saved only if a young man is willing to be walled up inside it.

This metaphor for a rich regional culture threatened by an oppressive larger one was surely not lost on Paradjanov's detractors, but the film, with its gorgeous Georgian landscapes and fantastic imagery, happily, has outlived its enemies.

Paradjanov's final film, *Ashik Kerib* (1988), was dedicated to his late friend and compadre Andrei Tarkovsky, who also suffered tremendously at the hands of reactionary Russian authorities. Based on a story by Mikhail Lermontov and shot in the Georgia/Azerbaijan area that was Paradjanov's inspiration, the film is a typical phantasmagoria of folkloric imagery whose power is heightened by a rich score of regional music.

Ashik is an impoverished minstrel (played by Yuri Mgoyan, a handsome petty criminal hired by Paradjanov). He must find "bride-money" to marry the daughter of a rich Turkish merchant.

This simple plot gives Paradjanov plenty of room to play as Ashik encounters a series of tests in the classic heroic mold; and play he does, in such unforgettable scenes as a "wedding of the blind, deaf, and dumb" at which Ashik's music entrances the participants.

Ashik's search is an immersion in the transcendent beauty and power of folk culture, which Paradjanov fleshes out with vivid colors, elaborate costumes and headgear, and riotous blends of music, dance, and movement. Even the simplest images show the director's constant theme of the triumph of nature over the temporal, as when falling rose petals replace the dowry of diamonds that Ashik cannot afford.

Some critics have seen *Ashik Kerib* as a parable for Paradjanov's oppression by the government, with the director himself represented by the hapless lute player wandering through a blasted landscape of lost souls. But this interpretation misses the celebratory, indeed transcendent, quality of image and sound that are the film's driving force. If Paradjanov was not reconciled to the political abuse he suffered, it would be impossible to tell this from his final film.

After Paradjanov's death on July 21, 1990, his home in Yerevan was converted into a museum containing some of his writings (Leonid Alekseychuk says he wrote twenty-three scripts and fifty volumes of diaries) and several hundred of his artworks, including some he made during his imprisonment.

—*Gary Morris*

BIBLIOGRAPHY

Alekseychuk, Leonid, "A Warrior in the Field." *Sight and Sound* 60 (Winter 1990–1991): 22–26.

Holloway, Ron. "Interview with Sergei Paradjanov." *Kinema* (Spring 1996): http://www.arts.uwaterloo.ca/FINE/juhde/hollo961.htm

Murray, Raymond. *Images in the Dark: An Encyclopedia of Gay and Lesbian Film and Video.* New York: Plume, 1996.

"Paradjanov, Sergei." *World Film Directors.* John Wakeman, ed. New York: H. W. Wilson Co., 1988. 2:735–739.

SEE ALSO

Film; European Film; Eisenstein, Sergei Mikhailovich

Pasolini, Pier Paolo   (1922–1975)

POET, ESSAYIST, JOURNALIST, PLAYWRIGHT, AND SOCIOPOlitical lightning rod, Pier Paolo Pasolini is unquestionably one of the most important cultural figures to emerge from post–World War II Italy. But it is with film that he made his greatest impact.

Born in Bologna in 1922, Pasolini grew up in Friuli. While openly gay from the very start of his career (thanks to a gay sex scandal that sent him packing from his provincial hometown to live and work in Rome), Pasolini rarely dealt with homosexuality in his movies.

The subject is featured prominently in *Teorema* (1968), where Terence Stamp's mysterious godlike visitor seduces the son of an upper-middle-class family; passingly in *Arabian Nights* (1974), in an idyll between a king and a commoner that ends in death; and, most darkly of all, in *Salò* (1975), his infamous rendition of the Marquis de Sade's compendium of sexual horrors, *The 120 Days of Sodom*.

None of them is the sort of work to inspire GLAAD awards. But then Pasolini never saw himself as a "gay artist." Indeed, he explicitly rejected the assimilated gay middle class he saw emerging just prior to his untimely death in 1975. And it is his death, apparently at the hands of a hustler (though there have been allegations of political assassination in which others were involved), that has frozen Pasolini's image in the popular imagination.

In a way, his was a terribly banal sort of death. As far as the heterosexual status quo is concerned, Pasolini, a wealthy, older, and therefore "corrupt" man, was killed by a poor and therefore "innocent" youth "disgusted" by his "advances." But, as every gay man knows, this homophobic scenario is never really the truth.

Pasolini's death (which involved the killer or killers' driving over the artist's head with his own car) was a gay-bashing as certainly as was that of Matthew Shepard. The difference is that in 1975 the cultural climate was not as sympathetic to the spectacle of the death of an intellectual as it proved to be in 1998 with the death of a gay college student.

In 2005, following the recantation of the confession by the man convicted of Pasolini's murder 30 years previously, Italian officials opened a new investigation into the director's death.

Still, no cultural context, past or present, would be amenable to Pasolini, whose commercial success as a filmmaker is as remarkable as it is ironic. For he was not a conventional "entertainer," and he despised the bourgeois intellectuals who were his most receptive viewers.

In the 1950s, Pasolini's novels of Roman slum life *Ragazzi di Vita* (1955) and *Un Via Violenta* (1959) marked him in the minds of Italian moviemakers as an "expert" on worlds they were chary of entering.

He began his career as a scriptwriter on such films as Fellini's *Nights of Cabiria* (1956) and Bolognini's *La Notte Brava* (1959). When he broke out on his own as a writer/director with *Accatone* (1961) and *Mamma Roma* (1962), he was apparently styling himself after the masters of Italian neorealism, especially Roberto Rossellini.

But in 1964, he found his moviemaking voice with *The Gospel According to St. Matthew*. With a nonprofessional cast and a quasi-documentary shooting style, Pasolini retold the familiar story of the life of Christ in the simplest, least Hollywood-like style imaginable.

While its musical score was fairly avant-garde, featuring as it did excerpts from the African "Missa Luba," Prokofiev's *Alexander Nevsky*, and Mahalia Jackson singing "Sometimes I Feel Like a Motherless Child," the movie was accessible to audiences of all kinds.

In fact, for a time, a Christian fundamentalist film distributor had the rights to the film in the United States and successfully exhibited it to church groups. One wonders how receptive the fundamentalist audience would have been to the movie had they known that its maker was a gay, atheistic Communist.

Gospel was followed by *The Hawks and the Sparrows* (1966), a comic fable about the adventures of a Chaplinesque father-and-son team, played by the great Italian star Toto and Ninetto Davoli, a young former lover of Pasolini's who was to appear in many of the filmmaker's works.

Not one to stick to the expected, Pasolini next turned to Sophocles's *Oedipus Rex* (1967), presenting the drama as a fable set in the wilds of North Africa and modern Rome, acted by a cast that included Franco Citti, Sylvana Mangano, Alida Valli, Carmelo Bene, and the Living Theater's Julian Beck.

After that came *Teorema* (1968), one of Pasolini's most controversial works, in which a sexual "exterminating angel" (Terence Stamp) has his way with an entire Italian family.

Porcile (1969), which, like Faulkner's *Wild Palms*, presents two contrasting stories, left audiences scratching their heads over what the adventures of a mute cannibal (Pierre Clementi) had to do with the melancholia of a bourgeois youth (Jean-Pierre Léaud).

More questions were raised when Pasolini cast Maria Callas in his rendition of *Medea* (1970), a film in which the legendary diva was not required to sing a note.

But a sudden turn of popular fortune came when Pasolini made *The Decameron* (1971), *The Canterbury Tales* (1972), and *Arabian Nights* (1974). They are as uncompromising as any of his films, but their comic spirit, frequent sexual interludes, and abundant nudity pleased moviegoers as no Pasolini work had done before.

And then came the posthumously released *Salò*. Most of the critics responded as though the horrors displayed in the film came directly from the gay Italian's feverish imagination. But all Pasolini did was extract selected passages of Sade and reset them in the last days of the fascist republic of Salò, the state-within-a-state established in the twilight of Mussolini's Italy.

Pasolini's most visually elegant and dramatically reserved work, *Salò* offers Sade's vision of old, wealthy, evil authorities (politicians, lawyers, and bishops) having their way with nude and compliant youths and maidens of the lower classes as simply standard operational procedure for the powers that be.

Despite the outrage of some critics who complained of the director's decadence and depravity, the film actually presents a scrupulous version of the everyday reality of man's inhumanity to man.

It is noteworthy that Ninetto Davoli does not appear in *Salò*. The embodiment of comic exuberance in so many of Pasolini's films, Davoli has no place in *Salò*, where he would be obliged to play either a victim or an executioner. And Pasolini could see his beloved friend as neither, even after the young man married and began a family of his own.   —*David Ehrenstein*

Bibliography

Indiana, Gary. *Salo*. London: BFI Modern Classics, 2000.

Pasolini, Pier Paolo. *Heretical Empiricism*. Louise K. Barnett, ed. Ben Lawton and Louise K. Barnett, trans. Bloomington, Ind.: Indiana University Press, 1988.

_____. *Lutheran Letters*. Stuart Hood, trans. London: Carcanet, 1987.

_____. *Theorem*. Stuart Hood, trans. London: Quartet Encounters, 1992.

Stack, Oswald. *Pasolini*. Bloomington, Ind.: Indiana University Press, 1969.

Willemen, Paul, ed. *Pier Paolo Pasolini*. London: British Film Institute, 1977.

See also

Film; European Film; Film Directors; Transvestism in Film; New Queer Cinema; Asian Film; Carné, Marcel

Porn Stars

PERFORMERS IN GAY PORNOGRAPHY HOLD A RELATIVELY esteemed position in gay culture, in contrast to their heterosexual counterparts. This is largely due to the fact that hard-core pornography itself is such an integral and accepted part of gay male life, especially in comparison to the marginalized position straight pornography holds for its audiences.

Gay porn performers are the idolized rock stars of the gay world, showing up for personal appearances and autograph sessions, participating in Gay Pride parades, and establishing a celebrity presence that permeates multiple levels of the gay subculture.

Lesbian Porn Stars

Because very little approaching a lesbian sex industry exists, gay porn stars are almost exclusively male. Although an enormous percentage of footage filmed in the adult industry features two women having sex, these scenes cannot be classified as lesbian. They are produced and directed by heterosexual men for the consumption of heterosexual men. A true lesbian identity can almost never be found in these scenes, many of which are only preludes to the appearance of one or more men. Instead, same-sex female activity is presented as an exotic diversion, doubling the erotic object of the straight male gaze.

While some porn by and for lesbians has been produced over the years, it has been relatively rare, making the emergence of lesbian porn stars unlikely.

Annie Sprinkle, a veteran of the heterosexual porn industry and today a self-identified lesbian, offers the closest approximation to a lesbian porn star. Although she has produced and acted in some lesbian-oriented features, her primary focus since leaving the mainstream adult industry has been on performance art and humorous theater pieces that espouse themes of sexual liberation and self-fulfillment.

Author Suzy Bright, perhaps better known as Suzy Sexpert, is a similar liberationist and proporn activist. Her public appearances consist of entertaining seminars about pornography and its history.

The 1970s: Casey Donovan, Al Parker, Jack Wrangler

Gay porn stars—referred to as "models" in the industry—were relatively rare until the early 1970s. Because the modern pornography industry has developed most extensively in the United States, and because Hollywood provided the template for notions of stardom, most gay porn stars—at least until recent years—have been American.

A number of print models for companies such as the Athletic Model Guild achieved a modest fame in the 1950s and 1960s through pictures printed in limited-circulation physique magazines. However, the first real gay porn star was Casey Donovan.

Donovan, an aspiring actor and successful fashion model, was the featured performer in the first big gay porn film, *The Boys in the Sand* (1971). The surprising commercial and popular success of this first attempt at a technically proficient gay porn film launched Donovan's career as a gay icon.

Through the 1970s and into the 1980s, Donovan not only acted in a series of pornographic films, but he also became a poster boy for the burgeoning gay movement—not through direct political activity, but because of his high profile as an unashamed, self-confessed gay man.

The same was true of another 1970s performer, Al Parker. Parker, whose dark good looks and beard contrasted with the blond, smooth Donovan, made his first hard-core feature in 1976 after starting out in print media. Whereas Donovan represented an earlier generation of gay men, Parker came to symbolize the late-1970s "clone" look—the macho, flannel-clad men often seen strolling the streets of San Francisco's gay Castro district. Both men had performing careers that lasted well into the 1980s.

Jack Wrangler was another gay porn icon of the 1970s, a convincing actor who later ended up in a heterosexual marriage with singer Margaret Whiting. Both Parker and Wrangler were especially qualified for their jobs because of their unusually large penises—an important attribute for those aspiring to gay porn stardom.

The 1980s: Jeff Stryker, Ryan Idol, Joey Stefano

As gay porn changed in the 1980s, so did the nature of gay porn stars. The opening years of the decade saw the decline of theatrical porn features as home video became increasingly common. Some of the biggest stars of these new videos were straight men who performed for money.

By far the most famous of these was Jeff Stryker. With sultry good looks reminiscent of Elvis Presley, and an endowment the equal of his predecessor Al Parker, Stryker epitomized the "gay-for-pay" mentality. He was exclusively the inserter, or the top, in all his sex scenes.

Similarly, the late 1980s saw the emergence of Ryan Idol, another young straight performer whose striking good looks led to a busy career of personal appearances and porn films that continued sporadically into the 1990s.

A self-identified gay performer, Joey Stefano, also came onto the scene in the 1980s. Unlike most of his predecessors (with the notable exception of Casey Donovan), Stefano made his career primarily as a bottom, taking the receptive role in anal sex. This contrast between straight-identified tops and gay-identified bottoms became a hallmark of 1980s porn.

Stefano's legendary problems with drugs led to his death from an overdose in 1994, but his troubled life and career only enhanced his romantic appeal for many viewers, making him the James Dean of the porn world.

The 1990s: Lukas Ridgston, Ken Ryker

Foreign-produced porn, especially from Eastern Europe, became increasingly common and popular during the 1990s. Sometimes produced or directed by Americans, these films featured attractive, young, athletic men.

The most famous of these was Lukas Ridgston. Ridgston's classic good looks and youthful innocence even led to occasional personal appearances in the United States. However, the geographic distance between these performers and their primary market in America meant that stardom was difficult to attain for most.

The 1990s saw yet another shift in gay porn stardom, perhaps best represented by Ken Ryker. In his first performances, during the mid-1990s, the strapping Ryker (his name undoubtedly chosen to echo Stryker's) was initially a straight-identified top. As the decade wore on and

his fame grew, he began to be more responsive in his roles, engaging in kissing and oral sex.

More important, in interviews Ryker hinted that he was not straight, without actually identifying himself as gay. This tactic was similar to the hedging of many mainstream Hollywood actors when queried about their sexuality. Ryker's fuzzy sexual identity heralded a gradual decline of interest in the straight top in favor of gay-identified stars.

The New Millennium

Tom Chase and Steve Cassidy have come to represent the new wave of gay porn stars in the new millennium: masculine and muscular, sexually versatile, and confidently gay. However, tastes in porn vary widely. Even as muscular men in their mid-to-late twenties and thirties currently dominate the pantheon of porn stars, more youthful and less muscular "twinks" also command the loyalty of a considerable segment of the current market for gay porn.

Gay porn stars are paid relatively little for their performances. Salaries, even for top-level models, rarely exceed several thousand dollars per scene. Instead, stars rely on personal appearances and engagements as club strippers for most of their money. Many also turn to prostitution—"escorting"—to boost their incomes. In addition, their faces appear in a vast array of advertising for gay products, from nightclubs to sexual aids.

Porn stars' presence in the gay subculture is ubiquitous—in entertainment, in advertising, and in Gay Pride parades everywhere. They represent the unashamed expression of gay identity through their open practice of the sexuality that defines that identity.

Considering pornography's accepted, even exalted, status in gay life and the shortage of visible gay role models in the broader culture, it should come as no surprise that porn stars are an important feature of gay culture.

—Joe A. Thomas

BIBLIOGRAPHY

Burger, John R. One-Handed Histories: The Eroto-Politics of Gay Male Video Pornography. Binghamton, N.Y.: Harrington Park Press, 1995.

Edmondson, Roger. Boy in the Sand: Casey Donovan, All-American Sex Star. Los Angeles: Alyson Publications, 1998.

———. Clone: The Life and Legacy of Al Parker, Gay Superstar. Los Angeles: Alyson Publications, 2000.

Isherwood, Charles. Wonder Bread and Ecstasy: The Life and Death of Joey Stefano. Los Angeles: Alyson Publications, 1996.

LaRue, Chi Chi [Larry Paciotti], with John Erich. Making It Big: Sex Stars, Porn Films, and Me. Los Angeles: Alyson Publications, 1997.

Wrangler, Jack, and Carl Johnes. The Jack Wrangler Story; or, What's a Nice Boy Like You Doing? New York: St. Martin's Press, 1984.

SEE ALSO

Pornographic Film and Video: Gay Male; Pornographic Film and Video: Lesbian; Dean, James

Pornographic Film and Video: Bisexual

As a genre, bisexual pornography began in earnest during the mid-1980s, shortly after the popularization of the concept of a bisexual identity during the previous decade. While the sexological concept of bisexuality may be defined simply as an erotic or romantic attraction to both sexes, within the pornography industry it has taken on a more circumscribed meaning: films that feature some type of male homosexual activity in addition to the usual heterosexual and all-female scenes.

Examples of same-sex activity mixed with heterosexual coupling are found as early as Etruscan tomb paintings. In the modern era, scenes of women together are found in pornography from its beginnings in nineteenth-century photography and the stag films of the early twentieth century—generally in conjunction with additional scenes of heterosexual intercourse.

During pornography's growth era in the 1970s and 1980s, sexual activity between two women became an expected component of mainstream pornographic film and video, and it is featured in such classics as *Deep Throat* and *Behind the Green Door*. However, these images were clearly designed for consumption by heterosexual male viewers. Male homosexual imagery was still off-limits outside gay pornography.

Partly as a result of the sexual revolution of the 1960s and 1970s, less restrictive notions of sexual identity began surfacing. By the late 1970s, readers' letters submitted to *Penthouse* and *Penthouse Forum*—relating various sexual escapades—began to include occasional forays into male bisexuality.

In 1984 and 1985, a few video companies, such as Catalina and Vivid, took the plunge into a new genre of porn: bisexual features that included not only the standard mix of heterosexual and all-female scenes but also scenes of men together.

Director Paul Norman was among the first to establish a reputation for these new bisexual videos. His "Bi and Beyond" series, which debuted in 1988, was among the most famous examples of early bisexual porn. Bisexual videos' titles almost always play on the prefix "bi," as in, for example, *Bi Dreams of Genie* (1994).

Frequently starring gay porn performers in the male roles, the sexual action is fairly evenly divided between heterosexual and same-sex activity. Bisexual videos offered heterosexual stars of gay pornography, such as Jeff Stryker, an opportunity to move toward the straight side of the industry.

What constitutes the exact audience and market for these videos is not completely clear. Certainly the idea was to tap into the new bisexual population, which the media was touting as a sizable and previously overlooked group.

While some free-thinking, self-identified bisexuals undoubtedly rented or bought these videos, perhaps a larger group of consumers was ostensibly heterosexual men who were curious about sex with other men, or who were coming to grips with their own burgeoning homosexual feelings. Straight women who enjoyed watching men together were also likely an (underappreciated) audience.

As the genre developed, however, bisexual videos became increasingly associated with the gay male porn industry. By the turn of the millennium, scenes with women together became increasingly rare in bisexual porn, and bisexual videos frequently resembled gay male videos with the addition of heterosexual scenes.

Perhaps partly a result of the AIDS epidemic, the performers, directors, and producers of bisexual videos were rarely active in the straight porn industry. This alienation increased to the point that in 1998, when straight performer Mark Slade performed in some gay videos, he was no longer able to find work in straight videos.

Thor Stephans, a veteran director of bisexual and gay videos, has reported that many women refused to perform in bisexual videos for fear of being stigmatized and prevented from returning to the straight business. As a result, the quality and number of bisexual videos has decreased dramatically since their heyday in the 1980s, and the genre faces an uncertain future.   —*Joe A. Thomas*

Bibliography

Flint, David. *Babylon Blue: An Illustrated History of Adult Cinema*. London: Creation Books, 1999.

See also

Pornographic Film and Video: Gay Male; Pornographic Film and Video: Lesbian; Pornographic Film and Video: Transsexual

Pornographic Film and Video: Gay Male

Pornographic film and video have played an important role in gay male culture. Whereas heterosexual pornography has been accompanied by a serious stigma in the straight world, gay pornography has been characterized partly by the high esteem in which it is held in the gay male subculture.

As a group that is both defined by its sexual activity and rejected by the majority culture for it, gay men have often seen in pornography an all-too-rare positive image of gay sexuality. Similarly, they have found in the exaggerated sexuality and marginal artistry of porn a campy rejection of the hierarchies of the heterosexual majority.

As with straight pornography, gay male pornography can be divided into two categories, hard core and soft core. Hard core is the genre commonly associated with the term *pornography*. It includes explicit imagery of actual sexual activity to the point of climax, including visible penetration and ejaculation.

Soft core is a less explicit alternative, generally focusing on nude or nearly nude bodies in sexual or sensual situations, but without views of penetration or visible climax. The sex is nearly always simulated in soft core, and it is often filmed with an emphasis on romance or mood. As porn diva Gloria Leonard once humorously proclaimed, "The difference between pornography and erotica is lighting."

Because both the production and consumption of pornographic film and video are dependent on relatively high levels of technology, the genre's development has taken place primarily in the industrialized West. The existence there of a large and economically advantaged gay community is another important factor.

Thus, Western Europe and especially the United States have been the centers of gay male porn production and its audiences, though in recent years South America and Eastern Europe have also figured as sources of pornography that is consumed mainly in the West.

As technology has spread, hard-core pornography has begun to be reported from such unexpected locations as India. However, the bulk of gay male film and video pornography continues to be made by and for white Western males.

Beginnings

While gay male pornography in literature and still images has a long history, gay male pornography in motion pictures really began in 1971 with the theatrical release of Wakefield Poole's *The Boys in the Sand*, a hard-core, ironic response to the groundbreaking play and film *The Boys in the Band*.

Before *The Boys in the Sand*, filmed images of same-sex activity were limited to a few examples in stag films (some dating to early in the twentieth century) and to the less narrative examples found in underground films of the 1960s such as Kenneth Anger's *Scorpio Rising* (1963).

In both cases, gay content had to be disguised or excused by some other aspect of the film. In the stags it was incidental to heterosexual activity, or involved a case of mistaken gender identity; in underground films the artistic content and context helped to justify the obvious same-sex activity.

The Boys in the Sand heralded a new era of openness and popularity in gay male pornography and introduced the first gay superstar, Casey Donovan. Grossing more than $800,000 shortly after its release, the film and its success helped create a new industry.

The production of gay pornographic films expanded during the 1970s, paralleling the simultaneous expansion of the straight porn industry following the huge success of *Deep Throat* in 1972–1973. Companies such as Jaguar and P.M. Productions began producing a stream of gay male hard-core features for release in a limited number of specialized gay porn theaters.

Simultaneously, short film loops also became common. These descendants of the old stag films consisted of hard-core scenes (often silent) run on projectors as continuous loops in adult bookstores and movie arcades for the entertainment of customers, who dropped coins or tokens into a coin box for a few minutes of viewing.

As the industry diversified during this period, it became more commercialized than previously. Gay male pornographic films lost their initial formal references to art films, and with them their aspirations to be something more than "just pornography." Increased explicitness gradually overwhelmed narrative and aesthetic content.

The Advent of Video

Theatrical films and loops, however, were soon to be replaced by a new medium: video. As the prices of home VCRs fell during the 1980s, the video market became increasingly lucrative. Producers of both gay and straight products gradually began to shoot their movies directly on video, aiming squarely at the target of the home viewer.

As gay male pornography made this transition, the initial videos were collections of earlier loops or theatrical releases transferred to video. By the mid-1980s, as the well-funded producers and distributors of straight pornography moved into the lucrative gay male market, features shot on video became standard; simultaneously, the old gay porn theaters disappeared, along with their straight counterparts.

A New Ideal of Male Beauty

The gay male pornography of the 1970s utilized a fairly wide variety of performers, from the beefy bodybuilders of Colt Studios to the young jocks of Nova and the variations of the "Castro clone"—the hypermasculine type—seen in P.M. Productions. During the early 1980s, however, a new ideal of male beauty overwhelmingly dominated gay male videos. Inspired by the example of the famous Calvin Klein underwear ads, the new performers were sleek and smooth, and rarely looked older than twenty-four.

The prolific French director Jean-Daniel Cadinot nearly always used boyish models as his stars, but he frequently paired them with more butch, often older, partners, sometimes from "exotic" locations and backgrounds such as North Africa.

Many of the classic American pornographic videos of the mid-1980s exemplify the trend toward youthful models, but without the diversity seen in Cadinot's productions: director William Higgins's *Sailor in the Wild* (1983); Matt Sterling's *The Bigger the Better* (1984); and John Travis's *Powertool* (1986), for example.

New superstars such as Jeff Stryker were often straight men in the business for the money, or "gay for pay," as those in the industry put it. Sexual roles in 1980s videos tended to be as tightly defined as the performers' musculature. The top took the inserter role in anal sex and often possessed bigger muscles (and a bigger penis) than the bottom. Producers and distributors often played up the heterosexual identity of some star tops, making them seem more virile and desirable than the gay-identified bottoms.

Changes in the Rules

By the late 1980s, however, the unwritten rules of the early years of gay video began to bend, largely due to the entry of a new player: Kristen Bjorn. A former porn model himself, Bjorn turned to photography in the 1980s, and then to live-action videos. *Carnaval in Rio* (1989) was his first full-length hard-core feature, after a series of videos with solo action only.

Bjorn's work is characterized by exotic settings, beautiful photography, ethnic diversity, and vastly improved production values (made possible partly by his unusually long and expansive shooting schedule). Whereas 1970s films had regularly—though infrequently—featured people of color, 1980s videos were largely racially segregated. Bjorn bucked this trend by featuring a veritable rainbow of ethnicities. His locales ranged from South America and the Caribbean to Australia, Canada, and eventually Eastern Europe. Bjorn threw down the gauntlet for the established video producers, who were compelled to deal with the popularity (and resulting profitability) of his stylish videos.

During the 1990s, gay male pornographic productions began to experiment, at least partly in response to Bjorn's challenge. Among the most obvious changes was the increased diversity of ages and body types in gay male videos. Performers in their forties began to reappear, as did body hair (exemplified by the 1990s star Zak Spears).

As the gay ideal of masculine beauty evolved in the 1990s, bulging bodybuilders began to be seen, along with the slimmer physiques of previous years. Simultaneously, the rigid definitions of sexual roles also began to relax as a number of this new, more diverse, crowd of performers took both the top and bottom roles in videos, often within a single scene ("flip-flopping," as it was called in the industry).

While racial segregation largely remained the norm, a few companies followed Bjorn's lead in offering videos with ethnic diversity. In addition, a significant specialty market developed for all-black and all-Latino features; a number of companies such as La Mancha Productions focused on "blatino" performers, frequently mixed-race street youths from New York.

Still, one can exaggerate the diversity that developed. After all, Falcon Studios, with its bevy of well-scrubbed, All-American, corn-fed, butch young men, became the industry sales leader in the 1990s—a position it held into the new century.

Overseas production was another important development. Eastern Europe and South America became new centers of pornographic production. Attractive models were available for a fraction of the cost of American performers. Budapest became one of the new capitals of porn production, both gay and straight.

Twenty-First-Century Pornography

As gay male pornography entered the twenty-first century, a number of new developments heralded further changes. The Internet was a burgeoning new market that could be exploited by both established and new pornographers. It became a significant presence as numerous companies and individuals established sex-oriented websites, including interactive, live-action performances.

DVD technology improved, and many companies began to rerelease older products in this new format (and to release newer features in both VHS and DVD formats).

Entire niche markets developed for specialized tastes. Fetish videos involving spanking or fisting became available. So did products focusing on older models, various ethnicities, solo videos, and bondage and discipline, among many others. Soft core gained a greater presence through the work of companies such as Greenwood-Cooper and 10% Productions.

Although for most performers pornography remained a brief sideline business in which they dabbled for only a couple of years, some, such as Eric Evans, Jake Andrews, and Chip Daniels, were able to maintain relatively long and stable careers in sex work, both in front of the camera and behind it.

For others, video porn was used as advertising for the prostitution (or "escorting," as it was euphemistically known) that was their primary source of income. Performing as a stripper in nightclubs was another profitable job that could develop from a career in pornography.

Moreover, the gay porn world became its own subculture within a subculture, boasting its own awards shows, pantheon of stars and directors, and a strong and open connection to the gay culture that was both its market and its source of inspiration.

By 2000, gay male pornography was thoroughly integrated into gay life in a way that straight pornography has never enjoyed in the majority culture. Gay porn actors became cultural heroes, their images sometimes gracing giant billboards in gay ghettos in Houston and Los Angeles. They made public appearances at important social functions, and organized and attended high-profile fund-raisers, especially for AIDS causes.

Today the gay subculture openly accepts—sometimes even revels in—pornography. Because gay sexual identity is already marked as deviant by the mainstream, it is hard for most gay men to see the enjoyment of pornography as marginalizing or problematic.

With the majority of gay men regarding pornography positively, the gay male community has not been polarized by the bitter debates over pornography that has sometimes divided lesbian communities.

Indeed, gay men at the beginning of the twenty-first century use pornography at least in part in a way similar to the way earlier generations of gay men used a camp sensibility: as a means of asserting their identity by flouting and mocking the arbitrary standards of the majority.

—*Joe A. Thomas*

BIBLIOGRAPHY

Burger, John R. *One-Handed Histories: The Eroto-Politics of Gay Male Video Pornography.* New York: Harrington Park Press, 1995.

Dyer, Richard. "Male Gay Porn: Coming to Terms." *Jump Cut* 30 (1985): 27–29.

Thomas, Joe A. "Gay Male Video Pornography: Past, Present, and Future." *Sex for Sale: Prostitution, Pornography, and the Sex Industry.* Ronald Weitzer, ed. New York: Routledge, 2000. 49–66.

Waugh, Thomas. *Hard to Imagine: Gay Male Eroticism in Photography and Film from Their Beginnings to Stonewall.* New York: Columbia University Press, 1996.

———. "Men's Pornography: Gay vs. Straight." *Out in Culture: Gay, Lesbian, and Queer Essays on Popular Culture.* Alexander Doty and Corey K. Creekmur, eds. Durham, N.C.: Duke University Press, 1995. 307–327.

SEE ALSO

Pornographic Film and Video: Bisexual; Pornographic Film and Video: Lesbian; Pornographic Film and Video: Transsexual; Porn Stars; Cadinot, Jean-Daniel

Pornographic Film and Video: Lesbian

PORNOGRAPHY HAS ALWAYS SPARKED A GREAT DEAL of controversy among lesbians. Traditionally rejected by lesbian feminists as an inherently male institution both violent and misogynistic, pornography has nonetheless been openly embraced by a faction of prosex lesbians (and so-called do-me feminists) for the past two decades.

At the same time, from its emergence only in the mid-1980s, there remains to this day a decided dearth of authentic lesbian pornographic film.

It is easy enough to find numerous woman-on-woman scenes in the majority of heterosexual pornographic films, of course; but these representations of all-female sexuality are generally so inaccurate, and so clearly geared toward a straight male audience, that very few could truly be considered lesbian.

The differences between lesbian-made and male-produced movies are easy to recognize: Most pornographic films made by and for lesbians are, first and foremost, noncommercial, often with amateur actors and makeshift sets.

These films feature women of different sizes, shapes, colors, and gender identities—butches, stone butches, femmes, androgynes, etc. Many of these lesbians have short nails, short hair, and modifications such as tattoos and body or facial piercings.

In contrast, most "lesbian" scenes in straight pornography feature stereotypical male-fantasy women with surgical enhancements, uniformly thin bodies, and long hair and nails. Despite the identification of many commercial porn actresses as bisexual or polysexual, there is never a butch in sight in these movies.

It was not until 1985 that the first pornographic film made entirely by and for lesbians appeared, well over a decade after the first gay male pornographic films emerged. The then brand-new technology of video facilitated the making of two short films, *Private Pleasures* and *Shadows*, which were released together on one tape.

These movies were the brainchild of Fatale Video, founded by Nan Kinney and Debi Sundahl—the same duo who launched *On Our Backs*, the first sex magazine created for lesbians by lesbians, in 1984.

Fatale went on to release other lesbian-made porn videos such as *Hungry Hearts* (1989); the infamous *Suburban Dykes* (1991), which starred Nina Hartley, a well-known, openly bisexual commercial porn actress; *Bathroom Sluts* (1991); and the instructional video *How to Female Ejaculate* (1992), among others.

Gay Male Porn vs. Lesbian Porn

In a culture that has long fostered the open expression of male sexuality while discouraging overt female sexuality and aggression, it comes as no surprise that pornography has historically been created by and for men, both gay and straight.

In addition, the longstanding "sex wars" between pro- and antiporn feminist camps also contributed to the scarcity of dyke-made porn. The sex wars, fought ferociously through the 1980s and made public by groups such as Women Against Pornography, have not yet ceased. In contrast, a loud outcry over pornography in the gay male community—or among straight men, for that matter—has yet to surface.

It is interesting to note, then, the disparity between the politics of gay male pornography and that of lesbian pornography. For example, gay male porn has found expression in a huge number of films and magazines, and gay porn theaters were at one time commonplace, at least in major cities. In terms of sheer quantity, there is simply no parallel in lesbian culture.

One reason for this is the economic situation of lesbians, who are in general a less economically prosperous group than gay men. Fronting the money to produce pornography has proven a challenge—especially when the lesbian market for explicit material remains tiny in comparison to the market for gay male or straight porn.

Very few lesbian sex magazines are published in the United States. (*On Our Backs* is the only one with which most lesbian readers are familiar.) Moreover, the small number of lesbian videos that do exist tend to embody political statements and emphasize issues such as diversity, safe sex, and varied expressions of sexual identity, which sometimes results in a less than truly titillating film for many viewers.

Interestingly enough, many lesbians regularly watch and appreciate gay male pornography, presumably because, among its other merits, it entails neither an overwhelming focus on political correctness nor the distracting and often disturbing heterosexual power dynamics found in straight porn.

Gay porn and lesbian porn have something important in common, however: They serve as positive, accurate representations of queer sexuality—a rare depiction in our society. As prosex lesbians and feminists point out, sexual material made by women and intended for a lesbian audience can be tremendously life-affirming in a world still permeated with heterosexism and lesbian exploitation.

Politically Correct Smut

Something of a lesbian film phenomenon, the safe-sex video gained popularity among lesbians in the early 1990s. Movies such as *Well Sexy Women* (The Unconscious Collective, 1992), *Safe Is Desire* (Debi Sundahl, 1993), and the compilation film *She's Safe!* (1993) have been marketed both as self-help tapes *and* as pornography.

Such videos make it acceptable for lesbians to watch smut because the smut has a greater social purpose: It teaches lesbians about AIDS prevention, rather than simply displaying activity between women that could be deemed exploitative (or could be co-opted by watchers of commercial straight porn).

Perhaps this focus on safety in women's sex videos can be attributed in part to the fact that the majority of HIV/AIDS research has not focused on woman-to-woman sexual activity and transmission.

In fact, little medical research into lesbian sexual practices has been done at all—somehow, the fact that lesbians really do have sex with each other, and in many different ways, has escaped the attention of many in the mainstream medical establishment.

However, the idea that women require videotaped instructions to figure out the proper use of latex gloves or dams lessens the credibility of these movies as educational materials—and may strike some viewers as downright silly.

Educational/erotic films for lesbians that do not stress latex include sex guru Annie Sprinkle's twenty-eight-minute "pornumentary" *Linda, Les, and Annie* (1989), which recounts Sprinkle's experiences with Les, a female-to-male transsexual lover who used to be a butch lesbian. The video, while perhaps not technically lesbian pornography, still proves of interest to sexually adventurous dykes.

Meanwhile, House of Chicks, a tiny lesbian production company, has produced a series of instructional videos such as *The Magic of Female Ejaculation* (1992) and *How to Find Your Goddess Spot* (1995). These are relatively small-scale projects, but have become easily available through the technology of the Internet.

Recent Developments

Although Fatale did not release any new films between 1993 and 2000, several other lesbian pornographic videos, aside from safe-sex instructionals, surfaced in the 1990s.

The "San Francisco Lesbians" movies, an extensive series of "real lesbian" sex videos, became available through mainstream channels, starting with *San Francisco Lesbians #1* in 1992 and continuing through an eighth installment in 1998.

Maria Beatty, with her company Bleu Productions, made numerous lesbian-themed S/M and fetish films, such as *The Boiler Room* (1998), *Doctor's Orders* (1998), and *Les Vampyres* (2000). However, while Beatty's films are highly artistic, they have a commercial bent that seems to appeal more widely to a heterosexual audience than to a lesbian one.

Christopher Lee's male-to-female transsexual porn film *Alley of the Tranny Boys* (1998) has proved to be of interest to many lesbians. In 1999, a Canadian lesbian pornographic film called *Classy Cunts*, made by Live Peach Productions, was screened to extremely limited audiences in Montreal. Unfortunately, this film, like some other wholly independent short films with very small budgets, is difficult to obtain.

The biggest breakthrough in the indie-porn industry came in 2000 with the release of S.I.R. Video's full-length tape *Hard Love/How to Fuck in High Heels*. Several years earlier, S.I.R. had coproduced, with Fatale Video, two films in the *Bend Over Boyfriend* series—which focused on unconventional heterosexual sex. But their 2000 release was something very new in dyke pornography.

The two films—one a narrative about a broken-up butch/femme couple who still cannot resist each other, the other a "mockumentary" based on a spoken-word piece by one of S.I.R.'s founders—won rave reviews among lesbian audiences for both their authenticity and their genuinely sexy content.

Unlike any other by-and-for-lesbians pornographic film, and despite the fact that it featured explicit depictions of butch sexuality, the video actually made enough of a crossover into the mainstream to win a 2001 AVN (*Adult Video News*) Award—the porn Oscar—for Best All-Girl Feature.

Jackie Strano and Shar Rednour, the couple who formed S.I.R., also write, direct, and star in the films. *Sugar High Glitter City*, S.I.R.'s 2001 release, is described by its creators as featuring "a fabulously diverse cast and multiple dyke sexualities"; it seems that even the hottest dyke videos still have politics somewhere in mind, which is only to be expected in an industry that has traditionally either ignored or exploited lesbians.

Conclusion

Despite continuing debates over pornography within the feminist and lesbian communities, lesbian indie-porn companies have emerged to enjoy considerable success. S.I.R. envisions creating a lesbian porn empire, and in 2001 Fatale Video—which is also launching an erotic book imprint—released a collection of shorts entitled *Afterschool Special.*

Groups such as Feminists for Free Expression and Feminists Against Censorship continue to fight for the right of women to make and watch pornography. It seems that, more than ever, lesbians are seizing that right.

—*Teresa Theophano*

BIBLIOGRAPHY

Califia, Pat. *Public Sex: The Culture of Radical Sex.* San Francisco: Cleis Press, 2000.

Henderson, Lisa. "Lesbian Pornography." *New Lesbian Criticism.* Sally Munt, ed. New York: Columbia University Press, 1992. 173–191.

Milliken, Christine. "Eroticizing Safer Sex: Pedagogy and Performance in Lesbian Video." *Lesbian Sex Scandals: Sexual Practices, Identities, and Politics.* Dawn Atkins, ed. Binghamton, N.Y.: Harrington Park Press, 1999. 93–102.

Taormino, Tristan. "Desperately Seeking Dyke Porn." *Village Voice,* April 26, 2000, 142.

www.bleuproductions.com

www.fatalemedia.com

www.sirvideo.com

SEE ALSO

Pornographic Film and Video: Gay Male; Pornographic Film and Video: Bisexual; Pornographic Film and Video: Transsexual

Pornographic Film and Video: Transsexual

EVEN THOUGH MOST OF THE PORNOGRAPHY THAT FEAtures transsexuals is made neither by nor for them and can be considered exploitative, in recent years trans porn activists have begun to produce pornography for transsexual and other queer audiences.

Most pornography is produced by and consumed by heterosexual men. In 1998, *Adult Video News* conducted a survey of adult video stores and found that a little over 90 percent of adult video consumers were heterosexual men, 20 percent of whom rented or bought pornographic videos with their female partners.

But as queer theorists and film critics have shown, it is unwise to assume that the type of sexuality depicted in pornography is a direct or necessary reflection of the consumer's identity or sexual practices. In *Hard Core: Power, Pleasure, and the "Frenzy of the Visible,"* Linda Williams cautions students of pornography that in the past decade, as the categories of pornography have proliferated, "it becomes difficult to describe the pleasures of sexual performances in any predictable binary terms."

For instance, straight men often enjoy viewing scenes that feature lesbian sex. Significantly, and perhaps more surprisingly, they are also the primary consumers of transsexual pornography.

The emergence of transsexuals in mainstream pornography undoubtedly has less to do with transsexuals' interest in seeing themselves as objects of desire and more to do with the fetishistic role such images play in the sexual imagination of heterosexual men.

The appeal of pornography that features "trannies," "chicks with dicks," or "she-males" lies in its blurring of conventional sexual boundaries and in the fantasies it offers viewers.

Transsexual pornography often features scenes in which male-to-female transsexuals penetrate the male performers. Such scenes allow straight male viewers to fantasize about their own penetration, while maintaining a semblance of heterosexual norms.

The *Bend Over Boyfriend* video series, popular among heterosexual couples, plays to this fantasy by showing these couples how a woman can use a strap-on dildo to penetrate her male partner.

Transsexual pornography also allows ostensibly straight men to explore bisexual fantasies without having to identify fully as desiring other men. As a quotation on the box of the latest *Dicks on Chicks* release suggests, "When you get the taste for meat but don't wanna cross the line, you take the middle ground and fuck with the Dicks on Chicks nasty crew."

Viewing scenes that feature men performing oral sex on male-to-female transsexuals who have penises permits men who identify as heterosexuals to satisfy their curiosity about bisexuality.

Transsexual Porn Produced by the Mainstream Pornography Industry

Transsexual pornographic films emerged in the 1970s, but did not become readily accessible and visible until the early and mid-1980s.

She-Male Encounters, Collections 1 and 2 (Caballero Productions, 1980) are early examples of transsexual pornography that was produced by the more mainstream heterosexual pornography industry. Titles by Bizarre Video Productions such as *Transsexual's Revenge, TV's Plaything,* and *TVs by Choice* were produced in the 1980s and are still available today.

As specialized pornography became more popular with mainstream heterosexual porn consumers in the late 1990s, a miniexplosion of transsexual pornography occurred.

In works such as *Trannie Love* (1995) and *The Princess with a Penis* (1996) from He-She Studios, transsexual porn also acquired a campy sense of humor. More recent series such as the *Rouge Adventures* and *Big Ass She-Male Adventures* have proven very successful and have won numerous adult video awards. Clearly, transsexual porn made for heterosexual men remains a viable market.

Trans Porn for Transsexuals

In spite of the fact that the overwhelming majority of transsexual pornographic videos are geared to straight men, a small number of trans activists have in recent years begun to produce trans porn for transsexuals and other queer audiences.

The best known of these videos is probably *Alley of the Tranny Boys* (1998). Directed by Christopher Lee, it was the first transsexual pornographic video featuring female-to-male (FTM) transsexual performers. Lee has gone on to make *Sex Flesh in Blood* (1999). Both works gleefully subvert the genre that most exploits transsexuals.

Lee prides himself on showing in his pornography sexual acts that have rarely been eroticized. In *Alley*, he uses the aesthetics of 1970s gay male porn to promote a hard-core FTM sexuality; transmen fuck and suck each other and biological men as well, thus challenging stereotypical assumptions about what FTMs can do in bed and in public-sex environments.

Lee's production staff for *Sex Flesh in Blood* was composed entirely of people of color. The video draws upon gothic images and mixes trans erotics with suggestions of raunchy sex and even necrophilia.

Rather than portray images of tranny passivity and submissiveness in the presence of biological, heterosexual men, Lee asks queer audiences to see transsexuals as sexual subjects with their own desires and the power to pursue them.

Other trans porn makers have employed similar strategies and have begun to change the way porn represents transsexuals. For example, *Dysfunctional* (Mirha-Soleil Ross, 1997) challenges assumptions that trannies should not enjoy their unaltered genitals, while *Look of Love* (Charles Lofton, 1996) remixes she-male porn in such an alluring way that it obliges viewers to rethink what turns them on.

Pansexual Porn (Del LaGrace Volcano, 1998) challenges not only heterosexual audiences but gay ones as well by showing FTMs with camcorders having sex with men in public-sex environments.

Collectively, these directors refuse to cater to sexual orientations and gender identities that fit into binary systems. Their pornography unsettles their audiences in order to suggest a new, more fluid, and freer sexual construct.

—*Geoffrey W. Bateman*

Bibliography

Dwyer, Susan, ed. *The Problem of Pornography.* Belmont, Calif.: Wadsworth Publishing, 1995.

"Marketing Specialty Porn to an Ever-Expanding Customer Base." *Adult Video News* (Dec. 2000): www.adultvideonews.com/archives/200012/cover/cover1200_01 .html

Sandler, Adam. "Adults Only, Big Business." *Variety*, January 19, 1998, 5.

Selke, Lori. "Trannyporn: Extreme Gender Cinema." *GettingIt.com* (January 19, 2000): www.fraudband.org/gettingit/article/521

Wilcox, Russell. "Cross-Gender Identification in Commercial Pornographic Films." *Porn 101: Eroticism, Pornography, and the First Amendment.* James Elias et al., eds. Amherst, Mass.: Prometheus Books, 1999. 479–491.

Williams, Linda. *Hard Core: Power, Pleasure, and the "Frenzy of the Visible."* Berkeley, Calif.: University of California Press, 1999.

See Also

Pornographic Film and Video: Bisexual; Pornographic Film and Video: Gay Male; Pornographic Film and Video: Lesbian

Praunheim, Rosa von   (b. 1942)

FILMMAKER ROSA VON PRAUNHEIM IS ONE OF GERMANY'S leading gay activists and chroniclers of queer life. In almost sixty films made over four decades, he targets the gay community through deliberate confrontation, provocation, and satire in order to foster self-examination by gay people and to advance gay rights.

Born Holger Bernhard Bruno Mischnitzky on November 25, 1942, in Riga, Latvia, he changed his name in the early 1960s. He took the name Rosa from *rosa Winkel,* the pink triangle of the Nazi era, and in a gesture of queer deviance adopted *von,* a sign of German nobility. The name Praunheim apparently comes from the Frankfurt suburb in which he grew up.

He studied painting, then began making films in the late 1960s. After an early success, *Die Bettwurst* (1970), a parody of heterosexual marriage, he began making films that featured gay subject matter and that advanced the goals of gay liberation.

Von Praunheim's first gay film, *It Is Not the Homosexual Who Is Perverse but the Situation in Which He Is Forced to Live* (1970), stirred controversy and met with harsh criticism from conservatives and liberals alike for its negative and degrading portrayal of irresponsible sexual behavior and narcissistic consumerism in the gay community.

Although publicly von Praunheim refers to it as his *Schwulenfilm*, or "faggot film," he is quick to add that the film started the gay rights movement in Germany and led to the formation of the Homosexual Interest Group.

Controversy and scandal are no strangers to von Praunheim, in any case. He courted controversy early in his career by outing politicians and businessmen on German television, a practice that he later came to regret.

One of his most controversial films is his nihilistic, strident, and comic depiction of AIDS in the gay community, *A Virus Has No Morals* (1985–1986), a combination musical and morality play. The film attacks the medical establishment, governments, journalists, charity organizations, and homosexuals for their complicity and passivity in the face of the epidemic. In this film, von Praunheim himself plays an HIV-positive bathhouse owner who equates sex with life.

Passionately committed to activism, von Praunheim frequently injects himself into his films, sometimes in ways that seem aimed at courting notoriety. In *Army of Lovers or Revolt of the Perverts* (1972–1976), for example, he filmed his students filming a gay porn star performing fellatio on him so they would have incendiary footage for a film project.

Decades of controversy and conflict with the gay community led to the self-deprecating and autobiographical film *Neurosia* (1995)—the title a combination of Rosa and neurosis—in which a drag queen investigates the murder of von Praunheim and digs into his past. While somewhat self-mocking, the filmmaker also mocks his detractors and reiterates his own accomplishments.

Critics have complained of the often chaotic and confusing structure of von Praunheim's films, overlooking their function as radical political tools. Adopting a style that often mixes fictional vignettes, old newsreel footage, stills, documentary film, and interviews, he eschews an entertaining narrative line. He opts, instead, for disjunctive and harsh argumentation.

A queer aesthetic is most evident in the nonfictional and quasi-fictional biographical portraits of outcasts struggling in a hostile environment, but refusing to relinquish their dignity. These affectionate and vivacious portraits of strippers, circus performers, transsexuals, and aging dancers and cabaret stars from pre–World War II Berlin stand in stark contrast to the targets of von Praunheim's films: weak, pensive, and assimilated middle-class gays.

I Am My Own Woman (1992) is von Praunheim's most successful portrait. It tells the remarkable story of Charlotte von Mahlsdorf, a homosexual transvestite who survived decades of indignities to receive the highest award bestowed by Germany, the Cross of the Order of Merit, for architectural and furniture restoration. In this film, von Praunheim uses nonfictional footage and interviews with von Mahlsdorf, as well as actors portraying her in brief vignettes.

Some of von Praunheim's films document queer activism. For example, films such as *Silence = Death* (1990) and *Positive* (1990) capture the voices of such AIDS activists as Larry Kramer, Michael Callen, Phil Zwickler, Keith Haring, and David Wojnarowicz, while *Transsexual Menace* (1996) reveals the complexity of the transgender community and documents transsexual activism in the United States.

In the 1990s, von Praunheim turned increasingly to "correcting historical awareness" with such films as *Gay Courage—100 Years of the Gay Rights Movement in Germany and Beyond* (1998). *Einstein of Sex* (1999) chronicles the life of Magnus Hirschfeld, a gay Jewish sexologist and pioneering advocate for homosexual rights.

In celebration of his sixtieth birthday, von Praunheim directed, produced and starred in *Pfui Rosa!* (2002). Attesting to von Praunheim's status in Germany as a provocative filmmaker and political activist, the West German Television Network aired the seventy-minute autobiography. Celebratory in nature, *Pfui Rosa!*, like *Neurosia*, is both self-indulgent and self-deprecating, and both irreverent and shocking.

In *Queens Don't Lie* (2003), an intimate portrait of the lives of four Berlin drag queens, whom he presents as important agents of social, cultural, and political change, von Praunheim returned to the documentary approach he perfected in *Anita—Dances of Vice* (1987), *I Am My Own Woman*, and *Wunderbares Wrodow* (1997).

In *Your Heart on My Mind* (2005), von Praunheim has galvanized public debate in Germany about cannibalism with a film based on the case of Armin Meiwes, a gay man recently convicted of manslaughter after using the Internet to find a consenting male to murder, dismember, and eat.

Von Praunheim is currently working on films—one a documentary, the other fictional—about gay Nazis, tentatively titled *Homosexuality and Fascism* and *Even Gay Nazis Like to Kiss*.

Von Praunheim has used his films to spark or reconfigure debates on a number of queer issues. A risk-taker both in terms of the images he creates and the subject matter he tackles, he has influenced such filmmakers as Michael Stock, John Greyson, and Monika Treut. He has provided visibility to topics, people, and history that most filmmakers have ignored.   —*Richard C. Bartone*

BIBLIOGRAPHY

Kuzniar, Alice. *The Queer German Cinema.* Stanford, Calif.: Stanford University Press, 2000.

Saunders, Michael William. *Imps of the Perverse: Gay Monsters in Film.* Westport, Conn.: Praeger Publishers, 1998.

SEE ALSO

Film; European Film; Documentary Film; Film Directors; Transvestism in Film; Greyson, John; Treut, Monika

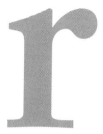

Richardson, Tony (1928–1991)

BRITISH FILM AND STAGE DIRECTOR TONY RICHARDSON was instrumental in challenging the censorship codes of the Lord Chamberlain's office, which—until the 1960s—held tremendous and repressive powers over the language and subject matter that was allowed to be presented on the British stage and screen.

While Richardson had a long history of controversies with this government office, one of his most notable victories resulted in the first sympathetic portrayal of a homosexual character in British film; indeed, one of the first in international cinema. Although Richardson himself was publicly heterosexual, he had a quiet—if not completely closeted—gay life as well.

He was born Cecil Antonio Richardson on June 5, 1928, in Shipley, Yorkshire, the son of a pharmacist. He was interested in the stage from an early age, and, as a student at Wadham College, Oxford, became involved with the Oxford University Dramatic Society.

At college, he also began to write for various drama and film journals and became acquainted with Lindsay Anderson and Gavin Lambert, who, like Richardson, would be instrumental in advancing British New Wave cinema (or Free Cinema)—film based in social realism and focusing on the lives of the lower classes.

After receiving a baccalaureate in English in 1952, Richardson became a television director for the British Broadcasting Corporation, and, even as he continued his career there, began as a stage director at the Royal Court Theatre and helped found the English Stage Company. In the latter capacity he directed the first performances of John Osborne's plays *Look Back in Anger* (1956) and *The Entertainer* (1957), which spearheaded the "Angry Young Men" trend that swept through British drama, film, and literature in the late 1950s and early 1960s.

In 1956, Richardson began his career in cinema with *Momma Don't Allow*, a short film about young people in a jazz club, which he codirected with Karel Reisz. Soon thereafter, Richardson and Osborne founded Woodfall Films, mostly for the purpose of filming *Look Back in Anger* (1958) independently.

The film's critical success led to more works of the New Wave genre, including *The Entertainer* (starring Sir Laurence Olivier, 1960), *A Taste of Honey* (1961), and *The Loneliness of the Long Distance Runner* (1962). Richardson's rise to acclaim culminated with *Tom Jones* (1963), which won Academy Awards for Best Picture and Best Director.

Of these works, *A Taste of Honey*, adapted from Shelagh Delaney's controversial play (1958), made film history by shattering many long-standing taboos regarding the representation of illegitimacy, miscegenation, and homosexuality.

In this film, Jo (Rita Tushingham), an unwed pregnant teenager, abandoned by her mother and separated from her black sailor boyfriend, is befriended by Geoff (Melvin Murray), a gay art student who, in spite of the abuse he receives from other characters, remains consistently kind and dignified.

Although Geoff might seem stereotypically effeminate by today's standards, it is a tribute to Richardson's determination in fighting censorship that so obvious a gay character was portrayed with complete sympathy.

From 1962 to 1967, Richardson was married to Vanessa Redgrave (whose father, Sir Michael Redgrave, was also bisexual) and had two children with her, the actresses Natasha Richardson and Joely Richardson. Even though he was married, and subsequently had a well-publicized affair with French actress Jeanne Moreau, he nonetheless had various relationships with men.

After a severe reversal of his previous successes, Richardson relocated to Southern California in the early 1970s, where fellow British expatriates Christopher Isherwood and David Hockney were among his closest friends.

His two French films with Moreau, *Mademoiselle* (1966) and *The Sailor from Gibraltar* (1967), were commercial and critical failures, as was his epic *The Charge of the Light Brigade* (1968), a ferocious deconstruction of military bravado and blind obedience.

None of Richardson's subsequent films, including *Ned Kelly* (starring Mick Jagger, 1969), *Joseph Andrews* (1977), *The Border* (1982), *Hotel New Hampshire* (1984), and *Blue Sky* (1994), achieved the acclaim of his earlier work.

Richardson died of AIDS-related illness in Los Angeles on November 14, 1991. His memoirs, discovered after his death by his daughter Natasha, were published in 1993.

—*Patricia Juliana Smith*

BIBLIOGRAPHY

Aldgate, Anthony. *Censorship and the Permissive Society: British Cinema and Theatre 1955–1965.* Oxford: Oxford University Press, 1995.

Radovich, Don. *Tony Richardson: A Bio-Bibliography.* Westport, Conn.: Greenwood Press, 1995.

Richardson, Tony. *The Long Distance Runner: A Memoir.* New York: William Morrow, 1993.

Welsh, James M., and John C. Tibbetts, eds. *The Cinema of Tony Richardson: Essays and Interviews.* Albany, N.Y.: State University of New York Press, 1999.

SEE ALSO

Film; European Film; Film Directors; Anderson, Lindsay

Riggs, Marlon   *(1957–1994)*

WRITER, DIRECTOR, AND PRODUCER MARLON RIGGS was an accomplished and outspoken activist whose efforts to promote black gay male visibility live on through his films and essays.

Born on February 3, 1957, into a Fort Worth, Texas, military family, Riggs was raised in Texas, Georgia, and Germany. He experienced the effects of racism throughout his life; as a gay man he also became acutely aware of homophobia as well.

Riggs's experience of racism began in his segregated childhood schools but continued even at Harvard, where he studied American history, graduating with honors in 1978. He earned an M.A. in 1981 at the University of California, Berkeley, Graduate School of Journalism, where he later taught documentary film courses.

Riggs first gained recognition for writing, producing, and directing the Emmy-winning, hour-long documentary *Ethnic Notions* (1987), which explored black stereotypes and stereotyping. The film helped establish Riggs's career as a producer of historical documentaries on subjects of contemporary relevance.

But most of his later films and writings probe the dichotomy Riggs perceived between the strong, Afrocentric black man and the black "sissy" gay man. As a "sissy" himself, Riggs felt deeply his status as a pariah within the black community.

Tongues Untied (1989), Riggs's most famous film, is an extensively reviewed and critically acclaimed documentary that met with controversy in conservative circles when it was aired on public television. Funded by a National Endowment for the Arts grant, it figured in the cultural wars over control of the NEA and the Public Broadcasting System.

But quite apart from the controversy it stirred when it was first broadcast, the film remains a groundbreaking exploration of black male sexuality, incorporating poetry, personal testimony, performance art, and rap as a means of exposing the homophobia and racism rampant in the lives of black gay men.

Riggs decided to make the film after almost dying of kidney failure, which turned out to be HIV-related; the experience helped him recognize the need to address sexuality as well as racism in his work. Making the film was truly cathartic, as it allowed him to express his long-pent-up anger and guilt over the black community's treatment of him as an outsider.

With *Tongues Untied*, Riggs's work had begun to benefit *him*, rather than instructing, entertaining, or enlightening only the public. The film was screened at Cannes and at the Berlin Film Festival, and won awards at several festivals, including the San Francisco International Lesbian and Gay Film Festival, the Atlanta Film Festival, and the New York Documentary Film Festival.

Later and lesser-known films that Riggs produced include *Color Adjustment: Blacks in Prime Time* (1991), which addresses images of black people on television, and *No Regrets (Non, Je Ne Regrette Rien*, 1993), which features interviews with HIV-positive black men.

His final film, *Black Is...Black Ain't,* is an examination of the diversity of black identities via music, history, and personal testimony. Released in 1995, it was completed posthumously.

Riggs's writings have been published in various arts and literary journals, such as *Black American Literature Forum, Art Journal,* and *High Performance,* as well as in the anthology *Brother to Brother* (1991).

His activism extended to writing on censorship issues and serving on PBS's national policy committee and panels such as the National Endowment for the Arts. He consistently criticized both the racism of the majority white gay community and the homophobia of the African American community.

Riggs died from AIDS complications in Oakland, California, on April 5, 1994. *—Teresa Theophano*

BIBLIOGRAPHY

Avena, Thomas. "Interview: Marlon Riggs." *Life Sentences: Writers, Artists, & AIDS.* Thomas Avena, ed. San Francisco: Mercury House, 1994. 258–273.

Hogan, Steve, and Lee Hudson. *Completely Queer.* New York: Henry Holt, 1998.

Riggs, Marlon. "Black Macho Revisited: Reflections of a SNAP! Queen." *Brother to Brother: New Writings by Black Gay Men.* Essex Hemphill, ed. Boston: Alyson, 1991. 253–257.

Simmons, Ron. "Tongues Untied: An Interview with Marlon Riggs." *Brother to Brother: New Writings by Black Gay Men.* Essex Hemphill, ed. Boston: Alyson, 1991. 189–199.

SEE ALSO

Film; Film Directors; Documentary Film; New Queer Cinema

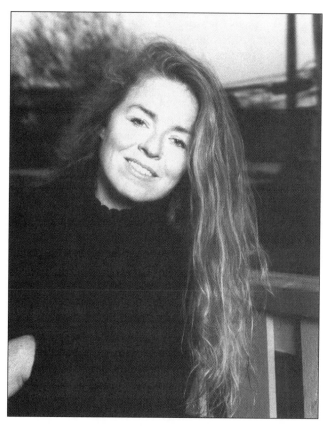

Patricia Rozema.

Rozema, Patricia   (b. 1958)

CANADIAN FILMMAKER PATRICIA ROZEMA IS KNOWN for imbuing her films, which she usually writes as well as directs, with feminist analysis and sensual cinematography.

Rozema was born on August 20, 1958, to Dutch immigrants in Kingston, Ontario, and raised in Sarnia, Ontario, in a strict Calvinist community. She did not see a film until she was a teenager.

She has identified herself as lesbian, although she has resisted being narrowly categorized as a lesbian filmmaker.

Rozema studied philosophy at Calvin College in Grand Rapids, Michigan. Upon her graduation in 1981, she intended to pursue journalism as a career. While working as a producer at CBC-TV in Toronto, however, she decided to leave journalism; and, after taking a course in film production, she made a short film in 16 mm,

Passion: A Letter (1985), and worked as an assistant director on several other film projects.

Made on a modest budget of $350,000, her first feature film, *I've Heard the Mermaids Singing* (1987), was warmly received at the Cannes Film Festival and went on to gross $6 million. The film focuses on the daydreaming assistant to a lesbian curator who yearns to be sophisticated and cosmopolitan.

As a result of this work, Rozema became the first female Canadian filmmaker to win significant international acclaim. *I've Heard the Mermaids Singing* also presented themes that Rozema, a magical realist, has continued to explore in many of her subsequent film projects: sublimated and realized desire, voyeurism, transcendence through love, the role of religion, and the desire to break free from restrictive situations.

Although her second film, *The White Room* (1990), received sharply negative criticism for being too bleakly melancholic, her third film, *When Night is Falling* (1995), demonstrated her growing maturity as a filmmaker.

Although earlier films such as *Personal Best* (1982), *Lianna* (1983), and *Desert Hearts* (1986) set precedents for lesbian romances, *When Night is Falling* is the first to present a lesbian romance in a rich and voluptuous production.

The film tells the story of a professor of mythology at a small Calvinist college who falls in love with a female circus performer while struggling with the inflexibility of her religion and her increasingly strained relationship with her fiancé.

Rozema's characteristically sensual cinematography reappeared in her brief film "Bach Cello Suite #6: Six Gestures" (1997), one of six works commissioned by Yo Yo Ma to interpret his performances of J. S. Bach's cello suites (*Yo Yo Ma: Inspired by Bach*).

Rozema layered sequences of Jayne Torville and Christopher Dean ice dancing with monologues by Tom McCamus as J. S. Bach. Using an approach from one of her earlier short films, "Desperanto" (1991), she included overlaid written text in the film, which resulted in a visually deft mix of music, spoken word, written word, and fluid movement.

Rozema's most mainstream film, *Mansfield Park* (1999), is an interpretation of Jane Austen's novel. It portrays the main character, Fanny Price, as a strong-willed, intelligent young woman struggling to find her place in the world. The film has been lauded for its portrayal of gender and class issues, but criticized for focusing on the autobiographical aspects of Austen's novel and for re-creating the main character with a feminist sensibility.

Rozema's misreading of Austen is deliberate and consistent with her desire to portray strong, self-realized female characters, regardless of whether they are heterosexual or lesbian.

Rozema's film *The Five Senses* (2000), explores the difficulties and problems of connection, as it examines the ways in which five individuals, whose lives run parallel and eventually intersect, cope with the loss of one of their senses.

Rozema has recently completed a filmed version of Samuel Beckett's play *Happy Days* for "The Beckett Film Project." (Other directors involved in the project include David Mamet, Neil Jordan, Anthony Minghella, and Atom Egoyan.) Presented at the Venice Film Festival and the Toronto International Film Festival in 2001, it was released on video and DVD in 2002.

Rozema has also recently written and directed a short film in honor of the twenty-fifth anniversary of the Toronto International Film Festival, *This Might Be Good*.

—Kelly A. Wacker

BIBLIOGRAPHY

Alemany-Galway, Mary. "Postmodernism in Canadian Film: 'I've Heard the Mermaids Singing.'" *Post Script: Essays in Film and the Humanities* 18:2 (Winter–Spring 1999): 25–36.

Crimmings, Emma. "Mansfield Park." *Cinema Papers* 132 (May 2000): 45.

Fleming, Bruce. "Exercises in Creative Misreading." *DanceView* 17:1 (Winter 2000): 45–47.

Guthmann, Edward. "A Fabulist Tale of Desire: Sexual Awakenings in 'Night is Falling.'" *San Francisco Chronicle*, November 24, 1995.

Johnson, Brian. "A High-wire Passion Play." *Macleans*, May 8, 1995, 95.

_____. "Sex and the Sacred Girl: Patricia Rozema Confronts Her Calvinist Roots in a Hot New Film about Lesbian Romance." *Macleans*, May 8, 1995): 93.

Johnson, Claudia L. "Run Mad, But Do Not Faint: The Authentic Audacity of Rozema's Mansfield Park." *Times Literary Supplement*, December 31, 1999, 16.

Lucia, Cynthia. "Communiqués: The Personal Becomes Political at the Montreal Festival." *Cineaste* 25:1 (December 1999): 36–38.

SEE ALSO

Film; Film Directors; Screenwriters

Rudnick, Paul   (b. 1957)

AMERICAN PLAYWRIGHT, NOVELIST, AND SCREENWRITER Paul Rudnick is a humorist who writes regularly for a variety of media, often on gay subjects. His subversive wit characteristically punctures pretensions and lays bare hypocrisies, yet it is also typically forgiving and healing.

Born in 1957 in the New York City suburb of Piscataway, New Jersey, to a father who was a physicist and a mother who worked as an arts publicist, Rudnick recalls his childhood as uneventful.

He had the advantage of frequent theater trips, which cemented his early goal to be a playwright, and a very funny family, which provided him with a great deal of source material and a comic outlook on life.

Rudnick knew he was gay by the time he went to Yale University, where he received a B.A. in theater. He considered further study in Yale's graduate program in drama, but soon decided he needed to move to New York to begin a career in writing.

In New York, he initially supported himself with a variety of odd jobs—copywriter, stage set painter, and the like—until his first play, *Poor Little Lambs*, a comedy recounting the antics of the all-male Yale singing group the Whiffenpoofs, was produced in 1982.

The play, which starred the young Kevin Bacon, received a mixed critical reception. Rudnick then turned to novel writing. He wrote two ruthlessly funny satires: *Social Disease*, concerning New York nightlife (1986) and *I'll Take It*, concerning the American obsession with shopping (1989). These novels received favorable reviews and marked Rudnick as a young writer with a gift for social comedy.

In 1991, Rudnick returned to the theater with *I Hate Hamlet*, a play about a struggling actor and his haunted apartment. The New York production was noted mostly for the tantrums thrown by actor Nicol Williamson as the ghost of John Barrymore. Although the original production closed after fewer than 100 performances, it has since enjoyed several successful revivals in regional theaters.

Rudnick came into his own with *Jeffrey* (1993), an ultimately life-affirming comedy about a gay man in New York City negotiating his need for love and commitment in the age of AIDS.

A nearly universally lauded play, *Jeffrey* has been produced throughout the United States and abroad. The original off-Broadway production won an Obie Award, an Outer Critics Circle Award, and the John Gassner Award for Outstanding New American Play.

In 1996, Rudnick premiered *The Naked Eye*, a comedy of manners that takes place at an exhibit of the homoerotic, sexually explicit work of a contemporary photographer: a funny character reminiscent of Robert Mapplethorpe.

In 1998, Rudnick produced *The Most Fabulous Story Ever Told*, a retelling of the Book of Genesis with same-sex couples, Adam and Steve and Jane and Mabel. Rebutting the fundamentalist Christian mantra "God didn't make Adam and Steve," the play has had several productions by regional theaters.

Rudnick has also written and doctored screenplays. He wrote the original version of the film *Sister Act* (1992), which he intended as a raucous Bette Midler vehicle. When the movie studio recast it as a Whoopi Goldberg showcase and tamed down his script, he insisted on using a pseudonym in the credits of the final version of the movie.

Rudnick also wrote or contributed to the screenplays for *The Addams Family* (1991, uncredited) and *Addams Family Values* (1993), both based on the macabre *New Yorker* cartoons by Charles Addams; as well as *The First Wives Club* (1996, uncredited).

Rudnick successfully adapted *Jeffrey* for the 1995 screen version directed by Christopher Ashley, starring Steven Weber, Sigourney Weaver, Patrick Stewart, and Nathan Lane. The gay romantic comedy became a great hit in the gay and lesbian community, but it failed to attract a large mainstream audience.

Not so Rudnick's most famous film, *In and Out* (1997), about the accidental outing of a small-town schoolteacher by a former student on national television. Loosely inspired by Tom Hanks's acceptance speech at the 1994 Academy Awards, in which he thanked a gay former teacher, the film has been lauded by critics and audiences alike.

Directed by Frank Oz, produced by Scott Rudin, and starring Kevin Kline and Tom Selleck, *In and Out* is particularly interesting for its approach to homosexuality (often a serious "problem" in films) via the conventions of screwball comedy. Although the homophobes are properly skewered, the film is suffused with good humor and good feeling. Indeed, the film is less a satire than a comic vision of a more relaxed and accepting middle America in which gay people are free to be themselves. This film is undoubtedly Rudnick's most popular work to date.

Rudnick also wrote the screenplay for *Isn't She Great* (2000), based on the life and career of novelist Jacqueline Susann and her need for celebrity. Despite its camp appeal, the film did not succeed at the box office.

He also contributed the screenplay to Richard Benjamin's disappointing *Marci X* (2003). More successful was the screenplay for Frank Oz's star-studded comic remake of the 1975 classic *The Stepford Wives* (2004).

As a journalist, Rudnick writes regularly for the movie magazine *Premiere* under the pseudonym Libby Gelman-Waxner, a fictional wealthy Long Island retail-store executive who mixes celebrity and family gossip with movie criticism and campy insights.

Rudnick also appears regularly on the gay TV newsmagazine *In the Life*. In his first appearance, soon after the September 11, 2001, World Trade Center attack, he hilariously deconstructed the homophobic remarks of Jerry Falwell and Pat Robertson, who attempted to blame gay men and lesbians for the outrage.

Rudnick writes for such diverse publications as *Vogue*, *The New York Times Book Review*, and *Interview*. He appears onscreen in Rob Epstein and Jeffrey Friedman's documentary *The Celluloid Closet* (1995), in which he discusses the disguised presence of homosexuality in the sex comedies of the 1950s.

Proudly open about his homosexuality, Rudnick is one of the most engaging comic writers at work today. He uses sharp wit and gentle satire to comment on contemporary mores. Unlike many satirists, his work is generally more positive than negative.

He lives and writes in his beloved New York City.

—*Robert Kellerman*

BIBLIOGRAPHY

"Paul Rudnick." *Contemporary Authors Online*. Reproduced in *Biography Resource Center*. Farmington Hills, Mich.: The Gale Group, 2002. http://galenet.galegroup.com/servlet/BioRC.

"Paul Rudnick." *Newsmakers 1994*, Issue 4. Reproduced in *Biography Resource Center*. Farmington Hills, Mich.: The Gale Group, 2002. http://galenet.galegroup.com/servlet/BioRC.

www.amrep.org/people/rudnick.html (American Repertory Theater).

SEE ALSO

Screenwriters; Lane, Nathan

RuPaul (RuPaul Andre Charles) (b. 1960)

A SIX-FOOT-FIVE-INCH-TALL AFRICAN AMERICAN DRAG queen who usually performs in a blonde wig, RuPaul has been responsible for giving drag a new visibility in American popular culture. He is one of the most famous drag queens in mainstream media history. RuPaul is credited with the statement "We're born naked, and the rest is drag."

RuPaul conveys a gentleness and an almost whole-some warmth that have made drag far less threatening to mainstream audiences. As a result, he has had not only a successful recording career as a disco diva, but also a wide variety of film roles, both in and out of drag, and has hosted a popular VH1 talk show.

In perhaps his most appropriate gender-bending career, he has been the "Face of M.A.C. Cosmetics": spokes-model for the Canadian cosmetics company and chair-person of the M.A.C. AIDS charity fund.

The concept of drag is all about manipulating surface images, and RuPaul's life has given him an intimate under-standing of the ways in which the surface can be deceptive.

Born into a working-class family in San Diego on November 17, 1960, RuPaul Andre Charles had an early fascination with things feminine. By the age of four, he was already an effeminate boy, imitating Diana Ross and Jane Fonda and beginning to be labeled a sissy.

His parents divorced when he was seven, and RuPaul was raised from then on in a household of strong women, consisting of his adored twin sisters, seven years older than he, and his mother, whom he describes in his autobi-ography as "the fiercest drag queen I've ever known."

By the time he was fifteen, RuPaul was ready to come out as a gay man, and he chafed under his mother's iron rule. He moved into his sister's house, and then moved with her to Atlanta.

There, free from parental constraints, he threw him-self into the gay life, performing in drag clubs and, briefly, with his own band, RuPaul and the U-Hauls.

In 1987, he relocated to New York and began the move into the big time. He landed roles in such films as Spike Lee's *Crooklyn* (1993), Betty Thomas's *The Brady Bunch Movie* (1995), Barry Shils's *Wigstock: The Movie* (1995), Wayne Wang's *Blue In The Face* (1995), Beeban Kidron's *To Wong Foo, Thanks For Everything, Julie Newmar* (1996), and Jamie Babbit's *But I'm a Cheerleader* (2000). In the latter film he appears sans drag, playing the part of a male, ex-gay camp counselor.

His albums, such as *Supermodel of the World* (1993) and *Foxy Lady* (1996), have received respectable reviews; and, from 1996 until September 1998, *The RuPaul Show* aired six days a week on VH1, featuring such guests as Cher, k.d. lang, Eartha Kitt, and Dennis Rodman.

In 2000, he narrated the acclaimed documentary *The Eyes of Tammy Faye*, about the evangelist Tammy Faye Bakker. His presence in the film is a poignant irony for those who recognize the clownishly made-up right-wing Christian Bakker as an unintentional drag icon herself.

After an extended sabbatical from performing, RuPaul returned to active duty in 2004. He signed a deal to

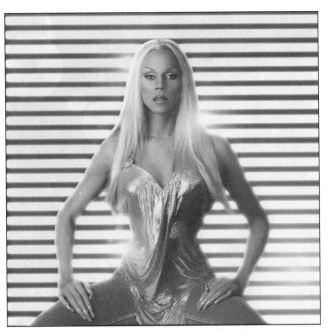

A portrait of RuPaul by Mathu Andersen.

cohost the morning show at adult-contemporary-format radio WNEW in New York and released a new album, *RuPaul: Red Hot*. A single from the album, "Looking Good, Feeling Gorgeous," enjoyed a brief stay at the top of the dance charts.

RuPaul enjoys playing with the contradictions of drag. As a black man, he is very conscious that most white people are much less threatened by him when he is dressed as a woman, even a six-foot-five woman.

However, though he cheerfully bends gender and challenges assumptions wherever possible, he is clear and irrepressible about his identity as a gay man. As he said to Maria Speidel in *People* magazine, "I never feel that I dress as a woman. I dress as a drag queen because, you know, women don't dress the way I dress. It's too uncom-fortable."

—*Tina Gianoulis*

BIBLIOGRAPHY

Charles, RuPaul Andre. *Lettin' It All Hang Out*. New York: Hyperion, 1995.

Feinberg, Leslie. *Transgender Warriors: Making History from Joan of Arc to Ru Paul*. Boston, Beacon Press, 1997.

Motsch, Sallie. "Dude Looks Like a Lady." *GQ*, June 1997, 198.

Speidel, Maria. "Happy Camper." *People*, September 23, 1996, 148.

Trebay, Guy. "Cross-dresser Dreams: Female Impersonator RuPaul Andre Charles." *New Yorker*, March 22, 1993, 49.

Yarbrough Jeff. "RuPaul: The Man Behind the Mask." *Advocate*, August 23, 1994, 64.

SEE ALSO

American Television: Talk Shows; Epperson, John

S

Sargent, Dick (1930–1994)

Actor Dick Sargent is most widely remembered as "the second Darrin" on the TV situation comedy *Bewitched*. He remained closeted for most of his career, but came out in 1991 and embraced gay activism as a "new mission in life."

Sargent was born Richard Cox in Carmel, California, on April 19, 1930. His mother, Ruth McNaughton Cox, had been an actress in silent films. His father, Colonel Elmer Cox, had served with distinction in World War I.

Sargent's relationship with his father was difficult. "I wanted him to love me, and I'm quite sure that he didn't," he commented in 1991.

Cox died of a stroke when Sargent was eleven, and afterward the boy was sent off to military school. He was so unhappy that he went on a crash diet to get himself expelled for poor health.

Once back home, he graduated from high school and entered Stanford University, where he studied acting and appeared in a number of student productions. During those years, he came to realize that he was gay, which filled him with anxiety and led him to "a couple of good college tries at suicide."

Sargent left Stanford to pursue a career as an actor. He did odd jobs to sustain himself while working onstage and eventually finding minor screen parts.

After appearances in several forgettable films, Sargent won roles—albeit still small ones—in more successful productions, including *The Great Impostor* (directed by Richard Mulligan, 1960) and *That Touch of Mink* (directed by Delbert Mann, 1962).

Sargent also did television work, including a recurring role on the situation comedy *One Happy Family* in 1961.

Sargent auditioned successfully for a lead role in the situation comedy *Bewitched* but was unable to accept it because of contractual obligations to Universal Studios. He eventually did take the part in 1969 when actor Dick York, who originally played the role, had to withdraw for health reasons.

Sargent took over the part of Darrin Stephens, an ordinary middle-class man who is married to a beautiful witch and has to put up with the shenanigans of her decidedly eccentric supernatural relatives. He joined a cast that included lesbian actress Agnes Moorehead and gay actor Paul Lynde.

Like many other actors, Sargent remained closeted, fearing that the revelation of his sexual orientation would spell ruin for his career. As other actors, including Raymond Burr, had done before him, he invented a former spouse, in Sargent's case a fictional divorced wife. In another timeworn move, he cooperated in fueling media speculation that he was romantically involved with women, escorting starlets to Hollywood parties. On one occasion, he posed with actress Connie Francis for pictures that appeared in a movie fan magazine. "We looked passionately at each other, but that was the only time I ever saw her," Sargent recalled in 1991.

Unbeknownst to audiences, Sargent was in a loving and stable relationship with another man, a television screenwriter whom he later identified publicly simply as Frank. It pained Sargent not to be able to speak openly about their bond and to have to call the love of his life a "business associate." The pair were together for twenty years until Frank died of a cerebral hemorrhage in 1979.

Among those who knew of the relationship was Elizabeth Montgomery, the star of *Bewitched*, who became a good friend to Sargent. She and her husband often socialized with Sargent and Frank.

After *Bewitched* ended its run in 1972, Sargent continued to work in television, appearing in a number of shows including *The Streets of San Francisco*, *Taxi*, *L.A. Law*, and *Murder, She Wrote*. He also played in both cinematic and television movies.

Sargent chose October 11, 1991, National Coming Out Day, to announce that he was gay. He stated that factors motivating his decision to come out included California governor Pete Wilson's veto of a bill to protect gay men and lesbians from job discrimination and also his concern about the rate of suicide among young gay people. But he was responding as well to his outing by a tabloid newspaper, the *Star*, which erroneously reported that he and a new lover had trashed a house and that the police had evicted them.

Sargent found coming out liberating. "It was such a relief. I lived in fear of being found out. Now it's given me a whole new mission in life," he commented.

Sargent—with his friend Montgomery at his side—served as Grand Marshal of the 1992 Orange County, California, Gay Pride parade. He also participated in the Lesbian and Gay Public Awareness Project and began speaking out on gay rights issues.

Sargent was gratified by the positive reaction he received from friends after coming out. He was especially pleased by the support of Eunice Kennedy Shriver, the founder of the Special Olympics, who assured him that she welcomed his continued participation in the organization, for which he had done work for two decades.

Sargent acted in a handful of movies—none of them particularly memorable—in the 1990s, but working became increasingly difficult because of his health. Diagnosed with prostate cancer in 1989, Sargent underwent extensive radiation treatment but finally succumbed to the disease on July 8, 1994.

—Linda Rapp

BIBLIOGRAPHY

"Bewitched TV Hubby Proudly Gay." *Toronto Star,* July 9, 1994.

"Dick Sargent, 64, Played Husband in TV's 'Bewitched.'" Obituary. *Cleveland Plain Dealer,* July 9, 1994.

Keehnen, Owen. "No More 'Straight Man'; Dick Sargent Is Out and Proud." www.harpiesbizarre.com/sargent_interview.htm

Podolsky, J. D., and John Griffiths. "It Was Like a Healing." *People,* December 2, 1991, 141.

SEE ALSO

American Television: Situation Comedies; Film Actors: Gay Male; Burr, Raymond; Lynde, Paul; Moorehead, Agnes

Schlesinger, John   *(1926–2003)*

A DIRECTOR OF NUMEROUS FILMS, STAGE PRODUCTIONS, television programs, and operas, John Schlesinger was one of the most influential figures in the post–World War II British entertainment industry. Always a daring innovator, Schlesinger was a significant force in introducing homosexual themes into mainstream British and American films.

Born on February 16, 1926, in London, Schlesinger attended Balliol College, Oxford, where he first became involved with acting and filmmaking. He directed a short film, *Black Legend* (1948), while a student.

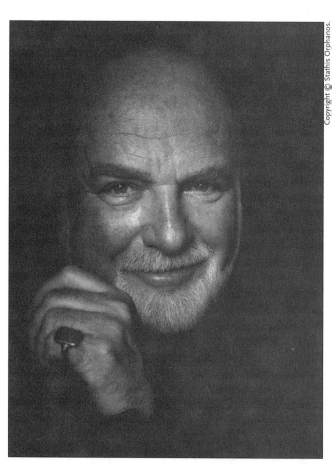

A portrait of John Schlesinger by Stathis Orphanos.

During the late 1940s and early 1950s, Schlesinger acted a number of small roles in films. His first significant success, however, came in television; between 1956 and 1961, he directed documentary films for the British Broadcasting Corporation.

His work for the BBC led to his first feature film, *Terminus* (1961), a documentary set in a London train station. Subsequently, he was selected by the producer Joseph Janni to direct a series of films that focused on the restlessness of young people coming of age at the beginning of the "swinging sixties."

Notable for their empathetic treatment of their youthful protagonists, these films featured such rising stars as Alan Bates, Tom Courtenay, and Julie Christie, and include *A Kind of Loving* (1962), *Billy Liar* (1963), and *Darling* (1965).

The latter film, although ostensibly concerned with the heterosexual adventures of its antiheroine Diana Scott, a model who sleeps her way to wealth and fame but fails to find love or happiness, is informed by gay sensibilities, not only through the introduction of a sympathetic minor character who is unambiguously homosexual, but also in its casting of the two male leads, Dirk Bogarde and Laurence Harvey.

Darling, which garnered a Best Actress Academy Award for Christie and a nomination for its director, established Schlesinger's international reputation. His newfound prestige allowed him to explore controversial themes, including homosexuality, more directly in his films.

Schlesinger's first American film, *Midnight Cowboy* (1969), which won the Academy Award for Best Picture despite an *X* rating, focuses on a relationship between two men, a male hustler (Jon Voigt) and an ailing con artist (Dustin Hoffman). It also features a disturbing scene in which the hustler beats up a client.

Released in 1971, only four years after homosexual acts between male adults in private were decriminalized in Britain, *Sunday Bloody Sunday* explores a romantic triangle with a different twist: an older gay man (Peter Finch) and a divorcee (Glenda Jackson) become rivals for the sexual attention of a younger man (Murray Head).

Schlesinger later directed numerous feature films, including *The Day of the Locust* (1975), *Marathon Man* (1976), *Yanks* (1979), *Honky Tonk Freeway* (1980), *The Falcon and the Snowman* (1985), *Madame Sousatzka* (1988), and *Pacific Heights* (1990).

A recent film, *The Next Best Thing* (1999), takes a wry look at a one-night stand (and an ensuing pregnancy) between a gay man (Rupert Everett) and a straight woman (Madonna).

Even as he continued his prodigious output as a director, Schlesinger also served, from 1973, as an associate director of the National Theatre, London, and was responsible for a number of opera productions at the Royal Opera House, Covent Garden, where his spectacular rendering of Jacques Offenbach's *The Tales of Hoffman*, first staged and televised in 1980, was revived once again in 2000.

Schlesinger never made a secret of his homosexuality, and he lived quite openly with his partner, Michael Childers, from the late 1960s until the end of his life in 2003.

He became publicly out, however, when, in 1991, Sir Ian McKellen, the first openly gay individual to be knighted by the British monarchy, was attacked in a public letter from filmmaker Derek Jarman for accepting the honor. Schlesinger was one of the dozen British gay and lesbian artists who signed a respectful response in McKellen's defense.

Schlesinger died on July 25, 2003, in Palm Springs, California, following a prolonged illness.

—*Patricia Juliana Smith*

BIBLIOGRAPHY

Brooker, Nancy. *John Schlesinger: A Guide to References and Resources.* Boston: G. K. Hall, 1978.

Philips, Gene. *John Schlesinger.* Boston: Twayne, 1981.

SEE ALSO

Film; Film Directors; European Film; British Television; Bisexuality in Film; New Queer Cinema; Anderson, Lindsay; Bogarde, Sir Dirk; Everett, Rupert; McKellen, Sir Ian

Screenwriters

A SCREENWRITER IS THE PERSON (OR GROUP OF PERSONS) who writes the script upon which a film is based. A script can be an original creation or an adaptation of previously published material.

However, it is important to note that most films involve a complex weave of talents, properties, and personalities. Moreover, film is usually considered a director's rather than a writer's medium; consequently, it is often the director's rather than the writer's vision that shapes a film. Therefore, the extent of a screenwriter's contribution to any given film can sometimes be difficult to ascertain. Nevertheless, gay and lesbian screenwriters have played significant roles in both mainstream and independent film.

The Hollywood Studio Era

During the Hollywood-studio era, roughly from the 1920s through the 1960s, homosexuality was rarely portrayed on the screen. When it did appear, it was typically depicted as something to laugh at or to scorn. As a result, gay and lesbian screenwriters learned to express their personal sensibilities discreetly, between the lines of a film script.

Perhaps the most significant and prominent lesbian filmmaker to function in the studio era was Dorothy Arzner. Although working within the constraints on form and content imposed by the studio system, Arzner nevertheless brought a distinctive, personal point of view to her films about strong-willed, independent women, within the context of such controversial subjects as extramarital sex, prostitution, and crossclass relationships.

Arzner began her film career as a stenographer in the script department of Famous Players–Lasky Corporation (later to become Paramount Studios) in 1919. She later advanced to writing scenarios for an assortment of silent features, including the Westerns *The No-Gun Man* (1924) and *The Breed of the Border* (1924); the drama *The Red Kimona* (1925), from a story on prostitution by Adela Rogers St. Johns; *When Husbands Flirt* (1925), a comedy; and the pirate adventure *Old Ironsides* (1926). In 1927, Arzner stopped writing scripts and turned her talents to directing; she completed nearly twenty films, spanning both the silent and sound eras, before retiring in 1943.

Notable gay male screenwriters of the studio era include Stewart Stern, Gavin Lambert, and Arthur Laurents.

A former stage actor, Stewart Stern turned to scriptwriting in the late 1940s, beginning with such television anthology shows as *Philco Television Playhouse* and *Playhouse 90*. He earned his first screenplay credit with the drama *Teresa* (1951), about a young war veteran struggling to adjust to civilian life. Stern went on to write scripts for such varied films as *The Rack* (1956), *The Outsider* (1962), *Rachel, Rachel* (1968), *Summer Wishes, Winter Dreams* (1973), and the television movie *Sybil* (1976), an award-winning story of a young woman with multiple personalities.

Stern's principal contribution to gay cinema is his screenplay for the classic alienated-teen drama *Rebel Without a Cause* (1955). The film features a gay-implied character, Plato, who is befriended by fellow high school students Jim and Judy. Although Plato's sexuality is never made explicit in the film, the character's yearnings were clear enough in the script for the Motion Picture Association of America (MPAA)—the governing board that determined what was and was not acceptable in films at the time—to send a memo to the filmmakers stating, "It is of course vital that there be no inference of a questionable or homosexual relationship between Plato and Jim."

Nonetheless, Plato's affectionate glances at Jim, and small details in the film, such as a photograph of the actor Alan Ladd taped to the inside of Plato's school locker, help to imply the character's feelings.

British-born writer Gavin Lambert began his screenwriting career with *Another Sky* (1954), which he also directed; the film concerns the sexual awakening of a prim Englishwoman in North Africa. Subsequent Lambert scripts include *Bitter Victory* (1958), *Sons and Lovers* (1960), based on the novel by D. H. Lawrence, and *The Roman Spring of Mrs. Stone* (1961), an adaptation of the Tennessee Williams novella, about an aging actress who becomes involved with a young Italian gigolo. Some critics have detected a homosexual subtext in the latter film, based primarily on a scene where the actress overhears herself being referred to as a "chicken hawk"—gay slang for an adult homosexual who is attracted to adolescents.

In 1965, Lambert adapted his novel *Inside Daisy Clover* for the screen. Set in the Hollywood studio system of the 1930s, the film tells the cautionary tale of a teenage movie star and her unhappy marriage to a closeted homosexual leading man. Lambert also wrote the scripts for made-for-television movies on transsexual tennis pro

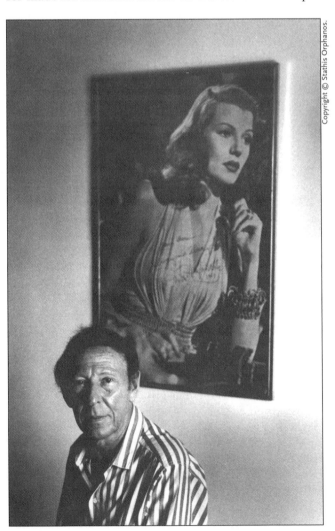

A portrait of screenwriter Gavin Lambert by Stathis Orphanos.

Renee Richards (*Second Serve*, 1986) and the gay, though closeted, performer Liberace (*Liberace: Behind the Music*, 1988).

Playwright, novelist, screenwriter, librettist, and stage director Arthur Laurents honed his writing skills on scripts for a variety of New York radio series in the late 1930s and early 1940s. In 1945, he wrote his first play, *Home of the Brave*, a wartime drama about a Jewish soldier confronting prejudice in the army. (When the play was adapted for the screen in 1949, with a screenplay by Carl Foreman, the Jewish character was changed to an African American.)

Laurents later went to work in Hollywood and wrote the scripts for such films as *The Snake Pit* (1948), *Caught* (1949), *Anastasia* (1956), and *Bonjour Tristesse* (1958), based on the best-selling novel by Françoise Sagan. Laurents again enjoyed popular success in the 1970s with the screenplays for *The Way We Were* (1973), a romance set mainly during Hollywood's anti-Communist blacklisting period, and *The Turning Point* (1977), an insider's view of the world of ballet.

In terms of gay cultural history, perhaps the most significant Laurents script is *Rope* (1948), an Alfred Hitchcock–directed film about two affluent young gay men who strangle an acquaintance merely as an intellectual challenge to commit the perfect murder. As a further display of arrogance and audacity, the two men hide the body in their apartment and proceed to host a small party, entertaining their guests around the concealed corpse.

The script was based on a play by Patrick Hamilton, which in turn was inspired by the notorious Leopold and Loeb murder case of 1924. Nathan Leopold Jr. and Richard Loeb were wealthy Chicago teenagers embroiled in a secret affair. The teens intellectualized their sexuality into a philosophical superiority and began to commit a series of crimes, escalating in seriousness to the eventual murder of fourteen-year-old Bobby Franks. Their defense attorneys successfully used the young men's homosexuality as a sign of their insanity; Leopold and Loeb escaped a death sentence and were instead sent to prison.

Laurents's screenplay, written in the late 1940s, was hampered by an inability to speak frankly about the conceptions of homosexuality that informed both the behavior of the two young men and the public's reaction to their crime. (The same is true for the 1959 film *Compulsion*, with a script by Richard Murphy, which explored similar territory.)

However, by the 1990s, with the release of *Swoon* (1992), the particulars of the Leopold and Loeb case finally could be explored unambiguously on film. *Swoon*, written by Hilton Als and Tom Kalin, outlines the facts of the murder case while also offering meditations on the philosophical, social, and aesthetic perceptions of homosexuality.

Capote, Vidal, and Williams

Truman Capote, Gore Vidal, and Tennessee Williams, three of the most prolific and honored gay male writers of the twentieth century, each made brief forays into screenwriting.

The novelist and short-story writer Truman Capote gained notoriety at the age of twenty-four with the publication of his first novel, *Other Voices, Other Rooms* (1948). Capote's reputation was enhanced by the novella *Breakfast at Tiffany's* (1958); he did not, however, write the script for the popular 1961 film version. The "nonfiction novel" *In Cold Blood* (1966), based on a six-year study of the brutal murder of a rural Kansas family by two young drifters, is considered by many critics to be Capote's best work.

Capote's ventures in screenwriting began with contributions to the film *Stazione Termini* (*Indiscretion of an American Wife*, 1953), directed by the renowned Italian neorealist Vittorio De Sica. Although a series of writers, including Alberto Moravia and Paul Gallico, also worked on the script, Capote received sole credit for the final screenplay. The story concerns the dissolution of a love affair between a married American woman and an Italian American professor who spend their last hours together in Rome's Termini Station.

Capote next worked on the script for the comic thriller *Beat the Devil* (1953), about a ragtag gang of criminals killing time in a small Italian seaport. The filmmakers have admitted to making up most of the script on the spot; director John Huston reportedly tore up the original screenplay on the first day of filming and flew Capote to Italy to work with him on writing new scenes each day.

Although a critical and commercial failure upon its first release, *Beat the Devil* has since become a cult classic and is often referred to as the first "camp" movie. The film is especially renowned for Capote's offbeat, eccentric dialogue.

Capote's final screenplay was the psychological horror film *The Innocents* (1961), based on the 1898 Henry James novella *The Turn of the Screw*. The subtle and cerebral screenplay, which Capote cowrote with William Archibald, is remarkably true to the mood and atmosphere of the James novella about a young governess who is either being haunted by malevolent spirits or slowly losing her grasp on reality.

Gore Vidal, the American novelist, playwright, and essayist, made his writing debut at the age of nineteen with the novel *Williwaw* (1946), based on his wartime experiences as an officer in the Army Transportation Corps. Key novels by Vidal in the history of gay culture include *The City and the Pillar* (1948), one of the first explicitly gay novels to be published in the United States, and *Myra Breckinridge* (1968), a sexually frank satire on gender identity with a male-to-female transsexual as its main character.

Vidal crafted dozens of one-hour original plays and adaptations for television anthology shows in the early 1950s. His most celebrated original teleplay is *Visit to a Small Planet*, which was first aired in 1955 and expanded and produced on Broadway two years later.

Vidal next worked as a contract writer for MGM and earned his first screenwriting credit for *The Catered Affair* (1956), based on a play by Paddy Chayefsky. Other Vidal screenplays from this period include *I Accuse!* (1958), a study of the Dreyfus case, in which a Jewish captain in the French army was falsely accused of treason, and *The Best Man* (1964), an adaptation of Vidal's own play, whose plot involves a presidential candidate's gay indiscretion. Vidal also worked, uncredited, on the script for *Ben-Hur* (1959), into which he infused a homosexual subtext.

Vidal's most noted contribution to gay cinema, however, is the script of *Suddenly, Last Summer* (1959). The film, based on a one-act play by Tennessee Williams (who also contributed to the screenplay), is a somewhat absurd and overheated melodrama of homosexuality, mental illness, and cannibalism. Although the MPAA initially objected to the film's content, the film's producer defended it by stating, "The story admittedly deals with a homosexual, but one who pays for his sin with his life." Perhaps due in part to its controversial subject matter, the film was a surprise commercial success.

Tennessee Williams, one of the world's foremost playwrights, created such renowned works as *The Glass Menagerie* (1945), *A Streetcar Named Desire* (1947), *The Rose Tattoo* (1951), *Camino Real* (1953), *Cat on a Hot Tin Roof* (1955), and *The Night of the Iguana* (1961), among others.

While nearly all of Williams's major plays have been brought to the screen, most were made with little or no input from Williams himself.

In the late 1940s, Williams contributed several one-hour plays for the television shows *Kraft Television Theatre* and *Actor's Studio*. He received his first screenwriting credit, which he shared with Peter Berneis, for the film version of his play *The Glass Menagerie* (1950). The screenplay is generally faithful to the original material, though slightly compromised by a more upbeat and hopeful ending.

Although *A Streetcar Named Desire* was a tremendous critical and commercial success on Broadway, Hollywood was initially reluctant to film Williams's play. Industry censors were concerned about the play's bold sexual subjects, especially Blanche's rape by her brother-in-law Stanley, her promiscuity, and her recollection of her husband's suicide after she finds him with another man. Among other edicts, the MPAA insisted that changes be made to the script that would "affirmatively establish that the husband's problem was something other than homosexuality."

Williams reluctantly labored to produce an acceptable screenplay, though he stated in a letter to the MPAA, "We will use every legitimate means that any of us has at his or her disposal to protect things in the film which we think cannot be sacrificed."

In the finished film, released in 1951, Blanche's speech about her husband's suicide was condensed significantly and the husband's homosexuality altered to an enigmatic "weakness of character," with implications of impotence. References to Blanche's promiscuity and attraction to young men were also removed.

In 1993, approximately five minutes of censored material, including references to Blanche's promiscuity and edited scenes from the rape sequence, were restored in a "director's version" rerelease. Nevertheless, even with these restorations, there is little homosexual content in the film version of *A Streetcar Named Desire*.

Williams wrote only one script expressly for the screen, *Baby Doll* (1956), a heterosexual gothic tale of two male rivals and the seventeen-year-old girl for whom they compete. Religious leaders in the United States fervently opposed its release, due in large part to the film's portrayal of an unconsummated marriage; many movie theaters were forced to cancel their showings. *Time* magazine wrote that the film was "just possibly the dirtiest American-made motion picture that has ever been legally exhibited." Despite such condemnation, *Baby Doll* did moderately well at the box office, no doubt bolstered by the film's themes of sexual repression, seduction, and infantile eroticism.

In 1967, Williams wrote a screenplay based on his 1945 short story "One Arm," about a boxer who, after losing an arm in an automobile accident, turns to hustling, only to murder a client and be sentenced to death. Undoubtedly because it was too daring for its time, the screenplay was never filmed, but it, along with the original story, forms the basis for a recent play by Moisés Kaufman.

The Boys in the Band and Beyond

In 1970, a watershed moment in the history of gay cinema occurred with the release of *The Boys in the Band*. Written by Mart Crowley, and based on his 1968 groundbreaking off-Broadway play, *The Boys in the Band* was the first mainstream Hollywood movie to focus exclusively on homosexual characters and issues. The story concerns a group of gay men, representing a cross section of emblematic gay types (a queen, a clone, a hustler, etc.), who meet to celebrate a friend's birthday in a Manhattan apartment.

Upon its release, *The Boys in the Band* was celebrated as bold and compassionate, a breakthrough work on a taboo subject. By today's standards, however, the attitudes of the characters, especially their self-loathing, seem somewhat archaic and even objectionable.

Written on the eve of gay liberation—the Stonewall riots occurred nearly one year after the play opened and preceded the film's release by nine months—*The Boys in the Band* is reflective of its times. "I knew a lot of people like those people," Crowley has said of his characters. "The self-deprecating humor was born out of a low self-esteem, from a sense of what the times told you about yourself." As one of the most famous lines from the work clarifies, "Show me a happy homosexual and I'll show you a gay corpse."

A less clichéd, and certainly more celebratory, view of same-sex desire is presented in the film *A Very Natural Thing* (1974), written by Christopher Larkin (who also directed) and Joseph Coencas. The screenplay focuses on a young seminarian, David, who leaves the church after acknowledging his sexuality and embarks on his first homosexual relationship. Reported to be the first American mainstream film made by an openly gay director (William Friedkin, who directed *The Boys in the Band*, is heterosexual), *A Very Natural Thing* is an insider's view of gay life, detailing the everyday events of David and his boyfriend.

Nearly ten years passed before Hollywood embarked on another mainstream film focusing on same-sex desire. Unlike *The Boys in the Band*, with its self-hating, archetypal characters, *Making Love* (1982) presents a nonstereotypical view of gay men attempting to deal honestly with their sexuality. Barry Sandler's screenplay utilizes elements of classic melodrama to tell a modern love story of a married couple forced to confront the husband's homosexuality when he becomes emotionally attached to an openly gay writer. Sandler has explained that the script was the direct result of his decision to write from his personal identity and experience.

Anglo-Pakistani novelist and screenwriter Hanif Kureishi first came to prominence with his Academy Award–nominated screenplay for *My Beautiful Laundrette* (1985), which presents a crossclass, crossracial homosexual relationship. Directed by Stephen Frears, and featuring excellent performances by Saeed Jaffrey and Daniel Day Lewis as the lovers, the film presents the homosexual relationship matter-of-factly even as it exposes the rapacity and inequities of Thatcherite Britain.

Other screenplays by Kureishi include *Sammy and Rosie Get Laid* (1988), *London Kills Me* (1991), *My Son the Fanatic* (1997), *The Escort* (1999), and *The Mother* (2003). Gay men, lesbians, and bisexuals frequently appear in Kureishi's screenplays and novels, though they often reject the categories of sexual identity politics, just as they frequently blur categories of nationality and ethnicity.

A defining moment in the history of lesbian cinema occurred with the sympathetic portrayal of lesbian characters in Natalie Cooper's screenplay for *Desert Hearts* (1985), adapted from the 1964 novel *Desert of the Heart*, by Jane Rule. The story concerns a married woman who has gone to Reno, Nevada, for a divorce and has taken up residence at a ranch to wait out the process. While at the ranch, she meets an open and self-assured lesbian, and the two women subsequently begin a relationship.

The film ends on a positive note, and offers the possibility that two women can end up in a happy, stable relationship—as opposed to the doomed lesbian couples portrayed in such earlier films as *The Children's Hour* (1962) and *The Killing of Sister George* (1968).

Another critically lauded film with nonstereotypical lesbian characters is *Go Fish* (1994), written by Guinevere Turner with the film's director, Rose Troche. The film tells, in a casual, meandering style, the story of an extended group of friends in Chicago. Shot in black and white with a minuscule budget and a cast of nonprofessional actors (including the film's cowriter, Turner), the film's frankness and feeling of everyday authenticity are perhaps its greatest virtues. *Go Fish* marked a breakthrough for young, urban lesbian women unused to seeing something approximating their lives on the big screen.

Turner also wrote the screenplay for *American Psycho* (2000), based on the novel by Bret Easton Ellis, and she has written several scripts for the television series *The L Word* (2004), about a group of lesbian friends in Los Angeles. Troche went on to direct *Bedrooms and Hallways* (1998), which focuses on a gay male relationship, and wrote and directed *The Safety of Objects* (2001), based on the collection of short stories by A. M. Homes.

The romantic comedy *Kissing Jessica Stein* (2001), another critically and commercially successful lesbian-themed film, concerns a straight young woman, frustrated with the heterosexual dating scene, who hesitantly embarks on a relationship with another woman. Heather Juergensen and Jennifer Westfeldt's script was adapted from their 1997 play *Lipschtick,* which was based on their own dating experiences and anecdotes culled from interviews. Several gay and lesbian groups objected to the film's sexual politics (the issue is addressed briefly in the film, when a gay male friend accuses one of the women of "trying lesbianism on as if it were the latest fashion"); many critics, however, championed the film for its very lack of political correctness.

Philadelphia and Other AIDS-related Films

Although not the movie industry's first foray into AIDS-related material, *Philadelphia* (1993), written by Ron Nyswaner, is significant for being Hollywood's first big-budget attempt to examine the subject. Nyswaner's script tells the story of Andrew Beckett, an attorney with AIDS, who is fired from his firm because of his illness; Beckett hires a homophobic lawyer who is the only willing advocate for a wrongful dismissal suit.

Primarily a courtroom drama, the script was somewhat sanitized, both politically and dramatically, for a mainstream audience. "Reaching a large audience, not just gays, was a prime consideration," Nyswaner explained when the film was released. "Our consuming goal was to make a movie that would play to the largest possible audience." Hence, Beckett's personal struggle with AIDS and his relationships with his lover and family are kept at a rather superficial level.

Nyswaner also wrote the script for the television movie *A Soldier's Girl* (2003), based on the true story of U.S. Army Pfc. Barry Winchell, who was beaten to death in 1999 after his fellow soldiers learned of his involvement with a transgendered nightclub performer.

A number of independent films have also explored the issue of AIDS, including Arthur J. Bressan Jr.'s *Buddies* (1985), the first American film to dramatize the AIDS crisis; *Parting Glances* (1986), written and directed by Bill Sherwood, about a group of New York friends and their responses to AIDS; *Longtime Companion* (1990), with a script by the noted playwright Craig Lucas, which also bore witness to the toll of AIDS on a circle of friends in the 1980s; *Together Alone* (1991), written and directed by P. J. Castellaneta; Gregg Araki's *The Living End* (1992); John Greyson's AIDS musical *Zero Patience* (1993); Randall Kleiser's *It's My Party* (1996), about the planned suicide of a man suffering from AIDS; and *Love! Valour! Compassion!* (1997), written by Terrence McNally and based on his Broadway success of the same name.

The Emergence of the Writer/Director

There is a long history of film directors serving as their own screenwriters. European auteurs, such as Pasolini and Visconti, often wrote—or at least collaborated on—their own scripts. This tradition has been continued by such contemporary glbtq directors as Pedro Almodóvar, Chantal Akerman, Monika Treut, and Rosa von Praunheim, among many others.

Since the late 1980s, with the emergence of gay and lesbian independent films and the New Queer Cinema movement, there has been a proliferation of glbtq-themed movies. This has been due in part to the economic viability of independent films, the growth of an audience responsive to queer-themed works, and the presence of openly gay and lesbian writer/directors who have brought their personal visions to the screen.

John Waters is one of the first openly gay writer/directors, and is in many ways a trailblazer for alternative films. Unreservedly embracing camp, kitsch, and graphic bad taste, his films have addressed such subjects as crime, religion, racism, and sexual subversion, and are notable for their audacious, willfully demented dialogue. Divine (born Harris Glenn Milstead), a 300-pound cross-dresser,

was the undisputed star of early Waters's movies until his death in 1988.

Waters began experimenting with 8 mm and 16 mm shorts in the 1960s; early feature-length films such as *Mondo Trasho* (1969) and *Multiple Maniacs* (1970) were rarely seen outside of Waters's hometown, Baltimore, Maryland. With *Pink Flamingos* (1972), a boldly transgressive film about two families fighting for the title of "Filthiest People Alive," Waters finally achieved critical acclaim and notoriety. In the film's final scene, which firmly established the reputations of both Waters and Divine as cultural icons of outrageousness, one family matriarch (played by Divine) proves herself the "Queen of Filth" by ingesting fresh dog excrement.

While his more recent films, such as *Hairspray* (1988), *Serial Mom* (1994), and *A Dirty Shame* (2004), have had increasingly bigger budgets and have shown greater technical proficiency, Waters's personal brand of absurdity has also been toned down to reach a broader, more mainstream, audience.

Gus Van Sant, a highly prolific and influential filmmaker, has worked both within and outside the Hollywood system. While he has directed films from other writers' scripts, including *Good Will Hunting* (1997) and a remake of the Alfred Hitchcock classic *Psycho* (1998), Van Sant's critical reputation derives mainly from those films he has both written and directed.

Van Sant's first feature-length film, *Mala Noche* (1985), based on an autobiographical novella by Walt Curtis, concerns the passionate, but unrequited, love of an openly gay liquor-store clerk for a teenage illegal alien from Mexico. The visually innovative, black-and-white film won nearly unanimous praise for the frank, nonjudgmental depiction of its marginalized characters.

Drugstore Cowboy (1989), cowritten with Daniel Yost and based on a novel by James Fogle, focuses on two young couples who rob pharmacies to support their drug addiction. Notably absent from the script is any moralizing about drug use.

My Own Private Idaho (1991), an ambitious film inspired by Shakespeare's *Henry IV*, focuses on the friendship between two teenage male hustlers. As with his two previous films, Van Sant artfully explores such concepts as unrequited love, alienation, and the concept of family.

Other films both written and directed by Van Sant include *Even Cowgirls Get the Blues* (1993), one of his rare artistic failures, based on the Tom Robbins cult novel; *Gerry* (2002), a minimalist experiment about two friends who get lost while on a hike in the California desert, with a script attributed to Van Sant in collaboration with the film's two stars Casey Affleck and Matt Damon; and *Elephant* (2003), inspired by the mass shootings at Columbine High School in 1999, which utilizes a loose, spontaneous narrative structure and visual style. Although Van Sant is credited with the script, the dialogue, similar to that of *Gerry*, seems mainly to have been improvised by the film's young actors.

Todd Haynes's complex and controversial experiments with genre, narrative, and character identification have earned him outstanding critical acclaim and positioned him as one of the leading figures of the New Queer Cinema. Haynes debuted in 1985 with the short film *Assassins: A Film Concerning Rimbaud*, a stylized study of the violent love affair between the French poets Arthur Rimbaud and Paul Verlaine. *Superstar: The Karen Carpenter Story* (1987), which Haynes cowrote with Cynthia Schneider, is a forty-three-minute film examining the career of 1970s pop singer Karen Carpenter as enacted not by actors but by a cast of Ken and Barbie–type dolls.

The writings of Jean Genet were the inspiration for Haynes's first feature-length film, *Poison* (1991). The film weaves together three seemingly unconnected stories (the first about a boy's murder of his abusive father; the second concerning a scientist who turns into a monster after ingesting the human sex drive in liquid form; and the final story an unrequited love affair between two men in prison), each told in its own distinctive style and juxtaposed so that they comment on one another.

Haynes has described *Poison* as "an attempt to link homosexuality to other forms that society is threatened by—deviance that threatens the status quo of our sense of what normalcy is." Although attacked by right-wing extremists as pornography, *Poison* is considered by most critics a defining work of the New Queer Cinema.

While *Safe* (1995), about a woman seemingly allergic to her very environment, is devoid of any overt gay content, some writers have interpreted the mysterious affliction in the film as a metaphor for the AIDS virus. Told in a visually austere style, the film is also notable for its dialogue, which Haynes consciously wrote to expose the way people speak to each other without actually communicating.

In *Velvet Goldmine* (1998), Haynes explores the glam rock scene of the early 1970s—a world of flamboyant theatrics and androgynous imagery. The film posits Oscar Wilde as the original "pop idol" and the self-consciously transgressive glam rock stars as Wilde's direct descendants; much of the film's dialogue directly refers to Wilde's writings.

Without resorting to either parody or camp, *Far from Heaven* (2002) pays tribute to, as well as deconstructs, Douglas Sirk's domestic melodramas of the 1950s, such as *Magnificent Obsession* (1954) and *All That Heaven Allows* (1955). Significantly, Haynes's film tackles social issues such as homosexuality and racism that Sirk's were never allowed to explore.

Another key figure in the New Queer Cinema movement, Gregg Araki, garnered praise for *The Living End*

(1992), the story of two young, HIV-positive gay men on a crime spree. Other films written and directed by Araki include the *ménage à trois* drama *Three Bewildered People in the Night* (1987); *The Long Weekend (O'Despair)* (1989), about a group of college graduates brooding over their future; the "teen apocalypse trilogy," which includes *Totally F***ed Up* (1993), *The Doom Generation* (1995), and *Nowhere* (1997), all of which focus on bored, alienated Los Angeles teenagers; the screwball comedy *Splendor* (1999); and *Mysterious Skin* (2004), a drama based on the novel by Scott Heim.

Lesbian writer and director Jane Anderson began her career scripting such mainstream films as *It Could Happen to You* (1994) and *How to Make an American Quilt* (1995). She went on to write and direct more groundbreaking films for television, including the first segment of *If These Wall Could Talk 2* (2000), which focuses on a woman coping with the death of her female partner of fifty years; *When Billie Beat Bobby* (2001), about the historic 1973 tennis match between Bobby Riggs and the young feminist Billie Jean King; and *Normal* (2003), the story of a married man who shocks his family and small-town community by revealing that he wants a sex change operation.

Lisa Cholodenko gained critical attention with her debut film, *High Art* (1998), and followed up with the equally ambitious *Laurel Canyon* (2002); both films concern reserved young women swept into the unconventional lifestyle of a charismatic older female artist.

Bill Condon is known principally as the writer/director of the biographical films *Gods and Monsters* (1998), an adaptation of Christopher Bram's novel *Father of Frankenstein*, focusing on the final days in the life of the gay, British-born film director James Whale; and *Kinsey* (2004), a study of the pioneer of human sexuality research Alfred Kinsey. Condon also wrote the screenplay for, but did not direct, the adaptation of the Kander-and-Ebb musical *Chicago* (2002).

Del Shores, producer and writer for the cable television hit *Queer As Folk*, who has also written for such other television shows as *Touched by an Angel, Ned and Stacey, Dharma and Greg,* and *Martial Law,* is the writer, director, and producer of the gay cult comedy *Sordid Lives* (2000).

Australian-born Stephan Elliott gained prominence with the exuberant drag-queen farce *The Adventures of Priscilla, Queen of the Desert* (1994). Elliott also wrote and directed the comedies of misadventure *Frauds* (1993) and *Welcome to Woop Woop* (1997), as well as the thriller *Eye of the Beholder* (1999), and, most recently, *Venetian Wedding* (2004), cowritten with Sheriden Jobbins, about a woman left at the altar when her fiancé runs off to Paris with his best man.

Andrew Fleming's semiautobiographical film *Threesome* (1994), which he both wrote and directed, concerns the romantic entanglements of three college roommates, one of whom is gay. Fleming also cowrote the screenplay (with Steven E. de Souza) for his feature-film directorial debut, *Bad Dreams* (1988), about a young girl who survives a cult group's mass suicide. He also directed and cowrote *The Craft* (with Peter Filardi, 1996), a stylish thriller about teenage witches, and *Dick* (with Sheryl Longin, 1999), a political satire about two high school girls who inadvertently become President Richard Nixon's secret advisors during the Watergate scandal.

The openly gay writer/director Scott McGehee codirected and cowrote (with his straight partner David Siegel) the atmospheric melodrama *The Deep End* (2001), about a mother's desperate attempt to cover up the murder of her young gay son's disreputable older lover. McGehee and Siegel based their script on the Max Ophüls cult noir *The Reckless Moment* (1949) and its original source, Elisabeth Sanxay Holding's 1947 novel *The Blank Wall*. McGehee and Siegel also codirected and cowrote the crime thriller *Suture* (1993).

The Hours and Times (1991), Christopher Munch's first feature, is a fictionalized account of what may have happened when the Beatles' John Lennon and the group's gay manager, Brian Epstein, went on holiday together to Barcelona in 1963. Münch also wrote and directed *Color of a Brisk and Leaping Day* (1996), a visually impressive account of a young Chinese American's attempt to revitalize a railroad built by his ancestors; *The Sleepy Time Gal* (2001), an elegiac film about a middle-aged woman coming to terms with cancer; and *Harry and Max* (2004), focusing on the relationship between two pop-star brothers.

The screenwriter Don Roos made his writer/director debut with the celebrated comedy *The Opposite of Sex* (1988), about a manipulative sixteen-year old girl who wreaks havoc on her extended family after seducing her stepbrother's boyfriend. Roos also wrote and directed the romantic comedy *Bounce* (2000), and the multilayered *Happy Endings* (2004).

Roos began his career writing scripts for such television series as *Hart to Hart* (1979 to 1984), *Paper Dolls* (1984), and *Casebusters* (1986). He eventually left television and wrote the screenplays for *Love Field* (1992), which focused on a housewife traveling to John F. Kennedy's funeral; *Single White Female* (1992), a psychological thriller based on the novel by John Lutz; *Boys on the Side* (1995), a female road movie whose characters include a lesbian singer and a young woman with AIDS; and *Diabolique* (1996), a remake of Henri-Georges Clouzot's classic 1955 mystery thriller.

Other key glbtq-themed films by noted writer/directors include *The Incredibly True Adventure of Two Girls in Love* (1995) by Maria Maggenti, the story of two young women of different social and economic back-

grounds who fall in love; Richard Kwietniowski's *Love and Death on Long Island* (1997), adapted from the novel by Gilbert Adair, about an elderly British writer's infatuation with a young American film actor; *Billy's Hollywood Screen Kiss* (1998), by Tommy O'Haver, about a young gay photographer who becomes infatuated with an aspiring musician of uncertain sexuality; *Boys Don't Cry* (1999), directed and cowritten (with Andy Bienen) by Kimberly Peirce, about the life and brutal death of a cross-dressing young woman; Greg Berlanti's *The Broken Hearts Club: A Romantic Comedy* (2000), focusing on a group of friends in Los Angeles; *Hedwig and the Angry Inch* (2001), John Cameron Mitchell's adaptation of his off-Broadway success about a German-born male-to-female transsexual punk-rock musician; *Party Monster* (2003), by Fenton Bailey and Randy Barbato, a true-crime account of the murder of a drug dealer by a club party organizer that the filmmakers based on their 1998 documentary of the same name; and *Monster* (2003) by Patty Jenkins, a study of Aileen Wuornos, one of the first female serial killers in the United States.

Other Significant Screenwriters

Larry Kramer, Derek Jarman, Harvey Fierstein, Craig Lucas, Paul Rudnick, Kevin Williamson, and Alan Ball have also made significant contributions to screenwriting.

Writer and AIDS activist Larry Kramer crafted the screenplay for *Women in Love* (1969), based on the D. H. Lawrence novel. Although the film has an ostensibly heterosexual plot, a palpable homoeroticism is evident throughout the film, especially in the famous wrestling scene, which contains full-frontal male nudity.

British filmmaker Derek Jarman, whose work reveals a fascination with gay history and gay representation, wrote many of his most acclaimed films, including *Sebastiane* (1975), *Caravaggio* (1986), *Queer Edward II* (1991), and *Wittgenstein* (1993). A painter and set designer as well as a director and writer, Jarman ensured that his works were always visually interesting and politically provocative. He died from complications of AIDS in 1994.

Harvey Fierstein, the playwright and actor, wrote the screen adaptation of his award-winning Broadway play *Torch Song Trilogy* (1988), which concerns a New York drag queen's search for love and respectability.

Fierstein also wrote the scripts for the made-for-television movie *Tidy Endings* (1988), about a man coming to terms with the death of his lover of AIDS; *The Sissy Duckling* (1999), an animated television cartoon about an effeminate duckling taunted by his schoolmates; and the segment "Amos and Andy," about a father's eventual acceptance of his son's marriage to another man, in the anthology film *Common Ground* (2000), which also contains segments written by the lesbian playwright

Paula Vogel ("A Friend of Dorothy's") and the noted gay writer Terrence McNally ("M. Roberts").

Playwright Craig Lucas, who wrote the screenplay for *Longtime Companion* (1990), also wrote the screen adaptations of his plays *Prelude to a Kiss* (1992), a fantasy romance about a young woman who inexplicably exchanges personalities with an elderly man she kisses at her wedding reception, and *Reckless* (1995), a dark comedy about a woman on the run from her husband who has contracted to have her killed.

Lucas also wrote the script for *The Secret Lives of Dentists* (2002), an adaptation of Jane Smiley's novella *The Age of Grief*, about a dentist's mounting suspicions of his wife's infidelities, and he has completed his first film as writer/director, the screen version of his play *The Dying Gaul* (2004), an examination of the relationship among a gay male writer, a bisexual film producer, and the producer's wife.

Playwright, humorist, and screenwriter Paul Rudnick's film scripts include such comedies as *Sister Act* (1992), under the pseudonym Joseph Howard; *The Addams Family* (uncredited, 1991) and *Addams Family Values* (1993), both based on the cartoons of Charles Addams; *Jeffrey* (1995), adapted from his own off-Broadway play; *In & Out* (1997), about a high school teacher inadvertently outed by one of his former students; *Isn't She Great* (2000), on the life and career of novelist Jacqueline Susann; *Marci X* (2003), set in the world of hip-hop and rap music; and *The Stepford Wives* (2004), a broad satire on suburban conformity based on the novel by Ira Levin.

Out director Kevin Williamson has written the scripts for the popular teen horror movies *Scream* (1996) and *Scream 2* (1997), *I Know What You Did Last Summer* (1997), and *The Faculty* (1998), and he both wrote and directed the comedy-thriller *Teaching Mrs. Tingle* (1999). Williamson is also the creator of the popular television series of teenage angst *Dawson's Creek* (1998 to 2003).

Alan Ball got his start writing television situation comedies, but went on to garner praise and several prestigious awards for his screenplay for *American Beauty* (1999), a darkly comic study of suburban despair. He is also the creator of the critically acclaimed television series *Six Feet Under* (2001), which prominently features several gay and lesbian characters. —*Craig Kaczorowski*

BIBLIOGRAPHY

Barrios, Richard. *Screened Out: Playing Gay in Hollywood from Edison to Stonewall.* New York: Routledge, 2003.

Clarke, Gerald. *Capote.* New York: Ballantine, 1988.

Ehrenstein, David. *Open Secret: Gay Hollywood, 1928–1998.* New York: William Morrow and Company, 1998.

Gever, Martha, John Greyson, and Pratibha Parmar, eds. *Queer Looks: Perspectives on Lesbian and Gay Film and Video.* New York: Routledge, 1993.

Mann, William J. *Behind the Screen: How Gays and Lesbians Shaped Hollywood, 1910–1969.* New York: Viking, 2001.

Nyswaner, Ron. "Leaving Philadelphia." *Advocate,* May 27, 2003, 36.

Russo, Vito. *The Celluloid Closet: Homosexuality in the Movies.* New York: Harper & Row, 1981.

Sandler, Barry. "Making Love." *Advocate,* November 12, 2002, 88.

Stephens, Chuck. "Gentlemen Prefer Haynes." *Film Comment* 31.4 (July/August 1995): 76–81.

Vidal, Gore. *Palimpsest: A Memoir.* New York: Random House, 1995.

Waters, John. *Shock Value.* New York: Thunder's Mouth, 1981.

Wyatt, Justin. "Cinematic/Sexual Transgression: An Interview with Todd Haynes." *Film Quarterly* 46.3 (Spring 1993): 2–9.

SEE ALSO

Film; Film Directors; New Queer Cinema; Akerman, Chantal; Almodóvar, Pedro; Araki, Gregg; Arzner, Dorothy; Condon, William "Bill"; Crowley, Mart; Cumming, Alan; Dean, James; Divine (Harris Glenn Milstead); Fierstein, Harvey; Greyson, John; Haynes, Todd; Laurents, Arthur; Liberace; Lucas, Craig; Mineo, Sal; Mitchell, John Cameron; Pasolini, Pier Paolo; Praunheim, Rosa von; Rudnick, Paul; Treut, Monika; Troche, Rose; Van Sant, Gus; Vilanch, Bruce; Visconti, Luchino; Waters, John; Whale, James

Set and Costume Design

SET AND COSTUME DESIGN AND PROPERTIES FOR STAGE and film are fields that have attracted many talented people, a large percentage of whom have been gay men. In fact, this field in the entertainment industry has often been identified specifically as "queer work."

While many heterosexuals have also been successful in the area of art direction, set design and decoration for stage and film have a distinctly gay cachet. Perhaps an even "gayer" field is that of costume design.

As William J. Mann has recently documented, even during the worst periods of repression, Hollywood offered opportunities of creative expression for gay men and lesbians, many of whom were open about their sexual orientation.

Opera and ballet also offered opportunities for gifted homosexuals. The trend here has been for painters to cross over from the fine arts to the applied arts, adding stage and design to their range. For many notable stage designers working in this field, their sexual orientation was never an issue in their professional lives.

Among the most significant gay and lesbian artists who are distinguished for their work as set designers are Charles Ricketts, Duncan Grant, Erté (Romain de Tirtoff), Pavel Tchelitchew, Oliver Messel, Cecil Beaton,

Léonor Fini, George James Hopkins, Robert Colquhoun, Robert MacBryde, Franco Zeffirelli, David Hockney, Derek Jarman, and Keith Haring, many of whom specialized in stage and opera rather than film design.

Many gay artists of Hollywood's golden age were extremely versatile, but openly gay men became especially associated with costume design. In some cases, Hollywood costume designers were considered on a par with world class couturiers and fashion designers and had a palpable influence on public taste. Among these designers, Howard Greer, Travis Banton, Adrian (Adrian Adolph Greenberg), Orry Kelly, and Walter Plunkett are best known.

Set Designers

In the first decades of the twentieth century, two significant factors influenced the development of set design, making it central rather than peripheral. The first was the massive impact of Sergei Diaghilev's lavish productions for the Ballets Russes. In particular, Leon Bakst's bold designs helped audiences appreciate the way color could be used to integrate an entire production. While the influence of the Ballets Russes was primarily on stage productions, it also influenced set design in the nascent film industry as well.

The second factor that altered the development of stage and set design was the impact of Robert Wiene's German Expressionist film *The Cabinet of Dr. Caligari* (1919), which set a precedent for using sets to express mood and theme. The film employs fantastic, stylized sets to capture the subjective perceptions of the main character. This cinematic innovation raised the status of sets to an importance comparable to that of characterization and narrative. Hence, it gave set designers a new prestige as significant collaborators in film and stage productions.

Erté

One of the most innovative and enduring designers of the twentieth century, Erté, or Romain de Tirtoff (1892–1990), earned fame for his sinuous and sophisticated Art Deco fashion designs, frequently featured on the covers of *Harper's Bazaar;* but he also designed sets and costumes for opera, theater, and ballet productions.

In 1925, Erté was transported from France by Louis B. Mayer to lend even more elegance and glamour to films at the MGM studios. Erté arrived in Hollywood with his lover Nicholas Ourousoff, under the lavish sponsorship of Mayer and in a blaze of publicity. He contributed work to *Ben Hur* (1925) and *La Bohème* (1926), but his stay in Hollywood ended after only a few months. He returned to Paris to design for the Music Hall.

Erté's drawings are intricate and highly detailed, creating an extravagant, exotic world of women dripping in pearls, covered in plumes, and wearing low-cut back lines. Erté treated costume design as a fine art, and his numerous designs, though often whimsical, were also slyly erotic and technically perfect.

Christian Bérard

A member of Jean Cocteau's circle, designer Christian Bérard (1902–1947), known simply as *Bébé,* made a name for himself in the French theater.

He was particularly known for his subtle, nostalgic use of color in designs for such works as *Cotillion* (1930) for George Balanchine and Molière's *Les fourberies de Scapin* (1947).

Bérard and his lover Boris Kochno (1904–1990), who directed the Ballets Russes and was cofounder of the Ballet des Champs Elysées, were the most prominent openly gay couple in French theater during the 1930s and 1940s. Perhaps Bérard's greatest achievement was his lustrous, magical designs for Cocteau's film *Beauty and the Beast* (1946).

Oliver Messel

For almost three decades, Oliver Messel (1904–1978) was Britain's most celebrated theatrical designer. He created lavish costumes and sets for ballet and stage productions in the country's most prestigious venues.

Messel first started out under the tutelage of the homosexual English painter and portraitist Glyn Philpot. He was then taken under the wing of French designer Christian Bérard, with whom he shared a similar sense of color and unerring use of fabrics.

Messel's first commission was to design the masks for a London production of Diaghilev's ballet *Zephyr et Flore* (1925). He then achieved great acclaim with his white-on-white set for Offenbach's comic opera *Helen* (1932). He won a Tony Award for *House of Flowers* (1935) on Broadway and received acclaim for the elaborate royal box decorations for the premiere of Benjamin Britten's opera *Gloriana* (1953), presented in the presence of the new queen, Elizabeth II.

Messel also designed the Royal Ballet's 1959 production of *The Sleeping Beauty*. In this work, which borrowed subtle nuances from the paintings of Antoine Watteau, the designer's innate sense of pomp and grandeur is evident. His work in opera at Glyndebourne and the Met was also notable.

In 1935, the gay film director George Cukor invited Messel to design the sets for *Romeo and Juliet*. Although Messel did not regard these designs as entirely successful, he subsequently designed numerous other Hollywood films, including *The Thief of Baghdad* (1940) and *Suddenly, Last Summer* (1959).

Cecil Beaton

Cecil Beaton (1904–1980) was Messel's principal rival as leading British designer. Although he is best known as a society photographer, after World War II Beaton designed extravagant stage sets and costumes for Broadway and London theater as well as opera and film.

Beaton's design for Lawrence Olivier's production of *The School for Scandal* (1947) was also notable. He won a Tony Award (1957) for his costumes for the Broadway production of *My Fair Lady*, and an Academy Award (1958) for sets and costumes for the film *Gigi*.

George James Hopkins

In 1916, the young George James Hopkins (1896–1988) was hired to do costumes for Theda Bara and set designs for her films. His set designs helped elevate the status of the profession in Hollywood, raising design beyond what was previously regarded as "glorified carpentry."

Hopkins executed a striking peacock throne for Bara's infamous film *Salome* (1919). *The Soul of Youth* (1920) included scenes set in a male whorehouse. *The Furnace* (1920) included an elaborate nude scene in hell.

But Hopkins's career was stalled for a while by an unresolved scandal involving his lover William Desmond Taylor, who died in 1922. In 1935, Hopkins joined Warner Brothers studios and went on to do the set designs for *Casablanca* (1942) and *Mildred Pierce* (1945), among others. He won Academy Awards for *A Streetcar Named Desire* (1951), *My Fair Lady* (1964), and *Hello, Dolly!* (1969).

Franco Zeffirelli

The Italian designer and director Franco Zeffirelli (b. 1923) studied architecture and acting as a young man. Under the tutelage of director Luchino Visconti, for whom he did set and costume designs, he gradually made the transition from protégé to hugely successful film and opera director.

Zeffirelli was nominated for a Tony Award for his scenic designs for the *Lady of the Camellias* (1963). His film *Romeo and Juliet* (1968) is remembered for its casting of unknown young actors to give authenticity and a fresh view to the production, as well as for its lush sets. His film and opera work, usually characterized by lavish and beautiful designs, still gains international attention, though he is sometimes criticized for allowing his designs to overpower other aspects of the productions.

Derek Jarman

Derek Jarman (1942–1994) was such a versatile artist that his work straddles many media, including gardening and political activism. However, he started out as a set designer at the Slade School of Art. His first break came when he was invited by Sir Frederick Ashton to design for the ballet *Jazz Calendar* (1968).

In the same year, Sir John Gielgud asked him to design *Don Giovanni* for the English National Opera. Jarman then met the director Ken Russell and designed

the monstrous set for *The Devils* (1970). He also worked on Russell's *Savage Messiah* (1971). While Jarman did not design the films that he directed, his design sense is palpable in them.

Other Designers

Artists not noted primarily for being designers but who nevertheless did sets and costumes include the film directors James Whale (1896–1957) and Vincente Minnelli (1910–1986).

One of the most productive art directors in Hollywood, Cedric Gibbons (1893–1960), was rumored to be homosexual. He won several Academy Awards over his long career.

Costume Designers

Costume design for stage and film has generally attracted a different kind of artist, designers often without a specific fine arts background. Nevertheless, their work has frequently reached pinnacles of stylishness and had a huge impact on the public taste and imagination.

Howard Greer

Howard Greer (1886–1964) started as a costume designer on Broadway and was one of the first to be appointed head of wardrobe at a major Hollywood studio. He worked on *Greenwich Village Follies* (1922) and *Jack and Jill* (1923) before moving to Hollywood to do set designs for Paramount Pictures. There he was responsible for such movies as *Bringing Up Baby* (1938).

Travis Banton

The most sought-after Hollywood costume designer of the 1930s and 1940s was Travis Banton (1894–1948). He is best remembered for creating the style of such actresses as Carole Lombard, Lilyan Tashman, Marlene Dietrich, and Mae West. His trademarks were understated elegance and luxurious fabrics.

Banton served as head designer at Paramount Studios for many years, but also designed for Fox and Universal Studios as well. Perhaps his most successful creations were the angled hat and veiled look that helped establish the onscreen charisma and mystery of Dietrich in such films as *Dishonored* (1931), *Shanghai Express* (1932), and *The Devil Is a Woman* (1935).

Orry Kelly

Australian-born Orry Kelly (1897–1964) emigrated to the United States as a young man. He found success as a costume and scene designer on Broadway before going to Hollywood during the Great Depression. His friend Cary Grant introduced him to the head of Warner Brothers' wardrobe department, where he stayed for eleven years.

Primarily associated with Warner Brothers, he designed costumes for a broad range of films in the 1930s, 1940s, and 1950s, including Busby Berkeley extravaganzas as well as gangster films and costume dramas. Near the end of his career he was especially associated with Hollywood musicals.

He designed for stars as various as Ingrid Bergman and Marilyn Monroe, but was especially close to Bette Davis. He won Academy Awards for his designs for *An American in Paris* (shared with Walter Plunkett and Irene Sharaff, 1951), *Les Girls* (1957), *Some Like It Hot* (1959), and *Gypsy* (1962).

Walter Plunkett

Walter Plunkett (1902–1982) is best known for his costume designs for *Gone with the Wind* (1939), but his long and distinguished career included many other triumphs. He came to Hollywood to become an actor, but gained an interest in costume design when he was invited to design costumes for the dancer Ruth St. Denis.

Plunkett worked for RKO from the late 1920s to the late 1930s, earning a reputation for the authenticity of his period costumes. He later worked primarily for MGM and designed for stars such as Irene Dunne, Judy Garland, Fred Astaire, Ginger Rogers, and Katharine Hepburn.

Although he did not receive an Academy Award for his designs for *Gone with the Wind,* he received numerous nominations and shared an Oscar with Orry Kelly and Irene Sharaff for their work on *An American in Paris* (1951).

Adrian

Adrian Adolph Greenburg (1903–1959) was one of the most flamboyant and successful costume designers of Hollywood's golden age. His first films were with Rudolph Valentino; then he moved to MGM, where he had the opportunity to design for some of Hollywood's biggest female stars, including Greta Garbo, Jean Harlow, Joan Crawford, and Norma Shearer.

Among the films for which he designed costumes are *The Wizard of Oz* (1939), *The Women* (1939), and *The Philadelphia Story* (1940). His work had an enormous influence not only on other designers, but also on the fashion world in general, as fans attempted to duplicate the glamorous style he created for Hollywood divas.

Arthur Freed and Roger Edens

Primarily a lyricist, choreographer, and producer, Arthur Freed (1894–1973) nevertheless exerted a massive influence on the design of some of Hollywood's most glamorous musicals. He, along with his assistant Roger Edens (1905–1970), reshaped this genre, taking it to new heights by unifying the designs of all the artists involved.

Freed himself was not gay, but his unit at MGM was known as "Freed's Fairies" because he had gathered so many talented gay designers, costumers, and other artists, including Roger Edens, whom he trusted implicitly. Among their most notable work are such classic film musicals as *The Wizard of Oz* (1939), *Meet Me in St. Louis* (1944), *Easter Parade* (1948), *Singin' in the Rain* (1952), and *Kismet* (1955).

Irene Sharaff

One of the few costume designers to have worked both on Broadway productions and on their film adaptations, Irene Sharaff (1910–1993) first developed a reputation in New York and then joined "Freed's Fairies" at MGM in 1942, an association that did not prevent her from continuing to design for Broadway.

Among the shows that she designed both for Broadway and for film are *The King and I* (1951/1956), *West Side Story* (1957/1961), *Flower Drum Song* (1958/1961), and *Funny Girl* (1964/1968).

She was nominated for Academy Awards nine times and won Oscars for five films: *An American in Paris* (1951), *The King and I* (1956), *West Side Story* (1961), *Cleopatra* (1962), and *Who's Afraid of Virginia Woolf?* (1966).

Equally adept at period or contemporary costume, Sharaff earned distinction for her attention to detail and for the elegance of her creations.

Although several other women achieved distinction in the fields of set and costume design—Edith Head, for example, who apprenticed with Howard Greer—openly lesbian women seem not to have found the same degree of success as gay men.

—*Kieron Devlin*

Bibliography

Castle, Charles. *Oliver Messel.* New York: Thames and Hudson, 1986.

Mann, William J. *Behind the Scenes: How Lesbians and Gays Shaped Hollywood, 1910–1969.* New York: Viking, 2001.

Pierpoint, Claudia Roth. "Bébé." *Ballet Review* 18.2 (1990): 23–27.

Saslow, James M. *Pictures and Passions: A History of Homosexuality in the Visual Arts.* New York: Viking, 1999.

Snow, Peter. "Designing for the Theatre and Cinema." *Derek Jarman: A Portrait.* Roger Wollen, intro. London: Thames and Hudson, 1996. 81–88.

Spencer, Charles. *Erté.* New York: Clarkson N. Potter, 1970.

See Also

Cocteau, Jean; Cukor, George; Dietrich, Marlene; Edens, Roger; Garbo, Greta; Garland, Judy; Gielgud, Sir John; Grant, Cary; Minnelli, Vincente; Visconti, Luchino; Warhol, Andy; Whale, James; Zeffirelli, Franco

Stereotypes

A STEREOTYPE IS A FIXED IDEA ABOUT THE CHARACTER-istics or qualities of a certain group (race, class, profession) of individuals. A stereotype about a group is usually created by people outside the group who make observations about some members of the group and then generalize that all its members behave in certain ways.

While many stereotypes may be rooted in more or less accurate observations, they often include a number of inaccurate and usually negative assumptions that are used not only to categorize members of the stereotyped group but also to condemn, dismiss, or trivialize them. Thus, stereotypes contribute to racism, classism, sexism, and other forms of oppression, including homophobia.

Members of different queer communities have not only been stereotyped by mainstream straight society, but they are often also stereotyped by each other, causing damaging divisions and misunderstandings.

In day-to-day interactions, people are constantly deluged with sensory input which we must quickly organize into manageable categories. While stereotyping evolves from this simple need for classification, the rigidity of the stereotyped ideas and facts that they so broadly generalize about people makes them counterproductive for dealing with real people in the real world. In fact, most observers of society agree that once stereotypes are in place, people tend to notice only those characteristics in others that agree with their preconceived notions and become oblivious to those qualities that do not fit the stereotypes.

Stereotyped Groups as Other

Although stereotyping represents a sort of cultural shorthand, enabling people to categorize other groups quickly, it also effectively distances us from those we stereotype by defining the stereotyped group as "other." Because it is based on characterizing a group through preconceived ideas, stereotyping fosters ignorance, and because stereotyping often traffics in negative generalities, it is frequently used to justify the oppression of stereotyped groups.

Another significant characteristic of the stereotyping of oppressed groups is that a wide variety of disenfranchised (and often despised) groups are stereotyped by mainstream society in remarkably similar ways. For example, Jews in medieval society, blacks in the post–Civil War South, and gay men in the twentieth century have all been stereotyped as sexual predators.

Jews, people of color, women, and the poor have shared many other stereotypically negative characteristics with queers. Gay men, lesbians, Jews, and outspoken women are often stereotyped as "pushy" and "shrill." Jews, blacks, gays, and poor people have also been seen as dirty carriers of disease.

Fear of the "other" has often caused members of dominant groups to see minorities as mentally unstable or threatening to women or children. These stereotypes have frequently been applied to members of queer communities as well as communities of color. In fact, one of the best-publicized antigay campaigns of the late twentieth century, Anita Bryant's "Save Our Children" crusade during the early 1980s, capitalized on the stereotype of gay men as child molesters.

Contradictory Stereotypes

Different queer groups have long been stereotyped in specific, if often contradictory ways. For example, gay men are just as often stereotyped as gentle sissies as they are dangerous, oversexed predators. Lesbians might be stereotyped as both the unattractive, masculine gym teacher type and the sultry, ultrafeminine seductress of straight pornography. Bisexuals are seen as both repressed and promiscuous. Transgendered people are assumed to be tricksters who deceive straights by impersonating the opposite sex as well as tortured misfits who have themselves been betrayed by mother nature.

Gay men and lesbians are affected by stereotypes of queers as depressed loners who cannot maintain relationships, though research and life experience has often proved those stereotypes untrue. Perhaps the predominant contradictory stereotypes for all queer groups are the conflicting assumptions that, on the one hand, queers are just the same as straight people, and, on the other hand, queers are totally different from straight people. While each of these stereotypes contains a germ of truth, neither encompasses the complexity of the queer experience within mainstream straight society.

Stereotypes within Queer Communities

Within queer communities, stereotypes also flourish. Lesbians may stereotype gay men as apolitical, wealthy, and misogynist, while gay men in turn stereotype lesbians as humorless, aggressive, and undersexed. Both gay men and lesbians may mistrust bisexuals because they accept the stereotype of the bisexual who abandons his or her same-sex lover in favor of a safer heterosexual relationship. These stereotypes, while sometimes used affectionately, like a community in-joke, can also create deep divisions within an oppressed group and prevent cooperation and unity.

Images in Popular Culture

Images of queers on television and in film tend to perpetuate the stereotypes that are found in the larger culture. For example, NBC's *Will and Grace*, which premiered in 1999, represents gay life as little more than a series of stereotypes, represented by the main gay characters, Will (played by Eric McCormack) and Jack (Sean Hayes).

Will is the masculine "just-the-same-as-straight" gay man who cannot seem to find a lover, while Jack is the frivolous "flaming queen" gay man who has slept with everyone. Neither character ever steps far enough away from stereotype to reveal a realistic individual who just happens to be homosexual.

On the ABC sitcom *Roseanne* (1988–1997), Sandra Bernhard played Nancy, a bisexual character who reinforced the stereotype of the fickle bisexual by first coming out as a lesbian, then switching back to men with little explanation, only saying glibly, "Don't label me." The Nancy character remained on the show as a humorous oddity, a token, rather than as a developed bisexual character.

Even a fairly gay-positive film like Mike Nichols's *The Birdcage* (1996) relies heavily on the humor of the stereotypically mincing, self-absorbed, effeminate, funny gay man played off against the masculine, gay "straight" man. Though there is enough reality behind the stereotypes to elicit laughs from gay audiences, neither image reflects much depth. Straight audiences learn little about the queer experience from these depictions, and too often the characters serve to perpetuate the stereotypes they demonstrate.

The good-natured stereotyping in a television show such as *Queer Eye for the Straight Guy* (2003–2005) is benign enough, but it plays off some unpleasant stereotypes of gay men as neat freaks and fashion mavens.

Conclusion

Stereotypes, in general, foster prejudice and discrimination. Decisions are often made about individuals based on their membership in groups. When the stereotypes of the group are negative and inaccurate, as they are for glbtq people, the potential for damage to individuals is all the greater.

Perhaps equally damaging, stereotypes may also be self-fulfilling prophecies, especially for young queers just coming out. Having internalized the stereotypes, they may think, for example, that to be a lesbian one must be hard and antimale or that to be a gay man one must be flighty and bitchy. Although such stereotypes are inaccurate and one-dimensional, many glbtq people have attempted to conform to them in efforts to find their niche in the queer subcultures.

—*Tina Gianoulis*

BIBLIOGRAPHY

"Debunking Stereotypes about Gay and Lesbian Relationships." *Argtocsexuality: Livin' da Life.* www.geocities.com/WestHollywood/Heights/5883/livindalife.html

Doty, Alexander. *Making Things Perfectly Queer: Interpreting Mass Culture.* Minneapolis: University of Minnesota Press, 1993.

Dyer, Richard. "Stereotyping." *The Columbia Reader on Lesbian & Gay Men in Media, Society, & Politics.* Larry Gross and James D. Woods, eds. New York: Columbia University Press, 1999. 297–300.

Link, Bruce G., and Jo C. Phelan. "Conceptualizing Stigma." *Annual Review of Sociology* (2001): 363–383.

Paul, Annie Murphy. "Where Bias Begins: The Truth About Stereotypes." *Psychology Today* (May–June, 1998): 52–57.

Troiden, Richard. *Gay and Lesbian Identity: a Sociological Analysis.* Dix Hills, N.Y.: General Hall, 1988.

Walters, Suzanna Danuta. *All the Rage: The Story of Gay Visibility in America.* Chicago: University of Chicago Press, 2001.

SEE ALSO

American Television: Situation Comedies; Bernhard, Sandra; Lane, Nathan

Stiller, Mauritz   *(1883–1928)*

SWEDISH FILM DIRECTOR MAURITZ STILLER'S PRINCIPAL claim to fame is his discovery of an unknown actress, Greta Gustafsson, whom he renamed Greta Garbo. However, this flamboyant gay Svengali to a legendary lesbian star also deserves recognition as a key figure in forging a national cinema that was eventually to become notable for its progressive treatment of sexuality and desire.

Born Moshe Stiller in Finland in 1883, the son of Polish Jewish parents who died when he was five, Stiller was raised by family friends, the Katzmans, who were haberdashers. As a youth, he attended Hebrew school, took violin lessons, and apprenticed at his foster parents' business until he was conscripted into the Russian Army. Rather than serve, he escaped to Sweden.

Suffering from tuberculosis and poverty, the young man used money offered for a health cure to travel to Stockholm, where, checking into a top hotel, he posed as a dapper, successful German director. The daring scam garnered the connections necessary to embark on a career as a director, writer, and occasional actor in the burgeoning Swedish film industry.

Over two decades, Stiller created works in various styles, from social realism to historical adventure and romance. Among his films are such titles as *Mother and Daughter* (1912), *The Modern Suffragette* (1913), *Alexander the Great* (1917), and *Erotikon* (1920).

Stiller's major triumphs, however, came in his innovative, poetic film versions of Swedish Nobel laureate Selma Lagerlöf's sweeping and intense epic novels. Lagerlöf voiced objections to Stiller's experimentalism, but the films are better for the director's resistance to slavishly literal adaptations.

Sir Arne's Treasure (1919) was followed by *Gunnar Hedes' Saga* (1923). In *Gösta Berling's Saga* (1924), Stiller cast as the heroine a shy, inexperienced ingenue who,

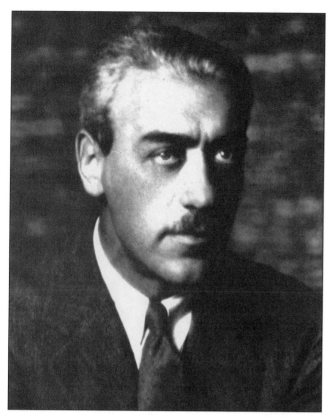

A portrait of Mauritz Stiller by Arnold Genthe.

under his guidance, gave a performance that caused a European sensation.

Seizing the moment, Stiller negotiated a contract for Garbo with MGM. He accompanied her to Hollywood, but constant bickering with studio bosses led him to be passed over as director of her first American film. He was sacked while directing her second, *The Temptress* (1926).

His fierce control over his once compliant protégée rapidly diminishing, a depressed Stiller returned to Sweden, where he died of pleurisy in 1928.

While playing on arrogant charm and sartorial elegance to manipulate his actresses (some of whom, including Garbo herself, he may have been romantically involved with), Stiller was also known for his homosexual liaisons, including a rumored failed affair with a Danish set designer, who committed suicide.

Although his films do not overtly reflect on same-sex desire, his technically innovative explorations of dark themes and emotions helped forge a film culture that was later to produce the likes of Ingmar Bergman.

Moreover, Stiller's role in shaping one of cinema's great queer icons should not be underestimated: "Don't bother about your friends," he advised Garbo at the outset of their association. "When I finish with you, you will have no friends, but rather admirers everywhere."

It is not difficult to discern, emerging from this almost Wildean *bon mot*, the Garbo who was to become legendary for wanting "to be alone." Despite some twinges of guilt for abandoning her mentor, she took his advice and learned not to bother about her friends, including, ironically, Stiller himself.

—*Deborah Hunn*

BIBLIOGRAPHY

Gronowicz, Antoni. *Garbo: Her Story*. New York: Viking, 1990.

Madsen, Axel. *The Sewing Circle: Hollywood's Greatest Secret, Female Stars Who Loved Other Women*. London: Robson Books, 1996.

Soila, Tytti, Astrid Soderbergh Widding, and Gunnar Iversen, eds. *Nordic National Cinemas*. London and New York: Routledge, 1998.

SEE ALSO

Film Directors; European Film; Garbo, Greta

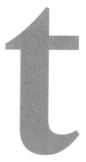

Tomlin, Lily (b. 1939)

COMEDIAN LILY TOMLIN IS PERHAPS LESS WELL KNOWN for being herself than for the many other memorable personages she "becomes" during her performances.

She first gained national fame on television, where she appeared regularly from 1969 through 1973 in the breakthrough comedy *Laugh-In*, portraying the goofily caustic telephone operator Ernestine and the plucky five-and-a-half-year-old philosopher Edith Ann.

As Tomlin's career has advanced, her characterizations have multiplied to include a wide variety of quirky personalities from all walks of society. From Crystal, the hang-gliding quadriplegic, to Trudy, the bag lady, to Agnes Angst, the fifteen-year-old punk performance artist, Tomlin's characters are all survivors of life, each with her or his own brand of pithy wisdom to share.

Rubber-faced and intensely focused, Tomlin manages to convey the universal silliness of the human condition while respecting the essential dignity of each of her characters.

Born Mary Jean Tomlin on September 1, 1939, in Detroit to parents Guy and Lillie Mae, who had immigrated there from the hills of Kentucky, Tomlin often refers to herself as having been "the best white cheerleader in Detroit." She began acting in plays while a premed student at Wayne State University, and soon left college for New York and a comedy career.

In New York, she studied acting with Charles Nelson Reilly. She was working days as a waitress and an office temp and evenings performing stand-up in nightclubs when she got her first television break in 1966 on *The Garry Moore Show*. Her appearance there led to her success on *Laugh-In*, which in turn led to television specials and film roles.

In 1975, she was nominated for an Academy Award for her work in Robert Altman's film *Nashville*. Although some of her films were widely panned (most notably, *Moment by Moment* in 1978 and *Flirting with Disaster* in 1996), she received good reviews in many, including *The Late Show* (1977), *9 to 5* (1980), *All of Me* (1984), *Big Business* (1988), *Tea with Mussolini* (1999), *Orange County* (2002), and *I "Heart" Huckabees* (2004). She also scored in recurring roles on television's *Murphy Brown* and *The West Wing*.

However, Tomlin's first love has been her one-woman comedy shows, which she has performed as television specials and on Broadway and other stages around the country. In such shows as *Appearing Nitely* (1977), *Lily— Sold Out* (1981), and the Tony-winning *The Search for Signs of Intelligent Life in the Universe* (1985, revived 2000), she has developed and refined her comedic style.

Equally important to the success of these productions have been the incisive scripts written by Tomlin's longtime partner, director, and collaborator, Jane Wagner. Wagner's words, channeled through Tomlin's chameleonlike performances, give the shows their power, not only to entertain, but also to unite the audience in delighted empathy.

From early in her career, many of Tomlin's gay fans recognized her as a lesbian. Their perceptions were boosted by a sketch in Tomlin's 1977 stage show *Appearing Nitely*, where she portrayed an inquisitive reporter interviewing Tomlin herself about her role in *Nashville*. How did it feel, the reporter wondered, to play a heterosexual woman in the film? Tomlin's tongue-in-cheek response, that she had been exposed to heterosexuals and observed them throughout her life, delighted the lesbians in the audience.

Many media-savvy dykes also chortled happily at the private joke when Tomlin was cast as Miss Hathaway in the 1993 film *The Beverly Hillbillies,* the same role played by lesbian actress Nancy Kulp in the 1960s television series. Others were pleased to see Tomlin in an overtly lesbian role as Georgie in Franco Zeffirelli's *Tea with Mussolini* in 1999.

However, Tomlin has never come out in a dramatic, public way. Rather, she has eased out of the closet with little fanfare. Magazine articles that used to refer to Jane Wagner as Tomlin's "best friend," now call her Tomlin's partner, and her queer fans continue to receive her warmly; but Tomlin herself does not often speak of her private life.

In early 2001, in an interview in the *Advocate*, Tomlin acknowledged her homosexuality, but pointedly remarked that she does not "want to become someone's poster girl."

She does, however, frequently put her body and talent where her politics are, supporting feminist and gay causes. For example, in a comfortably ironic voice, she narrates the acclaimed documentary *The Celluloid Closet* (Rob Epstein and Jeffrey Friedman, 1996), based on Vito Russo's history of gays in the cinema.   —*Tina Gianoulis*

BIBLIOGRAPHY

Allen, Jennifer. "Lily Tomlin: There are New Signs of Intelligent Life on Broadway." *Life,* November 1985, 17.

Burke, Tom. "Lily Tomlin: The Incredible Thinking Woman." *Cosmopolitan,* April 1981, 262.

"Lily Tomlin Sort of Comes Out." *Advocate,* January 12, 2001. www.advocate.com/html/news/011201/011201ent02.asp

Minkowitz, Donna. "In Search of Lily Tomlin." *Advocate,* November 5, 1991, 78.

Sorensen, Jeff. *Lily Tomlin: Woman of a Thousand Faces.* New York: St. Martin's Press, 1989.

Young, Tracy. "Tomlin-Wagner." *Vogue* (November 1985): 396.

SEE ALSO

Film Actors: Lesbian; American Television: Situation Comedies; Zeffirelli, Franco

Transsexuality in Film

REPRESENTATIONS OF TRANSSEXUALITY IN FILMS FALL along a spectrum from freak-show sexploitation to dramatic and documentary depictions of the struggles of transsexuals and, finally, to the metaphorical use of transsexuality in exploring borders, not only sexual borders but racial, religious, and political ones as well.

The Transsexual as Joke

Whereas transvestites have been depicted in film since the silent era, transsexuals (people who have undergone sex change surgery or who choose to live as the opposite gender) entered the movies only in the early 1950s. The earliest celluloid glimpses of transsexuality appeared shortly after news of George/Christine Jorgensen's 1952 sex change surgery shocked and mesmerized the world with headlines such as "Ex-GI Becomes Blonde Beauty," "Christine, by George!" and "Thousands in U.S. Don't Know Their True Sex."

The first movie attempting to capitalize on the story came from Ed Wood, a quirky filmmaker who was once named the "World's Worst Director." Wood's *Glen or Glenda (I Changed My Sex)* (1953) tells two stories, one about a transvestite, one about a transsexual. Ex-Dracula Bela Lugosi lurks between scenes delivering screwball pleas for tolerance: "Vat are little boys made ov? Ees eet puppy dog tails? Beeg fat snails? Or maybe brassieres!"

The result is pure camp, though Wood, a cross-dresser himself, flashed an intended moral across the screen in the film's opening frames: "Judge Ye Not!"

The filming of *Glen or Glenda* is depicted in Tim Burton's 1994 film biography *Ed Wood*. Wood's entourage includes a preoperative transsexual, Bunny Breckenridge, played for laughs by Bill Murray.

Bunny belongs to a cinematic convention—the transsexual as joke, a sleazy, decades-long parade that includes Bunny's namesake, Myron/Myra in Michael Sarne's *Myra Breckinridge* (1970), based on Gore Vidal's novel. Raquel Welch's Myra is a busty man-hating transsexual who moves to Hollywood to destroy The American Male by using men in the same ways men typically use women.

Mole McHenry, in John Waters's *Desperate Living* (1979), provides another transsexual parody. Hoping to please her curvy blonde girlfriend, Mole hijacks a surgeon, demands a sex change, and returns with a penis. When her lover rejects it, Mole cuts off the salamilike appendage and feeds it to a German shepherd.

Sometimes the transsexual caricature is more poignantly drawn, as with The Lady Chablis, a gutsy drag artist on preoperative hormones in Clint Eastwood's *Midnight in the Garden of Good and Evil* (1997), based on John Berendt's book; or John Lithgow's Roberta in

George Roy Hill's *The World According to Garp* (1982), based on John Irving's novel.

Roberta, a muscle-bound Amazon in a dress, dispenses friendship and wisdom but also reveals her former life with one of the film's biggest laugh lines: "I was a tight end with the Philadelphia Eagles."

Critics felt that Terence Stamp stole the show in Stephan Elliott's *The Adventures of Priscilla, Queen of the Desert* (1994) with his tragicomic portrait of the aging showgirl Bernadette. Bernadette's mournful, brave face is etched with the loss and rejection that has pervaded her transsexual experience as she confides to her two transvestite companions: "My parents never spoke to me again after I had the chop."

The Transsexual as Psychopathic Killer

Films have also asked what happens to the person who is denied "the chop." According to thrillers from Roy Ward Baker's low-budget horror film *Dr. Jekyll and Sister Hyde* (1971) to Jonathan Demme's Oscar-winning *Silence of the Lambs* (1991), that person becomes a psychopathic killer. *Dr. Jekyll and Sister Hyde* stars a transsexual madman in fogbound Victorian London, extracting hormones from freshly-killed women.

Brian De Palma's *Dressed to Kill* (1980) features Michael Caine as mad psychiatrist Dr. Elliot, denied surgery and locked in a life-or-death struggle with the female trapped inside him. When a woman arouses the doctor, his female alter ego slashes her to death with a razor.

This character prefigures Buffalo Bill, the serial killer in *Silence of the Lambs*. Also denied sex change surgery, "Billy" settles for flaying, tanning, and stitching together the skins of size-14 women. "He's making himself a woman's suit," the rookie FBI agent played by Jodie Foster explains, "out of real women."

Most of the whodunits and comedies that exploit transsexuality for its shock value also provide sober, if uninformed, "informational" segments delivered by a designated expert. A doctor solemnly recounts how his patient was "cured" by sex change surgery in *Glen or Glenda*.

In *Dressed to Kill*, a detective fields questions about the homicidal psychiatrist, explaining that Dr. Elliot was "a transsexual, about to take the final step, but his male side couldn't let him do it.... All they want to do is get their sex changed."

"How do they do that?"

"Penectomy."

"What's that?"

"Well, you know, when they take your penis and slice it down the middle."

True Stories of Transsexuals

Not until the late 1990s, with small-budget films such as Richard Spence's *Different for Girls* (1996), do we get reliable information about transsexuality delivered by insiders in drama. But almost a decade earlier, first-person accounts had already begun to appear in a number of documentaries that tell of the heavy price paid by transsexuals: the physical pain and financial drain of surgery, the loss of jobs, the incomprehension and rejection by family and friends.

For example, Jennie Livingston's *Paris is Burning* (1990), a documentary about the elaborate drag and voguing balls of gay Harlem, includes extensive interviews with a transsexual prostitute who was murdered shortly after the filming.

John Paul Davidson's *Boys from Brazil* (1993) captures the bittersweet lives of Rio de Janeiro's *travesti*, prostitutes who live their lives as women, taking hormones and injecting silicone into their breasts, buttocks, and hips.

Kate Davis's *Southern Comfort* (2001) follows the final year in the life of Robert Eads, a 52-year-old transsexual from the back hills of Georgia, who was diagnosed with ovarian cancer after having lived as a man for many years.

Josh Aronson's Showtime documentaries *The Opposite Sex: Rene's Story* (2004) and *The Opposite Sex: Jamie's Story* (2004) tell the stories of a female-to-male transsexual and a male-to-female transsexual, following them through their transitions and exploring the profound effects their decisions have on their families and friends.

True stories of transsexuals have also been dramatized, including Irving Rapper's *The Christine Jorgensen Story* (1970) and a made-for-television biography, Anthony Page's *Second Serve* (1986), the life of male surgeon turned women's pro tennis player Renee Richards.

Kimberly Peirce's acclaimed *Boys Don't Cry* (2000) is based on the life of Brandon Teena, formerly Teena Brandon, who moved to a small Nebraska town to live as a man. Perhaps it is telling that, in this rare depiction of a female-to-male transsexual, Brandon meets one of the most brutal ends in cinematic memory. He is brutally raped and murdered when revelations of his biological sex threaten the masculinity of his young male acquaintances.

Frank Pierson's television movie *Soldier's Girl* (2003), with a script by Ron Nyswaner, tells the true story of a young solider, Barry Winchell, beaten to death for falling in love with a transgendered nightclub performer.

Original Dramas

A few low-budget original dramas explore transsexuality with something other than the freakish curiosity of the thrillers and farces. John Dexter's *I Want What I Want* (1971), released the year after Christine Jorgensen's autobiography appeared, is a transsexual coming-of-age story. The film portrays a young person's painful development from a secret cross-dresser named Roy to a transsexual woman named Wendy, who falls in love with an abusive man.

The celluloid heir to Roy/Wendy's journey is Karl/Kim in *Different for Girls*, but Kim's story has a happier ending, as she refuses to be rejected or abused. Kim began life as Karl, an effeminate man whose only defender from schoolyard taunts was his male friend Prentice. When the two friends run into each other as adults, four years after Kim's sex change, Kim is a prim, defensive greeting card writer who hides from the world, while Prentice is a volatile, immature bike messenger. As their relationship blossoms, Kim learns to enjoy life, and Prentice's acceptance of Kim as a woman prompts his own growing up.

Additional films in which transsexuals are depicted as touchstones for other people's journeys toward tolerance and maturity include Tod Williams's *The Adventures of Sebastian Cole* (1998), in which a young man moves to New York to live with his stepfather, Hank, now Henrietta, and the two develop a positive relationship.

Armistead Maupin's two-part *Tales of the City* (1994, 1997), based on his series of novels and directed by Pierre Gang, depicts a group of San Francisco bohemians presided over by Olympia Dukakis's Mrs. Madrigal, a pot-smoking, transsexual landlady who serves as an unlikely mentor to her young tenants.

Robert Altman's *Come Back to the Five and Dime Jimmy Dean, Jimmy Dean* (1982) portrays the reunion of a group of friends in a small Texas town that leads to a sharing of their most painful secrets, including transsexualism.

Joel Schumacher's *Flawless* (1999) features Robert De Niro as a homophobic security cop who turns reluctantly to the preoperative transsexual next door for singing lessons as part of his therapy in recovering from a stroke.

In contrast to these stories of growth, Rainer Werner Fassbinder's *In a Year of Thirteen Moons* (1979) is a relentlessly pessimistic tale that evokes the continued suppression of difference in Fassbinder's postwar Germany. The film chronicles five days leading to the suicide of Elvira Weishaupt, born Erwin. Erwin had fallen in love with a man who said, offhandedly, "Too bad you're not a girl." After having a sex change, Elvira was rejected. Now she wanders through the slaughterhouse where Erwin once worked, recounting her history amid meat-hooked corpses of cattle that rain blood onto the floor.

The Transsexual as Metaphor

Unlike the dramas of Fassbinder and others, where such issues as essentialism and intolerance arise from narratives of transsexualism, Sally Potter's *Orlando* (1993)—

based on a novel by Virginia Woolf—features, rather than a clinical case, a more metaphoric transsexual character.

After two centuries of adventures—romance, war, a princely inheritance—ageless Orlando goes to sleep as a man, then wakes, lets down a cascade of red hair, and looks in the mirror. "Same person," she says. "No difference at all. Just different sex." Characters speak parables linking gender and ownership, as Orlando's personal journey spans four centuries and parallels the decline of the British Empire.

Liberation finally comes to Orlando when, as the parent of a young child, s/he no longer owns or is owned. And, as the child runs through a field of daisies, Orlando admits to no control over what it will do or be. In short, Orlando's transsexual experience has created a sexual escapee, "no longer trapped by destiny."

Neil Jordan's *The Crying Game* (1992) folds the tale of transsexuality into other kinds of stories in order to raise still broader questions, not only about gender but also about racial, religious, and political identities.

This artfully constructed film begins with a carnival scene by a bridge, evoking its preoccupation with borders and crossings. When Jody, a British soldier in occupied Ireland, is captured at the carnival and held hostage by the IRA, he points to the irony of his position as a black man representing a racist country. Before he is killed, Jody asks one of his captors, Fergus, to look after his girlfriend.

Deserting the IRA, Fergus crosses political, racial, and sexual borders to fall in love with Jody's girl, Dil, a beautiful, light-skinned black woman who turns out to be anatomically male.

Dil fools not only heterosexual Fergus, but the audience as well. She seems to be a blend of races and genders, confounding mainstream clarities, throwing all political, racial, and sexual identities in the film into doubt. Eventually, Dil kills one of Jody's former captors, and Fergus winds up in prison for the murder.

"Dil is Jody's revenge," writes critic Judith Halberstam. "Dil is the snare that awaits all literal readings of bodies, sexes, races, nationalities."

Reductive and literal readings of transsexualism have led to five decades of films preoccupied with "the chop." *The Crying Game* illustrates, perhaps more than any other exception, that cinematic exploitation of transsexuals as jokes or shock devices ignores a subject rich in human and symbolic complexity. —*Carolyn Kraus*

BIBLIOGRAPHY

Garber, Marjorie. *Vested Interests: Cross-Dressing and Cultural Anxiety.* New York: HarperCollins, 1992.

Guthmann, Edward. "Boys Will Be Girls." *San Francisco Chronicle,* September 7, 1997.

Halberstam, Judith. "The Crying Game." *PQ Movie Newsletter.* www.planetout.com/popcornq/db/getfilm.html?1900

Morris, Gary. "A New Kind of Tranny: Different for Girls." *Bright Lights Film Journal* 19 (July 1997): www.brightlightsfilm.com/19/19_different.html

Murray, Raymond. *Images in the Dark: An Encyclopedia of Gay and Lesbian Film and Video.* New York: Plume, 1996.

See also

Film; Documentary Film; Transvestism in Film; Fassbinder, Rainer Werner; Waters, John; Wood, Ed

Transvestism in Film

TRYING TO FIGURE OUT WHAT CINEMATIC TRANSVESTISM has meant for queer audiences is problematic not only because transvestism has never had a single meaning, but also because representations of transvestism have often fallen short of what we today consider queer.

While today we may take for granted the subversive possibilities of drag, it nevertheless remains true that actual representations of drag in film have reinforced conventional ideas of gender more often than they have challenged them.

The decorative, eye-catching, and parodic qualities of drag have made it the most easily appropriated and commodified facet of queer culture in mainstream films. Too often, however, cinematic drag is reduced to a mere joke, a harmless tease that tacitly reassures us that people can change their clothes but not their sexual identities.

Early Drag

In the silent era, drag was typically a ridiculous farce that only reinforced the "comical" discrepancy between a performer's biology and his or her costume. We may think of a young Harold Lloyd disguised as a female baseball pitcher in *Spitball Sadie* (1915), or Charlie Chaplin mischievously cross-dressed in *A Busy Day* (1914), *The Masquerader* (1914), and *The Perfect Lady* (1915).

A little more daringly, Al Christie's *Rowdy Ann* (1919) featured comedienne Fay Tincher as an ultra-butch cowgirl, the brawny equal of any man until she is "tamed" by the civilizing institution of marriage.

That early portrayals of drag were usually allowed only in slapstick comedies, where the sexuality of the drag performer is either neutered or denied altogether, reveals the built-in limitations of generic silent-film comedy.

This primitive, farcical aspect of drag—which, of course, still lingers today—may even be reducible to the familiar image of an insane, cross-dressed Bugs Bunny impishly smacking an infantile Elmer Fudd on the lips: both participants must be first desexualized in order for the farce to be clownishly effective.

In the slapstick era, we may remember Cary Grant "suddenly going gay" in a frilly bathrobe in Howard Hawks's *Bringing Up Baby* (1939), or the transvestite disguise plots of Arthur Leonard's *Boy! What a Girl* (1945), Hawks's *I Was a Male War Bride* (1949), or, most famously, Billy Wilder's later, oft-imitated *Some Like It Hot* (1959).

The Continuing Treatment of Transvestism as Comedy

What can be called the "transvestite plot," wherein a heterosexual character must temporarily cross-dress in accordance with a narrative contrivance, only to be happily unmasked at the conclusion—may be seen today as, by turns, quaint or coy, playful or conservative, potentially subversive or ultimately homophobic.

Indeed, we may think little has changed since Amos Vogel's 1974 critique of Wilder's *Some Like It Hot:* "The Hollywood view of transvestism: it must be portrayed flippantly or in jest to be acceptable. The titillation is built-in and sells tickets."

Thus, Wilder's film may not be ideologically very different from Gualtiero Jacopetti's sensationalist "shockumentary" *Mondo Cane 2* (1964), whose ad campaign promised its bourgeois ticket holders a peek into "the sexual ritual of British transvestites!"

Yet, when one surveys contemporary, mainstream, openly gay fare such as Eduoard Molinaro's *La Cage Aux Folles* (1978) or Stephan Elliott's popular *The Adventures of Priscilla, Queen of the Desert* (1994), it seems that the same campy, ticket-selling titillation can operate even when drag is framed within an out, progay context.

While we may be dismayed that the superficial aspects of drag are too easily mainstreamed for a straight audience, we should not forget that the majority of real-life transvestites are in fact heterosexual. It is therefore possible that within the conventions of the old transvestite plot mainstream drag films may offer covert and not necessarily homophobic pleasures to heterosexual audiences, even if politicized queer audiences may find such films stereotypical, tame, or simply uninteresting.

Issues of Queer Desire

Furthermore, because the standardized, apparently conservative transvestite plot is unlikely to come under much censorship, a few prequeer drag films have managed to raise issues of queer desire even if their formulaic plots eventually demand a safe return to heterosexuality.

Here, we may think of Ernst Lubitsch's then daring *I Don't Want to be a Man!* (1919), or the bisexual confusions generated by a cross-dressed Katharine Hepburn in George Cukor's *Sylvia Scarlett* (1935) and Renate Muller in Reinhold Schunzel's *Viktor und Viktoria* (1933), whose Berlin "decadence" the Nazis would soon extinguish.

On the other hand, queer postmodernism has appropriated iconic images of drag so wantonly that we tend to forget where they actually originate. For example, the indelible image of Marlene Dietrich performing cabaret in a man's top hat and tails has become retroactively synonymous with queer gender-bending, yet we should not conveniently forget that Josef von Sternberg's *Morocco* (1930) was, after all, a film about heterosexual masochism.

Gender and Sexual Polarities

Today, drag has become so commonplace in both straight and queer culture that it has become unwise—if not also impossible and simply tiresome—to try to pick out the "good" drag from the "bad," to distinguish proqueer from homophobic representations of drag in any binary way, which would be as primitive as the female/male polarity that drag is supposed to confuse.

Still, when it comes to a mainstream film like Sydney Pollack's *Tootsie* (1982), the jury seems split along lines of sexual preference: Whereas the straight establishment heaped it with awards, many gay and lesbian viewers criticized the film for perpetuating stereotypical definitions of what are essentially male and female characteristics.

In one sense, such a criticism of the *Tootsie*, or, if you prefer, *Mrs. Doubtfire* (1993) scenario, which supposes that a heterosexual male can become a better heterosexual by discovering his "inner" femininity, is certainly valid. But, while such films are easy to pick on, to insist that all transvestism must be ultimately queer is equally myopic.

Sexual transformations do not always follow from revelations of gender; and, because we cannot fairly delegitimize the identities of heterosexual transvestites, it is not unthinkable that certain acts of drag are indeed only about the heterosexual surfaces of gender and not the queer depths of sexuality.

Similarly, audiences disagree on whether or not the transvestism of Neil Jordan's overhyped *The Crying Game* (1993), which hinges on the revelation of a transvestite's penis, is an elaborate narrative metaphor for the unstable nature of sexual and national identity or a basically homophobic gimmick hiding beneath the trendy clothes of a middlebrow art film.

Still, an acute sensitivity to clichés or homophobias possibly underlying drag is understandable considering the history of silly, pseudo-Freudian, evil transvestites in film. Even acclaimed films such as Hitchcock's *Psycho* (1980) and Brian De Palma's *Dressed to Kill* (1980) place their fashionable transvestisms within a sophomoric understanding of Freud.

Avant-garde Cinema and Cult Films

Before the advent of today's openly queer cinema, the avant-garde cinema, and later the cult film, had offered select, marginal audiences less veiled and more clearly sexualized visions of drag, where cross-dressing was more often an active lifestyle than a passive pathology.

From Ed Wood's *Glen or Glenda* (1953), which provided an autobiographical account of the director's addiction to angora sweaters, to Jack Smith's once-banned underground classic *Flaming Creatures* (1963), from the endless parade of narcissistic drag queens that issued from Andy Warhol's "factory" to professional transvestite Divine's becoming a new definition of radical chic in John Waters's *Multiple Maniacs* (1970), *Pink Flamingos* (1972), and especially *Female Trouble* (1974), transvestism became synonymous not merely with camp but with a celebration of deviance and political marginality in themselves.

Meanwhile, semicommercial cult films such as Richard Benner's *Outrageous!* (1977) gradually pushed sympathetic (and gay) transvestite characters into a mainstream cinema that would in the 1980s embrace Hector Babenco's *Kiss of the Spider Woman* (1985), writer Harvey Fierstein's *Torch Song Trilogy* (1988), and Blake Edwards's *Victor/Victoria*, a campy remake of Reinhold Schunzel's celebrated 1933 classic.

But with the belated success of Jim Sharman's *Rocky Horror Picture Show* (1975), the mainstreaming of the transvestite cult film also brought with it a fallacious sense of democracy: The transvestite's nascent queerness was no longer a political statement automatically opposed to the mainstream, but now a user-friendly game of surfaces the middle class could temporarily engage in before returning to normal.

European Cinema

When we consider transvestite films internationally, however, we get quite a different picture from what North American cinema has, or has not, offered us.

European cinema, of course, has always presented the same farcical stereotypes as Hollywood—slapstick cross-dressing has been a staple of lowbrow comedy nearly everywhere. However, mainstream European films such as Claude Miller's *The Best Way* (1976) and Marco Risi's *Forever Mary* (1989) show that transvestism as a legitimate, if still troubled, representation of alternative desire was more allowable in European cultures whose homophobias were not quite as codified as those of Hollywood.

Elsewhere, in Rainer Werner Fassbinder's absurdist satire *Satan's Brew* (1976), we see that transvestism ultimately seems a far less neurotic practice than the mundane sadomasochisms we endure on a daily basis.

The image of the transvestite has also been used as a metaphorical figure in political films. Most radically, the infamous, coprophagic banquet scene of Pasolini's *Salò* (1975) offers the virginal young male transvestite as a perverse image of purity literally smeared by fascist power structures.

Complementarily, Rosa von Praunheim's fascinating semidocumentary *I Am My Own Woman* (1992) preserves the testimony of Charlotte von Mahlsdorf, a defiant, real-life, but hardly pure, transvestite survivor of Nazi terror.

Asian Cinema

In Asian cinema, we encounter national and historical tropes of theatrical transvestism entirely removed from Western gender binarism.

While Linda Hunt's male reporter in Peter Weir's *The Year of Living Dangerously* (1982) is a rare example of Western gender disguise not necessitated by a plot, this transvestism for its own sake is a staple of the operatic Hong Kong martial-arts films and the occasionally pornographic Japanese *anime*.

Yet, if we consider the political oppressions of the *kathoeys* of Thai cinema and the ostracized, "third-gender" *hijras* of Indian cinema, we see again that, depending on the social context, sexual emancipation does not always easily follow from the confusion of gender identity.

Queer Cinema

The queer American cinema of recent years has provided us with independent films whose transvestisms seem tailor-made for both queer audiences and queer analysis: Jennie Livingston's drag documentary *Paris Is Burning* (1990); Maggie Greenwald's female-to-male transvestite Western *The Ballad of Little Jo* (1993); and Kimberly Peirce's sensational *Boys Don't Cry* (1999), based on the true story of the murder of female cross-dresser Brandon Teena (given name Teena Brandon), also the subject of Susan Muska and Greta Olafsdottir's documentary *The Brandon Teena Story* (1998).

Likewise, European films such as Bettina Wilhelm's *All of Me* (1991) and Pedro Almodóvar's *All about My Mother* (1999) have both humanized the transvestite and rehumanized the camp sensibility, long gone stale, that enfolds her/him.

Recent Mainstream Films

Among recent mainstream films, however, perhaps the most exceptional is Alain Berliner's *Ma Vie en Rose* (1997), which might be called a drag film for children. Because it is the story of a prepubescent (seven-year-old) boy convinced he is a girl, cross-dressing occurs in the absence of the fully formed sexuality that would accompany an older, pubescent, psychically self-aware character.

Thus, while many commercial drag films tend to emphasize the surfaces of drag, pretending to be about sexuality when in fact they are concerned, at most, with the male–female duality of gender, *Ma Vie en Rose* is

perhaps the one film that manages to skirt the gender versus sexuality issue altogether. In this film, drag is not about surfaces diverting our attention from sexualities that may or may not exist; here, gender identity can exist only in terms of surfaces. —*Andrew Grossman*

BIBLIOGRAPHY

Garber, Marjorie. *Vested Interests: Cross-Dressing and Cultural Anxiety.* New York and London: Routledge, 1997.

Russo, Vito. *The Celluloid Closet.* New York: Harper and Row, 1987.

Suarez, Juan Antonio. *Bike Boys, Drag Queens, & Superstars: Avant-Garde, Mass Culture, and Gay Identities in the 1960's Underground Cinema.* Bloomington, Ind.: Indiana University Press, 1996.

Vogel, Amos. *Film as a Subversive Art.* New York: Random House, 1974.

SEE ALSO

Film; Transsexuality in Film; Documentary Film; European Film; Asian Film; Hong Kong Film; Japanese Film; Almodóvar, Pedro; Cukor, George; Dietrich, Marlene; Divine (Harris Glenn Milstead); Fassbinder, Rainer Werner; Fierstein, Harvey; Grant, Cary; Pasolini, Pier Paolo; Praunheim, Rosa von; Warhol, Andy; Waters, John; Wood, Ed

Treut, Monika (b. 1954)

FOR NEARLY TWO DECADES, GERMAN FILMMAKER MONIKA Treut's films have unselfconsciously depicted worlds that the mainstream media tends to treat as "deviant." Her work consistently explores challenging and controversial issues surrounding minority sexual and gender identities.

Born in Mönchengladbach, Germany, Treut studied literature and political science in Marburg/Lahn and wrote her doctoral dissertation on the Marquis de Sade and Leopold von Sacher-Masoch. It has been published as *The Cruel Woman: Female Images in de Sade and von Sacher-Masoch* (1984).

From 1978 until 1982, Treut was in charge of programming for media centers and art houses in Berlin and Hamburg. In 1984, Treut and Elfi Mikesch cofounded Hyena I/II, a film production company, in Berlin and Hamburg.

Mikesch and Treut's first film, *Verführung: Die Grausame Frau (Seduction: The Cruel Woman,* 1985) was inspired by the novel *Venus in Furs* by Leopold von Sacher-Masoch. *Seduction* examines the psychological aspects of sadism and masochism through the tale of Wanda (Mechthild Grossmann), a German lesbian dominatrix who runs a gallery where audiences pay for the privilege of watching her humiliate her slaves.

Treut's second feature film, *Die Jungfrauenmaschine (The Virgin Machine,* 1988) tells the erotic story of a young journalist, Dorothee (Ina Blum), who leaves Germany for

San Francisco. Her sexual adventures include encounters with a male impersonator, Ramona (Shelly Mars); a charming Hungarian bohemian, Dominique (Dominique Gaspar); and Susie Sexpert (Susie Bright), a barker for an all-girl strip show.

Treut's next film, *My Father Is Coming* (1991), continues her exploration of sexual subcultures. Vicky (Shelley Kastner) is a German actress in New York City who tries to impress her visiting father and hide her bisexuality by concealing her job as a waitress and by having her gay roommate pose as her husband. Meanwhile, her father explores a world of transgendered individuals and transsexuals, and has a fling with ex–porno queen turned performance artist Annie Sprinkle (playing herself).

Treut's best-known film, *Female Misbehavior* (1992), is a compilation of four shorts about "misbehaving" women: "Bondage" (1983) looks at the appeal of lesbian S/M, tit torture, and bondage; "Annie" (1989) showcases the performance art of Annie Sprinkle; "Dr. Paglia" (1992) is a portrait of the controversial critic Camille Paglia; "Max" (1992) documents the transsexual journey of Max Valerio from his former life as Anita, a lesbian Native American, to his new identity as a heterosexual male.

The director's most recent work includes shorts, documentaries, and feature films, but all are focused on aspects of sexuality.

In 1996, Treut directed the segment "Taboo Parlor" for the critically acclaimed collection of seductive vignettes, *Erotique.*

Didn't Do It for Love (1997) is a documentary that chronicles the flamboyant life of Eva Norvind. The Norwegian-born Norvind became a sex starlet in B movies in Mexico, then moved into prostitution, where she serviced some of the country's most prominent politicians. Years later, she became a professional dominatrix in New York City and a major player in the sex industry.

Treut's film *Gendernauts* (1999) won the Teddy Award at the 1999 Berlin Film Festival. *Gendernauts* explores gender fluidity at the end of the millennium in the Bay Area of California.

Among her most recent films are *Warrior of Light* (2003), which brings attention to Yvonne Bezerra de Mello, an artist and human rights activist who works with endangered children in the streets and slums of Rio de Janeiro; and *Jump Cut: A Travel Diary* (2004), a feature-length documentary.

Treut's career is profiled, along with those of six other prominent lesbian filmmakers, in Marc Maucerie's documentary *Lavender Limelight: Lesbians in Film* (1997). She currently lives in Hamburg and New York City.

—*B.J. Wray*

BIBLIOGRAPHY

Gemunden, Gerd. "How American Is It? The United States as Queer Utopia in the Cinema of Monika Treut." *A User's Guide to German Cultural Studies.* Scott Denham, Irene Kacandes, and Jonathan Petropoulos, eds. Ann Arbor, Mich.: University of Michigan Press, 1997. 333–353.

Klotz, Marcia. "The Queer and Unqueer Spaces of Monika Treut's Films." *Triangulated Visions: Women in Recent German Cinema.* Ingeborg Majer O'Sickey and Ingeborg von Zadow, eds. Albany, N.Y.: State University of New York Press, 1998. 65–77.

Knight, Julia. "The Cinema of Monika Treut." *Women and Film: A Sight and Sound Reader.* Pam Cook and Philip Dodd, eds. Philadelphia: Temple University Press, 1993. 180–185.

——. "The Meaning of Treut." *Immortal, Invisible: Lesbians and the Moving Image.* Tamsin Wilton, ed. London: Routledge, 1995. 34–51.

Treut, Monika. "Female Misbehavior." *Feminisms in the Cinema.* Laura Pietropaolo and Ada Testaferri, eds. Bloomington, Ind.: Indiana University Press, 1995. 106–121.

See also

Film; Film Directors; European Film; Praunheim, Rosa von

Troche, Rose   (b. 1964)

IN THE EARLY 1990S, WHEN ROSE TROCHE BEGAN HER professional filmmaking career with her then partner, Guinevere Turner, invisibility in the arts and media was one of the primary social issues affecting lesbians.

Thanks to *Go Fish* (1994), Troche's first feature film, in which Turner played one of the lead roles, lesbians have become more visible, not as women tortured by their sexuality, as they have traditionally been portrayed, but as individuals for whom female homosexuality is comfortable and, indeed, normal.

Rose Troche was born in Chicago in 1964 to Puerto Rican parents, and grew up on the city's North Side. While in her teens, she moved with her family to the suburbs, and there, while working part-time in a movie theater, she developed an interest in film. She studied at the University of Illinois, Chicago, where she was an undergraduate major in art history and later a graduate film student.

While in film school, she made several short films, including *Let's Go Back to My Apartment and Have Sex* (1990) and *This War Is Not Over* (1991). While making her *Gabriella* series of short films (1991–1993), Troche met Turner, and they began to plot a film based in part on their own experiences and those of their friends in the Chicago lesbian community. In this manner, the lesbian romantic comedy *Go Fish*, originally titled "Ely and Max," began.

While she was making the film, Troche was also teaching high school. A truly independent film, *Go Fish* was made on an incredibly low budget, financed by

Troche and Turner themselves; and during times when the cash ran out, filming stopped altogether—until the project was rescued by funding from generous producers.

The quirky girl-meets-girl story was premiered at the 1994 Sundance Film Festival, where it was met with considerable acclaim, and it was subsequently distributed by the Samuel Goldwyn Company as a feature film.

By 1993, however, Troche and Turner had ended their relationship, and Troche thereafter moved to New York, where she wrote several scripts.

In 1997, Troche met British producer Dorothy Berwin, who, along with her partner, Ceci Dempsey, asked Troche to direct *Bedrooms and Hallways* (1998), a sex farce that explores the romantic complications among a diverse group of characters—gay, straight, and undecided.

Troche moved to London to work on the film, which, unlike *Go Fish*, was backed by a major studio and completed quickly. It won the Audience Award at the 1998 London Film Festival.

Troche remained in England until 1999, when she returned to the United States to direct *The Safety of Objects* (2001), which she adapted from the short stories of A. M. Homes. Starring Glenn Close, it examines four days in the lives of several suburban families and the events that affect them during that period.

Troche has recently been active in teaching, as an adjunct faculty member at the New School in its film studies program and as a visiting lecturer at New York University and Columbia University.

Troche has also recently directed episodes of the television programs *Six Feet Under, Touching Evil*, and *The L Word*. For *The L Word*, which chronicles the interconnected lives of young lesbians in Los Angeles, Troche has also written several episodes.   —*Patricia Juliana Smith*

BIBLIOGRAPHY

Stukin, Stacie. "Rose to the Occasion: Director Rose Troche Has Moved from Go Fish Girl to Go-to Woman for Quality Mainstream Projects in Film and TV." *Advocate*, March 18, 2003.

SEE ALSO

Film; Film Directors; Screenwriters; Film Festivals; New Queer Cinema; Vachon, Christine

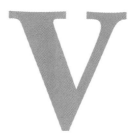

Vachon, Christine

(b. 1962)

Heralded as the most important producer in the history of queer cinema, Christine Vachon has become a driving force in independent film. Her dedication to making movies that matter—ones that broach contentious topics and require serious risk-taking—has brought her an unprecedented level of success in the independent film world.

Along with her own accomplishments, she has helped to bring talented filmmakers such as Kimberly Peirce, Tom Kalin, Mary Harron, and Todd Haynes into the public eye.

Vachon, born in Manhattan in 1962, developed a passion for the movies in early childhood; her parents contributed to her fascination by encouraging her to watch intelligent, mature films. While she was at Brown University, however, the only way for her to study film was to enroll in the semiotics department. She became immersed in theory rather than practice.

After graduation, she decided against going to film school. Instead, she took a series of jobs upon her return to New York City in 1983, in hopes of learning each step of making independent films.

Working as an assistant on the 1986 film *Parting Glances*, a matter-of-fact look at gay life in New York directed by Bill Sherwood, Vachon decided that the do-it-yourself attitude of the filmmakers would be a major influence on her own work.

With director Todd Haynes and another friend, Barry Ellsworth, Vachon formed her first filmmaking company,

Apparatus Films, in 1987. The company helped to lay the foundation for her current work by setting out to make films that were cutting-edge but genuinely entertaining.

At Apparatus, Vachon produced seven shorts in five years. These films dealt with African American life, women's issues, and gay themes. The most notorious of these was the first, Haynes's *Superstar: The Karen Carpenter Story* (1987), which uses Barbie dolls to tell the tragic story of the anorexic pop singer.

Vachon also produced two highly stylized features, Haynes's *Poison* (1991) and Tom Kalin's *Swoon* (1992). *Poison*, which won a prize at the Sundance festival, sparked controversy because of its graphic sex scenes and because it received partial funding from the National Endowment for the Arts.

But the controversy ultimately helped draw attention to the film and resulted in an unprecedented $50,000 opening weekend at the Angelika Film Center in New York City. *Poison*, along with Tom Kalin's *Swoon* (1992), helped gain Vachon notice.

Other films produced by Vachon in the early 1990s include Haynes's short *Dottie Gets Spanked* (1993) and his feature starring Julianne Moore, *Safe* (1995).

With her brand-new film company, Killer Films, Vachon produced the 1997 cult film *Office Killer*, directed by Cindy Sherman. Other titles of note from Vachon and Killer include queer-themed movies such as Kimberly Peirce's *Boys Don't Cry* (1999), Haynes's *Velvet Goldmine*

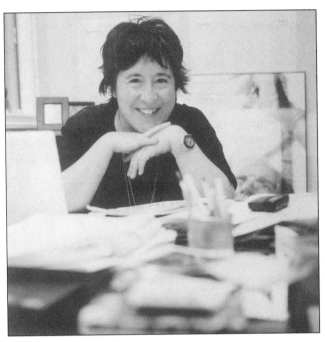

Christine Vachon.

(1998), and Tony Vitale's *Kiss Me Guido* (1997); as well as the highly controversial films *Happiness* (1998), directed by Todd Solondz, and *Kids* (1995), directed by Larry Clark; and Mary Harron's acclaimed *I Shot Andy Warhol* (1996). These works explore significant issues of transsexuality, homophobia, and pedophilia.

Vachon dislikes the "Queen of Queer Cinema" title often bestowed on her, and she does not want to be portrayed as the spokesperson for gay films. She has been criticized by both lesbians (for not making enough lesbian films) and gay men (for negative depictions of gay life). Nigel Finch's *Stonewall* (1996), loosely based on Martin Duberman's memoir, was particularly criticized for its fictionalization of the central event in the modern gay rights movement

Her lesbian audiences were somewhat mollified by the charming lesbian-themed film *Go Fish* (1994), directed by Rose Troche. Meanwhile, Vachon claims that she has never made, and never will make, a movie solely on the basis of its queer content or appeal to a queer audience. Yet neither will she tailor her work to straight audiences, and she is best known for her films that deal with American gay life in all its varieties.

Vachon received the 1994 Frameline Award for Outstanding Achievement in Lesbian and Gay Media, the Outfest Achievement Award for her dedication to queer film, and the 1996 Muse Award for Outstanding Vision and Achievement by New York Women in Film and Television.

Recent projects include her first movie with a big-name star, Robin Williams, in Mark Romanek's *One*

Hour Photo (2001); the film adaptation of John Cameron Mitchell's *Hedwig and the Angry Inch* (2001); Rob Schmidt's *Crime and Punishment in Suburbia* (2000); Haynes's acclaimed deconstruction of 1950s American life, *Far from Heaven* (2002); Rose Troche and Enrique Chediak's *The Safety of Objects* (2003); Fenton Bailey, Randy Barbato, and Teodoro Maniaci's *Party Monster* (2003); and Michael Mayer's *A Home at the End of the World* (2004), based on Michael Cunningham's novel.

Because Vachon is a producer rather than a highly publicized actress, her private life rarely comes up in interviews. Hence, she has felt no pressure to discuss her romantic life in the media. She is comfortably out as a lesbian and lives in New York City.   —*Teresa Theophano*

BIBLIOGRAPHY

Churi, Maya, and Mark Rabinowitz. "Christine Vachon—A Decade of Producing 'Movies That Matter,' Part 1." *indieWire* (December 23, 1999): www.indiewire.com

Vachon, Christine, with David Edelstein. *Shooting to Kill: How an Independent Producer Blasts Through the Barriers to Make Movies That Matter.* New York: Avon Books, 1998.

SEE ALSO

Film; New Queer Cinema; Film Festivals; Haynes, Todd; Mitchell, John Cameron; Troche, Rose

Valentino, Rudolph   (1895–1926)

THE MOST POPULAR OF SILENT-SCREEN STARS, THE darkly handsome Valentino gazed at his heroines with a mixture of passion and melancholy that sent chills down female (and some male) spines. To American women he represented mysterious, forbidden eroticism, the fulfillment of dreams of illicit love and uninhibited passion; but most male moviegoers found his acting ludicrous, his manner foppish, and his screen character effeminate.

His androgynous persona, at once assertively virile and gracefully sensitive, threatened traditional images of American masculinity in a crucial period of cultural change.

Born Rodolfo Alfonzo Raffaele Pierre Philibert Guglielmi in Castellaneta, Italy, in 1895, Valentino emigrated to New York in 1913. There he took a succession of jobs, including dishwasher and waiter, and was booked by the police several times on suspicion of petty theft and blackmail.

In 1917, he traveled to Hollywood, where he landed bit parts in the movies, mostly as an exotic dancer or villain. He married bisexual actress Jean Acker in 1920, but the marriage was probably never consummated.

Valentino's big break came in 1921, when Metro screenwriter June Mathis insisted that director Rex Ingram give him the lead in *The Four Horsemen of the Apocalypse.* The film catapulted Valentino to stardom.

He reached new heights with *The Sheik* (1921) for Paramount. During the film's exhibition, women fainted in the aisles. Such was the film's influence that Arab motifs suddenly pervaded American fashion and interior design.

Valentino also scored sensationally with *Blood and Sand* (1922) and *Monsieur Beaucaire* (1924); and in 1923 his small volume of mawkish poetry, *Day Dreams,* sold hundreds of thousands of copies. But soon his career began to turn downward.

While they have never been documented, rumors of Valentino's bisexuality have persisted. Certainly, it is true that the women in his life dominated him. His ambitious second wife, actress and set designer Natasha Rambova (born Winifred Shaunessy, 1897–1969), a former lover of Alla Nazimova, took charge and (mis)guided his career.

His screen image became increasingly effeminate, and Rambova's interference strained his relationship with studio executives. Just when he seemed to be recovering his popularity with *The Eagle* (1925) and *The Son of the Sheik* (1926), he was blasted in a venomous *Chicago Tribune* editorial, headlined "Pink Powder Puff." The writer lamented, "When will we be rid of all these effeminate youths, pomaded, powdered, bejeweled and bedizened, in the image of Rudy—that painted pansy?"

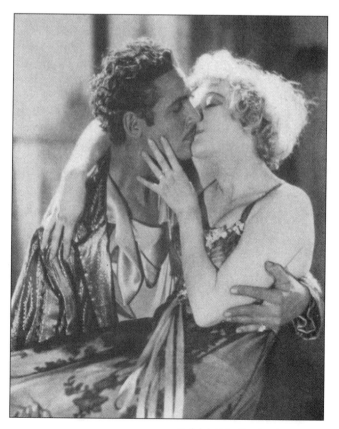

Rudolph Valentino in a love scene.

Valentino's death from a perforated ulcer in 1926, at the age of thirty-one, brought on a wave of mass hysteria among female fans.

Although the actor still commands a high position in American culture as an icon of the silent screen, film specialists hold him in rather low esteem. Kevin Brownlow, however, argues that though Valentino made more bad films than good, the force of his personality nevertheless transcended the "romantic kitsch" of his material.

Unlike those of a later screen icon, James Dean, Valentino's films are not well known today. His body of work died with silent pictures, and to the modern viewer, his acting style is incomprehensible.

Valentino's significance lies not in his having created an artistic legacy, but in how his dubious image—especially his dark sensuality and foreign, somewhat androgynous looks—challenged the way a parochial America looked at its heroes, both on and offscreen. Valentino opened the door for new models of masculinity.

John Dos Passos included a brief biography, "Adagio Dancer," in his trilogy *U.S.A.* (1936). Anthony Dexter portrayed the star in one film biography (1951) and Rudolph Nureyev in another (1977).   —*Peter J. Holliday*

BIBLIOGRAPHY

Bret, David. *Valentino: A Dream of Desire.* London: Robson Books, 1988.

Brownlow, Kevin, and John Kobal. *Hollywood: The Pioneers.* New York: Knopf, 1979.

Carroll, David. *The Matinee Idols.* New York: Arbor House, 1972.

Slide, Anthony. "Valentino, Rudolph." *International Dictionary of Films and Filmmakers. Vol. 3. Actors and Actresses.* Nicholas Thomas, ed. 2nd ed. Chicago and London: St. James Press, 1991. 993–995.

Studlar, G. "Discourses of Gender and Ethnicity: The Construction and De(con)struction of Rudolph Valentino as Other." *Film Criticism* 13.2 (1989): 18–35.

Walker, Alexander. *Rudolph Valentino.* New York: Stein and Day, 1976.

SEE ALSO

Film; Film Actors: Gay Male; Dean, James; Novarro, Ramón

Vampire Films

AN INVENTION OF THE NINETEENTH CENTURY, THE ARTISTIC vampire, as opposed to the vampire of folklore, is connected not with disease but with sexuality. For authors, artists, and filmmakers, artistic vampires represent a common sexualized metaphor—the release of insurgent passion and emotion—that includes such details as the erotic foreplay of vampires' attacks and the creatures' dependency on the bodily fluid of their victims.

From the inception of the type, as an outsider to polite society the artistic vampire has been linked consistently with homosexuality. Samuel Taylor Coleridge's "Christabel" (1797) portended a lesbian vampire, while John Polidori's "The Vampyre" (1819) depicted a young man's homosocial desire for the dominant male vampire.

While this association pervaded much of the Victorian era, by the beginning of the twentieth century the sexual vampire gave way to a more horrific image, and the first vampire films, F. W. Murnau's *Nosferatu* (1919) and Tod Browning's *London After Midnight* (1925), reflect this trend. Early vampire cinema is remarkably heterosexist, belying the literary tradition that spawned it.

The sexual revolution of the 1960s, coupled with the Stonewall riots of 1969 and a new public awareness of homosexuality, soon altered things, and gay and lesbian themes became commonplace in vampire cinema.

The first important homosexual vampire film was Roy Ward Baker's *The Vampire Lovers* (1970), an adaptation of J. Sheridan Le Fanu's "Carmilla." Other gay vampires appeared in Roman Polanski's *The Fearless Vampire Killers* (1967) and, almost simultaneously, in Lancer Brooks's *Sons of Satan* (1973), Ulli Lommel's *Tenderness of Wolves* (1973), and Jimmy Sangster's *Lust for a Vampire* (1973).

This marriage of metaphors—the vampire and the homosexual—remained a constant throughout the 1970s, culminating in Tony Scott's *The Hunger* (1983).

Now permanently linked with sexuality in such films as Neil Jordan's *Interview with the Vampire* (1994), Abel Ferrara's *The Addiction* (1995), Michael Almereyda's *Nadja* (1995), and David DeCoteau's *The Brotherhood* (2000), the vampire has come to be routinely represented as homosexual. In the vampire film genre, and in the arts generally, a sexual metaphor now binds vampires and homosexuals.

—*Michael G. Cornelius*

BIBLIOGRAPHY

Auerbach, Nina. *Our Vampires, Ourselves.* Chicago: University of Chicago Press, 1995.

Beebe, John. "He Must Have Wept When He Made You: The Homoerotic Pathos in the Movie Version of Interview with the Vampire." *The Anne Rice Reader.* Katherine Ramsland, ed. New York: Ballantine Books, 1997.

Benshoff, Harry M. *Monsters in the Closet: Homosexuality and the Horror Film.* Manchester, UK: Manchester University Press, 1997.

Melton, J. Gordon. *The Vampire Book.* Detroit: Visible Ink Press, 1994.

Weiss, Andrea. *Vampires and Violets: Lesbians in Film.* Kitchener, Ontario: Pandora Press, 2001.

www.queerhorror.com

SEE ALSO

Horror Films; Murnau, Friedrich Wilhelm

Van Sant, Gus   (b. 1952)

ONE OF THE MOST IDIOSYNCRATIC TALENTS TO HAVE emerged from the independent cinema over the past decade and a half, Gus Van Sant is matter-of-fact about his sexual orientation. More significantly, in his work he represents homosexuality matter-of-factly.

Back when Hollywood was still tip-toeing around the subject of homosexuality, Van Sant's low-budget feature *Mala Noche* (1985) burst onto the emerging gay and lesbian film festival scene with disarming frankness.

Based on the then unpublished writings of Portland, Oregon, poet Walt Curtis, the film told of the unrequited love of a skid-row liquor-store clerk (Tim Streeter) for a Mexican street hustler (Doug Coyote) and his more sexually available hustler pal (Ray Monge). Shot in 16 mm black and white, it evidenced a talent of remarkable assurance, as well as bravery.

Van Sant's confidence and courage have stood him in good stead in a career that has encompassed everything from films with high-profile superstars such as Sean Connery to music videos for groups such as the Red Hot Chili Peppers and Hanson, and from a thoroughly bizarre shot-for-shot remake of Alfred Hitchcock's 1960 classic film *Psycho* (1998) to such intensely personal short works as the ineffable *Five Naked Boys with a Gun* (1992).

Born in Louisville, Kentucky, on July 24, 1952, into a decidedly mainstream, business-oriented family (his father is responsible for the classic "Mac" raincoat), Van Sant is the perfect example of the American upper-middle-class black sheep. As a child, he evinced interest in artistic pursuits of all kinds and made a number of autobiographical Super 8 films.

At the Rhode Island School of Design, which he entered in 1970, Van Sant first fell in love with painting. But then he loved poetry and literature too, particularly the works of the blackest of all black sheep, William Burroughs, who later became a friend and collaborator. There he was also introduced to the work of such avant-garde filmmakers as Andy Warhol and Jonas Mekas.

Making Portland, Oregon, his home, Van Sant became part of its art and music scene, performing with a band named Destroy All Blondes; then he worked for some time in television. His adventures in television—particularly as they relate to the disadvantages of sleeping with your boss—are covered in his wry, self-starred short *Five Ways to Kill Yourself* (1987).

Van Sant's penchant for making experimental shorts—*My New Friend* (1988) and *Ken Death Gets Out of Jail* (1987) being the most remarkable of them—even after his career entered the mainstream, speaks volumes about his maverick nature.

Van Sant refuses to be pinned down. Instead of making a gay follow-up to *Mala Noche*, he turned to *Drugstore*

Cowboy (1989), his extraordinary drama of the life of a "functioning" drug addict (also based on then unpublished material, a novel by James Fogle). The gritty but tender film revitalized the careers of Matt Dillon and Kelly Lynch, while also introducing Heather Graham and James Le Gros.

But following that success, instead of continuing in a more heterosexual direction, he went on to make his gayest film to date, *My Own Private Idaho* (1991). Casting Keanu Reeves and River Phoenix as Portland street hustlers, it mixed Pasolini-style neorealism with a bizarre restaging of Shakespeare's *Henry IV*.

Idaho climaxes with one of the most memorable scenes in modern gay cinema, a fireside confession of love by one of the hustler heroes for the other. Interestingly, this scene was conceived not by Van Sant, but by his star, River Phoenix. It is a hallmark of Van Sant's directorial style that he creates an atmosphere that encourages such collaboration.

Still, there is such a thing as being too loose, as Van Sant learned the hard way with his adaptation of Tom Robbins's *Even Cowgirls Get the Blues* (1994). Lacking the dramatic coherence of *Drugstore Cowboy* or the playful spontaneity of *My Own Private Idaho, Cowgirls* simply never comes alive on the screen.

Van Sant lined up a more focused project for his next venture, *To Die For* (1995). This black comedy about a would-be news journalist (Nicole Kidman) who will not let a loving husband (Matt Dillon) stand in the way of her career was scripted by veteran writer/actor Buck Henry. It also gave Joaquin Phoenix (the former child actor Leaf Phoenix) his first important adult role.

Good Will Hunting (1997), Van Sant's most acclaimed mainstream effort, featured veteran comedian Robin Williams as the anticipated draw. But the stars of this tale of a blue-collar math genius proved to be its writer/performer wunderkinder, Matt Damon and Ben Affleck.

Instead of basking in this success or repeating himself, Van Sant followed *Good Will Hunting* with his *Psycho* remake, possibly the most ambitious piece of conceptual art since Warhol.

And then came *Finding Forrester* (2000), another "budding genius" tale starring Sean Connery as mentor to a teenage underdog. This commercial project is, however, filled with all sorts of personal touches, such as the lavishly orchestrated version of "Deep Night," the Rudy Vallee number used so hauntingly in *My Own Private Idaho*.

Van Sant followed *Finding Forrester* with a two-character film starring Matt Damon and Casey Affleck (who also share writing credit with Van Sant), *Gerry* (2002), and a film of teenage alienation set in a Portland high school, *Elephant* (2003).

Given the wide thematic range of his work, it is telling that Van Sant's visual style is equally broad. It encompasses both the swooningly romantic lighting style of cinematographer Jean-Yves Escoffier in *Good Will Hunting* and the edgy, color-saturated style of cinematographer Chris Doyle in *Psycho*.

Van Sant's breadth of style and range of interest are complemented by his quasi-surrealist penchant for making up his next move (be it highbrow or low) as he goes along. There is no way of knowing where Van Sant will find himself next. For this gay wild card in the Hollywood pack, being gay is simply one of many stories to be told.

—*David Ehrenstein*

BIBLIOGRAPHY

Ehrenstein, David. *Open Secret: Gay Hollywood, 1928–2000.* New York: HarperCollins, 2000.

Van Sant, Gus, "The Hollywood Way." *Projections* 3. John Boorman and Walter Donohue, eds. London: Faber & Faber, 1994.

_____. Pink. New York: Doubleday, 1997.

SEE ALSO

Film; Film Directors; Screenwriters; New Queer Cinema; Film Festivals; Warhol, Andy

Vilanch, Bruce   (b. 1948)

AN AWARD-WINNING COMEDY WRITER, BRUCE VILANCH has other strings to his bow. He has appeared onstage, on television, and in film, writes for the *Advocate* and other publications, and is a tireless proponent of glbtq causes.

Born in New York City on November 23, 1948, Bruce Vilanch was adopted at the age of four by Dr. Jonas Vilanch, an optometrist, and his wife, Henne Vilanch, a homemaker who loved show business and performed in charity shows.

Vilanch grew up in Paterson, New Jersey. As a child, he modeled, mainly in the "Charming Chub" division of Lane Bryant, and also did some acting in summer stock.

Vilanch realized early in life that he was gay and learned to use humor "partly to deflect peer-group persecution."

After high school, Vilanch enrolled at Ohio State University, where he appeared in student productions and wrote reviews in preparation for what he hoped would be a playwriting career. "I was going to be Neil Simon, batting out one Broadway show after another," he said in 1999.

As it turned out, his writing career began instead at the *Chicago Tribune*, where he got a job as a reviewer and columnist. After he reviewed a performance by Bette Midler, she called him, and in the course of their conversation Vilanch suggested that she ought to put more jokes into her act. When Midler asked him for some comic lines, Vilanch, who was then moonlighting as a cabaret performer, offered some, thus beginning a long professional relationship.

In addition to providing material for Midler's club act, he cowrote the 1980 film *Divine Madness* (directed by Michael Ritchie) for her as well as her television specials *Bette Midler: Ol' Red Head Is Back* (1978) and *Bette Midler in Concert: Diva Las Vegas* (1997).

Vilanch quit his newspaper job in 1975 and moved to Hollywood to do comedy writing full-time. He continued to write material for Midler and also for the variety shows that were popular at the time. He worked with stars like Carol Burnett and Dean Martin and wrote gags for *The Brady Bunch Variety Hour* (1977) and *The Donny and Marie Show* (1976–1979), where he faced, as Stephen Holden wrote, "the formidable task of making Donny and Marie Osmond sound semi-hip."

Vilanch's aspirations to become the next Neil Simon did not meet with success: his 1978 musical, *Platinum*, closed after only thirty-three performances.

The failure of the play was a great professional disappointment to Vilanch, but his comedy-writing skills were still much in demand.

Vilanch used his talents not only to earn a living but also to fight AIDS. He had experienced the devastation of the pandemic at first hand. "When you have to bury three or four friends a month, that's tough," he said of those grim days.

Vilanch began performing regularly at benefits, and he remains strongly committed to the cause of AIDS research and education.

Over the years, Vilanch has become recognized as the premier comedy writer for awards shows. His material has become a fixture of Oscar, Emmy, and Tony Awards telecasts. Vilanch has won two Emmy Awards himself for his work on the Academy Awards shows in 1991 and 1992.

Vilanch became an audience favorite when he joined the cast of the revival of the television game show *Hollywood Squares* in 1998. During his four-year stint with the program he was also head writer, providing witty banter for the celebrities who took part.

Vilanch was both the subject and the star of Andrew J. Kuehn's 1999 documentary *Get Bruce!*, which featured interviews with stars such as Midler, Robin Williams, Billy Crystal, and Whoopi Goldberg, who all benefited from Vilanch's comedy writing talents. Also appearing was Vilanch's mother, who stole all her scenes. Vilanch is extremely close to her and credits her with developing his sense of humor.

Vilanch took to the stage in 2000 with *Bruce Vilanch: Almost Famous*, a show about his life and career. After treating the spectators to behind-the-scenes tales of his work with performers on television shows and onstage—Tallulah Bankhead and Sophie Tucker among the latter—Vilanch fielded questions from the audience and responded with characteristic wit.

Vilanch has recently appeared in the musical *Hairspray* (book by Mark O'Donnell and Thomas Meehan, music and lyrics by Marc Shaiman and Scott Wittman) based on the 1988 John Waters film of the same name. Vilanch played Edna Turnblad, the role originated by Divine in the movie, with the show's national touring company in 2003, and the following year he replaced Harvey Fierstein in the Broadway production.

Despite his considerable girth, Vilanch had to don a "35-pound fat suit" to play Edna. He also had to sacrifice his beard, which for over thirty years had been part of his trademark look—along with large, colorful eyeglasses and one of the T-shirts in his collection (said to number well over 1,000). The departure of the (almost?) famous beard was televised on the *Live with Regis and Kelly* morning show.

Since 1980, Vilanch has been a reporter and columnist for the *Advocate*, for which he has written both humorous and serious pieces. A collection of his writings, *Bruce!: My Adventures in the Skin Trade and Other Essays* (2000), was nominated for a Lambda Literary Award.

Vilanch has been the recipient of a number of awards for his copious work in support of glbtq rights and AIDS charities. Among these are the Los Angeles Shanti Foundation's Daniel P. Warner Service Award (1990), GLAAD Media's Stephen F. Kolzak Award (1997), the Los Angeles Gay & Lesbian Center's Rand Schrader Distinguished Achievement Award (1998), the Outfest Honors Award for contributions to gay and lesbian visibility (2002), and the AIDS Project of Los Angeles Hero Award (2003).

—*Linda Rapp*

BIBLIOGRAPHY

Holden, Stephen. "The Man Behind the Naughty Chuckles." *New York Times*, September 17, 1999.

Isherwood, Charles. "Bruce Vilanch: Almost Famous." *Variety*, May 15, 2000, 37.

Preston, Rohan. "Large and in Charge; Gag Writer and 'Hollywood Squares' Veteran Bruce Vilanch Dares to Play Matriarch Edna Turnblad in the Touring Version of 'Hairspray.'" *Minneapolis Star Tribune*, February 13, 2004.

Tynan, William. "Roastmaster General: He Writes Brilliant Jokes for Celebrities. Can This Top Comic Writer Become Famous on His Own?" *Time*, September 13, 1999, 75.

SEE ALSO

American Television: Situation Comedies; Bankhead, Talluluh; Divine (Harris Glenn Milstead); Fierstein, Harvey; Waters, John

Visconti, Luchino   (1906–1976)

THE MOST CONTRADICTORY OF THE MAJOR ITALIAN filmmakers, Luchino Visconti was an aristocrat by birth, yet he is the progenitor of neorealism, the Italian cinematic movement dedicated to proletarian themes.

He was born Count Don Luchino Visconti di Modrone on November 2, 1906, a member of Milan's highest-ranking nobility and one of the leading aristocratic families in all of Italy.

He spent most of his youth as a dilettante, cultivating his interests in art, music, and racehorses. When he was thirty years old, he began his career in film, working as an assistant director and costume designer for French director Jean Renoir, whom he knew socially.

As a result of his association with Renoir, Visconti became a leftist in politics. Although he had close connections with Mussolini's son Vittorio, he became active in the antifascist movement and, during World War II, in the Resistance.

Also in his early thirties, he had his first serious homosexual affair, with a young German photographer named Horst (later known as Horst P. Horst), who became a well-known fashion photographer. The affair lasted three years, but their friendship endured until Visconti's death.

His first feature film, *Ossessione* (1942), with its insistence on location shooting, proletariat subject matter, and an unvarnished approach to reality, is acknowledged as the first manifestation of neorealism.

The sexual dynamics of the plot (derived from James M. Cain's *The Postman Always Rings Twice,* causing copyright problems that hindered international distribution) points to Visconti's tendency toward melodrama and operatic emotionalism. Centering on the relationships among two men and a woman, the friendship of the two leading male characters is subtly homoerotic.

In 1948, after a time directing in the theater, Visconti created *La terra trema,* a majestic examination of working conditions among the fishermen of Sicily, cast entirely with nonactors. This film ranks as one of the summits of the neorealist movement.

However, Visconti's next film, *Bellissima* (1951), with a brilliant star performance by Anna Magnani, is a satire of neorealism, as a working-class mother tries to get her little girl cast in a neorealist film.

Visconti followed *Bellissima* with the operatic costume drama *Senso* (1954), a study of sexual passion and betrayal set against the political and militaristic turmoil of the Risorgimento, the period of the late nineteenth century when Italy became a modern nation.

Le Notti bianche (1957; American title: *White Nights*) is a stylized adaptation of a Dostoevsky novella.

Rocco e i suoi fratelli (1960; American title: *Rocco and His Brothers*) is one of Visconti's most conflicted works.

Returning to the proletariat themes of *La terra trema,* Visconti traces a poor family as they travel to Rome to find work. But once in Rome, their travails become increasingly baroque, with the melodrama extending into operatic flourishes (such as the killing of the prostitute played by Annie Girardot).

Of all the Italian masters, Visconti was the most varied. He followed *Rocco* with the costume epic *Il Gattopardo* (1963; American title: *The Leopard*), the stylized family drama *Vaghe Stelle dell'Orsa* (1965; American title: *Sandra*), and a scrupulous adaptation of Albert Camus's *Lo Straniero* (1967; American title: *The Stranger*).

With *Götterdämmerung* (1969; American title: *The Damned*), Visconti moved into the most controversial phase of his filmmaking career. He wildly exaggerated the psychosexual posturings of *Götterdämmerung* in order to provide a rationale for fascism. After *Götterdämmerung,* in his adaptation of the Thomas Mann novella *Morte a Venezia* (1970; American title: *Death in Venice*), Visconti treated sexual obsession as a philosophical conceit.

His biographical film *Ludwig* (1972) takes his style of grand filmmaking to its extreme: Although initially released in a version almost three hours in length, it was later reassembled as planned, in its five-hour entirety.

His last two movies, *Gruppo di famiglia in un interno* (1974; American title: *Conversation Piece*) and *L'Innocente* (1976; American title: *The Innocent*), are the culminating movies of his career, with *Gruppo di famiglia* making overt the homoerotic tensions found beneath the surface of most of his movies; and *L'Innocente* taking his decorative tendencies to their logical conclusion.

Visconti died on March 17, 1976, during the editing of *L'Innocente*. His legacy also includes a distinguished career as a director of opera and theater.

Visconti's personal life was marked by tempestuousness and emotional upheavals. Early in his career, he maintained a scrupulous detachment from the actors and singers whose careers he helped to launch; but by the end of the 1960s he had become passionately involved with several young artists. This aspect of his life came to light when letters that he wrote to several young men, including the actor Helmut Berger, became public in the 1980s.

The arc of Visconti's film career mirrors his increasing openness about his homosexuality. His first proletarian epic, *La terra trema,* contained many stunningly composed images of young men at work, but no overt allusions of homosexuality; his later epic, *Rocco e i suoi fratelli,* constantly depicts Alain Delon in close-up, framed and lit in the most glamorous movie-star style, and includes a subplot involving a boxing promoter who pays young men for sex. In contrast to the subtlety with which homoeroticism is conveyed in the early and middle stages of Visconti's career, the homoeroticism of his later work, especially *Götterdämmerung, Morte a Venezia,* and *Ludwig,* is overt and configured in terms of obsession.

Critical opinion of Visconti's work remains sharply divided. But except for those critics who are totally dismissive (usually citing Visconti's decorative tendencies, which may be a coded term for his homosexual sensibility), most find at least one of his films praiseworthy, although each may cite a different one.

The divided response to Visconti's life and career points to a figure of great complexity, one of the towering figures of Italian culture in the twentieth century.   —*Daryl Chin*

BIBLIOGRAPHY

Leprohon, Pierre. *The Italian Cinema.* Roger Greaves and Oliver Stallybrass, trans. New York: Praeger, 1972.

Nowell-Smith, Geoffrey. *Visconti.* Garden City, N.Y.: Doubleday, 1968.

Servadio, Gaia. *Luchino Visconti: A Biography.* New York: F. Watts, 1983.

Stirling, Monica. *A Screen of Time: A Study of Luchino Visconti.* New York: Harcourt Brace Jovanovich, 1979.

SEE ALSO

Film; European Film; Film Directors; Bogarde, Sir Dirk; Zeffirelli, Franco

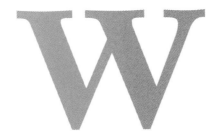

Warhol, Andy   *(1928–1987)*

AS A PAINTER, ANDY WARHOL (THE NAME HE ASSUMED after moving to New York as a young man) has been compared to everyone from Salvador Dalí to Norman Rockwell. But when it comes to his role as a filmmaker, he is generally remembered either for a single film—*Sleep* (1963)—or for works that he did not actually direct.

Born into a blue-collar family in Forest City, Pennsylvania, on August 6, 1928, Andrew Warhola Jr. attended art school at the Carnegie Institute of Technology in Pittsburgh. In 1949, he moved to New York, where he changed his name to Andy Warhol and became an international icon of Pop Art.

Between 1963 and 1967, Warhol turned out a dizzying number and variety of films involving many different collaborators, but after a 1968 attempt on his life, he retired from active duty behind the camera, becoming a producer/"presenter" of films, almost all of which were written and directed by Paul Morrissey.

Morrissey's *Flesh* (1968), *Trash* (1970), and *Heat* (1972) are estimable works. And *Bad* (1977), the sole opus of Warhol's lover Jed Johnson, is not bad either. But none of these films can compare to the Warhol films that preceded them, particularly *My Hustler* (1965), an unprecedented slice of urban gay life; *Beauty #2* (1965), the best of the films featuring Edie Sedgwick; *The Chelsea Girls* (1966), one of the few experimental films to gain widespread theatrical release; and **** *(Four*

Stars) (1967), the twenty-five-hour-long culmination of Warhol's career as a filmmaker.

Warhol's filmmaking career can be neatly divided into three parts. Between 1963 and 1964 he made silent films: black-and-white works shot with a newsreel camera capable of producing three and a half minutes of footage. In these films, movement on the part of his subjects was discouraged. *Sleep, Eat, Haircut,* and *Kiss* come from this period, along with the portrait films *13 Most Beautiful Boys* and *13 Most Beautiful Women*. But some liveliness breaks through in the Hollywood-shot film featuring Taylor Mead, *Tarzan and Jane Regained...Sort Of* (1964).

When Warhol secured a 16 mm synch-sound camera capable of holding thirty-five-minute-long reels in 1965, the second part of his filmmaking career commenced. Warhol discovered that two continuous shots could make for a feature-length film; and so with different collaborators he set about making them.

Off-off Broadway playwright Ronald Tavel supplied scripts for such deadpan satires as *Vinyl, Horse, The Life of Juanita Castro,* and *Screen Test* (all 1965). Chuck Wein, who codirected the *Poor Little Rich Girl* series starring Edie Sedgwick, contributed a different approach to cinema verité, attempting to use the camera to discover an "inner truth."

Paul Morrissey entered the picture in 1966, contributing a dramatic quality to certain sequences of *The Chelsea Girls,* which he codirected. This two-screen-projected, three-and-a-half hour work was hailed as the Greenwich Village answer to *La Dolce Vita* (1960) for its depiction of a variety of demimondaines.

The third and final stage of Warhol's filmmaking career began when he turned to color film. In color, with superimposed reels atop one another during projection, ***** (Four Stars)* is at once more ambitious and more experimental than the earlier works. Later broken up into several films including *The Imitation of Christ, The Loves of Ondine,* and *Tub Girls,* it represents Warhol at the apogee of creative freedom.

The Imitation of Christ is particularly noteworthy as an epic non–love story: the would-be lovers being too self-involved to take much notice of one another.

Warhol's contribution to gay cinema is of incalculable importance, and it is an artistic tragedy that his works (controlled as they are by his estate and not available for video release) are so little known today. Out before outness was a way of political life, Warhol was looked down upon by more conventionally masculine gays as too swish to "pass." Yet there seems to be an attempt to downplay his homosexuality and the homoeroticism of his work.

The casual homoeroticism of *Haircut,* little noted at the time of its first screenings, is unmistakable today.

My Hustler is particularly interesting. Part One consists of a conversation on the deck of a Fire Island cottage between acerbic sugar daddy Ed Hood, fag hag Genevieve Charbon, and semiretired hustler Joe Campbell, as they watch Hood's latest acquisition, Paul America, lie on the beach. Part Two is a long seduction scene in a bathroom as the older hustler seduces the younger. Toward the end, legendary wit Dorothy Dean also attempts to woo the younger man.

Shot two years before *The Boys in the Band* surfaced off-Broadway in 1968, *My Hustler* is a treasure trove of gay slang and attitude from the period. Moreover, it is also interesting as a historical footnote: At the time it was shot, Campbell was being kept by a well-heeled, deeply closeted investment banker named Harvey Milk.

Horse, a Western made four years before the Morrissey-helmed *Lonesome Cowboys* (1969), is far more homoerotic, dealing as it does with gay S/M rituals.

One of the most striking scenes in ***** (Four Stars)* finds actor (and Warhol impersonator) Alan Midgette falling in love on camera with a British youth identified

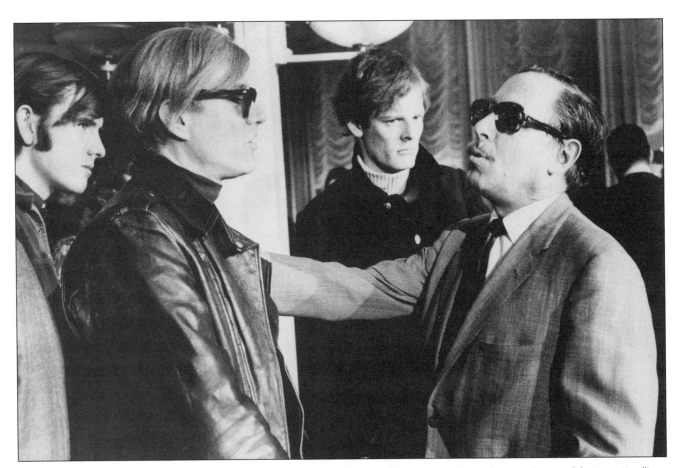

Andy Warhol (left) with Tennessee Williams in 1967. Photograph by James Kavallines.

only as Dingham. It is an utterly simple affair—like all of Warhol at his best, in the years prior to the attempt on his life and his later transmogrification into the first of the Reagan Democrats.   —David Ehrenstein

BIBLIOGRAPHY

Doyle, Jennifer, Jonathan Flatley, and Jose Esteban Muñoz, eds. *Pop Out: Queer Warhol*. Durham, N.C.: Duke University Press, 1996.

Ehrenstein, David. "An Interview with Andy Warhol." *Film Culture* 40 (Spring 1966): 41.

O'Pray, Michael. *Andy Warhol Film Factory*. London: The British Film Institute, 1989.

Smith, Patrick S. *Andy Warhol's Art and Films*. Ann Arbor, Mich.: UMI Research Press, 1986.

SEE ALSO

Film; Film Directors; New Queer Cinema; Transvestism in Film; Grinbergs, Andris; Kuchar, George; Morrissey, Paul; Van Sant, Gus

Waters, Ethel   *(1896–1977)*

ETHEL WATERS IS PERHAPS BEST REMEMBERED FOR THE depth and acuity she brought to her fat "mammy" roles in plays and films such as Carson McCullers's *Member of the Wedding* (1950, 1952) and television shows such as *Beulah* (1950), in the title role of which she replaced the redoubtable Hattie McDaniels. However, Waters had a long, varied, and colorful career.

She began as "Sweet Mama Stringbean," a slender and glamorous blues singer whose technical and emotional agility made her one of the major stars of the Harlem nightclubs of the 1920s.

Her ability to infuse dramatic meaning and intensity into her music made her a natural in musical theater as well, and for a time in the 1930s she was the highest-paid performer on Broadway, winning rave reviews for her roles in such plays as *Blackbirds* (1930) and *Mamba's Daughters* (1938).

She earned an Academy Award nomination for her supporting performance in the film *Pinky* (1949) and a New York Drama Critics' Circle Award as Best Actress of 1950 for her luminous performance on Broadway as the maid in *Member of the Wedding*, a role she reprised on film to further acclaim two years later.

Waters climbed to stardom from a childhood of crushing deprivation. Born on October 31, 1896, in Chester, Pennsylvania, the daughter of a twelve-year-old rape victim, Waters herself was married to her first husband by the age of twelve and divorced by fourteen.

In her autobiography, *His Eye Is on the Sparrow* (1950), she described her rough upbringing: "I never was a child…I just ran wild as a little girl. I was bad, always a leader of the street gang in stealing and general hell-raising. By the time I was seven I knew all about sex and life in the raw. I could out-curse any stevedore and took a sadistic pleasure in shocking people."

As a teenager, while working as a chambermaid in a Philadelphia hotel, Waters gathered her courage one Halloween and sang for the first time on a nightclub stage—behind a mask. Heartened by her success, she began to sing professionally in Philadelphia and Baltimore. Then she moved to New York to join the dynamic explosion of African American creativity that was the Harlem Renaissance.

Singing such trademark blues songs as "Dinah," "Heat Wave," and "Stormy Weather," Waters quickly became a

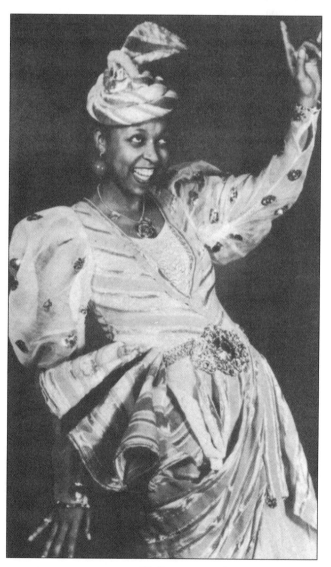

Ethel Waters in *As Thousands Cheer* (1933).

star in the Harlem clubs, and she also traveled a nightclub circuit from Chicago to St. Louis and throughout the South.

Marked by a vitality that gloried not only in black artistic achievement but also in black identity, the Harlem Renaissance also celebrated sexuality with a remarkable lack of censure. Like most blues singers of the time, Waters sang her share of raunchy, openly suggestive songs such as "Organ Grinder Blues" and "Do What You Did Last Night."

And, like many other women blues singers of the day such as Bessie Smith, Ma Rainey, and Alberta Hunter, she was known to have sexual relationships with other women.

Although she was not as open as Rainey about her same-sex relationships, Waters had at least one quite public affair, with a dancer named Ethel Williams, with whom she flirted from the stage and had notorious lovers' spats. She is also rumored to have had a brief liaison with the British novelist Radclyffe Hall, whom she mentions in her autobiography.

In the late 1920s and early 1930s, Waters was able to remake herself as an actress. She first appeared in several Broadway revues, then gradually garnered nonsinging dramatic roles on both stage and screen.

During her later years, Waters considerably toned down her "red hot mama" image and redefined herself as an evangelical Christian. Her last performances were as a member of Billy Graham's crusade. She died on September 1, 1977.

— *Tina Gianoulis*

BIBLIOGRAPHY

Antelyes, Peter. "Red Hot Mamas." *Embodied Voices: Representing Female Vocality in Western Culture.* Leslie C. Dunn and Nancy A. Jones, eds. Cambridge: Cambridge University Press, 1994. 212–229.

Garber, Eric. "A Spectacle in Color: The Lesbian and Gay Subculture of Jazz Age Harlem." *Hidden from History: Reclaiming the Gay and Lesbian Past.* Martin Baum Duberman, Martha Vicinus, and George Chauncey Jr., eds. New York: NAL Books, 1989. 318–331.

McCorkle, Susannah. "The Mother of Us All." *American Heritage* 45.1 (1994): 60–72.

Stryker, Susan. "Lesbian Blues Singers." www.planetout.com/news/history/archive/gladys.html

Waters, Ethel, with Charles Samuels. *His Eye Is on the Sparrow.* New York: Doubleday, 1950.

SEE ALSO

Film Actors: Lesbian

Waters, John   (b. 1946)

ADIRECTOR, WRITER, PRODUCER, AND PHOTOGRAPHER, Waters became well known in the early 1970s through his filmic collaboration with actor—and drag queen—Divine.

Influenced by Russ Meyer, Herschell Gordon Lewis, and the New York underground film scene of the late 1960s, Waters has infused into his uniquely American auteurist works a personal vision. His films constitute their own genre, combining as they do elements of dark comedy, melodrama, cult film, and exploitation film.

Waters was born on April 22, 1946, and has lived most of his life in Baltimore and its suburbs. When he was twelve years old and living in one of those suburbs, Lutherville, a new family moved into his neighborhood with a boy his age named Harris Milstead, who would become his friend and whom he would later rename Divine.

Generally set in Baltimore, Waters's films treat such diverse subjects as bad taste, Catholicism, racism, crime, violence, suburban values, early rock and roll, nonnormative sexual activity, big hair, high-impact modeling, and women in trouble. Campy, kitschy, and queer, Waters's movies—with their traditional narrative structures and hyperbolic dialogue—present hideously lovable characters in outrageous situations.

Moreover, as Waters tends to work with the same offbeat cast and crew, originally called Dreamlanders and based out of his own home, loyal viewers grow to love the performers, sets, and sleazy fictitious worlds from movie to movie in spite of the sometimes revolting onscreen antics.

For example, in *Pink Flamingos* (1972), Divine—in exaggerated drag—shoplifts meat by hiding it between her legs, engages in cannibalism, performs fellatio on her adult son, murders her rivals, and then eats real dog feces to prove she is "the filthiest person alive." Yet, viewers continue to root for her through the end of the story, as she remains the film's optimistic matriarch, innocent victim, and ultimate hero.

In the tamer *Polyester* (1981), Waters casts Divine as Francine Fishpaw, a suburban housewife continually tortured by her cheating husband, scheming mother, precocious daughter, sexually deranged son, and dishonest new boyfriend, Todd Tomorrow (former teen idol Tab Hunter).

With help from her upwardly mobile ex-maid, played by fellow Dreamlander Edith Massey, the Divine character uses her well-developed sense of smell—a gimmicky, mostly malodorous scratch-and-sniff card was provided to spectators at the original screenings—to "sniff" out her enemies while trying to create a pleasant family life.

The last shot of the film, a Waters-style happy ending, depicts Francine, having just witnessed both Todd's and

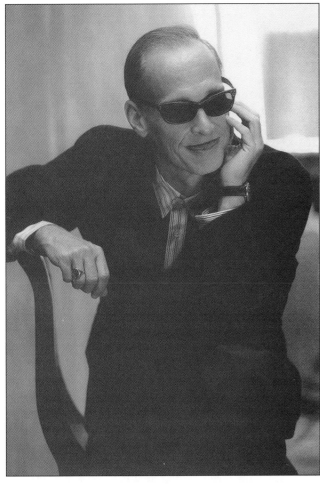

A portrait of John Waters by Greg Gorman.

recent films are more polished technically and less youthfully angry than Waters's earlier works. They are also visually and thematically toned down.

However, their bigger budgets have allowed Waters to explore more expensive filmmaking options, such as the use of better cameras, more sophisticated editing, larger crews and production facilities, and the casting of major stars such as Kathleen Turner, Johnny Depp, Edward Furlong, Rikki Lake, and Deborah Harry.

Formerly on the fringes, Waters today enjoys fame and professional respectability as both a filmmaker and an author.   —David Aldstadt

BIBLIOGRAPHY

Ives, John G. *John Waters*. New York: Thunder's Mouth, 1992.

Waters, John. *Crackpot: The Obsessions of John Waters*. New York: Vintage, 1986.

_____. *Shock Value*. New York: Thunder's Mouth, 1981.

SEE ALSO

Film; Film Directors; Screenwriters; New Queer Cinema; Transvestism in Film; Transsexuality in Film; Divine (Harris Glenn Milstead); Hunter, Tab; Kuchar, George; Wood, Ed

Webb, Clifton   *(1891–1966)*

A REMARKABLE CHARACTER ACTOR, CLIFTON WEBB WAS a familiar presence in American movies of the 1940s and 1950s. He is especially memorable for his transformation of the Hollywood sissy into a more serious—even threatening—figure.

Webb was born Webb Parmalee Hollenbeck in Indianapolis, probably on November 19, 1891, though various sources also give 1889, 1893, or 1896. He showed a theatrical bent early in his life, appearing at age nine with an opera troupe, quitting school at thirteen to study painting and music, and singing with the Boston Opera Company at seventeen.

Ambitious and self-assured, he became a leading New York ballroom dancer in his early twenties before moving into stage roles in both straight drama and musical comedy. He was a respected player on Broadway from the mid-1920s through the early 1940s. He acted in five forgotten films in the 1920s, but came into his own as a movie actor when director Otto Preminger signed him for the classic film noir *Laura* (1944).

Webb's portrayal of the murderous aesthete Waldo Lydecker not only made him a movie star, it was also at once a summation and expansion of Hollywood's sissy characters. Sissies were a popular fixture of 1930s comedies and musicals, where the presence of effeminate character actors such as Franklin Pangborn and Edward

her mother's gruesome deaths, spraying air freshener and hugging her children and friends.

For all the campiness and queerness of Waters's films, however, they only rarely include gay or lesbian characters; and when they do, the depictions are less than sympathetic. Rather than idealizing gay and lesbian characters, Waters usually portrays them in terms of the most ridiculous stereotypical behavior.

And despite the double entendres of some of his titles, Waters almost never includes erotic images, whether gay or straight, preferring to portray all sexual activity as inherently ludicrous.

Nonetheless, Waters's films are infused with a gay sensibility and awareness, a campy sense of humor, and an insistence on the inclusion of marginalized people of all kinds.

Waters continues to make films and to publish articles and essays. His recent mainstream works include *Hairspray* (1988), *Cry-Baby* (1990), *Serial Mom* (1994), *Pecker* (1998), *Cecil B. DeMented* (2000), and *A Dirty Shame* (2004). To the delight of his many new admirers but occasionally to the dismay of longtime fans, these

Everett Horton instantly signified to audiences a sophisticated, sexually ambiguous world. (The films of Astaire and Rogers abound with such characters.)

The sissy was usually a fussy foil to the heterosexual star, female or male; a sexless comic figure who popped up briefly to liven things up with a bon mot or a raised eyebrow or a dramatic exit.

In *Laura,* the sissy retains all the old characteristics—sophistication, brittleness, cynicism—while adding a new element of suppressed violence and sexual passion that threatens not only the other characters but also widely held cultural assumptions about the passivity of the effeminate male.

Webb played this role to perfection; as Waldo he is at once droll and scary, capable of enormous pathos and vicious vitriol ("I should be sincerely sorry to see my neighbors' children devoured by wolves"). He is both ridiculed and indulged by a straight policeman, standing in for society, who doesn't realize until it is almost too late that this sissy is also a killer.

Webb had the charisma and authority to single-handedly rescue the sissy from secondary roles; he is either the star or a major player in all of his films that followed.

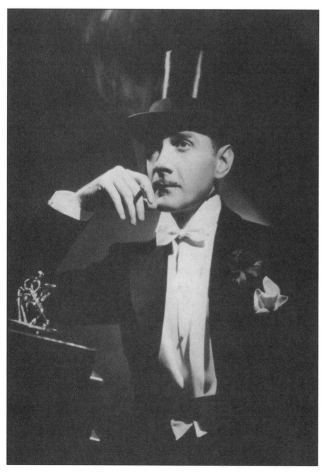

Clifton Webb.

The eternal puzzle of the sissy to straight society can be easily located in Webb's characterizations throughout his film career from 1944 to 1962.

Vito Russo reports in *The Celluloid Closet* that the preshooting script of *Laura* made Webb's Waldo Lydecker explicitly gay, a perverse Pygmalion to Gene Tierney's Galatea, but that many of these references were cut. Despite the film's conflicted view of Lydecker, Webb's nuanced portrayal makes it possible to read him equally credibly as both spurned heterosexual lover and woman-hating queen.

Webb played a similar role in *The Dark Corner* (1946) as the wealthy art dealer Hardy Cathcart. Like Waldo, despite his seeming prissiness, Hardy is a dandy obsessed with a glamorous woman and resorts to murder when she rejects him in favor of a more manly male.

In *Laura,* the audience doesn't see the pivotal murder; in *The Dark Corner,* Cathcart's crimes include luring a butch thug to a high-rise and stylishly pushing him out a window with his cane.

After *The Dark Corner* and his other homo-noir role in 1946's *The Razor's Edge* (which garnered him one of his three Oscar nominations), Webb moved into a variety of comic and dramatic roles, some of which seem strange indeed given his early persona as what critic Parker Tyler called "the lone high aristocrat of professional sissies."

He was cast in historical-iconic roles—as John Philip Sousa in *Stars and Stripes Forever* (1952); as a military intelligence officer in *The Man Who Never Was* (1956); and as a Catholic missionary in his last film, *Satan Never Sleeps* (1962).

Yet Webb always seemed to have the last gay laugh. Even in films where he is improbably cast as hyper-heterosexual—and there were several, including 1950's *Cheaper by the Dozen,* where he has twelve children, or 1959's *The Remarkable Mr. Pennypacker,* where he has two wives and two families—he never downplayed the bitchy evil queen that he perfected in his first roles.

In the huge mainstream hit *Sitting Pretty* (1948), which established a new identity for Webb as an unlikely parent figure, he plays an "eccentric" babysitter who, among other things, dumps a bowl of oatmeal on the head of one of his charges. Even in a serious thriller like *The Man Who Never Was,* when he is asked to pick a code name, he says coyly, "With your permission, sir, Mincemeat?"

Webb was apparently as much a dandy offscreen as on, and a noted tastemaker at that. His *New York Times* obituary gives him credit for "having introduced into the American man's wardrobe such items as the white mess coat dinner jacket, the double-breasted vest and the red carnation boutonniere."

Details of his personal life have not been widely reported. Rumors have surfaced that he "helped" some notable younger actors such as James Dean in their quest for stardom.

But his most crucial relationship appears to have been with his mother, Maybelle, to whom he was devoted. She was his secretary, business manager, and by all reports his constant companion at parties; when she died at age ninety, he was inconsolable. His seemingly bottomless grief inspired Noël Coward's famous remark that Webb was "the world's oldest living orphan."

He died on October 13, 1966.   —Gary Morris

BIBLIOGRAPHY

Howes, Keith. *Broadcasting It: An Encyclopedia of Homosexuality on Film, Radio, and TV in the UK 1923–1993.* London: Cassell, 1993.

Katz, Ephraim. *The Film Encyclopedia.* New York: HarperCollins, 1994.

Murray, Raymond. *Images in the Dark: An Encyclopedia of Gay and Lesbian Film and Video.* New York: Plume, 1996.

Russo, Vito. *The Celluloid Closet: Homosexuality in the Movies.* Rev. ed. New York: Harper & Row, 1987.

Tyler, Parker. *Screening the Sexes: Homosexuality in the Movies.* New York: Holt, Rinehart, Winston, 1972.

SEE ALSO

Film; Film Sissies; Film Actors: Gay Male; Dean, James; Haines, William "Billy"; Novello, Ivor

Weber, Bruce   (b. 1946)

ANYONE WHO HAS EVER GAZED UPON THE CHISELED models in an ad for Calvin Klein underwear has probably been experiencing a photograph made by Bruce Weber. Working for Klein, Ralph Lauren, and a slew of other designers, Weber became one of the preeminent photographers of the fashion industry in the 1980s and continues to be one of the world's most popular commercial photographers.

In addition to his advertisements, however, Weber has published several books of his photographs, made several films, and had his work widely exhibited in museums and galleries.

Weber's success is owed to his bold, sexy portrayal of the male body and an erotic, yet nostalgic take on American adolescence. The widespread resurgence of the male nude in photography and the pictorial ubiquity of the muscle hunk during the 1980s are due largely to Weber's influence.

Yet, ironically, the breadth of his contributions is perhaps best measured in its seeming invisibility: Weber has worked so widely within commercial photography and his signature style is so emulated that the reenvisioned male beauty for which he is credited may now seem commonplace.

Simply put, Weber's photographs are populated by beautiful people. Many of his subjects are celebrities and lend his images a glamorous, Hollywood appeal. But the vast majority of Weber's works feature amateur young men, a choice that reveals a key element of his visual world: a whole-milk, boy-next-door sensuality based on the idyllic, all-American white youth.

That is, Weber's images enlist those wholesome aspects of American culture that most resist—and therefore most compel—homoeroticism.

In 1987, for example, Weber produced *The Andy Book*, an entire volume of steamy photographs that worship the rough physicality of small-town high school boxer Andy Minsker.

Similarly, his 1991 book *Bear Pond*, which features young lads skinny-dipping and cavorting with the photographer's dogs, centers on a sort of erotic nostalgia: the comely wholesomeness of young bodies in old-fashioned summertime recreation, replete with Go Fetch and the backdrop of our beloved National Parks.

Weber typically works in black and white, which also contributes to the wistful, memoir-quality of his pictures.

But for all the calculated, layered homoeroticism in Weber's work, the homosexual act itself is keenly kept out of the picture: Weber is vigilant, even in his most explicitly homoerotic works, about leaving narrative room for platonic brotherhood, no matter how incredulous we may be.

This feature is especially evident in Weber's recent commercial work for Abercrombie & Fitch, a trendy American clothier. The pictures for the company's print ads and lavish catalogs (which, after some controversy, one must now be eighteen to purchase) idolize a sort of collegiate sexual culture in which young men are everywhere on display: the indomitable prowess of the captain of the football team; the anything-goes debauchery of Spring Break; the sweaty camaraderie of team sports; or the sadomasochistic hazing of fraternity pledges.

Despite the mainstream pretenses of the Abercrombie campaign (and its mainstream target demographic), Weber's tantalizing, over-the-top depictions of homoerotic possibility have lent these ads widespread gay currency and, not incidentally, have gained the company entrée into a lucrative gay consumer base.

Much as Weber's pictures for Calvin Klein underwear made that designer's white briefs the signifier par excellence of ideal gay male physicality in the early 1990s, Weber's work for Abercrombie has launched their merchandise into gay consciousness; A&F regalia surfaces in gay street culture, gay pornography, and many places in between.

It is difficult to say for certain whether Weber's pictures, by introducing the potential for man-to-man lust, further advance or subtly undermine the idol status of the muscle-bound white men he so loves to photograph. However, the fact that the A&F campaign's homoerotic texts go largely unnoticed by straight consumers—and must for the campaign to be effective—speaks to the subversive limitations of Weber's art.

Born on March 29, 1946, in rural Greensburg, Pennsylvania, Weber has attributed his interest in photography to his father's tradition of taking family pictures every Sunday and his photographic style to the all-American aesthetics of his pastoral childhood home.

Weber first studied theater in Ohio, then went on to pursue filmmaking at New York University in the 1960s. While in New York, he studied photography under Lisette Model and was also influenced by his friend, the photographer Diane Arbus.

Although Weber is best known for his advertising photography, he has also earned acclaim for his filmmaking. His first film, *Broken Noses* (1987) is a documentary about boxer Adam Minsker, the subject of *The Adam Book*. His documentary focusing on the life of jazz trumpeter Chet Baker, *Let's Get Lost* (1989), was nominated for an Academy Award.

His most recent feature, *Chop Suey* (2001), highlights one of Weber's "discoveries," a gorgeous hunk named Peter Johnson who became a highly paid photographic model; but it is also an autobiographical work in which Weber examines his own career and interests, including his passion for legendary lesbian cabaret performer Frances Faye.

Weber has also directed music videos for Chris Isaak and the Pet Shop Boys.

Although Weber is widely credited with elevating advertising photography to an art form, a more compelling effect of his practice may be the way in which it collapses, rather than elevates, the ad with the artful photograph.

The erotic traits so celebrated in Weber's images are themselves readable as market commodities. His privileged, youth-only world of smooth white skin on seething, untouchable bodies partakes of the formal language of advertising; Weber's men are redolent, seductive, and too perfect, partly accessible through the act of consuming, but ultimately unattainable.

Like any good advertisement, his pictures incite, but never fully quench, the viewer's desire.   —*Jason Goldman*

BIBLIOGRAPHY

Hainley, Bruce, and David Rimanelli. "Shock of the Newfoundland: Bruce Weber's Canine Camera." *Artforum International* 33 (April 1995): 78–81.

Leddick, David. *The Male Nude.* New York: Taschen, 1998.

Weber, Bruce. *Bruce Weber.* New York: Knopf: 1988.

———. *Hotel Room with a View.* Washington, D.C.: Smithsonian Institution Press, 1992.

SEE ALSO

Documentary Film

Weiss, Andrea   (b. 1956)

ANDREA WEISS IS AN AWARD-WINNING WRITER AND documentary filmmaker whose innovative work has provided many unique insights into lesbian and gay life in the twentieth century.

Any serious account of Weiss's work must acknowledge the crucial role of her collaborative partner, director/producer Greta Schiller, with whom Weiss founded Jezebel Productions, a New York–based nonprofit film production company, in 1984.

Weiss, a New Yorker now resident in London, was born in 1956, and completed a Ph.D. in cultural history before moving into film work. In 1984, she was research director on Schiller's documentary *Before Stonewall*, winning an Emmy Award for Best Historical Research. The film—a pioneering study of pre-Stonewall gay and lesbian life in the United States—won an Emmy as Best Historical and Cultural Program.

Three subsequent Jezebel projects, produced in association with Britain's Channel 4, successfully explored marginalized women jazz musicians. *International Sweethearts of Rhythm* (1986) focused on the multiracial all-woman band of the 1940s; *Tiny and Ruby: Hell Divin' Women* (1988) explored the partnership of trumpeting legend Tiny Davis and pianist/drummer Ruby Lucas; and *Maxine Sullivan: Love to Be in Love* (1991) recounted the fluctuating fortunes of 1930s jazz diva Maxine Sullivan.

The challenge of representing minorities—lesbians and gays, blacks, Jews, and women—led Weiss and Schiller to forge experimental documentary techniques to overcome a paucity of archival footage. *Tiny and Ruby*, for example, skillfully utilizes superimposed images, video animation, and the narrative poetry of black lesbian writer Cheryl Clarke.

The politics and poetics of lesbian representation also preoccupy Weiss as a critic. In 1992, she published *Violets and Vampires: Lesbians in Film*, an acclaimed study of films by or about lesbians. Her next book, *Paris Was a Woman* (1996), is a companion piece to her research and writing for a 1995 documentary of the same name.

Directed by Schiller, the film *Paris Was a Woman* is a stylish study of the lesbian coterie associated with the Paris Left Bank in the 1920s and 1930s, offering insights into such modernist luminaries as Gertrude Stein and Djuna Barnes.

Skillfully chosen archival footage, a stylish and informative script, and pertinent interviews garnered *Paris* the audience award for Best Documentary at the Berlin Film Festival, and led the *New York Times* to comment: "Time travel to golden ages doesn't exist…but *Paris Was a Woman* is the next best thing."

Weiss has continued her exploration of hybrid forms through her work as a director. *A Bit of Scarlet* (1997), a

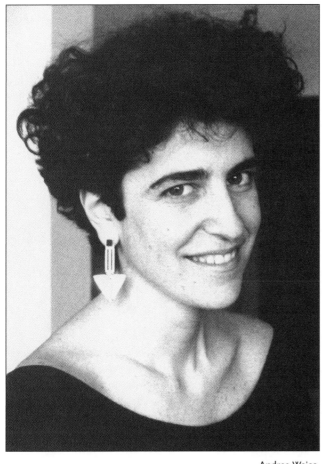

Andrea Weiss.

BIBLIOGRAPHY

Van Gelder, Lawrence. "Paris Was a Woman." *New York Times*, November 8, 1996.

Weiss, Andrea. *Violets and Vampires: Lesbians in Film*. New York: Penguin, 1993.

www.jezebel.org

SEE ALSO

Film; Film Directors; Documentary Film

"collage" documentary, addresses the history of lesbian and gay representation in British cinema, while *Seed of Sarah* (1998) melds video collage and archival material with Mark Polishook's electronic chamber opera to convey the wartime memories of Hungarian holocaust survivor Judith Magyar Isaacson.

Recent Weiss ventures include *Escape to Life: The Erika and Klaus Mann Story* (2000), codirected with German filmmaker Wieland Speck and featuring Vanessa and Corin Redgrave as the voices of Erika and Klaus, the dissident queer children of acclaimed writer Thomas Mann; and *Recall Florida* (2003), a documentary road movie following former Attorney General Janet Reno's botched campaign for Governor of Florida, which Weiss directed and coproduced (with Schiller and Hunter Reno).

Speck and Weiss's joint directorial statement of purpose eloquently sums up Weiss's contribution to contemporary gay and lesbian culture, particularly in its reference to a "seemingly contradictory commitment to art and political action without sacrificing one for the other; a strong sense of the individual's responsibility to society; the search as a gay/lesbian person to find one's own way in the world."

—*Deborah Hunn*

Whale, James (1889–1957)

DIRECTOR JAMES WHALE IS BEST REMEMBERED FOR HIS four stylish horror films: *Frankenstein* (1931), *The Old Dark House* (1932), *The Invisible Man* (1933), and *The Bride of Frankenstein* (1935). Today these are still recognized as outstanding examples of the genre, noted for their semiexpressionistic mood and understated black humor.

Whale's dramatizations have been interpreted, by film historian Vito Russo, for example, as compelling allegories of a man grappling with his homosexuality. Perhaps equally important, Whale's career demonstrates that it was possible for an openly gay man to achieve success in 1930s Hollywood, at least behind the camera.

Whale was born into a working-class family in Dudley, England, probably on July 22, 1889. Growing up poor deeply affected him, as did the fact that he found little support within his family for his artistic leanings and ambitions. Later in his life he would sometimes give the impression that he was of the British upper class or aristocracy, but he never forgot his humble beginnings.

He first pursued a career as a newspaper cartoonist, but was drafted for service in World War I. During the war, Whale earned a commission as second lieutenant and was captured by the Germans. While a prisoner of war, he learned to stage plays.

After the war, he pursued a career in the theater, first as an actor, then as a set designer, and, finally, as a director. In 1929, Whale won notice for his direction of the R. C. Sheriff play *Journey's End*. He was promptly imported to Hollywood in 1930 to direct the screen version. Enthralled by Hollywood and the opportunities it represented, he never left.

In addition to his horror classics, Whale also directed refined and intelligent films in other genres, usually adaptations from literature or the stage. His films are marked by fluid camera movement, leisurely pace, emphasis on detail, and discriminating restraint.

Among his films are the highly regarded *Show Boat* (1936), perhaps the best version of the musical; a pair of highly sophisticated comedies, *Remember Last Night?* (1935) and *The Great Garrick* (1937); and several sharply crafted melodramas, including *Waterloo Bridge* (1930) and *The Man in the Iron Mask* (1939).

Coming on the heels of *Show Boat*, *The Road Back* (1937), Whale's film of Erich Remarque's sequel to *All Quiet on the Western Front*, was expected to secure his growing reputation as one of Hollywood's most important directors.

But the Laemmle family, who helmed Universal and had given Whale carte blanche in the past, had lost control of the studio by the time production began. When the Nazi government objected to the film's supposedly anti-German elements, the studio's new owners took Whale off the project, and "comic relief" scenes shot by another director were inserted to tone down the elements the Nazis found objectionable. The result was a critical and commercial disaster.

Whale worked out his Universal contract with second-rate material, eventually walked off the set of his last contracted Universal film, and never directed again.

Wise investments allowed Whale to retire in comfort. Relieved of the necessity to earn a living, he returned to his first love, painting, occasionally directed plays, and often entertained young men at swimming parties.

In 1929, Whale and David Lewis, a young story editor and later a producer, began a relationship that lasted more than two decades. Although their sexual relationship was an open secret, they lived rather circumspect lives in the English colony in Hollywood.

The sexual component of their relationship ended in the early 1950s, but they remained friends until Whale's death. In the early 1950s, Whale began a relationship with Pierre Foegel, a Frenchman working as his chauffeur.

After a series of strokes left Whale physically and spiritually depleted, he committed suicide by throwing himself into his swimming pool on May 29, 1957. Because his suicide note was withheld until after Lewis's death (and first published in James Curtis's biography of the director), Whale's death was shrouded in mystery for many years.

Christopher Bram's excellent novel *Father of Frankenstein* (1995) offers a fictional account of Whale's final days. The novel was adapted to film by Bill Condon as *Gods and Monsters* (1998, produced by Clive Barker), in which Ian McKellen gives a stunning performance as Whale.

—*Peter J. Holliday*

BIBLIOGRAPHY

Curtis, James. *James Whale.* Metuchen, N.J.: Scarecrow, 1982.

————. *James Whale: A New World of Gods and Monsters.* Boston: Faber and Faber, 1998.

Ellis, Reed. *A Journey into Darkness. The Art of James Whale's Horror Films.* New York: Arno Press, 1980.

Gattis, Mark. *James Whale, a Biography. Or, The Would-be Gentleman.* New York: Cassell, 1995.

Russo, Vito. *The Celluloid Closet: Homosexuality in the Movies.* New York: Harper & Row, 1981.

Slide, Anthony. "Whale, James." *International Dictionary of Films and Filmmakers.* Vol. 2. Nicholas Thomas, ed. 2nd ed. Chicago and London: St. James Press, 1991. 913–914.

SEE ALSO

Film; Film Directors; Horror Films; Set and Costume Design; Barker, Clive; Laughton, Charles; McKellen, Sir Ian

Williams, Kenneth   *(1926–1988)*

THE ACTOR, RACONTEUR, AND WRITER KENNETH WILliams was beloved by the British public as much for his outrageously camp persona as for his considerable comedic gifts.

British audiences had long tolerated gay stereotypes in comedy, but Williams "pushed the envelope," especially on radio, at a time when homosexuality was only just becoming acceptable to a wider public. His popularity on chat and game shows—where he often displayed a highly amusing, acidulous, and somewhat hysterical temperament—could also be said to have helped to widen general acceptance of nonstraight behavior.

The son of a London hairdresser, Williams was born on February 22, 1926. He studied lithography before the war, but was evacuated during the blitz. He performed briefly with the Tavistock Players, an amateur dramatic troupe, but was inducted into the army in 1944.

He began his professional performing career in Singapore just after World War II, as a member of Combined Services Entertainments.

In 1948, having returned to Britain, he embarked on a career that would encompass theater, film, cabaret, television, and radio.

After a spell in repertory theater, Williams enjoyed critical acclaim as the Dauphin in a London production of George Bernard Shaw's *Saint Joan* (1954) and popular success in three celebrated revues, commencing with *Share My Lettuce* in 1957.

Beginning with *Carry On Sergeant* in 1958 and continuing through the late 1970s, he appeared in twenty-six of the slapstick, innuendo-filled "Carry On" films. In these he played characters that were, to a degree that varied from film to film, camp, knowing, and sarcastic. The "Carry On" films were lucrative for Williams, but they stereotyped him as a campy queen and eventually limited his career.

A gifted actor, Williams periodically attempted to play roles more challenging than the campy ones with which he was associated, but audiences seemed uncomfortable with this. Even his turn as Inspector Truscott in the original production of his close friend Joe Orton's *Loot* (1965) was not well received by the audiences to whom he had become a household name.

Williams's vocal talents brought him fame through two comedy radio shows of the 1950s and early 1960s: *Hancock's Half Hour* and *Beyond Our Ken*. His ability to create vivid comic characters through voice alone was never put to better use than in another radio show, Kenneth Horne's *Round the Horne* (1965–1968).

Especially memorable, considering prevailing attitudes to homosexuality at the time, were the "Julian and Sandy" sketches. Here, Williams played Julian to the actor Hugh Paddick's Sandy: a pair of screaming queens who burbled on cheerfully and provocatively in the gay argot called *Polari* to a middle-class audience of millions.

Williams was homosexual by inclination but avoided sexual relationships. From his astonishingly frank diaries (published posthumously), it seems clear that he felt safer with the satisfaction afforded by masturbation rather than in an encounter with someone else.

By turns outrageous and conservative, he was plagued by disgust for what he considered to be typical gay lifestyles (promiscuous, disordered, camp, in some way sinful) and he admired heterosexual family life. He wrote in his diaries of wanting to find his perfect companion, but carefully avoided involvement with any possible candidates.

Despite the ambiguity he felt about his sexuality, Williams supported the Albany Trust, which aimed to decriminalize sexual relationships between consenting male adults, a reform that was not adopted until 1967.

Williams suffered from bouts of depression throughout his life. In his final years, these bleak periods were made worse by his own poor health and that of his mother, to whom he remained very close.

On April 15, 1988, he was found dead in his London flat. He had taken an overdose of barbiturates, washed down with alcohol. The coroner recorded an open verdict on Williams's death.   —*Chantal Stoughton*

BIBLIOGRAPHY

Freedland, Michael. *Kenneth Williams: A Biography*. London: Weidenfeld and Nicolson, 1990.

Williams, Kenneth. *Just Williams*. London: Dent, 1985.

_____. *The Kenneth Williams Diaries*. Russell Davies, ed. London: HarperCollins, 1993.

_____. *The Kenneth Williams Letters*. Russell Davies, ed. London: HarperCollins, 1994.

SEE ALSO

British Television; Film

Winfield, Paul   *(1941–2004)*

THE THEATER ALWAYS HAD A SPECIAL PLACE IN THE heart of actor Paul Winfield, but his career included numerous film and television roles. He was nominated for several acting awards and won an Emmy in 1995.

Paul Edward Winfield was born in Los Angeles on May 22, 1941, to Lois Beatrice Edwards, a garment-industry worker and union organizer. When Winfield was eight, his mother married Clarence Winfield, a construction worker.

The family moved to Portland, Oregon, for a time. One of Winfield's vivid memories from those years was seeing Mark Robson's 1949 film *Home of the Brave*, in which African American actor James Edwards played a leading part rather than the role of servant to which actors of color were typically confined.

When the family returned to Los Angeles, Winfield attended Manual Arts High School, where he excelled in both music and acting. He was named Best Actor in the Speech and Drama Teachers Association Drama Festival for three consecutive years.

Because of these achievements, he was offered a scholarship to Yale but, apprehensive about fitting in there, chose to accept a two-year scholarship at the University of Portland. He subsequently attended other colleges on the West Coast, including UCLA, which he left in 1964, six credits short of a degree, when professional opportunities beckoned.

In addition to appearing onstage, he served as artist in residence at Stanford University during the 1964–1965 academic year.

Winfield became a contract player for Columbia Pictures in 1966. Initially, he continued his stage work and played minor parts on television, but in 1969 Sidney Poitier chose him for a role in Robert Alan Arthur's film *The Lost Man*.

Winfield also became familiar to viewers of the small screen with a regular role as Diahann Carroll's boyfriend on the situation comedy *Julia* (1968–1970), a groundbreaking series that many consider to have been influential in increasing opportunities for African American actors on television.

Winfield turned in a memorable performance in Martin Ritt's 1972 film *Sounder*, which earned him a nomination for an Academy Award as Best Actor.

Sounder came out when many films starring African Americans were of the so-called blaxploitation variety that featured comic-book-style action heroes. Winfield's portrayal of Nathan Lee Morgan, a Louisiana sharecropper jailed for stealing a ham to feed his starving family during the Great Depression, was a radical departure from what audiences had come to expect.

Of Winfield's performance, Stephen Bourne wrote, "A black father had never been depicted in an American movie in such a personal and intimate way, and with such humanity." He added that Winfield's finest moment in the film came when he expressed his love for his son.

Winfield lived with his *Sounder* costar Cicely Tyson for about a year and a half, but the relationship failed. In 1975, Winfield left Hollywood for San Francisco, which he described in a 1990 interview as a place where "a lot of people go to find themselves. There's a lot of introspection, a lot of social and sexual and interpersonal experimentation."

These comments are undoubtedly an oblique reference to his personal life, for there he began a lifelong relationship with San Francisco native Charles Gillan Jr., a set designer for television shows and a partner in the design firm TECTA Associates, which specialized in architectural restoration. The couple remained together until Gillan's death of a bone disease on March 5, 2002.

Following the brief sojourn in San Francisco, Winfield returned to Los Angeles, where he amassed a long string of credits in film and television. He was honored with Emmy nominations for his 1978 portrayal of Martin Luther King Jr. in Abby Mann's miniseries *King* and for his role in Georg Stanford Brown and John Erman's *Roots: The Next Generations* in 1979. He finally won an Emmy in 1995 for his work as a guest star on the series *Picket Fences*.

The versatile Winfield appeared in a wide variety of other screen projects, from the science-fiction classic *Star Trek II: The Wrath of Khan* (1982, directed by Nicholas Meyer) to James Cameron's 1984 action picture *The Terminator* and a comedy series spoofing the Cinderella story, *The Charmings* (1987), on which he played a wisecracking mirror.

Winfield also had a starring role in gay filmmaker James Bridges's *Mike's Murder* (1984), in which he portrayed a gay man distraught over the death of his former lover.

In addition to on-camera work, Winfield also did voice-overs. After playing boxing promoter Don King in the HBO movie *Tyson* (1995, directed by Uli Edel), he voiced the King-inspired character Lucius Sweet on the cartoon series *The Simpsons* (1996 and 1998). Beginning in 1998, he narrated the A&E cable television series *City Confidential*, which deals with crimes and their impact on the cities in which they occur. Winfield's narration for this series was highly melodramatic.

Winfield was happiest performing onstage, particularly in the works of Shakespeare. He also appeared in numerous plays by modern writers.

Winfield's avocations included home renovation, an interest that he shared with Gillan; playing the cello; and raising champion black pug dogs, which he named after characters from his beloved Shakespeare. He also became an avid collector of objects depicting the breed,

accumulating hundreds of bronze and ceramic figures, including a 600-year-old sculpture from China.

While at a dog show in Denver in the late 1990s, Winfield fell into a diabetic coma and required three weeks of hospitalization. This caused him to "take [the disease] seriously" and to speak out publicly to make African Americans more aware of the dangers of diabetes and obesity. He was also a vocal proponent of civil rights. Within the entertainment industry he worked tirelessly to promote cultural diversity.

Winfield did not, however, play an active role in the gay rights movement. His friend actor/producer Jack Larson described him as "openly gay in his life if not in the media." Indeed, in a 1990 article in *People* Tim Allis wrote that Winfield "mentions no current relationship," though he and Gillan had by then been partners for well over a decade.

One cannot say with certainty why Winfield chose to maintain public silence regarding his sexual orientation. It may be noted, however, that many actors of his generation, such as Rock Hudson and Richard Chamberlain, long concealed their homosexuality for fear of losing employment.

Larson stated that Winfield had been distraught in his final years due to Gillan's death. Winfield died of a heart attack on March 7, 2004, in Los Angeles.   —*Linda Rapp*

BIBLIOGRAPHY

"Academy Award-nominated Actor Paul Winfield Dead at 62." *Advocate* (online edition) (March 10, 2004): www2.advocate.com/news_detail.asp?id=03912

Allis, Tim. "On Charges of Stealing the Show, Paul Winfield Is Presumed Guilty." *People*, August 20, 1990, 61.

Bourne, Stephen. "Obituary: Paul Winfield; Actor Nominated for an Oscar for His Role in 'Sounder.'" *Independent* (London), March 12, 2004.

Hall, Ken. "Paul Winfield." *Antique & Collecting Magazine* (November 2003): 31.

King, Susan. "Paul Winfield, 62; Actor Catapulted to Fame in 'Sounder.'" *Los Angeles Times*, March 9, 2004.

Sullivan, Patricia. "Acclaimed Actor Paul Winfield Dies at 62." *Washington Post*, March 11, 2004.

Trescott, Jacqueline. "The Worries of Paul Winfield; Back on Stage as Falstaff, the Actor on His Struggle to Find Other Weighty Roles." *Washington Post*, June 4, 1991.

SEE ALSO

Film Actors: Gay Male; Chamberlain, Richard; Hudson, Rock

Wong, B. D. (b. 1960)

THE ONLY ACTOR TO WIN THE TONY AWARD, THE Drama Desk Award, the Outer Critics Circle Award, the Clarence Derwent Award, and the Theater World Award for the same performance, Asian American actor B. D. Wong came to prominence with his extraordinary performance in the title role of David Hwang's *M. Butterfly* (1988).

While few of his subsequent roles have been as challenging, Wong has since established himself as a talented character actor in film and television, as well as onstage, and as a champion of glbtq causes.

Born Bradley Darrell Wong on October 24, 1960, in San Francisco, Wong is a fourth-generation Chinese American. He was raised in the San Francisco Bay Area. Following high school graduation, he traveled to New York to pursue his dream of becoming an actor.

In New York, he studied acting, accepted dinner theater and summer stock opportunities, and appeared in off-Broadway productions and in small television and film roles.

His career did not shift into high gear until he returned to the West Coast as a member of the cast of the Los Angeles production of the Jerry Herman–Harvey Fierstein musical *La Cage aux Folles*. His adeptness at playing a female impersonator prepared him for the lead in *M. Butterfly*.

Wong's performance as Song Liling in his Broadway debut was no less than mesmerizing. Playing a male Chinese spy who successfully poses as a woman in a twenty-five year relationship with a French male diplomat, Wong not only convincingly portrayed the fluidity of gender, but also brought to the role a rare humanity and complexity.

He conveyed the racialized stereotype of the Asian man as an emasculated sissy and the Asian woman as a submissive object of desire, while also turning the stereotypes on their heads. In his role as Song, Wong was at once a "Cio-Cio San," or abandoned and exploited lover, and a manipulative spy. He vividly brought to life the themes of sexual and political imperialism and gender fluidity at the heart of Hwang's play.

Wong also gave a highly acclaimed performance as Kico Govantes, the lover of activist Bill Kraus, played by Ian McKellen, in the HBO television production of *And the Band Played On* (1993), the adaptation of Randy Shilts's searing account of the first years of the AIDS epidemic.

He was also memorable in the New York Shakespeare Festival's production of gay Singapore playwright Chay Yew's *A Language of Their Own* (1995), a play that explores a gay interracial relationship.

Wong costarred as Margaret Cho's brother in the short-lived ABC situation comedy *All American Girl* (1994–1995), the first situation comedy on American network television to deal with the Asian American experience.

From 1997 until 2002, Wong had a recurring role as a priest in the gritty HBO series *Oz*, which was set in a maximum-security prison.

In 2002, Wong joined the cast of NBC's *Law and Order: Special Victims Unit*, playing Dr. George Huang, a forensic psychiatrist.

Wong is a notably versatile actor. Hence, despite the paucity of roles specifically written for Asian Americans, he has kept busy on both the large and small screens.

Wong's film roles have varied from a campy caterer in *The Father of the Bride* (1991) to a geneticist in *Jurassic Park* (1993) and a member of an elite antiterrorist unit in *Executive Decision* (1996). He was happy to supply the voice of Captain Li Shang in the Disney animated feature *Mulan* (1998), because the story was one Wong had learned as a child from his parents. He repeated the role in the 2004 sequel *Mulan II*.

Wong has also appeared in the off-Broadway production of the Irving Berlin–Moss Hart musical *As Thousands Cheer* (1998) and as Linus in the Broadway revival of the musical *You're a Good Man, Charlie Brown* (1999). He has made dozens of guest appearances on television series such as *Law and Order: Special Victims Unit, Chicago Hope, Sesame Street,* and *The X-Files.*

He has recently scored in the Roundabout Theatre Company revival of the Stephen Sondheim musical *Pacific Overtures* (2004), about America's 1853 mission to Westernize Japan, and has directed his first feature-length film, *Social Grace*, a comedy about a high-profile interracial romance, due to be released in 2005.

Wong has taken seriously his status as one of the few well-known Asian American actors in Hollywood. He told an interviewer that he is very much connected to his Chinese heritage, "but in a very American way." He frequently lectures on diversity issues, particularly on the problem of racial self-hatred and rejection.

Wong also very strongly identifies as a gay man. Hence, he has been a visible presence at AIDS-related charity functions and in gay and lesbian community events, as well as at events sponsored by the Asian and Pacific Islander communities.

Wong has appeared at the GLAAD Awards, made promotional spots for the gay and lesbian television newsmagazine *In the Life*, and worked in various ways to further understanding among both Asians and non-Asians, gays and nongays, about the experience of being both gay and Asian.

In 2003, Wong published a memoir, *Following Foo*, which tells the story of how he and his life partner, talent agent Richie Jackson, created their family. They became the fathers of premature twins via a surrogate mother in 1999. One of the twins, Boaz Dov Wong, weighed only two pounds, five ounces and died quickly. The other twin, Jackson Foo Wong, nicknamed "Chestnut Man," was eight ounces heavier and, after a number of close calls, finally prevailed. The book is an inspirational account of the support Wong and his partner received during their ordeal.   —*Claude J. Summers*

Bibliography

Barney, Brian. "B. D. Wong." *Online Directory of Asian Pacific American Artists.*
    www.public.asu.edu/~dejesus/210entries/bdwong/bdwong.htm

Hobson, Louis B. "Man on a Cultural Mission." *Calgary Sun,* June 18, 1998.

Wong, B. D. *Following Foo: (The Electronic Adventures of the Chestnut Man).* New York: HarperEntertainment, 2003.

See also

Film Actors: Gay Male; Cho, Margaret; Fierstein, Harvey; *In the Life;* McKellen, Sir Ian

Wood, Ed   (1924?–1978)

DURING HIS LIFETIME, 1950S TRANSVESTITE DIRECTOR Edward D. Wood Jr., known as Ed Wood, worked diligently—if sometimes despairingly—at the margins of Hollywood, making bizarre low-budget films that went almost entirely unnoticed.

He died in 1978, a penniless alcoholic, but posthumously became the center of one of cinema's most enduring cults. Opposing camps celebrated and reviled him, using the same epithet: "the world's worst director."

Born in Poughkeepsie, New York, on October 10, 1924 (some sources give 1922), Wood served in the U.S. Marine Corps from 1942 to 1946. According to legend, he stormed the beaches of Tarawa wearing women's underwear beneath his uniform.

After the service, he moved to Hollywood, where he made his first film, the no-budget Western *Crossroads of Laredo* (1948). Five years later, collaborating with producer George Weiss, he directed his breakthrough film, *Glen or Glenda,* also known as *I Changed My Sex,* which would start his fitful career and his reputation as a hack of prodigious proportions.

This "torn-from-the-pages-of-life" story, based on the then scandalous sex change of Christine Jorgensen, became a fractured but compelling exercise in autobiography, as Wood himself played the lead roles of Glen and his cross-dressing alter ego, Glenda. With its narrative ruptures, genre melding, split-screen effects, sudden insertions of stock footage and pornographic tableaux, and consistently surprising imagery, *Glen or Glenda* bolsters the case for Wood as an early postmodernist constantly at war with his own narrative.

A cult favorite with little critical following, Wood has nonetheless been defended by some critics, including Danny Peary, as among the most interesting directors of the post–World War II film scene.

In addition to being a transvestite, Wood was an alcoholic, a writer of pornographic novels, and a habitué of Hollywood's seedier bars and demimondes. *Glen or Glenda,* masquerading as a plea for tolerance, is in fact a tour of the director's fevered psychic landscape, complete with cut-rate cheesecake and bondage imagery and a view of deviance at once empathetic and lurid.

Notwithstanding his cross-dressing, Wood was in some ways the quintessential "American"—an ex-soldier, buoyant, creative, charismatic, and resourceful—but he attracted an entourage that included some of Hollywood's most unusual personalities.

Among Wood's collaborators were such artists and misfits as horror hostess Vampira, psychic Criswell, the hyperdramatic Dudley Manlove, horror-movie has-been Bela Lugosi, Swedish wrestler Tor Johnson, and drag queen Bunny Breckenridge.

Wood's willingness to accept, embrace, and display these eccentrics alongside himself made them both his friends and, for works such as *Bride of the Monster* (1956) and *Plan 9 from Outer Space* (1958), a seedier version of the kind of stock company that major directors such as John Ford and Orson Welles cultivated.

Plan 9 is formally less extreme than *Glen or Glenda,* but is perhaps the classic Wood film, the apotheosis of 1950s exploitation camp. Its amusing crudities include startling continuity gaps, hubcaps doubling for spaceships, tombstones made of paper, and actors clearly reading their lines from cue cards in front of them.

In a legendary conceit, Wood replaced Bela Lugosi, who died midproduction, with a blond chiropractor and drinking buddy, who holds his cape over his face to prevent the audience from verifying the obvious.

Wood, and *Plan 9* specifically, was memorialized in Tim Burton's feature *Ed Wood* (1994). Burton takes the Wood cult's view that *Plan 9,* like all of the director's oeuvre, is, unmistakably, naive art, purveyed to an unsuspecting culture by an endearing misfit whose sheer tenacity would inspire many future independent filmmakers.

Wood's unapologetic transvestism—it fueled novels with titles such as *Death of a Transvestite* (1967) and caused considerable grief in his personal life—was radical for its time; and his films wittily portend, consciously or not, the trash camp of later masters such as John Waters and the Kuchar brothers.   —*Gary Morris*

Bibliography

Grey, Rudolph. *Nightmare of Ecstasy: The Life and Art of Edward D. Wood.* Los Angeles: Feral House, 1992.

Hoberman, J. "Bad Movies." *Vulgar Modernism.* Philadelphia: Temple University Press, 1991. 13–21.

McCarty, John. *The Sleaze Merchants: Adventures in Exploitation Filmmaking.* New York: St. Martin's Press, 1995.

Okuda, Ted. "Remembering Ed D. Wood Jr., a Moviemaker." *Filmfax* 6 (March–April 1987).

Peary, Danny. *Cult Movies: The Classics, the Sleepers, the Weird, and the Wonderful.* New York: Dell, 1981.

Wood, Edward D. Jr. *Death of a Transvestite.* 1967. New York: Four Walls Eight Windows, 1999.

SEE ALSO

Film; Film Directors; Transvestism in Film; Transsexuality in Film; Kuchar, George; Waters, John

Z

Zeffirelli, Franco   (b. 1923)

For half a century, Franco Zeffirelli has been in the spotlight for his visually extravagant opera, stage, and film productions. While his self-proclaimed "crusade against boredom" in the dramatic arts and his emphasis on spectacle have brought him considerable acclaim, they have also been the target of significant critical derision.

The controversial Italian director has also been lambasted by religious groups for his supposedly blasphemous representation of biblical figures, yet he has also provoked the ire of many gay men and lesbians for siding publicly with the Roman Catholic Church on homosexual issues.

Zeffirelli was born on February 12, 1923, in Florence, the son of Ottorino Corsi, a wealthy businessman, and his mistress Adelaide Garosi, a fashion designer. Through his father, Zeffirelli was related to the family that centuries before had produced Leonardo da Vinci.

He was originally Gianfranco Corsi, but his mother subsequently followed the Florentine tradition of naming a child born out of wedlock with a created name beginning with the letter Z. After his mother's death, he was placed in the care of an English governess, from whom he learned the English language and its literature.

Zeffirelli graduated from art school in 1941 and, following his father's plan, became an architecture student at the University of Florence. While at the university, he became active in directing student theatrical productions, including stagings of operas under the tutelage of his aunt Ines Alfani Tellini, a retired soprano.

In 1943, he left college to join the Partisans and fight against the Nazi occupation of Italy. Subsequently, he became an interpreter for the British Army after the Allied invasion.

As a result of meeting British troops who shared his dramatic interests, Zeffirelli abandoned his plans for a career in architecture and, after the war, became a theatrical set and costume designer.

During the late 1940s, he worked as an assistant to director Luchino Visconti, whose attention to realistic detail and action profoundly influenced the young apprentice's own work.

Through the 1950s and 1960s, Zeffirelli firmly established his reputation as a drama and opera director. In the former capacity, he presented highly naturalistic stagings of Shakespeare at London's Old Vic.

Simultaneously, he was responsible for noted productions at Milan's La Scala, London's Covent Garden, and New York's Metropolitan Opera, starring the leading divas of the period, particularly Maria Callas, Joan Sutherland, and Leontyne Price.

His lavish visual appeal created greater mainstream interest in legitimate theater and opera, but Zeffirelli's characteristic style—which he likened to that of the Hollywood epics of Cecil B. De Mille, "but in good taste"—did not meet with universal acclaim.

Many found his productions overdone to the extent that the sets and stage action drew attention away from the actual performance. Indeed, this was the case with the 1966 world premiere of Samuel Barber's *Antony and Cleopatra*, which was commissioned for the opening of the new Metropolitan Opera House in Lincoln Center. The technology operating the prodigious stage machinery malfunctioned, the spectacle was almost unanimously panned, and Barber's career was effectively ended.

His detractors notwithstanding, Zeffirelli continued to expand his audience during the mid-1960s with his debut as a film director. His first feature film, *The Taming of the Shrew* (1967), featured the most discussed theatrical couple of the day, Elizabeth Taylor and Richard Burton. As a cinematic rendering of a traditional work of English literature, it set the tone for many of his subsequent screen productions.

His best-known film, *Romeo and Juliet* (1968), soon followed. It was controversial for his casting of unknown and inexperienced (if highly attractive) teenaged actors in the title roles. He would again present such adolescent sensuality and sexual awakening in *Endless Love* (1981), which tells the story of an obsessive teen romance set against the backdrop of parental prohibition.

Zeffirelli's later films have received widely mixed reviews and are generally regarded as uneven in quality. These include *Brother Sun, Sister Moon* (1973), *Jesus of Nazareth* (television miniseries, 1977), film versions of Verdi's operas *La Traviata* (1982) and *Otello* (1986),

Hamlet (with Mel Gibson and Glenn Close, 1990), *Jane Eyre* (1996), the autobiographical *Tea with Mussolini* (1999), and *Callas Forever* (2001).

Although Zeffirelli is openly gay and has frankly discussed his sexuality in his autobiography, he is nonetheless somewhat paradoxical in this regard. Some critics have noted a "homosexual gaze" in his films, particularly in their lingering and erotically tinged close-up shots of the seminude male body. In *Tea with Mussolini*, moreover, he cast Lily Tomlin as an unambiguously lesbian character.

At the same time, however, his advocacy of Catholic dogma in opposition to gay activism has not gone unnoticed, particularly his backing of Vatican efforts to thwart the inception of a Gay Pride parade in Rome.

Yet this seeming contradiction is, perhaps, characteristic of Zeffirelli's career and work, for which he has long been regarded with extreme degrees of reverence and revilement, in almost equal measure.

— *Patricia Juliana Smith*

BIBLIOGRAPHY

Zeffirelli, Franco. *Zeffirelli: The Autobiography of Franco Zeffirelli*. New York: Weidenfeld & Nicolson, 1986.

SEE ALSO

Film Directors; Set and Costume Design; Tomlin, Lily; Visconti, Luchino

Notes on Contributors

DAVID ALDSTADT is a doctoral candidate in French cinema, modern French literature, and French culture at Ohio State University. His dissertation examines cinematic collaboration, authorship, and star personae in films by Marcel Carné with Arletty and by Jean Cocteau with Jean Marais. Entries: Cocteau, Jean; Divine (Harris Glenn Milstead); Waters, John

RICHARD C. BARTONE, Professor in the Department of Communication at William Paterson University of New Jersey, teaches a course in Media Representation of Lesbian, Gays, Bisexuals, and the Transgendered. He has worked as a documentary film and news archivist for CBS News and served as Senior Associate Editor of the journal *Film & History: An Interdisciplinary Journal of Film and Television.* Entries: Araki, Gregg; Documentary Film; Everett, Rupert; Film Actors: Gay Male; Haynes, Todd; Laughton, Charles; Ottinger, Ulrike; Praunheim, Rosa von

GEOFFREY W. BATEMAN is the Assistant Director for the Center for the Study of Sexual Minorities in the Military, a research center based at the University of California, Santa Barbara, that promotes the study of gays and lesbians in the military. He is coeditor of *Don't Ask, Don't Tell: Debating the Gay Ban in the Military,* as well as author of a study on gay personnel and multinational units. He earned his M.A. in English literature at the University of California, Santa Barbara, in eighteenth-century British literature and theories of genders and sexuality, but now lives in Denver, Colorado, where he is coparenting two sons with his partner and a lesbian couple. Entries: O'Donnell, Rosie; Pornographic Film and Video: Transsexual

JENNIFER BURWELL, Assistant Professor of English at Ryerson University, teaches communications and cultural studies with an emphasis in television studies. She is author of *Notes on Nowhere: Feminism, Utopian Logic, and Social Transformation.* Entry: Canadian Television

DARYL CHIN is an artist and writer based in New York City. Associate Editor of *PAJ: A Journal of Performance and Art,* he is the author of a monograph on the video artist Shigeko Kubota. Entries: Carné, Marcel; Eisenstein, Sergei Mikhailovich; Murnau, Friedrich Wilhelm; New Queer Cinema; Visconti, Luchino

BUD COLEMAN, Associate Professor in the Department of Theater and Dance at the University of Colorado at Boulder, is a former dancer with Les Ballets Trockadero de Monte Carlo (as Natasha Notgoudenuff), Fort Worth Ballet, Kinesis, and Ballet Austin. He has directed and choreographed numerous productions and published in several journals and encyclopedias. Entry: Liberace

MICHAEL G. CORNELIUS is a doctoral student in early British literatures at the University of Rhode Island. He is the author of a novel, *Creating Man.* Entries: LaBruce, Bruce; Vampire Films

KIERON DEVLIN studied Art & Design at Manchester Art School, England. He holds a Master's degree from Leicester University and an M.F.A. in Creative Writing from New York City's New School. He is working on a novel and a collection of short stories. Entry: Set and Costume Design

DAVID EHRENSTEIN is author of *The Scorsese Picture: The Art and Life of Martin Scorsese* and *Open Secret: Gay Hollywood 1928–1998.* He has contributed to numerous journals, newspapers, magazines, and television shows. Entries: Pasolini, Pier Paolo; Van Sant, Gus; Warhol, Andy

JIM ELLIS is Assistant Professor of English at the University of Calgary, where he also teaches in the film program. He has published essays on gender and sexuality in early modern literature and a series of essays on the work of Derek Jarman and his contemporaries. Entries: Davies, Terence; Julien, Isaac

BRETT FARMER is Senior Lecturer in Cultural Studies at the University of Melbourne, Australia. He is the author of *Spectacular Passions: Cinema, Fantasy, Gay Male Spectatorships* and numerous essays in cultural, film, and queer studies. Entry: Film Spectatorship

EUGENIO FILICE is a doctoral student in art history at McGill University. He is currently preparing a dissertation on representation of gay men in contemporary Canadian art, and on the revival of figurative painting that occurred during late 1970s and 1980s. Entry: Greyson, John

MARK FINCH, former Exhibitions and Festival Director for Frameline and the San Francisco International Lesbian & Gay Film Festival, was a seminal figure in international gay and lesbian cinema. A native of Manchester, England, he worked for the British Film Institute and programmed the London Gay and Lesbian Film Festival before moving to San Francisco in 1991. He wrote extensively about film for a number of publications, both mainstream and gay and lesbian. He ended his own life, jumping from the Golden Gate Bridge, in 1995. Entry: Film

RAYMOND-JEAN FRONTAIN is Professor of English at the University of Central Arkansas. He has published widely on seventeenth-century English literature and on English adaptations of biblical literature. He is editor of *Reclaiming the Sacred: The Bible in Gay and Lesbian Culture.* He is engaged in a study of the David figure in homoerotic art and literature. Entry: Laurents, Arthur

TINA GIANOULIS is an essayist and freelance writer who has contributed to a number of encyclopedias and anthologies, as well as to journals such as *Sinister Wisdom.* Entries: American Television: Soap Operas; Borden, Lizzie; Clift, Montgomery; DeGeneres, Ellen; Dietrich, Marlene; Garbo, Greta; Garland, Judy; Minnelli, Vincente; RuPaul (RuPaul Andre Charles); Stereotypes; Tomlin, Lily; Waters, Ethel

JASON GOLDMAN is currently pursuing a Ph.D. in Art History at the University of Southern California. His academic interests include the history of photography, twentieth-century art, pornography, contemporary art, and contemporary visual culture. Entry: Weber, Bruce

ANDREW GROSSMAN is the editor of *Queer Asian Cinema: Shadows in the Shade,* the first full-length anthology of writing about gay, lesbian, and transgender Asian films. His writings on film and queer issues have also appeared in *Bright Lights Film Journal; Scope: The Film Journal of the University of Nottingham; Senses of the Cinema; American Book Review;* and elsewhere. Entries: Asian Film; Hong Kong Film; Japanese Film; Transvestism in Film

PETER J. HOLLIDAY, Professor of the History of Art and Classical Archaeology at California State University, Long Beach, has written extensively on Greek and Roman art and their legacies and on issues in contemporary art criticism. Entries: Mineo, Sal; Novarro, Ramón; Valentino, Rudolph; Whale, James

KEITH G. HOWES has been researching, writing, and speaking about gay film, radio, and television for twenty-five years. He lives in Sydney, Australia, where he is employed as a bush regenerator, helping to restore native flora and fauna. Entries: Australian Television; British Television; Hudson, Rock

DEBORAH HUNN is a Lecturer in Communication and Cultural Studies at Curtin University of Technology, Western Australia. She has taught English, Media Studies, and Women's Studies in several Australian universities. Entries: Australian Film; Film Directors; Stiller, Mauritz; Weiss, Andrea

JACQUELINE JENKINS teaches Medieval Literature and Culture as well as Film and Gender Studies at the University of Calgary. Her research interests include vernacular book production and the reading habits of late medieval laywomen; women's spirituality and late medieval religiosity; Saints' legends and performance; medieval and contemporary popular culture. Entry: Arzner, Dorothy

CRAIG KACZOROWSKI writes extensively on media, culture, and the arts. He holds an M.A. in English Language and Literature, with a focus on contemporary critical theory, from the University of Chicago. He comments on national media trends for two newspaper-industry magazines. Entries: Barker, Clive; European Film; Screenwriters

ROBERT KELLERMAN holds a doctorate in English literature from Michigan State University. Entry: Rudnick, Paul

MATTHEW KENNEDY teaches anthropology at City College of San Francisco and film history at the San Francisco Conservatory of Music. A film critic for the *Bay Area Reporter,* he has also written for such publications as *Performing Arts,* the *San Francisco Chronicle,* and *Bright Lights Film Journal.* He is author of *Marie Dressler* and a biography of film director Edmund Goulding. Entries: Goulding, Edmund; Novello, Ivor

GEORGE KOSCHEL is a writer of short fiction and the contact person for Frontrunners New Orleans. Entry: Cadinot, Jean-Daniel

CAROLYN KRAUS is Associate Professor of Communications at the University of Michigan–Dearborn, where she teaches journalism and creative nonfiction. She has written for a variety of publications, including the *New York Times*, the *New Yorker*, and *Partisan Review*. Entry: Transsexuality in Film

CHARLES KRINSKY teaches in the Liberal Studies and Ethnic and Women's Studies Departments of California State Polytechnic University, Pomona. His research focuses on the construction of masculinity and male sexuality in Post–World War II American films and culture. Entry: Marais, Jean

RICHARD G. MANN is Professor of Art at San Francisco State Univerity, where he teaches a two-semester multicultural course in queer art history. Entry: Flynn, Errol

JOHN McFARLAND is a Seattle-based critic, essayist, and short story writer. He is author of the award-winning picture book *The Exploding Frog and Other Fables from Aesop*. He has contributed to such anthologies as *Letters to Our Children: Lesbian and Gay Adults Speak to the New Generation*, *The Book Club Book*, *The Isherwood Century*, and *Letters to J. D. Salinger*. Entry: Lucas, Craig

GARY MORRIS is the editor and publisher of *Bright Lights Film Journal*, now online as www.brightlightsfilm.com. Author of *Roger Corman*, he writes on film regularly for the *Bay Area Reporter* and *SF Weekly*. He serves on the editorial advisory board of www.glbtq.com. Entries: Bartel, Paul; Broughton, James; Cukor, George; Film Noir; Film Sissies; Hammer, Barbara; Horror Films; Kuchar, George; Morrissey, Paul; Paradjanov, Sergei; Webb, Clifton; Wood, Ed

JENNI OLSON is one of the world's leading experts on glbtq cinema. She is the director of entertainment and e-commerce for PlanetOut.com and Gay.com, and is the founding producer of PlanetOut's PopcornQ, a massive film website based on her book, *The Ultimate Guide to Lesbian & Gay Film and Video*. Codirector of the San Francisco International Lesbian & Gay Film Festival from 1992 to 1994, Olson continues to be a consulting programmer to the Minneapolis/St. Paul Lesbian, Gay, Bi & Transgender Film Festival. Her first feature film as writer/director is an experimental documentary, called *The Joy of Life*. Entry: Film Festivals

JULIA PASTORE is a New York–based freelance writer who works in book publishing. Entry: Grant, Cary

JIM PROVENZANO, a sports columnist for the *Bay Area Reporter*, is also a fiction writer. He is the author of the novels *Pins* and *Monkey Suits* and of numerous short stories. Entry: Dean, James

LINDA RAPP teaches French and Spanish at the University of Michigan–Dearborn. She freelances as a writer, tutor, and translator. She is Assistant to the General Editor of www.glbtq.com. Entries: Almendros, Néstor; Burr, Raymond; Butler, Dan; Callow, Simon; Chamberlain, Richard; Chapman, Graham; Cheung, Leslie; Condon, William "Bill"; Crowley, Mart; Cumming, Alan; Davis, Brad; Edens, Roger; Epperson, John; Fernie, Lynne; Fierstein, Harvey; Hunter, Tab; Iglesia, Eloy de la; Jeter, Michael; Jones, Cherry; Lane, Nathan; Moorehead, Agnes; Nader, George; Sargent, Dick; Vilanch, Bruce; Winfield, Paul

MIGUEL A. SEGOVIA was born in Monterrey, Mexico, and raised in Houston, Texas. He is a doctoral student in Religious Studies at Brown University. Entry: Cho, Margaret

PATRICIA JULIANA SMITH is Assistant Professor of English at Hofstra University. With Corinne Blackmer, she has edited a collection of essays, *En Travesti: Women, Gender Subversion, Opera*. She is also author of *Lesbian Panic: Homoeroticism in Modern British Women's Fiction* and editor of *The Queer Sixties* and *The Gay and Lesbian Book of Quotations*. She serves on the editorial advisory board of www.glbtq.com. Entries: Anderson, Lindsay; Asquith, Anthony; Bogarde, Sir Dirk; Flowers, Wayland; Fry, Stephen; Gielgud, Sir John; Hawthorne, Sir Nigel; Ivory, James, and Ismail Merchant; Lynde, Paul; McDowall, Roddy; McKellen, Sir Ian; Richardson, Tony; Schlesinger, John; Troche, Rose; Zeffirelli, Franco

CHANTAL STOUGHTON graduated from Corpus Christi College, Cambridge, and has worked as a writer and subeditor for newspapers and magazines in Japan, Hong Kong, and the United Kingdom. Entry: Williams, Kenneth

CLAUDE J. SUMMERS, William E. Stirton Professor Emeritus in the Humanities and Professor Emeritus of English at the University of Michigan–Dearborn, is General Editor of www.glbtq.com. He has published widely on seventeenth- and twentieth-century English literature, including book-length studies of E. M. Forster and Christopher Isherwood, as well as *Gay Fictions: Wilde to Stonewall* and *Homosexuality in Renaissance and Enlightenment England: Literary Representations in Historical Context*. He lives in New Orleans. Entries: Condon, William "Bill"; Crisp, Quentin; *In the Life*; Wong, B. D.

MARK ALLEN SVEDE is a historian and curator whose work often addresses marginalized artists and communities. He publishes extensively about Latvian visual culture, ranging from nonconformist art and underground film to hippie fashion and dissident architecture. He also works as a residential architect. Entries: Anger, Kenneth; Fassbinder, Rainer Werner; Grinbergs, Andris

TERESA THEOPHANO, a freelance writer, is a social worker who specializes in community organizing with glbtq populations. She is also the editor of *Queer Quotes*. Entries: Bernhard, Sandra; Collard, Cyril; Film Actors: Lesbian; Pornographic Film and Video: Lesbian; Riggs, Marlon; Vachon, Christine

JOE A. THOMAS is Associate Professor and Chair of the Art Department at Clarion University of Pennsylvania. His research focuses primarily on issues of sexuality and representation, but also digresses into American Pop Art and Italian Mannerism. Entries: Porn Stars; Pornographic Film and Video: Bisexual; Pornographic Film and Video: Gay Male

NATHAN G. TIPTON is a Ph.D. candidate in Textual Studies at the University of Memphis. He has published critical articles on Robert Penn Warren, Martha Stewart, and the "Batman" comics, and is a long-standing reviewer for *Lambda Book Report*. He is writing his dissertation on queer eccentricity and gay identity in 1950s Southern fiction. Entries: American Television: Drama; American Television: Reality Shows; American Television: Situation Comedies; American Television: Talk Shows

BENJAMIN TRIMMIER is a painter and installation artist affiliated with the Lower East Side Tenement Museum in New York City. Entries: Bankhead, Tallulah; Haines, William "Billy"

GREG VARNER was arts editor of the *Washington Blade* from October 1997 until September 2001. He earned an undergraduate degree in writing at Oberlin College, and a master's degree at the University of Virginia. He lives in Washington, D.C. Entries: American Television: News; Dong, Arthur; Mitchell, John Cameron

KELLY A. WACKER is Assistant Professor of Art History at the University of Montevallo in Alabama. She earned her Ph.D. at the University of Louisville, where she wrote her dissertation on Land Art and the work of Alice Aycock, Nancy Holt, and Mary Miss. She served as Editor in Chief of *Parnassus: The Allen R. Hite Art Institute Graduate Journal*. Entry: Rozema, Patricia

CARLA WILLIAMS is a writer and photographer from Los Angeles who lives and works in Santa Fe. Her writings and images can be found on her website at www.carla-girl.net. Entry: Bisexuality in Film

B.J. WRAY lectures in the Department of English at the University of California, Davis. She is revising her dissertation on nationalism and sexuality in English-Canada lesbian cultural texts into a book-length study of the performance of sexual citizenship in the United States and Canada. She has published on lesbian performance art and queer choreography. Entry: Treut, Monika

JOYCE M. YOUMANS is Curatorial Assistant in the Department of African Art at the Nelson-Atkins Museum of Art in Kansas City. She curated the exhibition Another Africa. Her article "African Art at the Nelson-Atkins Museum of Art" appears in *African Arts*. Her research interests include contemporary Western and African art, the abject in visual art, and pragmatist aesthetics. Entry: Akerman, Chantal

ANDRES MARIO ZERVIGON earned his Ph.D. in the History of Art from Harvard University and now teaches at Rutgers University. He specializes in the art and design of Germany's Weimar period and in the painting of Britain's post–World War II era. Entry: Almodóvar, Pedro

Index of Names